COCHLEAR PROSTHESES

AN INTERNATIONAL SYMPOSIUM

ANNALS OF THE NEW YORK ACADEMY OF SCIENCES

Volume 405

COCHLEAR PROSTHESES

AN INTERNATIONAL SYMPOSIUM

Edited by Charles W. Parkins and Samuel W. Anderson

The New York Academy of Sciences
New York, New York
1983

Library of Congress Cataloging in Publication Data

Main entry under title:

Cochlear prostheses.

(Annals of the New York Academy of Sciences; v. 405)

Papers presented at a conference entitled Cochlear Implants, held on April 14–16, 1982 by the New York Academy of Sciences.

Bibliography: p.

Includes index.

1. Cochlear implants—Congresses. 2. Electrocochleography—Congresses. I. Parkins, Charles W., 1937– . II. Anderson, Samuel W., 1929– . III. New York Academy of Sciences. IV. Series. [DNLM: 1. Auditory prosthesis—Congresses. W1 AN626YL v. 405/ WV 274 C6615 1982]

Q11.N5 Vol. 405 [RF305] 500s [617.8′82] 83–4263

ISBN 0–89766–202–4

ISBN 0–89766–203–2 (pbk.)

PCP

Printed in the United States of America

ISBN 0–89766–202–4 (cloth)

ISBN 0–89766–203–2 (paper)

ANNALS OF THE NEW YORK ACADEMY OF SCIENCES

VOLUME 405

June 6, 1983

COCHLEAR PROSTHESES: AN INTERNATIONAL SYMPOSIUM *

Editors and Conference Chairmen
Charles W. Parkins and Samuel W. Anderson

CONTENTS

* This volume is the result of a conference entitled Cochlear Implants, held on April 14–16, 1982 by The New York Academy of Sciences.

Part IV. Electrode Fabrication Techniques

Part V. Cochlear Implants and Histologic Damage

Part VI. Perceptions from Electrical Stimulation

Part VII. Clinical Results with Cochlear Prostheses

Part VIII. Pre- and Postoperative Evaluation of Patients

Part IX. Potential Coding Solutions for Electroneural Speech Discrimination

Financial assistance was received from:

- BIOSTIM INC.
- SURGICAL PRODUCTS DIVISION/3M
- WORLD REHABILITATION FUND

PREFACE

Charles W. Parkins

Division of Otolaryngology
University of Rochester
School of Medicine and Dentistry
Rochester, New York 14642

Samuel W. Anderson

Department of Psychiatry
College of Physicians & Surgeons of
Columbia University
New York, New York 10032

The earliest attempts at electrical stimulation of hearing have been credited to Volta, who in 1790 connected his own ears to his newly discovered voltaic cell and described the auditory sensation. It was not until 1957, however, that serious attempts at electrical stimulation of the auditory nerve as a treatment for sensorineural deafness began. In 1957, Djourno and Eyries reported that one of their patients experienced auditory sensations when his auditory nerve, which had been uncovered by disease and surgery, was stimulated electrically. This led to separate efforts by three different investigators in California (Drs. House, Simmons, and Michelson) to develop an implantable cochlear prosthesis. As is true in any new frontier, early work was frequently founded on an inadequate and sometimes poorly understood data base, and some misconceptions. Despite these valid criticisms the pioneers in this field demonstrated the early potential of the cochlear prosthesis, namely, its ability to alert the wearer to environmental noises and warning sounds, to provide auditory feedback which allowed the wearer to appropriately modulate the intensity of his own voice, and to function as a very acceptable lipreading aid for those patients who had lost their hearing after having acquired normal speech.

It soon became apparent that multidisciplinary teamwork would be essential if a cochlear prosthesis were to be developed that would provide the wearer with intelligible speech perceptions. Engineers (electrical, mechanical, and chemical) are essential to the development of a miniaturized multichannel stimulating electrode which may have to coil itself through two turns of the cochlea without producing additional damage to this already compromised miniature structure. The problems of mechanical damage, chemical toxicity, and electrochemical damage must all be addressed and solved. Miniaturization of the implanted and external electronics and the development of a reliable transcutaneous transmission system for data and power for multiple channels also require their maximum efforts. So far, there has been a suboptimal input from the speech science field. Since speech perception is the ultimate goal for the cochlear prosthesis, the appropriate type of electrical stimulation to achieve this goal must be developed. Speech science has long been involved with the acoustic signals produced by speech and the relative importance of the various components of this signal to the perception and understanding of speech. In developing the electrical stimulus code for the successful cochlear prosthesis, the most important information in the acoustic signal must be presented to the auditory neurologic system (the auditory nerve) in a manner that will produce auditory nerve responses that will be most easily decoded by the higher neurologic portions of the system as intelligible speech.

Cochlear prosthesis investigators are now developing a second generation of cochlear prostheses using information from a larger and better data base. This development is taking place in at least seven different countries and includes a number of disciplines. This conference was established to allow this international group of multidisciplined investigators to meet, to exchange ideas, and to publish in one volume papers reflecting the current state of the art for cochlear prostheses. Efforts were made to include each of the related disciplines with the aim of stressing the coding necessary for a successful cochlear prosthesis. Towards this aim, papers from the fields of speech and auditory physiology are presented first. Investigators in the field of speech science have generally not yet shown much interest in the cochlear prosthesis and it is hoped that their inclusion in this conference will serve to arouse their interest and activity in this area.

As with all conferences, the quality of the papers establishes the quality of the conference. We wish at this time to thank the authors for the quality and timeliness of their papers and for their cooperation with the editors. We are also deeply indebted to The New York Academy of Sciences: to Dr. M.H. Shamos, President; to Ellen Marks, Renée Wilkerson, and Erna Levine of the Conference Department for their skilled administration in making all of the arrangements for this meeting; and to Bill Boland, Executive Editor of the Editorial Department, Joyce Hitchcock, Managing Editor, and Justine Cullinan, Associate Editor, for their careful work in the production of this book. Finally, we would like to thank Dr. Elaine Reiman Fenton of the Advisory Committee of the Linguistics Section, Dr. Juergen Tonndorf of the College of Physicians & Surgeons of Columbia University, and Richard Bernard for their encouragement and support of this endeavor.

Part I. Acoustic Coding of Speech and Normal Limits on Transfer of Information

INTRODUCTION

Samuel W. Anderson

Department of Psychiatry
College of Physicians & Surgeons of Columbia University
New York, New York 10032

It is quite proper for us to begin this conference with a session devoted to the acoustic characteristics of speech reception by subjects with normal hearing. There are at least three reasons for this: First, and most obvious, is to provide an adequate description of the normal process that cochlear prostheses are intended to restore. Second, we need to extract from the normal acoustic waveforms the properties of the speech code itself—that essential subset of primary signal characteristics that maximizes communicative efficiency. It is of more than passing interest to observe that we can imagine any and all of the acoustic waveforms to be discussed in this session in terms of their electromagnetic power spectral analogs in real time. Thus, each acoustic manipulation has a corresponding hypothetical pattern of stimulation that might be delivered directly to the cochlea by an experimenal implant. I am quite sure that the optimal electroneural stimulus code will not be discovered as easily as this, but it is easy to envision a program of research that would compare normal limits on transfer of information with the power of resolution for corresponding electrical stimuli in transmitting not only individual phonemes, but also the temporal structures of words and phrases that may directly facilitate decoding at these higher levels of language organization. Third, we shall hear papers that remind us of how multifarious the signals that pass between speaker and hearer during normal communication really are. I have in mind the more or less redundant features that conspire to conserve the integrity of message transmission, especially under less than optimal conditions. Such features also may be possibly utilized in designing a prosthesis for cases in which cell loss or other impairment has rendered the primary signal code incapable of satisfactory restoration alone.

ACOUSTIC PROPERTIES USED FOR THE IDENTIFICATION OF SPEECH SOUNDS [a]

Kenneth N. Stevens

Research Laboratory of Electronics and
Department of Electrical Engineering and Computer Science
Massachusetts Institute of Technology
Cambridge, Massachusetts 02139

Phonetic Segments, Features, and Properties

An essential step in the process of understanding a spoken utterance is to identify words within the stream of sound. We usually think of words as being composed of sequences of speech sounds or phonetic segments. The concept of a phonetic segment (such as the vowel *ee* or the consonant *p*), however, is somewhat abstract, since it is not possible to divide up the stream of sound into individual sound segments, with sharp boundaries that separate adjacent segments. Some parts of the sound wave may show the influence of more than one phonetic segment and thus a particular section of the sound wave often cannot be associated exclusively with one speech sound.

Each phonetic segment is manifested in the sound wave by a set of acoustic properties, and these properties are, for the most part, independent of the context in which the segment occurs. There is an inventory of a relatively small set (probably 15–20) of these properties that are used to characterize different speech sounds.[1] Each property may be present or absent in a segment (or may be unspecified). Thus a relatively small set of properties can be combined in a large number of ways to produce a large number of different speech sounds. These properties can, in effect, organize phonetic segments into classes such that the segments in each class have one of the properties in common. Such a class of phonetic segments is said to have a phonetic *feature* in common, and a particular acoustic property is present in the sound wave whenever this feature is marked in a segment within a word.

Words can be regarded, therefore, as complexes of acoustic properties that occur in particular time relations to one another. Words are distinguished from one another on the basis of the difference between one or more of these properties. The acoustic information needed by a listener to identify a word is presumably contained in these properties that are distributed throughout the word.

In order to gain insight into this inventory of properties, it is often useful to construct pairs of words that are minimally different, in the sense that they are distinguished on the basis of just one (or just a small set) of these properties. Thus, for example, for the two utterances *a tot* and *a dot*, spectrograms of which are shown in Figure 1, most of the acoustic properties are the same, except that in one case the initial stop consonant [t] is voiceless, and in the other the consonant [d] is voiced. For the voiced consonant, there is periodic

[a] This work was supported in part by Grant NS–04332 from the National Institutes of Health and by Grant MCS–8112899 from the National Science Foundation.

low-frequency sound during the time the tongue blade forms a closure of the vocal tract, whereas there is no such low-frequency energy for the [t].

The inventory of properties that are available to make phonetic distinctions in language seems to be determined in part by the way in which the auditory system responds to sound, and in part by the capabilities of the speech-generating system for producing sounds with particular attributes. The sounds that are used in language have probably evolved to provide an optimum match with the sound-processing and sound-generating characteristics of the human auditory and articulatory systems.

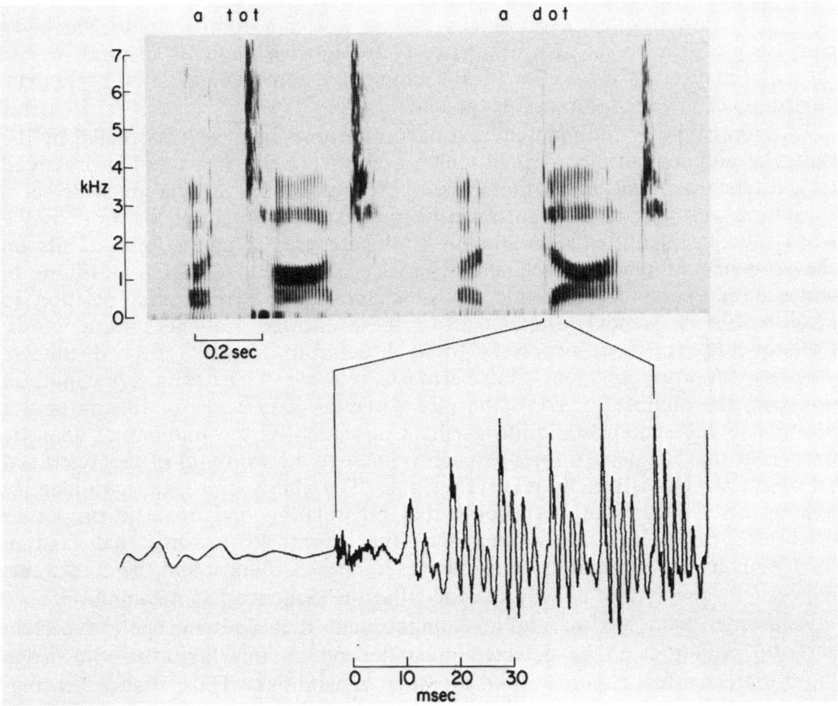

FIGURE 1. (*Top*) spectrograms of the utterances *a tot* and *a dot*. The low-frequency periodicity corresponding to vocal-fold vibration can be seen in the stop gap for [d], but not for [t]. (*Bottom*) segment of the waveform near the release of the [d].

DISTINCTIVE AND REDUNDANT FEATURES

In a given language (such as English) not all properties are fully utilized for making phonetic distinctions. If each sound could be characterized by the presence or absence of fifteen-odd acoustic properties, we would have the capability of producing and receiving 2^{15} or about 30,000 distinctive sounds. This is clearly more than is utilized in practice, by a factor of 100 to 1,000. Thus, for any distinction we want to make, we have available extra, unused properties, and we often recruit these properties to enhance the distinction, that is, to make it "easier" for a listener to distinguish one word from another. These properties are in some sense redundant, since they are not strictly needed to make a phonetic distinction, but they are available to assist the listener and to reinforce the main, distinctive property.

In the example given above (FIG. 1) for English, the distinction between the [t] and the [d] is carried not only by the low-frequency periodicity during the closure interval for the stop, but also by the presence of aspiration noise following the release of the [t], and a consequent delay in the onset of vibration of the vocal folds. In fact, there are some phonetic environments for which the distinction between [t] and [d] is carried only by the aspiration noise and not by the low-frequency periodicity. Thus we have a situation in which we can use more than one acoustic property to signal a phonetic distinction, but the combination of properties that is employed may depend on the phonetic environment in which the segment appears.

Another type of redundancy that occurs in running speech is created by the syntactic and semantic context in which a word occurs. If a word is presented to a listener in isolation, in the absence of context, the listener must detect a substantial number of different acoustic properties throughout the word if the word is to be identified unambiguously. There are, of course, constraints on the sequence of phonetic segments that are allowed at different positions in words (for example, the sequence *sp* is allowed in word-initial position in English, but *vn* is not), and not all of these allowed sequences form words. Consequently it is not necessary for a listener to identify every distinctive property for every segment. Furthermore, if a word occurs in a meaningful sentence, the number of words that are potential candidates for this particular position in the sentence is quite small. Consequently, the number of acoustic properties that are needed for a listener to identify the word out of this restricted set of alternatives is usually relatively small. The ability of a listener to identify a word on the basis of both contextual information and acoustic properties requires a knowledge of the language—the inventory of words that exist in the language, the constraints on sequences of speech sounds, and the constraints imposed by the syntax and by the fact that the sentence has meaning.

A listener who has an auditory impairment that does not permit certain acoustic properties to be detected must depend on this linguistic knowledge more than a listener with normal auditory capabilities. Thus, such a hearing-impaired listener is doubly handicapped if he or she has limited proficiency with the language, as is often the case with those who have hearing impairments from a very early age.

Some Universal Properties of Sequences of Speech Sounds

We turn now to examine some of the acoustic properties that are used for making phonetic distinctions. Before we comment on these properties in detail, however, we first look at some properties that all sequences of speech sounds have in common. In a sense, these properties provide us with a baseline against which we can begin to look at more detailed attributes associated with particular classes of phonetic segments. Some of these universal properties are illustrated in FIGURE 2.

One basic property of running speech is that there are rises and falls in amplitude, corresponding roughly with the alternating vowels and consonants in a sequence of syllables. These changes in amplitude are illustrated at the bottom of FIGURE 2. During the vowel portion of a syllable, the size of the opening in the air passage that forms the vocal tract is a maximum, and the amplitude of the sound reaches a peak around this point. In the region of the consonant or consonants that precede or follow the vowel, there is a narrowing of the vocal tract, leading to a minimum in the amplitude of the sound. The

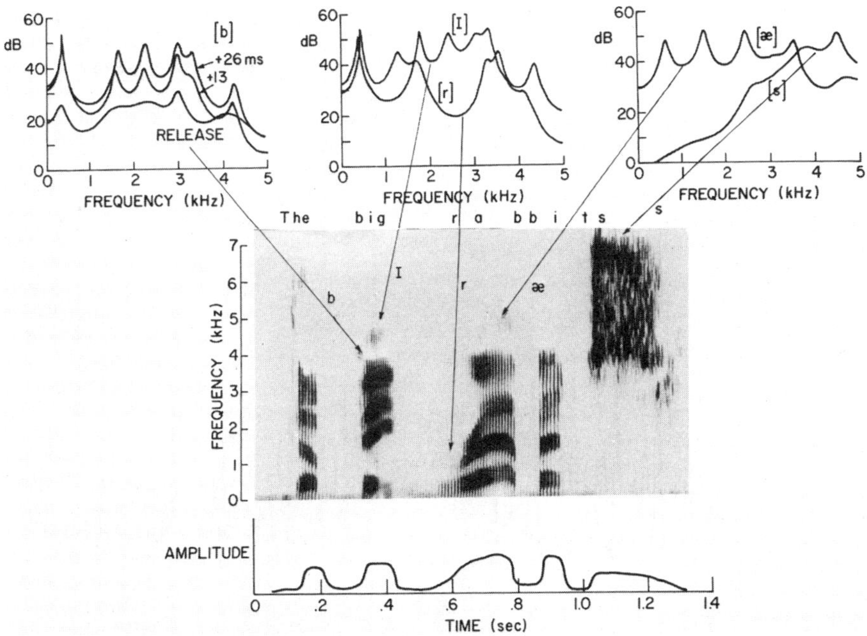

FIGURE 2. Several representations of the acoustic attributes of an utterance in the frequency and time domains. (*Middle*) spectrogram of the utterance "The big rabbits." (*Bottom*) variation of amplitude versus time during the utterance. (*Top*) spectra sampled at various points throughout the utterance as indicated. In the case of [b] at the left, three spectra are shown, and these are obtained by sampling at three points in time 13 msec apart. The spectra are computed for the preemphasized waveform, and are smoothed using a linear prediction procedure. (From Stevens and Blumstein.[4] Reproduced by permission.)

amplitude of the sound in running speech rarely remains constant over a time interval of more than a few tens of milliseconds.

During the time intervals when the amplitude is a maximum, in the vowel portions of the syllables, the vocal folds are almost always vibrating, and the frequency of vibration will vary depending upon the stress that is to be placed on the syllable, the way the speaker wishes to group words together, and the position of the syllable in the sentence. Within a given utterance, this frequency can vary over half an octave or more. An example of this is shown in FIGURE

3. Here we see the contour of fundamental frequency versus time for the sentence "We take a winding path to the pond." The waveform of the sound is illustrated for two selected brief time intervals within the sentence. The fundamental frequency begins low on the initial unstressed word, it is a maximum on *take*, it falls on the next few syllables, has a maximum on *path*, which is given emphasis here, and again has a maximum on *pond*, following which there is a fall to the end of the utterance. The waveforms show the more closely spaced glottal pulses for the word *take*, and the more widely spaced pulses corresponding to the lower fundamental frequency near the end of *pond*. No contour is shown during time intervals when the vocal folds are not vibrating.

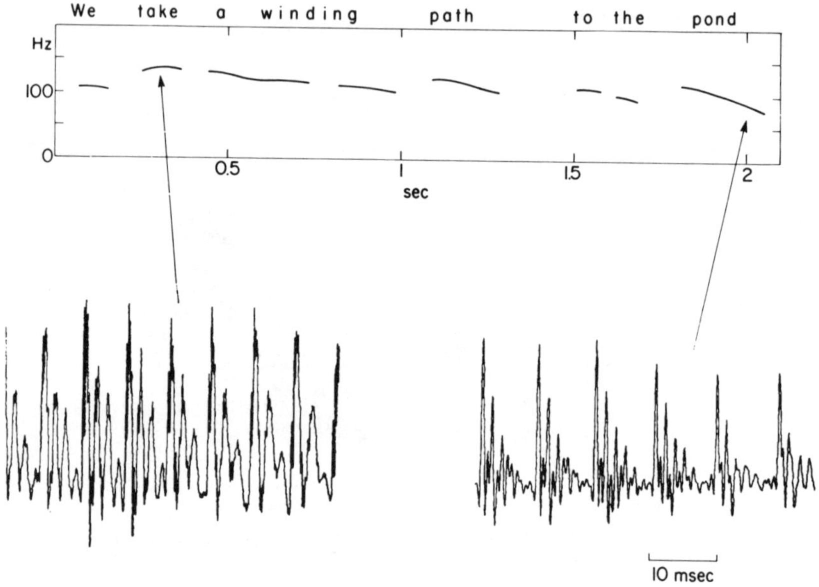

FIGURE 3. (*Top*) fundamental frequency versus time for the voiced portions of the sentence "We take a winding path to the pond." (*Bottom*) brief segments of the speech waveform sampled in two different vowels.

These two basic parameters—the rises and falls in amplitude for each syllable, and the rises and falls in fundamental frequency—already provide a listener with substantial information. The short, function words can be located, some idea of word grouping can be gained, and the end of the utterance or of a phrase or sentence can be identified. These parameters represent a rather gross kind of acoustic analysis. For a severely hearing-impaired listener, these fluctuations in loudness and pitch can often be heard even when a number of other more subtle properties cannot be detected.

But a listener needs much more information than these gross changes in amplitude and frequency in order to understand an utterance. This additional information must come from the spectral characteristics of the sounds and the time variation of these spectral characteristics, some of which can be seen in FIGURE 2.

An attribute that characterizes most speech sounds is the presence of significant peaks and valleys in the spectra, particularly in the frequency range below about 2500 Hz. The ratio of the spectrum amplitude at a peak to that in an adjacent valley can be 20 dB or more. The peaks arise from vocal-tract resonances or formants, and these resonances are usually narrower than the bandwidths of the analyzing filters in the peripheral auditory system. Consequently, the time response of these auditory filters is usually dominated by the frequencies of the spectral peaks rather than by the filters themselves.[2, 3] Individual units in the auditory nerve tend to respond synchronously to the frequencies of these spectral peaks up to about 2500 Hz, and there are usually two or three such peaks in this frequency range for nonnasal vowels. For frequencies above about 2500 Hz, the peaks and valleys in the spectrum are not so prominent, particularly if the spectrum is examined with filters that simulate the filtering in the peripheral auditory system.

The peaks that are observed in the short-time spectrum change with time as the shape of the vocal tract changes during the production of speech. Sometimes these changes are quite rapid, with significant movements of peaks over time intervals of 10–20 msec, as shown in the successive spectra sampled following the release of [b] in FIGURE 2. Several acoustic properties that are used to distinguish among speech sounds may be packaged in the sound wave in the vicinity of these time intervals. These are times when the vocal tract is moving away from or towards a constricted configuration associated with a consonant.

SOME SELECTED PROPERTIES OF SPEECH SOUNDS

With these general properties of speech as a background, we now examine some of the more detailed acoustic properties that listeners appear to use in making phonetic distinctions. We shall consider only a subset of the total number of properties that are used in various languages, and we shall concentrate on properties that seem to be utilized across many languages, including English.

Low-Frequency Periodicity

The example in FIGURE 1 illustrates a phonetic distinction that is made by detecting the presence or absence of low-frequency periodicity or *voicing* in the sound. The frequency of this periodicity is usually in the range 80–350 Hz for adult speakers, and may be higher than this for children. This periodicity can be detected by a listener even if no energy is present in the sound at the fundamental frequency, since the periodicity can be produced in the sound by the higher harmonics of the spectrum without the fundamental component. In the case of consonants that are produced with a narrow constriction in the vocal tract, the low-frequency periodicity may occur over only a portion of the constricted interval—either just after the constricion is produced or just before it is released. For example, in the closure interval of [d] in FIGURE 1, the spectrogram and the waveform show that the low-frequency periodicity seems to disappear (or at least becomes very weak) in the 10–20 msec preceding the consonant release, but is present throughout the earlier part of the closure interval. FIGURE 4 shows additional examples of sounds with no low-frequency periodicity (*f*in), and those with periodicity (k*n*ot and *w*in).

Presence of Aperiodicity in the Sound

Some aperiodicity or noise appears in the sound whenever the vocal tract is constricted to produce a consonant in such a way that pressure builds up behind the constriction. When air flows through the constriction, turbulence is generated in the flow, and noise is produced in the vicinity of the constriction. Examples of utterances that are distinguished on the basis of a consonant produced with or without this noise are given in FIGURE 4. For the utterance *a knot,* there is no pressure buildup behind the alveolar constriction, and hence no aperiodicity in the sound, whereas in *a dot* (FIG. 1) noise is generated at the instant of consonantal release. For both of these utterances there is complete closure of the vocal tract during the consonantal interval, but the buildup of pressure is prevented in the case of the nasal sound by allowing air to flow through the velopharyngeal opening and the nasal passages. In the case of the pair *a win* and *a fin,* the closure during the consonant is not complete. Noise is continuous during the closure interval for [f] because there is pressure behind the constriction, whereas there is no pressure buildup and no noise for [w]. Of course, [f] and [w] are distinguished on the basis of the voicing property as well as the property of aperiodicity in the sound.

Abrupt Rise in Amplitude

In the course of generating some speech sounds, a complete closure is made at some point along the vocal tract, whereas for other sounds there is only a partial constriction. When a complete closure is made, as in [t] and [d] in FIGURE 1 and [n] in FIGURE 4, the amplitude of the sound during the closure is quite low, so that when the closure is released there is an abrupt increase in amplitude over the entire frequency range. This abrupt rise in amplitude, preceded by an interval of low amplitude, distinguishes noncontinuant or abrupt segments from continuant segments. In the examples in FIGURE 4, the segments [f,w] are continuant.

Among the five consonants illustrated in the spectrograms of FIGURES 1 and 4, we can observe several combinations of the three properties of low-

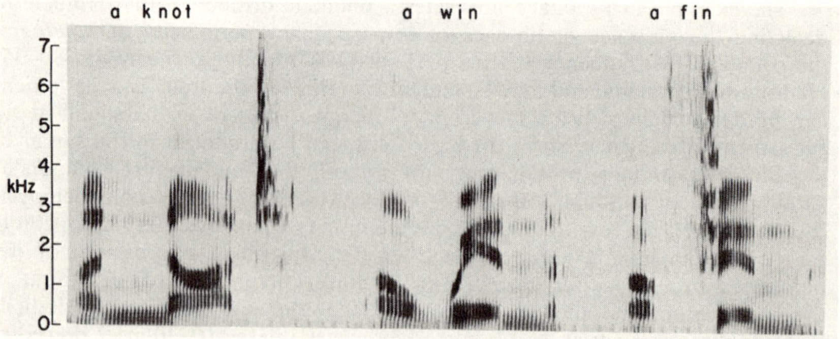

FIGURE 4. Spectrograms of the utterances *a knot, a win,* and *a fin.* For the first two utterances, there is no aperiodicity in the waveform in the intervocalic consonants, whereas the [f] exhibits aperiodicity or noise.

TABLE 1

	Low-Frequency Periodicity	Presence of Aperiodicity	Abrupt Rise in Amplitude
d	+	+	+
t	—	+	+
f	—	+	—
w	+	—	—
n	+	—	+

NOTE: The +'s and —'s indicate the presence or absence of three different properties corresponding to the phonetic segments in the left column.

frequency periodicity, presence of noise or aperiodicity, and abrupt amplitude rise. These combinations are summarized in TABLE 1. On the basis of these few simple properties, then, it is possible for a listener to make a partial identification of a word.

Stridency

Certain consonants in English and in other languages are produced by generating turbulence in the airstream, and this turbulent flow results in a source of noise or aperiodic sound in the vocal tract. The amplitude of this noise can be controlled by appropriate manipulation of the airstream. If the airstream is directed against an obstacle, such as the lower teeth, then the noise has a relatively large amplitude, whereas if the airstream is directed in such a way that it does not impinge directly on an obstacle, then the noise is much weaker. Consonants produced with greater noise amplitude are called *strident,* and two of these ([s] and [š] as in *shin*) are illustrated in FIGURE 5. For these consonants, the amplitude of the noise in the high-frequency region of the spectrum is well above that of the adjacent vowel in the same frequency region. For a nonstrident consonant (such as [θ] in the word *thin* in FIGURE 5), on the other hand, the spectrum amplitude of the noise is less than that of the vowel over most of the frequency range. Other examples of strident consonants in English are [z], [ž] (a*z*ure), [č] (*ch*ur*ch*), and [ǰ] (*j*ump).

Place of Articulation for Consonants

As we have already observed, the properties of the sound in the vicinity of points where there is a rapid change in the spectrum are often used to distinguish one class of speech sounds from another, particularly for consonant sounds. One set of such properties is used to make distinctions between consonants produced with constrictions at different places along the vocal tract. For example, in English we distinguish between consonants produced with a constriction at the lips (such as [p b f v m]), consonants with a constriction formed by the tongue blade (such as [t d s z n]), and those produced by raising the tongue body against the palate (such as [k g ŋ], an example of the last of these being in si*ng*).

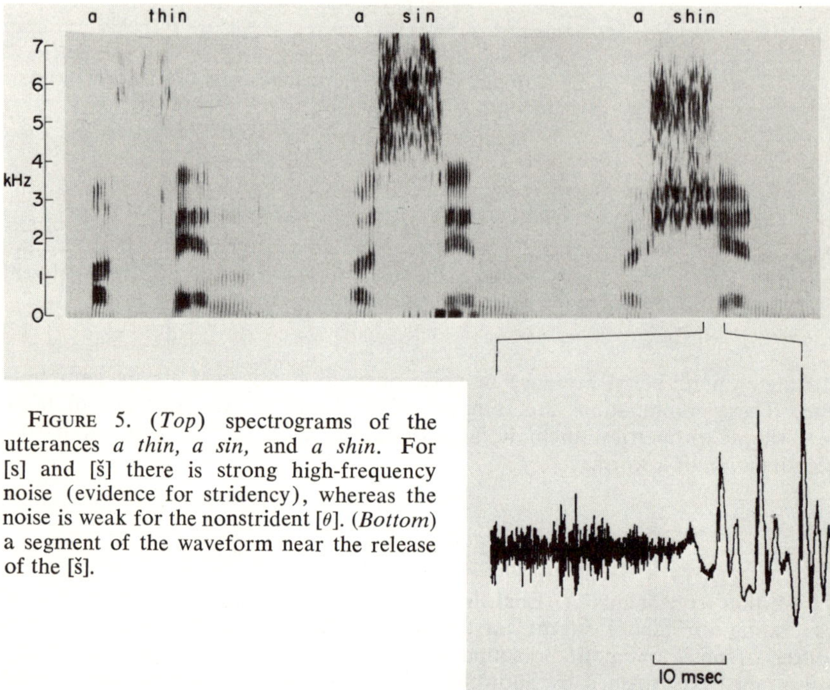

FIGURE 5. (*Top*) spectrograms of the utterances *a thin, a sin,* and *a shin.* For [s] and [š] there is strong high-frequency noise (evidence for stridency), whereas the noise is weak for the nonstrident [θ]. (*Bottom*) a segment of the waveform near the release of the [š].

One of the properties that helps to distinguish among these groups of consonants examines whether the spectrum of the sound has a prominent or compact spectral peak in the midfrequency range, or whether the spectral peaks are more diffuse, either distributed throughout the auditory frequency range or concentrated at one end or the other of this range. These contrasting properties of spectral compactness versus diffuseness are illustrated in FIGURE 6. This figure shows spectrograms of the utterances *a gap, a bat,* and *a dad,* together with spectra sampled in the vicinity of the release of the consonant. The prominence of the midfrequency spectral peak for [g] contrasts with the more diffuse spectra for [b] and [d]. The midfrequency range, where the prominent spectral peak occurs, is generally between 1000 and 3000 Hz. This property of compactness is evident in consonants produced with a constriction in the velar region, that is, the consonants [k, g, η].

If we examine further the distinction between the labial [b] and the alveolar [d], we observe that the spectrum for [d] at the release tends to be sloping upwards with increasing frequency, whereas the spectrum at onset for [b] tends to be flat or sloping downwards. The principal attribute that distinguishes a labial from an alveolar consonant, however, seems to be determined by the way in which the spectrum amplitude at high frequencies changes immediately following the release of the consonant. In each panel of FIGURE 7 we show the spectrum sampled close to the release, together with the spectrum sampled at the beginning of the vowel. For the alveolar consonants, the amplitudes of the spectral peaks at high frequencies in the burst are just as high as or higher than the corresponding amplitudes in the immediately following vowel. In the case of the labials, however, the burst amplitude at high frequencies is generally not as great as in the following vowel, so that full amplitude at high frequencies is not reached until slightly after the onset of voicing for the vowel. In other words, for the alveolar the rise in amplitude at high frequencies is very abrupt, reaching full amplitude in a few milliseconds, whereas for the labial the rise at high frequencies is less abrupt, and is, in effect, somewhat delayed. The manner in which the high-frequency amplitude changes with time immediately following the release for each class of consonant is illustrated schematically at the bottom of FIGURE 6. These contrasting properties are a direct consequence of the place in the vocal tract where the consonant constriction is made. These classes of consonants, then, are distinguished in terms of abruptness of amplitude rise in particular frequency ranges. These attributes involving the time course of rapid amplitude changes in different frequency ranges can also be applied to distinguish place of articulation for fricative consonants ([f v] versus [s z] and for nasal consonants ([m] versus [n]) as well as for stop consonants.

The distinction between labials and alveolars in English is also carried by the trajectories of the formants immediately following the consonantal release—particularly that of the second formant. In FIGURE 6, for example, we observe

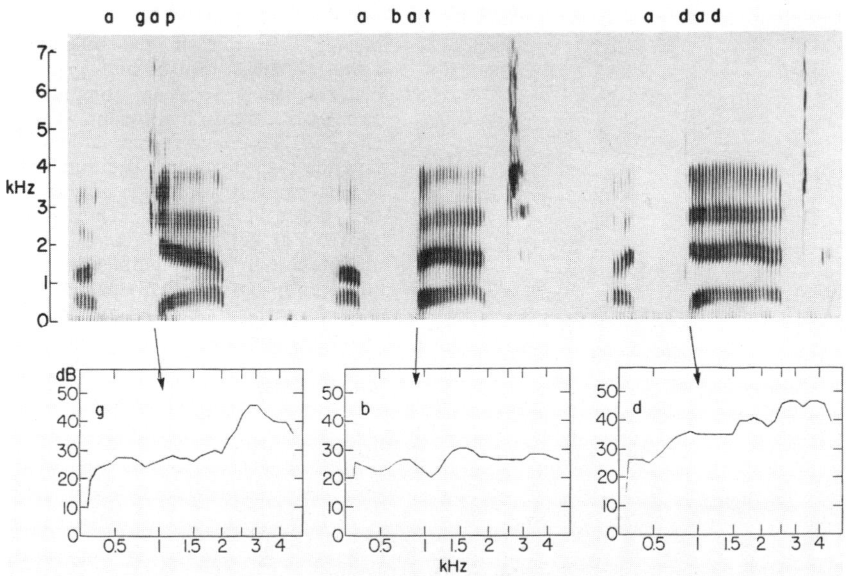

FIGURE 6. (*Top*) spectrograms of three utterances containing the stop consonants [g b d]. (*Bottom*) under each spectrogram is a spectrum sampled at the consonant release, indicating the spectrum shape of the burst. The spectrum is calculated in critical bands, which represent an approximation to the filtering at the cochlea. The spectra illustrate the prominent spectral peak for [g] (at about 2900 Hz in this example), and the diffuse spread of spectral energy, without a prominent peak, for [b] and [d].

that there is a large separation between first and second formants just after the release of [d] (spectrogram at the right), whereas immediately following the [b] release, these two formants are much closer together (middle spectrogram). These two properties—the time course of the spectrum amplitude at high frequencies, as in FIGURE 7, and the starting frequency of the second formant in relation to the first—provide an example of the redundancy that can be used to indicate a phonetic distinction in language.

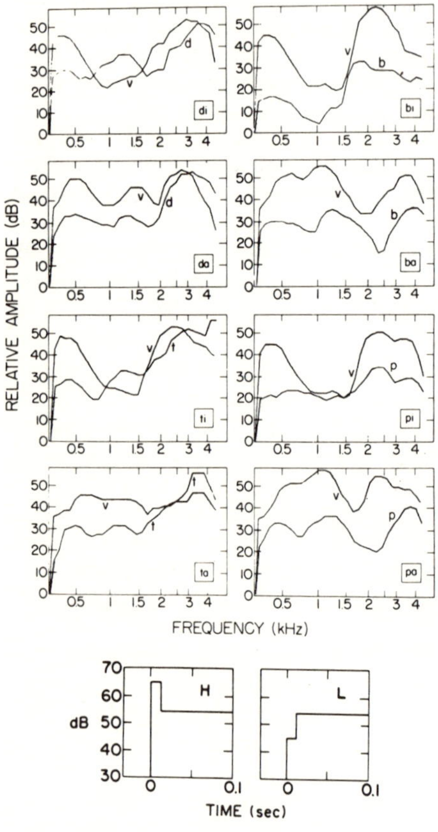

FIGURE 7. (*Top*) two spectra are shown in each panel: one is sampled at the release of the stop consonant in the syllable indicated, and the other (v) is sampled after the onset of voicing in the vowel. The consonants [d] and [t] are represented at the *left*, and [b] and [p] at the *right*. In the high-frequency region (above 2.5 kHz), the average spectrum amplitude at onset for [d] and [t] is equal to or greater than that in the following vowel, whereas for [b] and [p] the high-frequency spectrum amplitude at onset is less than that for the vowel. (*Bottom*) schematic representation of how the high-frequency spectrum amplitude changes with time for these two classes of sounds represented above. For [d] and [t] there is an abrupt rise to an amplitude that is equal to or greater than that of the vowel, whereas for [b] and [p] there is an initial rise at the onset, followed by a later rise in amplitude as the vowel begins.

Vowel Distinctions

When the vocal tract is relatively open, the source of acoustic excitation of the tract is in the vicinity of the glottis, and the changes in the spectrum of the sound are not very rapid. The sound that results from this configuration always has a series of spectral peaks corresponding to the natural frequencies or formants of the vocal tract. The frequencies of these spectral peaks are determined by the shape of the vocal tract, which in turn is determined by the position of the tongue and the configuration of the lips. Different classes of vowels are characterized by different patterns of these formant frequencies, particularly the lowest two or three formants, which usually lie in the frequency range up to about 3 kHz.

Examples of some basic vowel distinctions are illustrated by the spectrograms and spectra in FIGURE 8. One such distinction is determined primarily by the frequency of the first formant. For one class of vowels—the high vowels such as [i] (beat) and [u] (boot)—the lowest spectral peak is at a low frequency, such that there is very little drop in the amplitude spectrum for frequencies below this peak. These vowels are produced by elevating the tongue body to a relatively high position in the mouth. The contrasting class of vowels—the low vowels such as [*a*] (father) and [æ] (bat)—has a first formant peak at a much higher frequency, such that there is a significant "valley" in the spectrum below this peak.

Another basic distinction is determined by the position of the second formant in relation to the first and third formants. The class of back vowels, such as [u] and [*a*], is characterized by a second formant that located close to the first formant, so that the valley in the spectrum between the two formant peaks is very small. This proximity of the first two formants dominates the spectrum, so that higher formants play a negligible role in shaping the vowel quality. Back vowels are produced with the tongue body displaced in a posterior direction in the mouth. For front vowels such as [i] and [æ], on the other hand, the second formant is well separated from the first, and is located relatively close to the third formant. The second and third formant (and sometimes also the fourth formant) combine to form a broad spectral prominence that is separated from the first formant by a relatively deep valley in the spectrum. When the first formant is low (that is, for high front vowels), it is possible to displace the second and third formants to relatively high frequencies, so that the high-frequency spectral prominence includes the fourth formant as well as the second and third. For low vowels, however, fronting of the tongue body does not produce such a high frequency for the second formant.

In addition to the two vowel classes defined by these adjustments of the first and second formants (giving rise to four different vowels), it is possible to generate other classes of vowels either by modifying the configuration of formant frequencies relative to that for the four basic vowels, or by changing the formants in particular ways throughout the time course of the vowel. For example, diphthongization helps to create additional vowel contrasts, as can be seen in the spectrograms in FIGURE 9. In this figure we show the time course of the movements of the formants for the three pairs of words *beet–bit, bait–bet,* and *who'd–hood.* We observe that the vowel in the second member of each pair is shorter, and that there are differences in the way the formants move throughout the vowel. For the longer vowel, the first formant always moves down in frequency, and the second formant moves up for [i] and [e] and down for [u]. For the shorter vowel of each pair, on the other hand, the formant trajectories move in different directions so that the contrast between the members of each pair is accentuated. Thus, for example, for [I] the second formant moves down and the first formant increases during the vowel, in a way that is just opposite to the movements for [i].

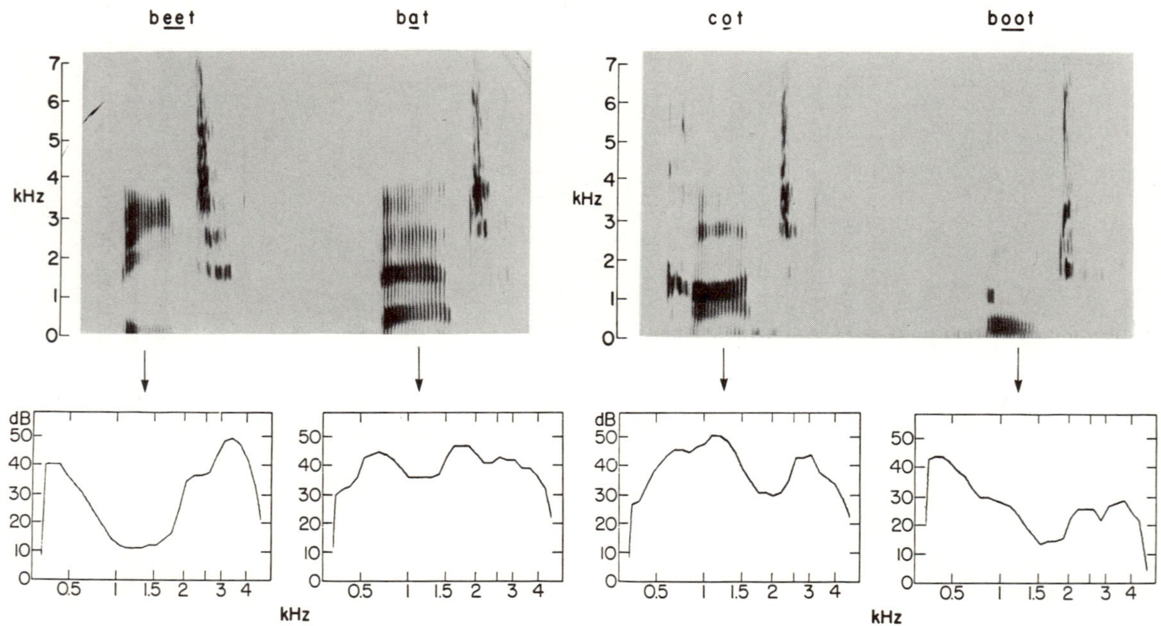

FIGURE 8. Spectrograms and spectra illustrating the acoustic properties corresponding to several vowel categories. The vowels in *beet* and *boot* are high vowels, and are characterized by a low first formant, whereas the vowels in *bat* and *cot* are low vowels, and have a high first formant. For the back vowels in *boot* and *cot*, the second formant is close to the first, whereas for *beet* and *bat* there is a substantial difference between these two formants.

Identification of Words in Sentences

With this brief survey of some of the acoustic properties that a listener needs to detect in order to distinguish between words, let us examine the task that the listener is faced with when presented with the acousic pattern for a

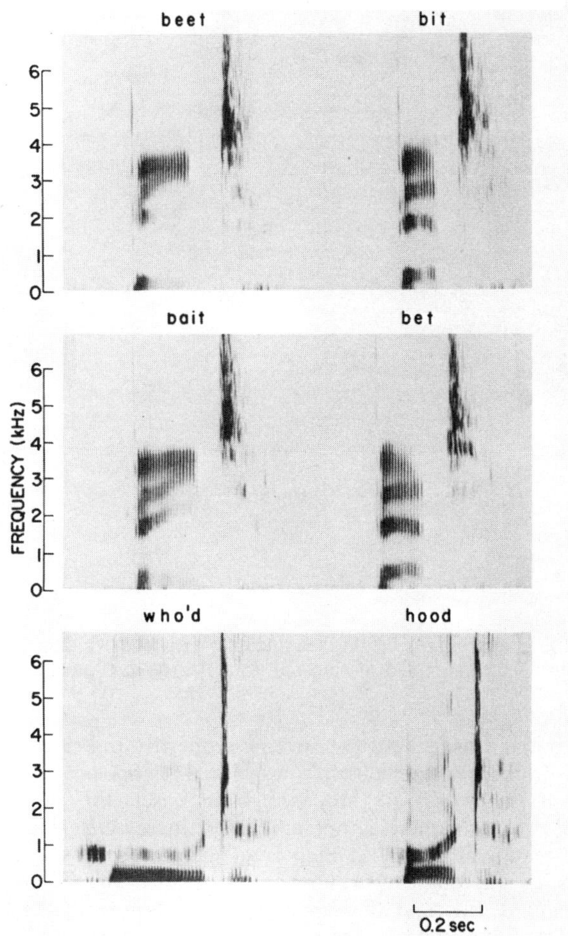

FIGURE 9. Spectrograms illustrating differences between long and short vowels in English. For each pair, the tense or long vowel is on the *left* and the lax or short vowel is on the *right*. The vowels show differences not only in length but also in the formant trajectories.

sentence. As an illustration, we use the sentence "We take a winding path to the pond," discussed earlier. A spectrogram of the sentence is shown in FIGURE 10, together with the spectra sampled at selected times throughout the sentence.

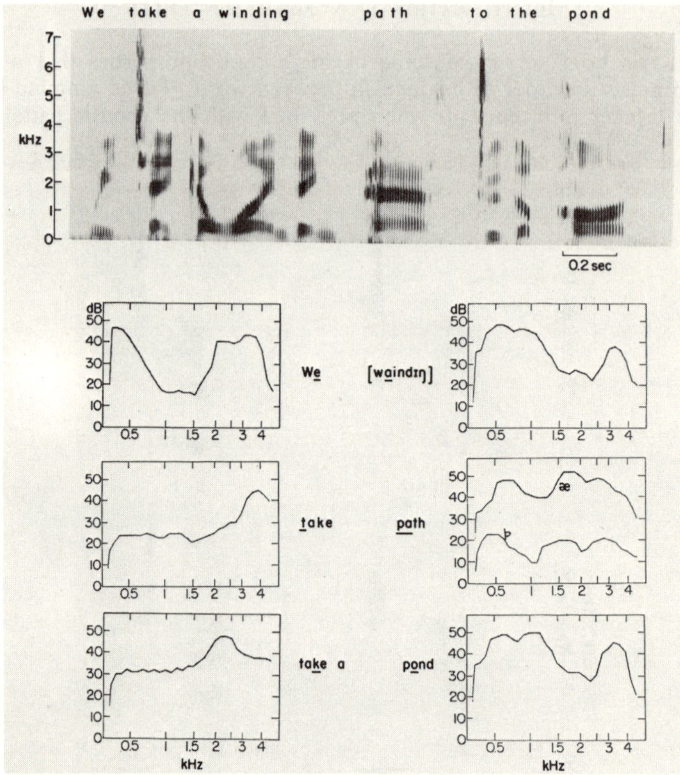

FIGURE 10. Spectrogram of the sentence "We take a winding path to the pond," together with spectra sampled at selected points through the sentence.

In the initial word, there are several properties that identify the word and distinguish it from other possible words: (1) no noise is present at the beginning of the word; (2) following the onset, the spectral peaks move relatively slowly, and there is not an abrupt increase in amplitude; (3) there is very little spectral energy at high frequencies and substantial energy at low frequencies at the onset; (4) later in the word, the first spectral peak or formant remains low, and there is a broad minimum in the spectrum in the midfrequency range with a spectral peak at high frequencies, as shown by the spectrum of this vowel [i] in the figure. These and other properties are used by the listener to search his internal lexicon and to identify the word that is characterized by this array of properties. It is assumed that different lexical items are represented in the memory of the listener by arrays of properties or features of this kind. Following this vowel [i], the relevant properties that the listener must detect include the abrupt onset of silence, the lack of low-frequency periodicity during this closure interval, the abrupt onset of energy at the release of [t] closure, the presence of noise immediately following the release, and a spectrum near onset that is diffuse and rising, as shown in the panel for [t] in the figure. After the onset of the noise burst, the listener must be sensitive to the fact that there is a delay of more than 20-odd milliseconds before voicing begins. After the onset of voicing, the first formant (F1) is in the middle of its range, and the second formant (F2) is relatively high, indicating a front vowel that is nonlow. The trajectories of the formants (downward movement of F1 and upward movement of F2) also provide cues for identification of the word *take*. The vowel is followed by an abrupt offset or reduction in amplitude, an interval of silence, an abrupt onset that is characterized by noise, and a noise spectrum that has a dominant peak in the midfrequency range, as shown in the spectrum at the [k] onset in the figure. This sequence of properties is sufficient for the listener to search his lexicon and identify the word *take*.

A similar analysis of the relevant acoustic properties could be carried out for subsequent words in the sentence. Examples of spectra sampled at selected points of these words are given in the figure. Thus, in each of the three words *winding, path,* and *pond,* the vowel spectrum shows a relatively high F1 with a substantial drop in spectral energy below F1, indicating a low vowel. For the vowel in *path,* there is a space between F1 and F2, whereas for [*a*] in *winding* and in *pond*, F2 is close to F1. A listener must be sensitive to these different spectral patterns in order to identify these words. Also shown in the panel giving the spectrum for [æ] is the spectrum sampled near the release of the initial consonant in *path,* indicating a spectrum amplitude that is weak compared with that of the vowel.

Concluding Remarks

We have described a few of the acoustic properties that must be identified by a listener in order to distinguish between words. These properties include the presence of low-frequency periodicity, the presence of noise or aperiodicity, a high versus a low amplitude of turbulence noise, an abrupt as opposed to a gradual rise in amplitude, certain gross characteristics of the spectrum sampled near the release of a consonant, and the relative positions of spectral prominences for vowels. A distinctive response is assumed to occur in the auditory system of the listener at a particular point or region in time when one of these properties is present in a word. Words are presumably stored in memory in terms of patterns of these acoustic properties. Thus, when a particular pattern of properties is detected in the speech wave during an utterance, the listener is able to search the lexicon and identify which word best fits this pattern.

References

1. Jakobson, R., G. Fant & G. Halle. 1963. Preliminaries to Speech Analysis. MIT Press. Cambridge, MA.
2. Sachs, M. B. & E. D. Young. 1980. Effects of nonlinearities on speech encoding in the auditory nerve. J. Acoust. Soc. Am. **68:** 858–875.
3. Delgutte, B. 1980. Representation of speech-like sounds in the discharge patterns of auditory-nerve fibers. J. Acoust. Soc. Am. **68:** 843–857.
4. Stevens, K. N. & S. E. Blumstein. 1981. The search for invariant acoustic correlates of phonetic features. *In* Perspectives on the Study of Speech. P. D. Eimas and J. L. Miller, Eds.: 1–38. Lawrence Erlbaum Associates. Hillsdale, NJ.

SPEECH CODING: RECOGNIZING WHAT WE DO NOT HEAR IN SPEECH

Bishnu S. Atal

Bell Laboratories
Murray Hill, New Jersey 07974

Introduction

Human speech production is a complex process.[1] The acoustic speech signal is produced as a result of a sequence of transformations occurring at many different levels: semantic, linguistic, articulatory, and acoustic. Each stage of transformation involves extensive coding (putting information in a form that facilitates its transmission over a communication channel) to arrange the signal for transmission to the next stage. Speech is thus a code for transmitting ideas from one person to another through acoustic channels. It is a very robust code capable of providing reliable transmission of information between two persons even in the presence of considerable noise and distortion in the transmission path. The robustness is achieved by introducing appropriate redundant structure in the signal in the encoding process.

Speech coding aims at minimizing the information rate needed to reproduce a speech signal with specified fidelity on a given communication channel.[2] There are three important points to know for efficient coding of speech signals. First, we must understand the nature of the human speech generation process and the constraints it imposes on the speech signal. Second, we must have an understanding of various sources of redundancies in the speech signal. These redundancies are present in the speech signal to cope with noise and distortion in the air pathways between the speaker's lips and the listener's ears and may not be appropriate for handling the noise present in the digital communication channel. Third, and most important, we must understand what our ears can hear and cannot hear in the speech signal. The inability of the human ear to perceive certain distortions in the reproduced speech signal must be recognized and exploited to achieve coding efficiency.

How much information does a speech signal carry? There is really no good answer to this question. The acoustic signal representing the sound pressure variations in front of speaker's lips is a continuous signal which can assume an infinite number of different values at any instant of time. The information rate of a continuous signal, in principle, is unbounded. However, the capabilities of human speech perception in detecting small differences are limited. Two speech signals need not be mathematically identical for us to say that they are perceptually identical. A properly chosen *fidelity criterion* is essential in deciding how accurately we must reproduce a speech signal to avoid hearing any distortion.

The speech signal can be carried over many different types of communication channels. The exact nature of speech coding depends upon the properties of the channel. The focus of the paper is on digital transmission of speech. A digital channel can transmit only integer values. The speech signal must be quantized and sampled prior to digital transmission. The

0077–8923/83/0405–0018 $01.75/0 © 1983, NYAS

simplest digital channel is a binary channel capable of transmitting either a +1 or a −1, that is, one bit of information at any instant of time. The information rate of a digital channel is expressed in bits/sec. This paper will discuss procedures for minimizing the bit rate needed to achieve high-quality speech reproduction.

Properties of Speech Signals

For efficient coding, it is necessary to gain a proper understanding of the nature of the signal to be coded. Although our knowledge of vocal tract acoustics has increased significantly in recent years, very little is known quantitatively about the signal transformations occurring at other levels. We will briefly discuss some of the properties of the speech signal at the acoustic level.

Speech sounds are produced as a result of acoustical excitation of the vocal tract, which consists of the cavities in the pharnyx and the mouth.[1, 3, 4] The entire vocal tract can be thought of as an acoustic tube terminated by the lips at one end and by the vocal cords at the other end. The shape of the vocal tract is changed continually during speech production by the movement of different articulators such as the tongue, the jaw, and the lips. It is customary to classify sounds according to their mode of excitation. There are three important modes of exciting the vocal tract. Voiced sounds are produced as a result of excitation by a series of nearly periodic wave shapes generated by the vocal cords. Examples of voiced sounds are vowels, semivowels, voiced stops, and nasals. Unvoiced sounds are produced when the vocal tract is excited by a noise-like turbulent flow of air at a point of constriction. The resulting excitation has a relatively uniform spectrum. Examples of unvoiced sounds are fricatives, such as */f/*, */s/*, and */sh/* and voiceless stop consonants like */p/*, */t/*, and */k/*. Finally, the plosive sounds are produced by making a complete closure, building up pressure behind the closure, and abruptly releasing it. Examples of plosives are stop-consonants like */b/*, */d/*, */g/*, */p/*, */t/*, and */k/*. Continuous speech uses combinations of these different types of excitation. Some examples of speech waveforms are shown in FIGURE 1. The first two waveforms show examples of voiced and unvoiced speech, respectively. The third waveform includes mixtures of both voiced and unvoiced speech.

A simplified model of speech production can be made by representing the vocal tract as a linear time-varying filter excited either by a periodic source or by a white-noise source, as shown in FIGURE 2. The output of the vocal tract is then expressed as a convolution between the excitation function and the impulse response of the time-varying linear filter. Often, the shape of the vocal tract changes slowly compared to the variations in the excitation waveforms. Then speech production can be considered to be a quasi-stationary process. The quasi-stationarity of the model permits us to look at speech characteristics in the frequency domain. For voiced speech, the vocal excitation has a nearly periodic waveform whose period varies slowly with time. Its spectrum consists of a series of harmonics whose amplitude falls off at approximately 12 dB per octave. The spacing between adjacent harmonics is determined by the period of the vocal cord vibrations. The spectrum of the

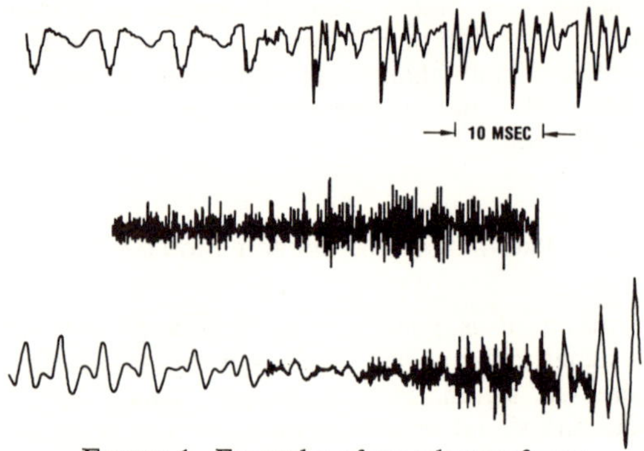

FIGURE 1. Examples of speech waveforms.

vocal tract response consists of a number of resonances whose locations depend upon the vocal tract shape. The voiced speech spectrum is thus composed of harmonically related frequency components whose amplitudes are determined both by the wave shape of the vocal cord vibrations and the vocal tract shape. For unvoiced speech, the excitation spectrum is uniformly distributed over a wide frequency range; the speech spectrum for these sounds is primarily determined by the vocal tract shape. Such idealized representations of spectra for voiced and unvoiced speech are given in FIGURE 3.

A useful concept for describing properties of nonstationary signals such as speech is the time varying or "short-time" spectrum.[4] In such a short-time representation, only a portion of the signal in the neighborhood of any given time is considered in computing the spectrum. The frequency range of interest in speech usually extends from about 100 Hz to 10 kHz. The short-time spectrum of speech contains nearly all of the important information relating to intelligibility of speech and has formed the basis for most of the present methods of characterizing speech in the parametric form. In the earlier days before the availability of fast digital computers, the short-time power spectrum was obtained by passing speech through a bank of bandpass filters. On digital computers, the short-time power spectrum is obtained directly by using Fourier transforms. An example of the spectrum of a short segment of a vowel */e/* excerpted from the word "may" spoken by a male speaker is shown in FIGURE 4. The fine structure corresponding to the regularly spaced peaks in the spectrum is due to the periodicity of voiced speech; the frequency spacing between the peaks is the pitch frequency. The range of pitch fre-

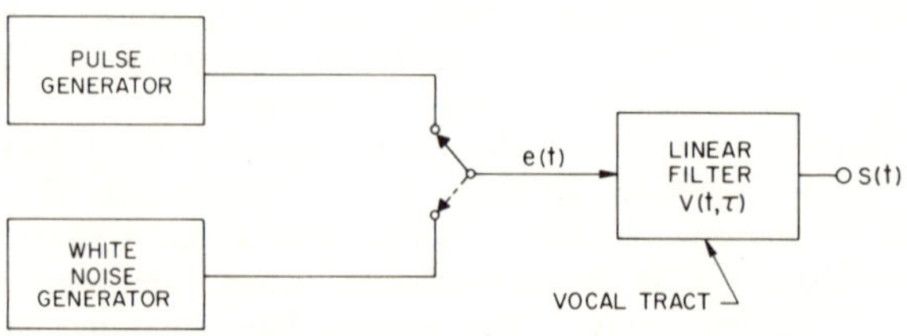

FIGURE 2. Simplified model of speech production.

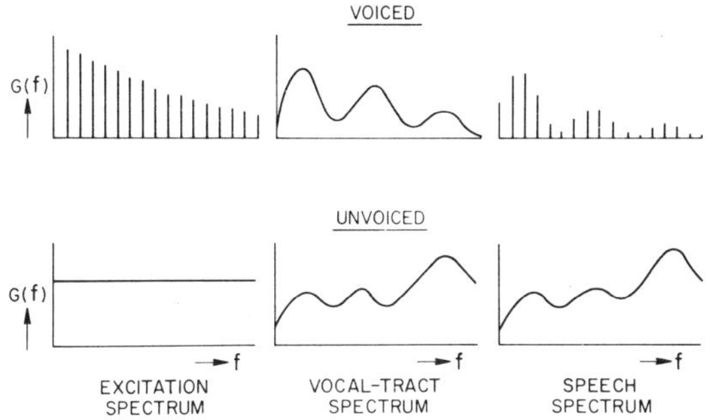

FIGURE 3. Source-filter characterization of speech spectra.

quency in speech for a normal adult is 60 to 400 Hz. The amplitude of the peaks—often described as the spectral envelope—is a function of the vocal cord wave and the vocal tract shape. It is often desirable to separate the fine structure of the spectrum from the envelope. Such a decomposition leads to a compact description of the power spectrum.[4]

SPEECH CODING BY PULSE CODE MODULATION

The simplest digital representation of speech is obtained by sampling followed by quantizing. A speech signal limited to a frequency range of 4 kHz can be sampled at a rate of 8 kHz without any loss of information. Quantization forces each sample of the signal to assume only one of a set of preassigned values. The process of quantization introduces additional noise in the signal. In a simple PCM (pulse code modulation) system, the quanti-

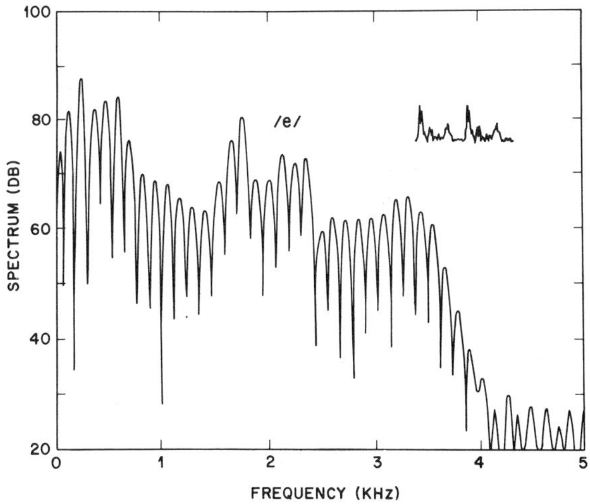

FIGURE 4. Example of a vowel spectrum.

zation levels are uniformly spaced. The power in the speech signal varies over a considerable range. With uniformly spaced quantization levels, the quantization noise power stays constant independent of the signal level. This is not a good idea, because speech segments with low power levels, such as consonants, are reproduced with poor accuracy. One is likely to hear noise in the quantized speech signal during such segments. FIGURE 5 shows a plot of the power levels (expressed in dB) in the speech signal and the quantization noise as a function of time for a sentence-length utterance. The speech signal was sampled at a rate of 8000 samples/sec and each speech sample was quantized by a 7-bit (128 levels) quantizer. The signal-to-noise ratio (SNR) varies considerably from one part of the utterance to another over a range of 0 to 30 dB.

A better procedure is to have nonuniformly spaced quantization levels—small spacing for low amplitudes and large spacing for large amplitudes. An example of nonuniform quantization is logarithmically companded PCM.[5] Such a companded PCM system indeed provides improved speech quality. A plot of the power levels for the speech signal and the quantization noise for the PCM system with nonuniform quantization levels is shown in FIGURE 6. As expected, the noise is decreased considerably (by about 18 dB) during low-level speech segments. Improved performance is achieved even at higher amplitudes. In practice, a logarithmically companded PCM system (LOGPCM) with 7 bits per sample sounds as good as a linear PCM system with 10 bits per sample. What is the reason for this improvement? First, the linear PCM cannot accommodate the large dynamic range of the speech signal. Second, the probability density function of speech amplitudes is not uniform; lower amplitudes occur with much greater probability than higher amplitudes.[4] The linear PCM would have been the right choice if all amplitudes occur with equal probability. Third, our perception of noise is *not* independent of the signal level. Indeed, we tolerate more distortion for speech segments with higher amplitudes than for those with lower amplitudes. What we have said so far applies only for acoustic signals. For example, it would be a mistake to suggest that the LOGPCM system is also effective for quantizing video signals meant to be seen by human eyes.

So far, we have looked at the SNR as a function of time. Let us look at the distribution of signal and noise powers as a function of frequency. FIGURE 7 shows spectra of speech and noise for a 7-bit companded LOGPCM system. The speech spectrum shows peaks at various pitch harmonics and at various formants. Although the noise spectrum shows considerable random behavior, the distribution is approximately uniform. A similar situation is illustrated in FIGURE 8, where only the spectral envelopes are shown for clarity. In both examples, the SNR is very high in the formant regions and poor in the frequency regions between the formants. A uniform spectrum of the noise is not the optimum choice for proper subjective performance. Most of the audible distortion comes from those frequency regions where the signal power is low. A better choice for the noise spectrum would be that shown in FIGURE 9. The noise power is higher in the formant regions and lower in between the formants, providing a more uniform distribution of SNR than the case shown in FIGURE 8. What is the optimum noise spectrum? We will discuss various factors governing the choice of optimum noise spectrum in the next section.

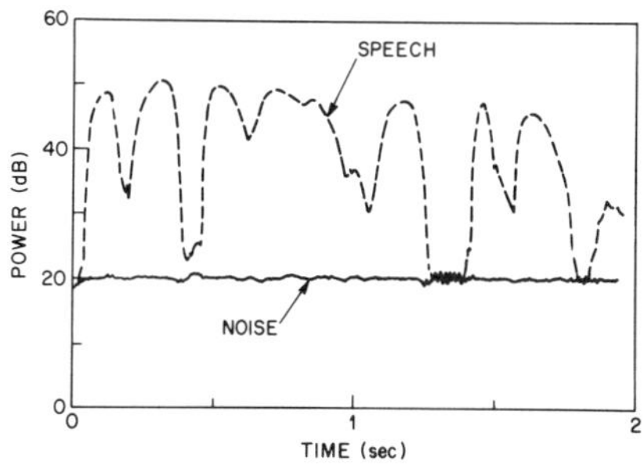

FIGURE 5. Power levels of speech and noise in a linear PCM system.

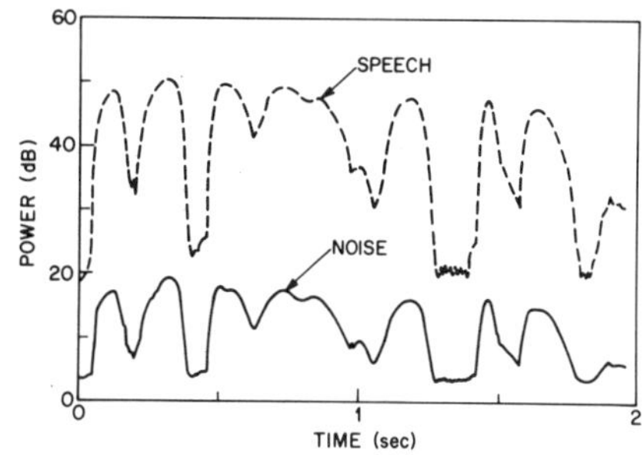

FIGURE 6. Power levels of speech and quantizing noise in a LOGPCM system.

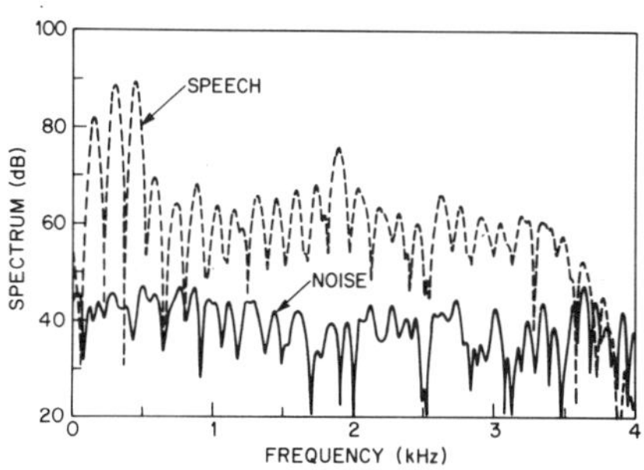

FIGURE 7. Spectra of speech and noise in a LOGPCM system.

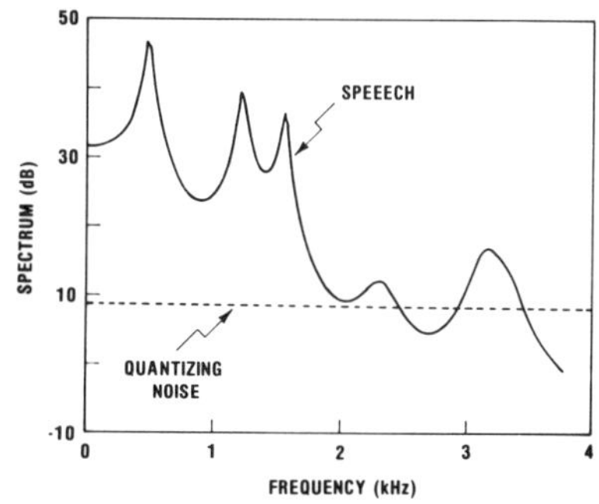

FIGURE 8. Another example showing the spectral envelopes of speech and noise.

PERCEPTUAL CRITERIA FOR OPTIMUM NOISE SPECTRUM

Human speech perception is as complex as human speech production and consists of a sequence of transformations occurring at several levels. An important transformation occurs in the cochlea, where the acoustic signal is converted into neural signals for transmission to the higher auditory centers in the brain. In recent years, our understanding of cochlear mechanics has improved significantly, but we understand very little, if any, of what goes on beyond the cochlea. For efficient coding, we ought to know what kind of information about the speech signal is retained in the acoustic-to-neural transformation. There is no point in transmitting through the digital communication channel information which would be lost in the acoustic-to-neural conversion. We summarize some of the important features of this transformation.

A change in the ambient pressure at the ear drum causes it to move. The movement of the ear drum is transmitted to the stapes and then to the inner ear, causing the basilar membrane to vibrate. The basilar membrane performs a kind of short-time Fourier analysis in which the frequency is represented by distances along the membrane. An important point about motion of the basilar membrane is that a single frequency component in the signal produces a displacement over a wide region on the basilar membrane. The peripheral auditory analyzer, represented by the basilar membrane, can be thought of as a bank of bandpass filters with bandwidths of about 100 Hz below 500 Hz and bandwidths of one-sixth the center frequency above 1 kHz. Like any other physical device, the frequency resolution of our hearing is limited. This limitation can be exploited to gain coding efficiency.

Masking is another property of our auditory system that we must consider in designing speech coders. Masking represents the inability of our hearing mechanism to hear one sound in presence of another. Typically, one considers the problem of a signal being masked by noise. In speech coding, the problem is just the reverse. Every coder introduces errors during the encoding and decoding processes. It is interesting to find out if these errors (or noise) could be masked by the speech signal itself.

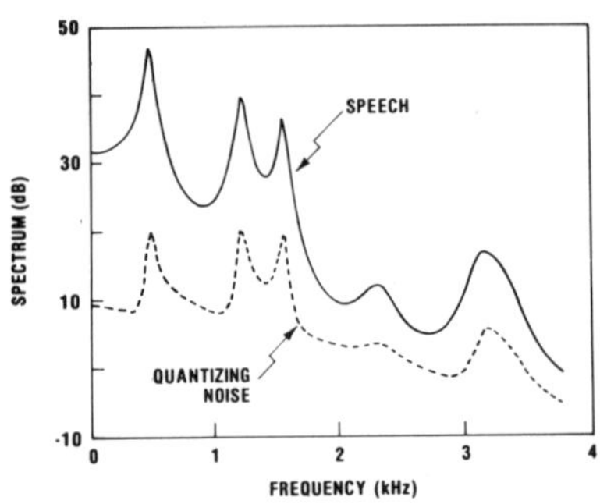

FIGURE 9. An example of the noise spectrum that provides better subjective performance.

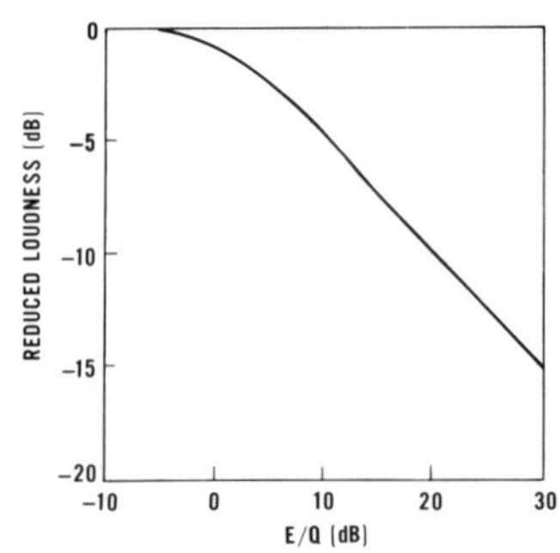

FIGURE 10. Reduced loudness due to auditory masking as a function of the ratio E/Q of signal-to-noise excitations on the basilar membrane.

The audibility of quantization noise depends upon the excitation pattern on the basilar membrane of *both* the speech signal and the quantization noise. In general, the loudness of the noise is reduced by the presence of the speech signal. Quantitative results for accurate computation of loudness of noise in the presence of masking signals are sparse.[6, 7] Recent studies by Hall[8, 9] suggest that the masking effect can be described as a function of the ratio of the signal (E) and noise (Q) excitations on the basilar membrane, as shown in FIGURE 10. This figure shows a plot of reduced loudness due to the masking effect as a function of the ratio E/Q. These results suggest that the loudness of the noise increases by 5 dB for a 10-dB increase in the ratio of signal excitation to noise excitation. Another illustration of masking from the recent studies by Hall is shown in FIGURE 11, which shows the variation of noise intensity at threshold as a function of the frequency of a masking tone. The noise was centered at 1 kHz with a bandwidth of one critical band (160 Hz at 1 kHz). The intensity of the masking tone was 80 dB SPL.

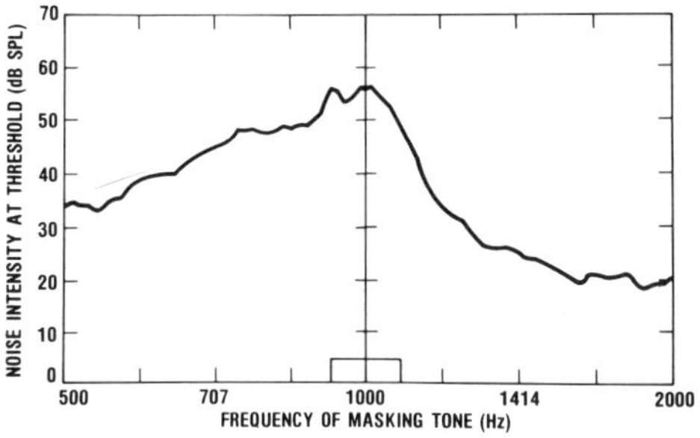

FIGURE 11. Variation of noise intensity at threshold as a function of the frequency of a masking tone. The noise band was centered at 1 kHz with a bandwidth of one critical band at 1 kHz. The intensity of the tone was 80 dB SPL.

As pointed out earlier, linear PCM does not take advantage of auditory masking and, consequently, suffers from poor subjective performance. The logarithmically companded PCM takes advantage of the masking phenomena and thus provides superior performance.

How do we use auditory masking and limited-frequency resolution of our hearing to achieve superior speech quality at a given bit rate? One possibility is to minimize the subjective loudness or audibility of the quantizing noise in the coder. Because of the nonstationary nature of the speech signal, its short-time spectrum and therefore its excitation pattern along the basilar membrane vary continuously with time. Detailed procedures for computing the time-varying loudness of speech signals and noise are described by Schroeder *et al.*[10, 11] An efficient procedure for minimizing the subjective loudness of the quantizing noise is described in Atal and Schroeder.[12]

MODELS OF SPEECH PRODUCTION

Development of accurate models of speech production is essential for efficient encoding of speech signals. A simplified model of speech production using a time-varying linear filter to represent the vocal tract was discussed earlier. There are several equivalent ways of specifying a linear filter. For example, a linear filter is completely specified by the location of poles and zeros of its transfer function. The general problem of determining parameters of a linear filter that accurately define the shapes of the time-varying vocal

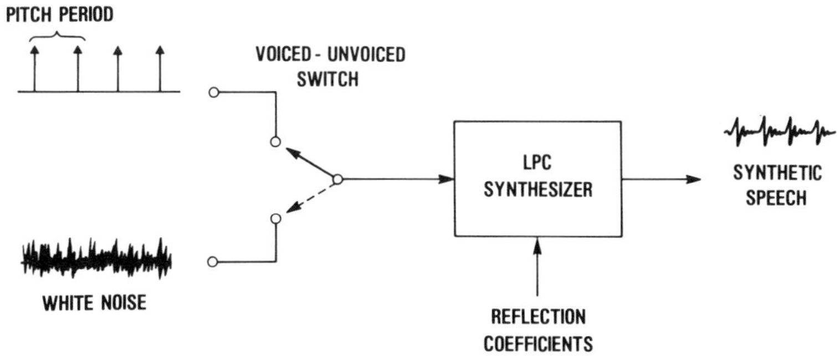

FIGURE 12. Block diagram of an LPC synthesizer using periodic pulse train for synthesizing voiced speech and white noise for synthesizing unvoiced speech.

tract during speech production is still unresolved. A mathematically tractable way of defining the linear filter is to represent it as an all-pole filter.[13] Such an approximation is quite reasonable for vowels and similar sounds. Linear predictive coding (LPC) analysis techniques provide a very simple method of determining the parameters of an all-pole model of the vocal tract.[13, 14]

A model of speech production for synthesizing speech at low bit rates is shown in FIGURE 12. The model performs two basic functions. It has an all-pole filter to model the characteristics of the vocal tract and the spectral shaping of the vocal source. The second part provides the excitation to the all-pole filter. The model assumes that the speech signal can be classified into one of two classes, voiced and unvoiced, and that the pitch period of the voiced speech segment is known. For voiced speech, the excitation is a quasi-periodic pulse train with delta functions located at pitch-period intervals. For unvoiced speech, the excitation is white noise. This model of speech production is widely used for synthesizing speech at low bit rates—particularly below 4.8 kbit/sec. The model is capable of producing highly intelligible speech, but, the speech often does not sound as natural as human speech. The exact reasons for the unnaturalness of the speech synthesized from speech production models such as the one shown in Figure 12 are not completely understood. The reasons may lie in some of the imperfections of LPC analysis techniques in representing the vocal tract accurately or in the idealized model of excitation in terms of pitch pulses and white noise used in the synthesis.

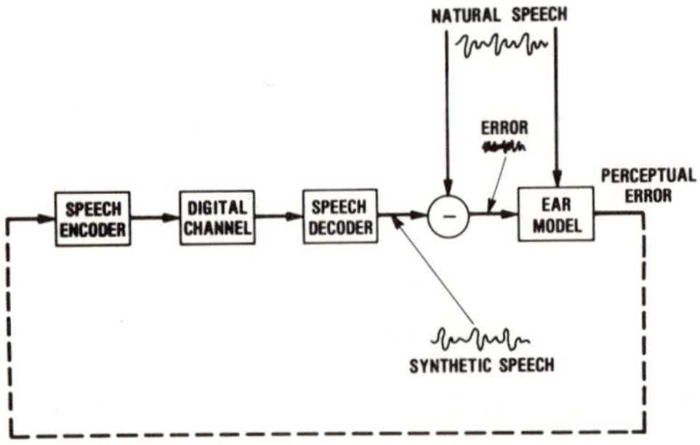

FIGURE 13. Block diagram of a speech coder using an ear model.

Speech coders that use a parametric model of speech production are often called vocoders.[3, 4] Vocoders typically analyze the speech signal into a set of time-varying parameters and then attempt to synthesize speech from these parameters. They make no attempt to ensure that the characteristics of the synthesized speech follow closely those of the natural speech signal. Of course, there is some correspondence between the natural and synthetic speech signals because the synthesis parameters are derived from natural speech. A better way of coding speech would be to incorporate a model of auditory perception explicitly in the encoding process to determine how close the synthesized signal is to the natural speech signal. Such a speech coder is illustrated in the block diagram shown in FIGURE 13. Our knowledge of both human speech production and perception is limited. However, the configura-

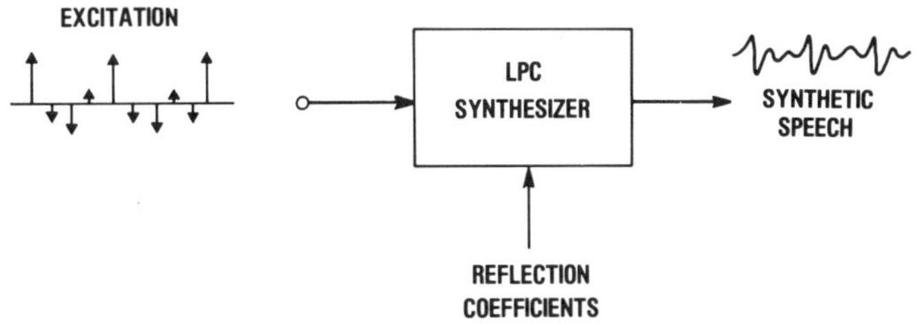

FIGURE 14. Multipulse excitation of a LPC synthesizer.

tion in FIGURE 13 allows one to improve the performance as we gain better understanding of human speech production and perception processes.

The quality of synthetic speech can be improved considerably by eliminating the pitch pulse and white-noise excitation used in the synthesizer shown in FIGURE 12. An improved model [15] using multi-pulse excitation is shown in FIGURE 14. It is quite similar to the traditional LPC synthesizer except for the absence of the pulse and white-noise generators and the voiced–unvoiced switch. In this model, no *a priori* assumption is made about the nature of the excitation signal; the excitation is assumed to be a sequence of pulses for all speech classes, including voiced and unvoiced speech. No attempt is made to produce either a periodic or a nonperiodic excitation.

Of course, if the number of pulses is increased to arbitrarily large value so that there is a pulse at every sampling instant, it should be possible to duplicate the original speech waveform (at the expense of a high bit rate). What we find interesting is that only a few pulses (typically 4 pulses every 5 msec) are sufficient for generating different speech sounds, both voiced and unvoiced, with little audible distortion. Thus, we do not need any prior knowledge of either the voiced–unvoiced decision or the pitch period for synthesizing speech. The periodic (or nonperiodic) nature of the speech signal does not play a crucial role in analysis or synthesis, although the periodicity could be used to decrease the bit rate to lower values.

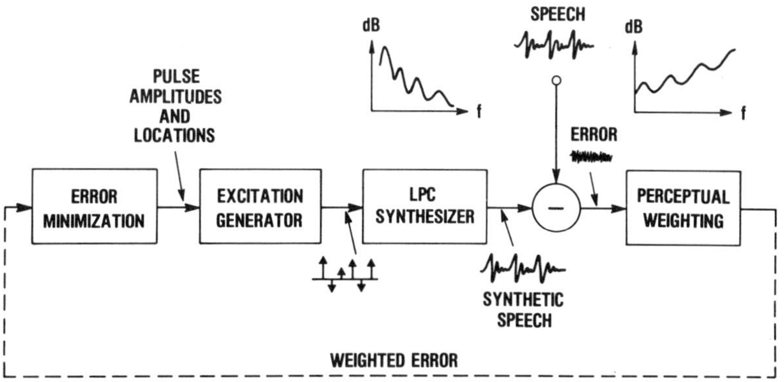

FIGURE 15. An analysis-by-synthesis procedure for determining the optimum pulse locations and amplitudes in multipulse excitation.

An analysis-by-synthesis procedure for determining the locations and the amplitudes of the pulses is shown in the block diagram in FIGURE 15. The LPC synthesizer produces samples of synthetic speech signal in response to the excitation pulses. The synthetic speech samples are compared with the corresponding speech samples of the original (natural) speech signal to produce an error signal. This error is not very meaningful and must be modified to take account of how the human perception treats the error. Broadly speaking, the error in the formant regions must be de-emphasized. This is done by a linear filter which suppresses the energy in the error signal in the formant

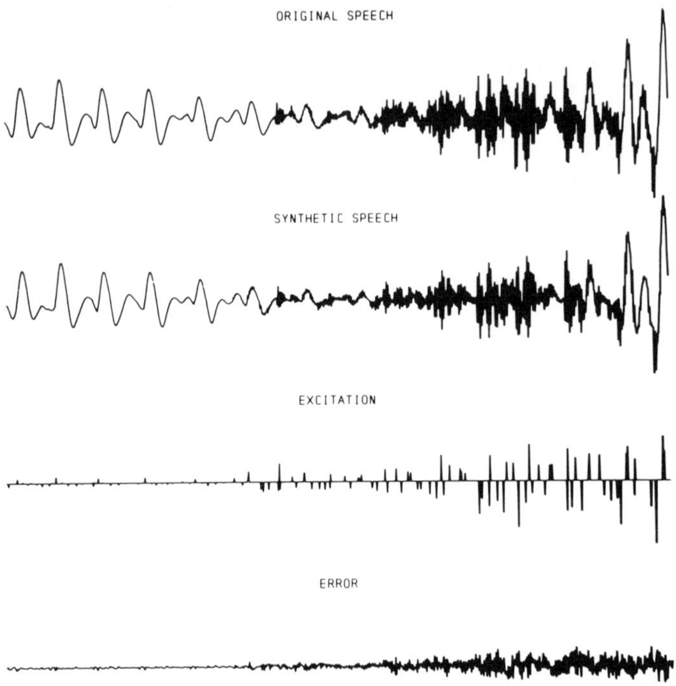

FIGURE 16. Typical examples of original and synthetic speech waveforms. The corresponding multipulse excitation and the error between the original and synthetic signals are also shown.

regions. The error signal is thus weighted to produce a subjectively meaningful measure of the difference between the natural and synthetic speech signals. The weighted error is squared and averaged over a short time interval 5 to 10 msec in duration to produce the mean-squared weighted error. The locations and amplitudes of the pulses are chosen to minimize this error.

Several examples of original and synthetic speech waveforms are shown in FIGURES 16 and 17. The duration of the speech segment is 0.1 sec in each figure. Four pulses every 5 msec were used in the excitation. The figures show the waveforms of the original speech signal, the synthetic speech

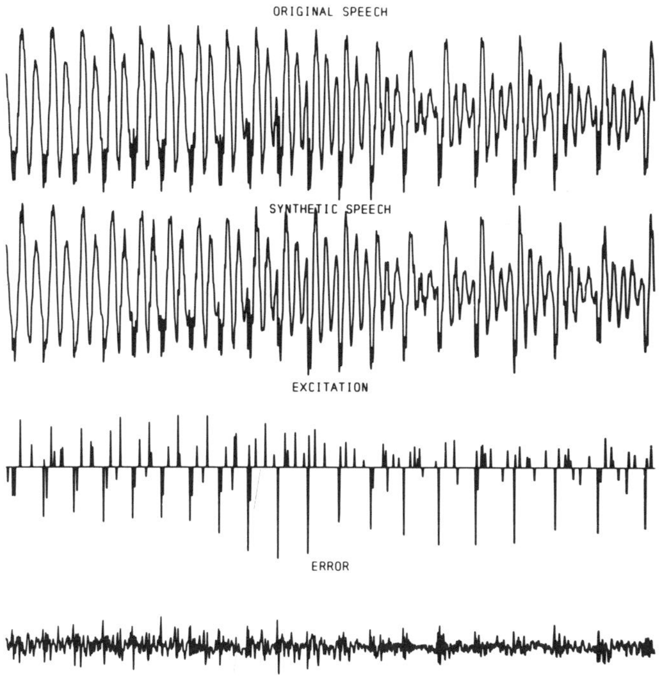

FIGURE 17. Another example of original speech, synthetic speech, multipulse excitation, and error waveforms.

signal, the excitation signal, and the error between the original and the synthetic waveforms. As can be seen, the multi-pulse excitation is able to follow rapid changes in speech waveforms, such as those occurring in rapid transitions. For voiced speech, the quasi-periodic nature of the excitation is produced by the error-minimization procedure without any knowledge of whether the segment is voiced or unvoiced and what its pitch period is.

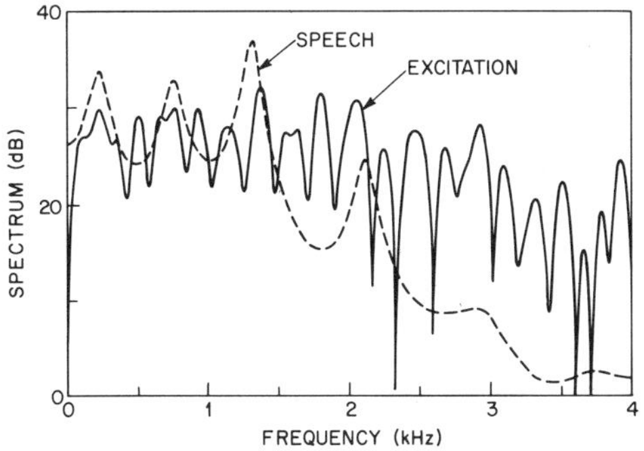

FIGURE 18. Spectra of multipulse excitation and speech signals.

Similarly, the random excitation pattern is also produced automatically by the matching procedure. Mixed excitation comes out automatically, depending upon the nature of the speech signal.

Informal listening tests show that the synthetic speech signal is perceptually close to the original speech signal. The synthetic speech signal from the multi-pulse excitation model does not have the unnatural or buzzy characteristics so often associated with synthetic speech from vocoders.

What is the influence of the excitation pulses on the speech spectrum? FIGURE 18 shows an example of the spectrum of the excitation signal for a single pitch period. As expected, the excitation spectrum has many peaks and valleys—the range of variations often exceeds 10 dB. The speech spectrum is shown also on the figure by a dashed curve. We do not know yet what role the secondary pulses in the excitation play in producing natural-sounding speech.

What kind of bit rate can one expect for this coder? It depends upon the number of pulses used in the excitation signal. With 4 pulses every 5 msec, a bit rate of 6 kbit/sec is needed to encode the pulses. If we combine the bit rate needed to encode the vocal tract parameters, which is approximately 2 kbit/sec, we get a bit rate of approximately 8 kbit/sec. This bit rate represents a substantial reduction over the straight PCM quantization of the waveform.

Discussion

In this paper we have discussed many factors that influence the design of efficient speech coders. We have seen that the inability of the ear to hear certain kinds of distortions in the speech signal plays a crucial role in producing high-quality speech at low bit rates. Analysis-by-synthesis techniques, which include a parametric model of speech production, are very effective in maximizing the perceptual similarity between the natural and synthetic speech signals at a fixed bit rate. The physical difference between the waveforms of a given speech signal and its coded replica generally does not tell us much about the subjective quality of the coded signal. A signal-to-noise ratio as small as 10 dB can be tolerated in the coded signal, provided the errors are distributed both in time and frequency domains where they are least audible.

Speech is a highly redundant signal. The redundant nature of speech is important for providing reliable communication over air pathways. A large part of this redundancy is useless for speech communication over digital channels. The redundancy, unless removed, is a waste of channel capacity. Present speech coders exploit mostly the redundancy apparent at the acoustic level. To achieve even lower bit rates, we must improve our understanding of what goes on beyond the acoustic level in the vocal tract. The acoustic parameters defining the time-varying shapes of the vocal tract vary smoothly as a function of time. An accurate model of these variations in terms of more basic speech parameters is fundamental to further reduction of bit rates.

Although our qualitative understanding of the various steps in the acoustic-to-neural conversion has improved considerably in recent years, we still lack accurate quantitative models. Proper understanding of what is transmitted over the neural pathways to the higher centers is crucial for achieving higher coding efficiency. We have just scratched the surface in speech coding. Future speech coders will use accurate models of both human speech production and perception.

Summary

Speech is a highly redundant signal. The redundant nature of speech is important for providing reliable communication over air pathways. A large part of this redundancy is useless for speech communication over digital channels. Speech coding aims at minimizing the information rate needed to reproduce a speech signal with specified fidelity. In this paper, we discuss factors that influence the design of efficient speech coders. The encoding and decoding processes invariably introduce error (noise and distortion) in the speech signal. Inability of the human ear to hear certain kinds of distortions in the speech signal plays a crucial role in producing high-quality speech at low bit rates. The physical difference between the waveforms of a given speech signal and its coded replica generally does not tell us much about the subjective quality of the coded signal. A signal-to-noise ratio as small as 10 dB can be tolerated in the coded signal provided the errors are distributed both in time and frequency domains where they are least audible. Recent work on auditory masking has provided us with new insights for optimizing the performance of speech coders. This paper reviews this work and discusses new speech coding methods that attempt to maximize the perceptual similarity between the original speech signal and its coded replica. These new methods make it possible to reproduce speech signals at very low bit rates with little or no audible distortion.

References

1. Denes, P. B. & E. N. Pinson. 1973. The Speech Chain: The Physics and Biology of Spoken Language. Anchor Press/Doubleday. New York, NY.
2. Flanagan, J. L., M. R. Schroeder, B. S. Atal, R. E. Crochiere, N. S. Jayant & J. M. Tribolet. 1979. Speech coding. IEEE Trans. Comm. COM-27(4): 710–737.
3. Flanagan, J. L. 1972. Speech Analysis, Synthesis, and Perception, 2nd ed. Springer-Verlag. New York, NY.
4. Rabiner, L. R. & R. W. Schafer. 1973. Digital Processing of Speech Signals. Prentice-Hall. Englewood Cliffs, NJ.
5. Smith, B. 1957. Instantaneous companding of quantized signals. Bell Syst. Tech. J. **36:** 653–709.
6. Zwicker, E. 1963. Ueber die Lautheit von ungedrosselten und gedrosselten Schallen. Acustica **13:** 194–211.
7. Hellman, R. P. 1972. Asymmetry in masking between noise and tone. Percept. Psychophys. **11:** 241–246.
8. Hall, J. L. Unpublished work.
9. Hall, J. L. Unpublished work.

10. SCHROEDER, M. R., B. S. ATAL & J. L. HALL. 1979. Optimizing digital speech coders by exploiting masking properties of the human ear. J. Acoust. Soc. Am. **66:** 1647–1562.
11. SCHROEDER, M. R., B. S. ATAL & J. L. HALL. 1979. Objective measure of certain speech signal degradations based on properties of human auditory perception. *In* Frontiers of Speech Communication Research. B. Lindblom and S. Ohman, Eds.: 217–229. Academic Press. London.
12. ATAL, B. S. & M. R. SCHROEDER. 1979. Optimizing predictive coders for minimum audible noise. Proceedings of the 1979 International Conference on Acoustics, Speech, Signal Processing. Washington, DC.: 453–455.
13. ATAL, B. S. & S. L. HANAUER. 1971. Speech analysis and synthesis by linear prediction of the speech wave. J. Acoust. Soc. Am. **50**(2): 637–655.
14. ATAL, B. S. 1982. Predictive coding of speech at low bit rates. IEEE Trans. Comm. COM-30 (4): 600–614.
15. ATAL, B. S. & J. R. REMDE. 1982. A new model of LPC excitation for producing natural-sounding speech at low bit rates. Proceedings of the 1982 International Conference on Acoustics, Speech, Signal Processing. Paris, France.: 614–617.

LIMITS ON ALTERNATIVE AUDITORY REPRESENTATIONS OF SPEECH [a]

Michael Studdert-Kennedy

Queens College and Graduate Center
City University of New York
Flushing, New York 11367; and
Haskins Laboratories
New Haven, Connecticut 06510

The history of attempts to construct reading machines for the blind may guide us in our attempts to devise speech-listening aids for the deaf. The goal of the early reading machine work was to construct an acoustic alphabet, that is, to find a set of discrete, discriminable acoustic patterns that might substitute for the visual alphabet. To devise such a set—of tones, chords, bursts of filtered noise, perhaps varying in amplitude or duration—was not difficult, and, if the patterns were presented one at a time in a comfortable test format, listeners readily learned to identify them. However, if patterns were presented in rapid sequence, listener performance dropped precipitously. In fact, no one has yet devised an acoustic alphabet more effective than the dots and dashes of Morse code, with which highly skilled operators may reach a rate of 30–40 words a minute—roughly one-fifth of the rate at which we typically follow spoken language. Not surprisingly, the search for an acoustic alphabet for reading machines has been largely abandoned in favor of synthetic (or compiled) speech.

The failure to devise a viable acoustic alphabet seems all the more surprising when we consider the success of the visual alphabet. On the face of it, one might have expected that transposition into another sensory modality would have been more damaging—certainly more "unnatural"—than remaining within the biologically given modality of sound. But, as we all know, that is far from the case. Even without benefit of special "speed-reading" instruction, reading rates of 300–400 words a minute are commonplace.

What are we to make of this paradox? Why do speech and a visual alphabet succeed where a sound alphabet fails? The answer seems to lie, first, in certain properties of the visual and auditory systems, and second, in the different types of information that speech and alphabets convey.

Although the temporal distribution of light carries important information for the perception of an event as it develops in time, the spatial distribution of light at any instant is sufficient to specify a stationary object. In fact, the eye is particularly sensitive to spatial patterns of contour and it is this sensitivity that writing systems exploit: we read by a series of static fixations during which information from many points in the visual field is gathered simultaneously. By contrast, sound is never static; we perceive auditorily by virtue of the way in which events structure the spectrum over time. Recent studies of the response to speech of auditory nerve fibers in cat [1-3] have demonstrated that the nerve

[a] This work was supported by Grant HD 01944 from the National Institute of Child Health and Human Development of the National Institutes of Health.

0077-8923/83/0405-0033 $01.75/0 © 1983, NYAS

is particularly responsive to abrupt discontinuities in amplitude and frequency: at such instants of discontinuity, there occurs a rapid increase or decrease in firing rate, reflecting an increase or decrease in the number of fibers sampling the input. Such on- and off-responses may serve as a first stage in segmenting the speech signal.[7] Moreover, the spectral structure [4] or shifts in spectral structure [5] in the tens of milliseconds following an abrupt onset may carry important acoustic–phonetic information. Of course, more gradual shifts in spectral structure with transitions into and out of relatively steady-state portions of the signal are also reflected in the temporal structure of cat neural response [2,6] and, in the human, presumably serve to specify phonetic elements.[7] My point here is simply that the dynamic structure of speech seems nicely tuned to evade (or exploit) the limits imposed by refractory neural response and by neural adaptation and masking. We may suspect then that the failure of acoustic alphabets in reading machines stemmed, in part, from their use of static segments modeled on those of the visual alphabet: the repeated abrupt breaks in acoustic pattern, inevitable in a sequence of arbitrary static elements, ran foul of the refractory, adaptive and masking characteristics of the auditory system. There would seem to be no reason, in principle, why an acoustic alphabet more shrewdly tailored to the requirements of the auditory system should not work. But then, of course, it might be simpler to use a facsimile of the acoustic structure that evolution has prescribed: synthetic speech.

We come now to a second and deeper reason for the differences between speech and an acoustic alphabet: The information conveyed by speech is quite different from the information conveyed by an alphabet (or by any other secondary mode of representation such as a syllabary or logographic system). Speech conveys information about the gestures that produced it. There is nothing intrinsically linguistic in these gestures. They have, of course, been selected by a long process of evolution and historical development to answer the motoric and perceptual demands of linguistic communication. But the linguistic value of the gestures is available only to the listener (or viewer) who knows something of the language being spoken. The gestures themselves are simply a complex, coordinated pattern of articulatory activity, and the function of the speech signal is to specify this activity. By contrast, the elements of an alphabet specify nothing. Their structure is arbitrary, constrained only by the perceptual capacities of their users. Their structure can be arbitrary precisely because their function is not to specify, but to indicate (or symbolize) something other than themselves, namely, the elements of a language.[8]

What does all this have to do with listening aids for the deaf? Let me begin by justifying the claim that the function of the speech signal is to specify articulation. The value of lip-reading for the deaf is well known, but the implications of this skill for an understanding of normal speech perception have only recently begun to emerge. McGurk and MacDonald [9] discovered that listeners' perception of a spoken utterance can be altered if they simultaneously watch a videotape of a speaker articulating a different utterance. For example, if subjects are presented with four spoken repetitions of the syllable [ba], while watching a synchronized videotape of a speaker articulating the sequence [ba, va, ða, da], it is the latter sequence that they will typically report. Or again, if subjects are presented with audio [ba] in synchrony with video [ga], they will typically report [bga], [gba] or [da]. Here the integrated percepts are either clusters corresponding to both the acoustical and the optical patterns presented, or a merged segment [da], corresponding to neither.[10,11]

Roberts and Summerfield [12] took advantage of this last effect to demonstrate the distinction between surface acoustic structure and the phonetic percept in a study of audio-visual adaptation. The standard adaptation procedure calls for forced-choice, two-category identification of items drawn at random from a synthetic speech continuum, along which some acoustic correlate of a single phonetic feature has been systematically varied, as from [ba] to [da] or from [da] to [ta]. Subjects make their judgments both before and after being exposed to (that is, adapted with) many repetitions of a good exemplar from one or other of the two endpoint categories. The effect of this adaptation procedure is a significant drop in the frequency with which subjects assign ambiguous items from the continuum to the category from which the adapting syllable was drawn.

Roberts and Summerfield [12] gave a novel twist to this paradigm. On a [bϵ-dϵ] continuum they compared the effect of a standard auditory adaptor, [bϵ], with that of an audio-visual adaptor, auditory [bϵ], visual [gϵ], intended to be perceived as [dϵ]. Of their twelve subjects, six reported the audio-visual adaptor most of the time as [dϵ] or [ðϵ], four as [klϵ], one as [flϵ], and one as [ma]. Not one of the subjects reported the auditory syllable actually presented, namely, [bϵ]. Yet the adaptation effect was purely auditory: every subject displayed a drop in the number of items identified as [bϵ], roughly equal to the drop for the control condition in which auditory [bϵ] was presented alone. Thus, while listeners' auditory systems were normally adapted by the acoustic input, their conscious phonetic percepts were specified by a blend of acoustical and optical information.

The basis of this acoustical–optical blend is not understood. The acoustical information is presumably carried by the familiar pattern of formants, friction noise, plosive release, harmonic variation, and so on; apparently, the optical information is carried by varying configurations of the lips and, perhaps, of the tongue and teeth.[11] But how these qualitatively distinct patterns of light and sound are combined to yield an integrated percept is not obvious. We can certainly point to covarying properties in, for example, the opening of the mouth and a pattern of formant movement, or in the rounding of the lips and a downward shift in spectral structure. But these are mere correlations: They are not directly given in perception—unless we adduce an *ad hoc* theory of learned association. And this seems implausible, in light of the discovery that 6-month-old infants recognize structural correspondences between patterns of speech and facial movement.[13, 14] What we need is some deeper, underlying metric, common to both the light reflected and the sound radiated from mouth and lips.

Insight into the nature of this metric may come from the phenomenon of imitation. We are not surprised that if someone pouts her lips, someone else can pout in imitation, because the capacity to imitate seems "natural," so natural, in fact, that even 36-hour-old infants can do it.[15, 16] Nonetheless, there is a puzzle here. How does the imitator transpose a pattern of light into a pattern of movement? Or, as Gibson's followers ask, how do we get light into a muscle? What seems to be required is that we perceive in a movement not simply its surface kinematics (such as displacements, velocities, and accelerations), but also the biophysical forces that define the structure to be moved and that produce the movement, in other words, the underlying dynamics (mass, elasticity, force, and momentum, for example). Notice that we require an equivalent (and, surely, no less biologically specialized) perceptual capacity to account for our ability to repeat a spoken utterance. The "kinematics" of the utterance, that is, the changes and rates of change in sound source and spectral structure, as illustrated in the spectrogram, are incommensurate with the muscular controls that produce them. How do we get sound into a muscle? We are led, it seems, by the facts of imitation to suppose that we perceive in both the sound and the sight of speech not only the surface kinematics, but also the underlying dynamics of articulation.[17-19]

For present purposes, the import of this brief discussion is simply that the forces controlling articulation are not revealed in the static spectral sections of the spectrograph. Therefore, if the speech percept is, indeed, properly specified in a ". . . metric closely related to that of articulatory dynamics," [11] as the facts of imitation seem to require, then any viable alternative auditory representation of speech must, first and foremost, preserve the information that makes these dynamics available to the listener: not the static spectral patterns putatively corresponding to the static elements of phonetic description, but the subtle patterns of changing spectral structure.

The point is vividly illustrated by the phenomenon of sinewave speech.[20] Here the spectral structure is drastically reduced. The speech signal is whittled down to a temporal pattern of change in three (or even two) sinewaves, roughly following the center frequencies of the first three (or two) formants. Yet the speech remains surprisingly intelligible: Many listeners (perhaps most listeners, with practice) can understand unknown sentences—even, incidentally, when all amplitude changes corresponding to syllabic rise and fall have also been eliminated.[21] In effect, the sinewave transformation removes all information concerning the sound source (voicing, frication, plosive release), but retains (sharply reduced) information concerning instants of silence (for example, stop closure) and the partially reciprocal variations in size and shape of the front and back cavities of the vocal tract.[22] However, what is crucial here is that the information preserved is not simply some trace of the formant structure, sufficient to specify instantaneous cavity relations, but the temporal patterns of spectral change that specify the forces controlling the movements by which cavity shapes are determined.

The nature of these temporal patterns may be clarified if we consider another, closely related study. Risberg and Agelfors [23] report the results of an experiment in which the speech signal was reduced to a single sinewave modulated in frequency to match the center of gravity, and in amplitude to match the total energy, of the spectrum. With practice, subjects were able to identify up to nearly 90% of a closed set of twelve Swedish spondee words and up to 50% of the Swedish numerals from 13–99. The authors suggest that, while their minimal spectral display evidently preserved enough information for the identification of fricatives and certain vowels, subjects may have relied largely on the timing of word or syllable onsets and offsets. It would seem that these timing patterns may have sufficed to distinguish among the elements of a closed set, very much as some arbitrary, unique property of a word may serve for artificial machine recognition.

My point here is not that a single sinewave representation might not, by judicious weighting of its spectral determinants, be made to specify the phonetic structure of unknown sentences. That might very well be the case. My point is rather to distinguish between temporal patterns of syllable onsets and offsets, which may serve to distinguish among a closed set of words or word sequences, and a temporal pattern of spectral change that specifies the dynamics of articulation. The latter entails rates of change in overall structure, as well perhaps as delicate shifts in the temporal alignment of formant movement that reflect interarticulator timing. It is something of this that the earlier sinewave studies [19] seem to have preserved, if we may judge from their subjects' success in identifying unknown phonetic sequences.

In conclusion, the movements of speech are not disembodied. They are the movements of a biologically given articulatory system with characteristic configurations. At any instant, the configuration may be described in terms of articulator placement (as in traditional phonetics) and may be specified, in principle, by the static morphology of lips and mouth or by the spectral structure of sound. But speech only emerges from systematic changes in articulator placement and interarticulator organization. It is to change that the auditory system is particularly sensitive, and it is in spectral change that the prepared observer finds the dynamic patterns that specify the phonetic event. The limits on an alternative auditory representation of speech would seem then to be that it preserve some minimal, perhaps grossly transposed, spectral structure, sufficient to specify instantaneous articulator placement, and that this structure be such that it can be modulated over time to specify the underlying articulatory dynamics.

Acknowledgments

My thanks to Robert Remez and Philip Rubin for useful discussion.

References

1. Delgutte, B. 1980. Representation of speech-like sounds in the discharge patterns of auditory-nerve fibers. J. Acoust. Soc. Am. **68:** 843–857.
2. Delgutte, B. 1982. Some correlates of phonetic distinctions at the level of the auditory nerve. *In* The Representation of Speech in the Peripheral Auditory System. R. Carlson and B. Granstrom, Eds.: 131–149. Elsevier Biomedical Press. New York, NY.
3. Kiang, N. Y. S. 1980. Processing of speech by the auditory nervous system. J. Acoust. Soc. Am. **68:** 830–835.
4. Stevens, K. N. & S. E. Blumstein. 1978. Invariant cues for place of articulation. J. Acoust. Soc. Am. **64:** 1358–1368.
5. Kewley-Port, D. 1980. Representations of spectral change as cues to place of articulation in stop consonants. Unpublished Ph.D. dissertation, City University of New York, New York, NY.
6. Sachs, M. B., E. D. Young & M. I. Miller. 1982. Encoding of speech features in the auditory nerve. *In* The Representation of Speech in the Peripheral Auditory System. R. Carlson and B. Granstrom, Eds.: 115–130. Elsevier Biomedical Press. New York, NY.
7. Chistovich, L. A., V. V. Lublinskaya, T. G. Malinnikova, E. A. Ogorodnikova, E. I. Stoljarova & S. Ja. Zhukov. 1982. Temporal processing of peripheral auditory patterns of speech. *In* The Representation of Speech in the Peripheral Auditory System. R. Carlson and B. Granstrom, Eds.: 165–180. Elsevier Biomedial Press. New York, NY.
8. Carello, C., M. T. Turvey, P. N. Kugler & R. E. Shaw. Inadequacies of the computer metaphor. *In* Handbook of Cognitive Neuroscience. M. S. Gazzaniga, Ed. Plenum Press. New York, NY. In press.

9. McGurk, H. & J. MacDonald. 1976. Hearing lips and seeing voices. Nature **264:** 746–748.
10. MacDonald, J & H. McGurk. 1978. Visual influences on speech perception processes. Percept. Psychophys. **24:** 253–257.
11. Summerfield, Q. 1979. Use of visual information for phonetic perception. Phonetica **36:** 314–331.
12. Roberts, M. & Q. Summerfield. 1981. Audiovisual presentation demonstrates that selective adaptation in speech perception is purely auditory. Percept. Psychophys. **30:** 309–314.
13. Kuhl, P. K. & A. N. Meltzoff. 1982. The bimodal perception of speech in infancy. Science **218:** 1138–1141.
14. MacKain, K., M. Studdert-Kennedy, S. Spieker & D. Stern. Infant intermodal speech perception is a left hemisphere function. Science. In press.
15. Field, T. M., R. Woodson, R. Greenberg & D. Cohen. 1982. Discrimination and imitation of facial expressions by neonates. Science **218:** 179–181.
16. Meltzoff, A. N. & M. K. Moore. 1977. Imitation of facial and manual gestures by human neonates. Science **198:** 75–76.
17. Fowler, C. A., P. Rubin, R. E. Remez & M. T. Turvey. Implications for speech production of a general theory of action. *In* Language Production. B. Butterworth, Ed.: 373–420. Academic Press. New York, NY.
18. Runeson, S. & G. Frykholm. 1981. Visual perception of lifted weight. J. Exp. Psychol.: Hum. Percep. & Perform. **7:** 733–740.
19. Summerfield, Q. 1980. The structuring of language by the requirements of motor control and perception: Group Report. *In* Signed and Spoken Language: Biological Constraints on Linguistic Form. U. Bellugi & M. Studdert-Kennedy, Eds.: 89–114. Verlag Chemie. Deerfield Beach, FL.
20. Remez, R. E., P. E. Rubin & D. B. Pisoni. 1983. Coding of the speech spectrum in three time-varying sinusoids. This volume.
21. Remez, R. E., P. E. Rubin & T. D. Carrell. 1981. Phonetic perception of sinusoidal signals: effects of amplitude variation. J. Acoust. Soc. Am. **69**(S1): 114(A).
22. Kuhn, G. M. 1975. On the front cavity resonance and its possible role in speech perception. J. Acoust. Soc. Am. **58:** 428–433.
23. Risberg, A. & E. Agelfors. 1982. Speech perception based on non-speech signals. *In* The Representation of Speech in the Peripheral Auditory System. R. Carlson and B. Granstrom. Eds.: 209–215. Elsevier Biomedical Press. New York, NY.

TECHNIQUES FOR COMPUTER RECOGNITION OF SPEECH [a]

Roberto Bisiani

Department of Computer Science and Robotics Institute
Carnegie-Mellon University
Pittsburgh, Pennsylvania 15213

Introduction

Although computers are now a necessary tool providing the basis for many of the functions of modern society, the quality of interaction between persons and computers is lower than one would expect. One reason for this is that it is impossible for computers to perform most of the sensory-based tasks on which human interaction rests. Speech communication is one of the tasks that are natural for humans and very difficult for machines.

Since machine understanding of fluent, unrestricted speech is difficult, researchers have investigated subtasks that compromise on some of the capabilities that humans have. For example, number of words (vocabulary size), structure of sentences (syntax), naturalness of speech (for example, fluent speech rather than one word at a time), and independence from speaker differences have been restricted to cope with machine inadequacies. Most of these characteristics present rather different research problems that are most conveniently tackled individually, and we are thus confronted with a very large range of existing research and commercial speech systems.

This paper will not present an exhaustive taxonomy of recognition systems because in-depth presentations of the complete spectrum of solutions are available in the literature.[8, 15] The paper will instead focus on the current most promising techniques and the difficulties that hinder the implementation of more powerful systems.

Speech Recognition as an Encoding Process

At first approximation, speech recognition systems can be viewed as a sequence or pipeline of independent modules each performing a transformation over the input signal and delivering it to the next module. This process continues until the signal becomes a sequence of words. Two considerations that apply to all the modules can be made. Firstly, the "bandwidth" of the

[a] This research was sponsored in part by Grant MCS–7825824 from the National Science Foundation, and in part by the Defense Advanced Research Projects Agency (DOD), ARPA Order No. 3597, monitored by the Air Force Avionics Laboratory under Contract F33615–78–C–1551.

The views and conclusions contained in this document are those of the author and should not be interpreted as representing the official policies, either expressed or implied, of the Defense Advanced Research Projects Agency or the United States government.

0077–8923/83/0405–0039 $01.75/0 © 1983, NYAS

signal keeps decreasing, that is, the symbols used to encode the speech signal are more and more concise and powerful. Secondly, the data reduction techniques that are applied become less and less "localized." In other words, the first modules process small "segments" of signal independently of the rest of the information, while the subsequent modules take into account how the segment being processed interacts with other parts of the signal. The most commonly used modules are described in the following paragraphs.

The simplest digital representation of speech is pulse-code modulation. The changes in air pressure caused by speech are sampled by using an analog to digital converter. The sampling frequency can vary between 8,000 to 20,000 samples per second, each sample represented by 9 to 16 bits (about 500 to 16,000 quantization levels).

Most of the compression techniques that are applied to the raw speech signal are based on the assumption that the signal will remain constant for a short period of time. One of the most common representations is the so-called *short-time spectrum* that can be obtained either by using an (analog or digital) filter bank or by computing a DFT. A viable alternative to the short-time spectrum is the linear predictive coding (LPC) parameters.[1, 5] The LPC parameters are based on the facts that: (a) the vocal tract can be modeled as an acoustic tube whose input is impulses or noise; (b) such model is mathematically tractable. A third and rather crude way of coding speech is to represent it by the signal amplitude and number of zerocrossings.[2]

Further reduction of the signal bandwidth goes often under the generic term of *phonemic labeling*.[15] This includes a complex set of techniques that: (1) splice the signal in fixed length units or variable length segments either separated by silence or having some acoustic similarity; (2) extract a few features such as voicing, stress, or pitch; and (3) label segments with a symbol from a limited (a few tens to a thousand) set of "typical" symbols.

It should be noted that the compression techniques described so far become more and more specific and limited to a given domain when they get closer to the final recognition: pulse code modulation can be used for any signal, LPC works for speech only, and phonemic labeling is based on typical speech sounds and is therefore language-dependent. The next compression steps are even more restrictive because they collapse sequences of phonemic labels into words and words into utterances. Most of these operations require the availability of some task-dependent knowledge such as the set of legal words (vocabulary), the grammatical structure of legal sentences (syntax), the meaning of words within a sentence (semantics), and the restriction imposed by the conversation context (pragmatics).

The boundary between data compression and recognition is often not well defined since most of the data compression performed after the very first few steps involves some kind of recognition and, at the end, some task-specific knowledge. By strongly constraining the discourse alternatives (for example, the number of legal words, the syntax), some of the final more elaborate compression steps can be avoided and the recognition obtained with a pattern matching process. This approach can be successful only in very restricted domains.

REVIEW OF THE STATE OF THE ART

Initial research in man–machine communication via speech focused on *isolated word recognition.* Systems have been constructed with recognition error rate of 1% (that is, one error every 100 utterances processed) on tests using small vocabularies (30–200 words) and a known speaker.[5, 18, 19] Most of these systems use one of many variations of the dynamic programming (DP) time normalization algorithm. In essence, the DP algorithm finds the best frame-by-frame spectral match between a test and reference pattern by stretching or folding the temporal axis of either the test or the reference in a nonlinear fashion. For a single speaker, Itakura obtained 2.7 error rate on a 200-word vocabulary of Japanese geographical names using telephone speech (3 kHz) and 8 LPC coefficients. These results demonstrated that DP template matching can produce high recognition scores for some vocabularies.

Itakura's research, and many subsequent studies, have shown that DP template matching will produce high recognition accuracies *as long as the vocabulary items are acoustically distinct.* For example, substituting the English alphabet and digits for the Japanese geographical names and leaving everything else equal yields an error rate of 11.4 percent. Moreover, almost all of the errors occur among a few confusable items: for example, the letters B, D, E, P, T, V were only recognized about 50% of the time.

There is an enormous variation in the acoustic realization of the same words across speakers due to different speech habits and vocal tract sizes. Approaches to speaker-independent recognition using dynamic programming have applied a number of techniques, such as frequency warping and the use of multiple templates. In general, speaker-independent systems produce substantially lower performance for acoustically confusable vocabularies, but high recognition accuracies for acoustically distinct vocabularies. For example, Rabiner, Levinson, Rosenberg and Wilpon [13] used a statistical clustering technique to derive an average of 13 templates for each of the items in the alphadigit vocabulary from templates produced by 100 different talkers. Using a different set of talkers, they obtained 21% overall recognition error rate, and 2% speaker-independent error rate for the digits.

The problem with isolated word recognition systems is that the speaker must pause before and after each word. Such artificial pauses greatly reduce the naturalness of communication. *Connected word recognition* systems eliminate the pause constraint and allow the user to communicate by fluent speech, which introduces two major problems caused by the absence of physical cues to word boundaries and the variability of words at junctures. Coupled with speaker variability and semantic ambiguity, connected speech recognition is beyond classical pattern recognition techniques. The solution to the problem is to use all available sources of knowledge to reduce ambiguity in the transcription process.[15] Knowledge of segmentation, phonetics, prosodics, syllables, lexicon, syntax, semantics, and pragmatics must be brought to bear during the recognition process.

A number of connected speech-understanding systems have been developed in recent years. These include the IBM system, the Harpy and Hearsay-II systems developed at Carnegie-Mellon University, the HWIM system developed at BBN (Bolt, Beranek & Neuman), and two-level DP connected digit systems developed by NEC (Nippon Electric Co.), Verbex, and Bell Labs.

Connected Digit Recognition

A number of connected-speech-recognition systems have been developed, both as laboratory tools and for commercial use, that are based on the principles of DP matching.[10, 11, 14, 16] Since DP template matching is best suited for vocabularies with acoustically dissimilar items, most of these systems have been tested with digits.

Sakoe's system,[16] which has been implemented in the commercially available NEC system, is called two-level DP matching. On the first pass, the reference templates are exhaustively matched to each subsection of the input string. The second pass uses the distance scores generated in the first pass to determine the best overall match to the spoken string. Rabiner and Schmidt [14] use a similar procedure in which the DP algorithm is used to "spot" digits. The boundary of a word with a high score, defined as the termination point of the warp, is used to start successive warps. The recognizer keeps track of all candidate strings, and the one with the lowest cumulative score is chosen.

A number of connected-word-recognition systems have recently been developed for use in grammatically well-defined task domains with vocabularies of about 100 words. Meyers and Levinson [11] have extended the level-building DP algorithm of Meyers and Rabiner [10] for use with an airline information and reservation task with a vocabulary of 127 words. Speaker-dependent recognition scores of 6% word error and 13% sentence error were reported.

Shikano [17] has developed a speaker-independent phoneme-based connected-speech-recognition system which produces 3% wrong phrase recognition on a train reservation task with a 112-word vocabulary. The system uses vowel templates averaged across speakers and extracts a number of acoustic features to perform consonant identification. The phoneme recognition results are represented in a phoneme lattice so that ambiguous segmentation and labeling can be made, and a linguistic processor interprets the sentence. The linguistic processor also composes a response sentence, which is automatically transmitted as voice output.

Harpy

Harpy [8, 9] extracts 14 LPC coefficients every 10 msec. Adjacent frames are combined into segments on the basis of similarity. Each segment is compared to spectral templates using the Itakura [5] minimum residual error metric. All knowledge (lexical, syntactic, semantic) is precompiled in a state transition network. The network includes (*a*) all possible paths through a finite-state grammar (that is, a graph representation of all possible sentences), (*b*) alternate representations of all words as sequences of spectral templates, and (*c*) a set of rules for expected acoustic changes at word boundaries. The recognition strategy consists of matching the acoustic segments in the input utterance to 98 speaker-dependent templates, and finding the lowest scoring path through the network.

Harpy provided 95% correct semantic interpretation of 100 sentences on a document retrieval task having a vocabulary of 1011 words. All of the words in a sentence were recognized 90% of the time. The success of the Harpy system is due largely to the constraints built into the state-transition network. Word-level recognition errors of 10% were achieved even though the top scoring template was wrong more than 50% of the time.

Hearsay-II

In Hearsay [4, 8] the signal is divided into 10-msec frames based on smoothed and differenced amplitude and zero-crossing parameters. Frames are combined into segments on the basis of similarity, and segments are then assigned to manner of articulation classes on the basis of a decision tree of logical thresholds (10% wrong). Labels based on LPC spectra are assigned to templates (51% wrong first-choice error).

Knowledge is represented in Hearsay-II as a set of independent processes that communicate with each other through a global data base or "blackboard." Knowledge sources are activated by the appearance of new information on the blackboard; when activated, they try to extend the analysis. Knowledge sources predict, verify, or concatenate words on the basis of acoustic or syntactic data. Recognition proceeds in Hearsay-II by finding a lexical description that is compatible with all of the knowledge sources.

On the document retrieval task Hearsay-II achieved 9% wrong semantic interpretation of a set of test utterances. Twenty-seven percent were not recognized correctly word-for-word.

HWIM

BBN's HWIM [8] estimates formant frequencies, extracts energy as a function of time in different frequency bands, computes zerocrossing, and estimates fundamental frequency every 5 msec. This information is used to derive a set of phonetic transcription alternatives that are stored in a lattice representation which allows for multiple choices. Knowledge about the phonological structure of words is represented in HWIM as a lexical decoding network which contains the expected phonetic realizations of each word in all possible phonetic contexts (these realizations are generated automatically by using phonological rules).

Recognition proceeds in HWIM by searching through the derived segmental representation for good word matches. Word hypotheses are verified using an analysis by synthesis procedure, and if the verified score is high enough, they are sent to the syntactic prediction component to hypothesize words to the right and left of the high scoring word. This process of verification and hypothesis continues until a complete sentence is found.

The BBN system provided a correct semantic interpretation of a set of test sentences 44% of the time. However, the task domain chosen required a much less constraining grammar than that used in the Carnegie-Mellon systems, so it is difficult to compare results across systems. Performance of the segmentation and labeling components of HWIM were evaluated by using 124 sentences read by three speakers. When following the most correct path through the lattice, only 1.6% of the segmentation points were missed, and an extra segment was added 1.8% of the time. Labeling performance was also evaluated for the most correct path through each lattice. With 71 possible labels, the wrong label was produced 49% of the time.[7]

IBM

The IBM system[6] employs a multi-pass approach. In one of its most recent implementations[12] a discrete Fourier transform is computed every 10 msec using a 20-msec sliding window to produce vectors of 80 spectral amplitudes ranging from 0 to 8 kHz in bands of 100 Hz each. For each vector, the acoustic processor outputs the label of the closest phonetic prototype. In earlier IBM systems, prototypes were selected manually, but they are now selected automatically by using clustering techniques,[12] with little loss in recognition accuracy, using 5 minutes of continuous speech for a given speaker. In current system versions, 200 prototypes are used to account for acoustic variability due to the phonetic context.

Lexical knowledge is represented in a network structure called a "directed-graph lexical entry." Initially, each word is described by a set of pronunciations. These standard pronunciations are altered by phonological rules. The probabilities and parameters of the graph models are estimated from about 2 hours of training data. Each phone is in turn characterized by a finite-state acoustic graph, and each arc of the graph corresponds to a vector output of the acoustic processor. Conceptually, the appropriate acoustic graphs are embedded in the phonological graph. This composite graph models the possible sequence of outputs and the probabilities with which they are produced. Syntactic knowledge is incorporated as a probabilistic function of a Markov process.

Using "centisecond modeling," the IBM system has achieved extremely good word recognition accuracy. For example, on the document retrieval task (on which Harpy and Hearsay-II were evaluated), word recognition error of less than 1% has been obtained. This improvement in performance is due mainly to the precise extraction of spectral information every 10 msec. By comparison, the Harpy system forms templates from spectrally similar centisecond frames (average duration 5 csec) and retains only the 14 LPC coefficients at the center of each frame. The use of 80-point spectral resolution every 10 msec produces a substantially better performance on the same set of test data.

Recent tests of the IBM system have been performed on a laser-patent corpus, which consists of sentences from descriptive portions of patents in laser technology. Tests have used sentences composed of the 1,000 most frequently occurring words in this corpus. Word recognition error rates of 8.7% have been reported. When sentences were spoken with pauses between the words, error rates fell to 3.1%.

Discussion and Prediction of Future Trends

The state of the art in computer speech recognition can be summarized as follows:

1. Isolated word recognition systems can perform with error rates of less than 1% with vocabularies of several hundred words, as long as the words are not acoustically confusable. For smaller vocabularies of acoustically distinct words, such as the digits, speaker-independent systems achieve equivalent performance.

2. Connected digit recognition systems perform with error rates of less than 2% in both speaker-dependent and speaker-independent modes.

3. Connected speech understanding systems with vocabularies from 100 to 1000 words perform with word error rates of 10% to 1% on task domains in which word choice is highly constrained, and alternatives are acoustically dissimilar. These systems are able to integrate diverse sources of knowledge to constrain word choice, and are able to deal with errorful input and ambiguity in a graceful manner.

Given that we can build systems that accept connected speech and recognize more than 1,000 words with less than 1% word error rate in limited task domains, what prevents us from building systems that can recognize conversational speech? One of the factors that hinder recognition is that computers cannot make *fine phonetic distinctions.* In conversational speech, it is often the case that, at a particular point in a sentence, several words which differ by a single phonetic segment are plausible. In these cases, recognition depends entirely on the ability of the system (human or machine) to discriminate between two or more phonetic segments. Present recognition systems can discriminate among acoustically simliar segments with no greater than about 50% error rate. In fact, the problem of performing fine phonetic discrimination is so difficult that no one has yet devised a speaker-dependent system that can discriminate among the confusable letters B, D, E, P, T, G, V, Z, and C, spoken in isolation, with better than about 30% error rate averaged over a number of different speakers.

In limited task domains, where word choice is highly constrained, knowledge of these constraints can be used to compensate for poor "acoustic" performance. Thus, Harpy recognizes 9 of every 10 words on the document retrieval task, even though the correct phone template is identified less than 50% of the time. In more natural situations (such as conversational speech), where word choice is less highly constrained and word alternatives are likely to be acoustically similar, the performance of the system depends entirely on its ability to discriminate among phonetic segments. In other words, when vocabulary items are acoustically confusable, it is not possible to compensate for poor phonetic discrimination through the use of higher-order knowledge to constrain word choice. This was demonstrated most dramatically when the Harpy system was tested with connected letters. After several months of tuning the system, the best performance on a single speaker was 20% word level errors (where a word is now a letter), with an average error rate of 40% over several speakers.

The other major factor that prevents us from building human-like recognition machines is the lack of computer algorithms that can cope with all the knowledge involved in speech recognition. Even if we had a good "phonetic analyzer," the recognition of fluent speech would be hindered by the difficulty that current machines have with certain kinds of "information" like the context, which very often serves the purpose of improving the recognition between humans.

Speech recognition research makes a large number of speech-coding techniques available, whose effectiveness under different conditions has already been evaluated in detail. Cochlear implant experiments such as those mentioned by Eddington [3] seem to indicate that some of the cues and techniques that recognition systems have been using are also useful for cochlear implant stimulation. It seems therefore promising to attempt using some machine coding techniques for this purpose.

Summary

This paper provides a review of the state of the art in speech recognition by machine. Although many speech recognition systems have been demonstrated and several commercial products are currently being used in selected environments, computer speech recognition has still very limited capabilities when compared with human performance. Typical component subsystems at the acoustic, phonetic, syntactic, and semantic level are described. The major problems in developing recognition systems and their performance under various conditions are presented.

References

1. Atal, B. S. & M. R. Schroeder. Predictive coding of speech signals. Proceedings of the 1967 Conference on Speech Communication and Processing, IEEE, November, 1967.
2. Baker, J. M. A New Time-Domain Analysis of Human Speech and Other Complex Waveforms. Ph.D. thesis, Computer Science Department, Carnegie-Mellon University, 1975.
3. Eddington, D. K. 1980. Speech discrimination in deaf subjects with cochlear implants. J. Acoust. Soc. Am. **68**(3): 885–891.
4. Erman, L. D., F. Hayse-Roth, V. L. Lesser & D. R. Reddy. 1980. The Hearsay II speech understanding system: Integrating knowledge to resolve uncertainty. Computing Surveys **12**(2): 213–253.
5. Itakura, F. 1975. Minimum prediction residual principle applied to speech recognition. IEEE Trans. Acoustics, Speech, Signal Processing ASSP-23 **1:** 67–72.
6. Jelinek, F. 1976. Continuous speech recognition by statistical methods. Proc. IEEE April **64:** 532–556.
7. Klatt, D. H. 1977. Review of the ARPA speech understanding project. J. Acoust. Soc. Am. **62:** 1345–1366.
8. Lea, A. W. 1980. Trends in Speech Recognition. Prentice-Hall. Englewood Cliffs, NJ.
9. Lowerre, B. T. The Harpy Speech Recognition System. Ph.D. thesis, Computer Science Department, Carnegie-Mellon University, 1976.
10. Meyers, C. S. & L. R. Rabiner. Connected word recognition using a level building dynamic time warping algorithm. Proceedings of the IEEE International Conference on Acoustic, Speech and Signal Processing, 1981.
11. Meyers, C. S. & S. E. Levinson. Connected word recognition using a syntax-directed dynamic programming temporal alignment procedure. Proceedings of the IEEE International Conference on Acoustic, Speech and Signal Processing, 1981.
12. Nadas, A., L. R. Mercer, L. R. Bahl, R. Bakis, P. S. Cohen, A. G. Cole, F. Jelinek & B. L. Lewis. Continuous speech recognition and automatically selected acoustic prototypes obtained by either bootstrapping or clustering. Proceedings of the IEEE International Conference on Acoustic, Speech and Signal Processing, 1981.

13. RABINER, L. R., S. E. LEVINSON, A. E. ROSENBERG & J. G. WILPON. 1979. Speaker-independent recognition of isolated words using clustering techniques. IEEE Trans. Acoustics, Speech, Signal Processing ASSP-27 **4** (August): 336–349.
14. RABINER, L. R. & C. E. SCHMIDT. 1980. Application of dynamic time warping to connected digit recognition. IEEE Trans. Acoustics, Speech, Signal Processing ASSP-28 **4** (August): 377–388.
15. REDDY, D. R. 1976. Speech recognition by machine: A review. Proc. IEEE **64** April: 501–531.
16. SAKOE, H. 1979. Two-level DP-matching—A dynamic programming based pattern matching algorithm for connected word recognition. IEEE Trans. Acoustics, Speech, Signal Processing ASSP-27 **6** (December): 588–595.
17. SHIKANO, K. Acoustic processing in the conversational speech recognition system. Proceedings of the IEEE International Conference on Acoustic, Speech and Signal Processing, 1981.
18. WAIBEL, A. & B. YEGNANARAYANA. 1981. Comparative Study of Nonlinear Time Warping Techniques in Isolated Word Recognition Systems. Tech. Rep. CMU-CS-81-125. Department of Computer Science, Carnegie-Mellon University.
19. WHITE, G. M. & R. B. NEELY. 1976. Speech recognition experiments with linear prediction, bandpass filtering, and dynamic programming. IEEE Trans. Acoustics, Speech, Signal Processing ASSP-24 April: 183–188.

THE PERCEPTION OF FLUENT SPEECH [a]

William E. Cooper

Department of Psychology and Social Relations
Harvard University
Cambridge, Massachusetts 02138

Introduction

Listening to speech typically engages two major types of information, one provided by the acoustic signal, the other by the listener's knowledge of the language and real-world context. It is relatively simple to demonstrate the critical role played by each source of information. As for the acoustic signal, precise comprehension is simply impossible unless the listener receives at least some portion of the acoustic input. On the other hand, without possessing a working knowledge of the language being spoken, the listener cannot correctly segment the speech stream into words. Given the importance of both acoustic-driven and knowledge-driven sources of information, a major task becomes figuring out how these two sources are utilized in combination by the listener in perceiving fluent speech. In this presentation, I will attempt to address aspects of higher-level decision processes in human speech recognition, including processes that involve a bottom-up, acoustic-driven flow of information as well as those that involve a top-down, knowledge-driven flow. While considering these processes in light of research with listeners having normal hearing, suggestions will be made about possible guidelines for the testing and improvement of speech perception in the hearing-impaired.

Acoustic-Driven Processes

The use of acoustic information in decoding segmental aspects of the phonetic structure of an utterance has been reviewed in this volume by Stevens and Studdert-Kennedy, and we shall consider here how acoustic information also serves as a cue to both higher-order linguistic information and the speaker's nonlinguistic characteristics. One type of acoustic information that directly conveys clues to such higher-order elements involves the suprasegmental aspects of speech, associated commonly with the acoustic cues of duration, intensity, and fundamental voice frequency (hereafter F0). From the standpoint of work on cochlear prostheses, interest in listeners' perception of these suprasegmentals is heightened by the fact that these properties of speech are typically among the best preserved sources of speech information in the sensorineural hearing-impaired, with or without prosthetic aids.[4, 12] Unfortunately, only a small amount is known about the utilization of suprasegmentals among normal listeners, and appreciably less so for the hearing-impaired. It appears that research on this topic has lagged behind work on segmental aspects of speech perception for two related reasons. For one, perceptual research

[a] This work was supported by Grant NS 15059 from the National Institutes of Health.

0077–8923/83/0405–0048 $01.75/0 © 1983, NYAS

can only be relevant to normal listening circumstances if the acoustical variables being tested are actually produced in a similarly distinctive manner by speakers, and research on the production of suprasegmental aspects of speech has only recently reached the stage where it can provide strong constraints on the kinds of perceptual studies that might be worthwhile.[10] Relatedly, the lag in research on both the production and perception of suprasegmentals is partly attributable to the fact that such research requires the use of fluent speech contexts, typically rendering a highly complex experimental situation from the standpoint of stimulus materials, testing procedures, and data analysis.

Cues to Word Stress

In one of the earliest perceptual studies of suprasegmentals, Fry[19] tested the influence of variations in F0, duration, and intensity on listeners' perception of stress patterns in words like *convict* and *permit,* which contain the same sequence of phonetic segments, but are normally produced with differing stress pattern when intended as noun versus verb. Fry found that each of the three sugrasegmental cues served to produce systematic variations in listeners' perception of the stress patterns, with greater perceived stress on a syllable associated with higher F0, longer duration, and greater intensity. Thus, a word like *convict* is more likely to be perceived as a noun to the extent that these suprasegmental cues are carried on the first syllable.

Cues to Word Boundaries

When listening to fluent speech in our native language, we perceive a series of crisply demarcated words, and only when confronted with an unfamiliar language does one realize that the acoustic stream of speech does not provide reliable cues to the boundaries between adjacent words. The segmentation of speech into words is particularly aided by knowledge-driven information (see later), but segmental and suprasegmental cues can also play a role. At the segmental level, word boundaries may be marked by the insertion of a glottal stop.[51] Some word boundaries are also delimited by pauses as well as by abrupt shifts in intensity and F0. The precise role of these acoustical cues in aiding segmentation under normal listening circumstances has not yet been determined. Yet a large percentage of the word boundaries in fluent speech are not accompanied by any of these cues. It is the listener's knowledge of the language's acoustic–lexical relationships and information provided by prior context that are required to accomplish the segmentation of speech.

Cues to Syntactic Structure

Suprasegmental information provides a variety of reliable cues to the syntactic structure of an utterance, although relatively little is known about whether and how listeners utilize such information. In speech production, the boundaries between major clauses are typically demarcated by segmental lengthening of the clause-final word[9, 25] and a fall–rise pattern of F0.[10, 30, 36, 50]

Less reliably, but prominent when it occurs, is the appearance of optional pausing at the same locations.[2, 9, 20] These same prosodic effects are also present at phrase boundaries within clauses, and detailed studies of their magnitudes at various types of boundaries have permitted inferences to be made about the precise form of syntactic representation that the speaker might compute.[9, 10, 20]

For present purposes, however, it is simply relevant to observe that the consistency and magnitude of segmental lengthening and F0 fall–rise patterns, in particular, are sufficiently great to warrant their careful consideration as candidates for perceptual cues to syntactic structure. Indeed, a machine recognition program by Lea [31] has included F0 fall–rise patterns as a primary means of determining phrase boundaries in speech, achieving a recognition accuracy of about 85%. The question remains, however, whether human listeners typically utilize such information to decode syntactic structure.

In the case of segmental lengthening, one attempt to test perceptual cue value has been made by Lehiste, Olive, and Streeter.[33] These researchers utilized structurally ambiguous sentences like "The hostess greeted the girl with a smile," in which the prepositional phrase "with a smile" modified either "the girl" or the entire verb phrase, referring to the hostess's manner. When each segment of the string "girl with a smile" was lengthened electronically, listeners were more likely to perceive the latter reading. Lehiste *et al.*[33] claim that this effect is due to an increase in the interval between stressed syllables,[32] although it is conceivable that the listeners' judgments were guided more by the absolute lengthening of a particular segment within the manipulated string, most probably lengthening of the word "girl."

Other studies of segmental timing have tried to determine how small a change in segmental duration is detectable by listeners when perceiving fluent speech.[24, 27, 47, 48] These studies suggest that listeners are capable of detecting durational differences on the order of one or two glottal cycles (approximately 8–16 msec for a male voice). This capability would almost certainly be less finely tuned in normal conversation, however, when the listener is more actively engaged in extracting meaning from the utterance. Typically, the experiments on detectability for segment durations involved only a small set of similar utterances, and listeners were asked to make direct judgments of segment duration, quite unlike the circumstances of natural listening. It does seem likely, however, that listeners could readily detect and utilize differences in segment duration on the order of 20% or more under normal circumstances, and many of the clause- and phrase-boundary influences on segment duration are sufficiently large to be perceived on the basis of this estimate.

In the case of F0, there exists some evidence that listeners can utilize fall–rise patterns to detect major syntactic boundaries.[13, 60] For example, Streeter demonstrated that variations in F0 alter listeners' perception of ambiguous algebraic expressions of the form "(A plus E) times O" versus "A plus (E times O)." However, the acoustical properties of the F0 variations were not described in her study, so it is not possible to determine whether a fall–rise pattern per se, some portion thereof, or a related F0 cue provided the listeners with a basis for their judgments (see also Wales and Toner [63] and Larkey.[28]

Pausing has also been the object of a few perceptual studies. For example, Reich [55] found that listeners were better able to categorize words and to recall propositions from utterances that contained pauses between clauses rather than within the clauses. However, it is difficult to determine whether the advantage accorded to between-clause pauses is attributable to a cue value of the pause or simply to the fact that these utterances conformed more closely to a natural overall suprasegmental pattern.

In conclusion, studies of speech production indicate that the suprasegmental characteristics of segmental lengthening, F0 fall–rise patterns, and pausing accompany many syntactic boundaries. A variety of studies have been conducted on listeners' ability to detect small changes in one or another of these prosodic parameters, and the results suggest that, indeed, listeners *ought* to be capable of detecting and using the kinds of variations in suprasegmentals that accompany fluent speech. But perceptual studies have yet to assess adequately the degree to which such acoustic information provides the listener with cues to syntactic structure in normal listening circumstances. (For further discussion and proposals, see Cooper and Paccia-Cooper.[9])

From the standpoint of the hearing-impaired listener, it seems that the cue value of F0 fall–rise patterns might be particularly salient, since the relatively low frequency range of speaker's F0 values (rarely exceeding 300 Hz for adult voices) is relatively well perceived by most hearing-impaired listeners suffering sensorineural impairment.[3,4,12,35,57,62] Fortunately, fall–rise patterns of F0 appear to be among the most reliable indicators of syntactic structure.[10,31] In addition, these patterns offer some advantage over segmental lengthening and pausing as cues to syntactic structure inasmuch as the influencing source of F0 fall–rise patterns is not as readily confused as in the other two cases. As pointed out by Klatt,[26] segmental duration varies with the inherent phonetic segment, speaking rate, and other factors to a great extent, while pausing may also be produced by word-finding hesitation or more global backtracking of the speaker. While extrasyntactic factors also influence F0, such factors rarely camouflage the fall–rise patterns that accompany syntactic boundaries.

Cues to Semantic Interpretation

Aside from providing cues to syntactic structure, which in turn disambiguate the meanings of structurally ambiguous strings, suprasegmentals and, in particular, F0 patterns appear to provide essential cues to semantic information in certain renderings of an utterance. The utterance "I'm ecstatic," when spoken with different F0 contours, can signify meanings varying from the true ecstasy to just the opposite. Ordinarily, pragmatic circumstances conspire with the F0 pattern to provide unambiguous information about the intended meaning.[52]

Perceptual studies have shown that English-listeners utilize variations in F0 to interpret a given utterance as a statement versus a question, with a falling F0 on the last word of an utterance yielding the perception of a statement and a rising F0 on the same word yielding the perception of a question.[61] This perceptual finding is consistent with evidence from speech production showing that English-speakers typically produce a terminal fall in F0 at the end of the declarative, whereas they produce a terminal rise in F0 at the end of a question.[50]

Cues to Speaker Characteristics

The suprasegmental aspects of speech also provide a number of cues about characteristics of the speaker, including sex, age, and personality. Again F0 seems to provide the most distinctive information of the suprasegmental cues. In adults, females generally have higher F0 than males, and listeners are appropriately influenced by F0 in making judgments about a speaker's gender.[8] In addition, F0 provides the listener with cues to a speaker's sexual characteristics. Among a group of males, speakers with relatively high average F0 are judged to be more effeminate than speakers with relatively low average F0.[67] Among females, speakers with relatively low average F0 are judged more virile than those with relatively high average F0.[11] Although these studies do not indicate whether the listener's judgments in these cases correlate with independent measures of the speaker's sexual characteristics, it does appear that listeners judge speakers' sexual characteristics in part on the basis of mean F0. Interestingly, a study of actual F0 production in homosexual versus heterosexual males showed no systematic difference,[34] suggesting that listeners' judgments of F0 may, in certain circumstances, provide unreliable information about the sexual preference of speakers.

Average values of F0 also provide listeners with cues to the speaker's age. Here again, however, the listeners' use of F0 as a cue may not accurately reflect the speaker's actual characteristic. In speech production, mean F0 correlates positively with adult age only in the range from 60 through the 80s.[21] But listeners perceive adults to be older to the extent that they exhibit a higher mean F0, regardless of whether the speakers are older or younger than 60.[22]

The mean F0 of a speaker also influences listeners' judgments about the speaker's personality. Apple, Streeter, and Krauss [1] raised or lowered the F0 of male speakers' voices by 20% electronically and found that listeners perceived the speech having higher F0 values as being uttered by a speaker who was less truthful, less persuasive, more nervous, and weaker than normal. Similar effects were obtained when the speech was electronically slowed in tempo, except that the speakers were perceived as being less nervous than normal.

There remains a need for further work to examine the possible influence of F0 and other suprasegmentals on listeners' judgments about other speaker characteristics, including physique and emotions. Intuition suggests that such characteristics may be inferred in part on the basis of F0, as when one is talking to someone for the first time over the phone, and it will be informative to find out whether one's perceptual judgments correlate highly with actual speaker characteristics.

To conclude, F0 is utilized by listeners in making a variety of judgments about a speaker's characteristics. In ordinary listening, perceptual judgments about such traits appear to be made automatically and without any serious disruption in the listener's processing of the speaker's linguistic content. While this automatic assessment of speaker characteristics is often not a primary goal of the listener, there exist circumstances in which it becomes crucial, as in cases of trying to discern a speaker's emotional tone when linguistic content is intentionally vague (for example, in certain diplomatic conversations). A case in point was provided by John F. Kennedy's insistence on having his Russian translator attempt to decode Nikita Khrushchev's emotional tone, presumably via suprasegmental cues, during phone conversations amidst the 1962 Cuban missile crisis.

In research with hearing-impaired listeners, little attention has been devoted to perceptual cues to speaker characteristics, probably because of the pressing concerns of linguistic decoding. It would be interesting to find out, however, whether hearing-impaired listeners make automatic perceptual judgments about speaker characteristics in a manner similar to that of normal listeners, how such judgments might differ from normal because of loss of acoustic information, and whether such judgments deplete any of the processing resources that are otherwise needed for decoding linguistic information.

Conclusion

In summary, acoustic-driven information from the suprasegmental aspects of the speech wave provides cues to higher-order factors, such as word stress, word boundaries, syntactic structure, semantic interpretation, and nonlinguistic characteristics of the speaker. In some cases, perceptual experiments have demonstrated the cue value of these acoustical features for listeners, although in most instances the perceptual role of these traits in normal listening circumstances can only be surmised on the basis of inferences from related studies of speech production. Because hearing-impaired listeners are often capable of perceiving suprasegmental aspects of speech, particularly F0, it seems worthwhile at even this early stage of knowledge to explore the possible ways in which supresegmental information can be used to full advantage by such listeners.

Knowledge-Driven and Contextual Processes

As noted in the Introduction, knowledge-driven processes refer to the listeners' use of linguistic and real-world knowledge in decoding utterances. This knowledge, stored in the listeners' long-term memory, should be distinguished from short-term contextual information, derived from the listener's decoding of recent portions of an utterance, with such decoding typically engaging acoustic-driven and knowledge-driven sources and with subsequent use of such contextual information relying more exclusively on knowledge-driven processes. In the case of hearing-impaired listeners, the use of short-term contextual information may be impaired under many circumstances because the acoustic-driven processes were not sufficiently capable of decoding such information when it originally appeared in the speech stream.

Segmentation

As observed earlier, the acoustic stream often lacks clear cues to the boundaries between words. Cole and Jakimik [6] estimate that less than 40% of all word boundaries are acoustically marked. Thus, our perception of speech as a stream of well-defined word units must derive in large part from the knowledge of the language that we bring to bear on the listening task.

This knowledge includes a mental lexicon, allowing the listener to distinguish plausible words from nonwords, as well as a variety of linguistic and pragmatic contextual rules that help guide the perception of fluent speech. When words are excised from conversation and presented individually to listeners, correct recognition may be as low as 50%.[53] The segmentation problem for listeners would be overwhelming if they relied solely on acoustic–lexical information to define word boundaries, and errors in segmentation would readily cascade into subsequent errors. To illustrate this point, Reddy[54] asked listeners to comprehend utterances like "In mud eels are, in clay none are," in which normal contextual cues to word meaning are absent. Sample responses of four different listeners appear below:

in mud eels are	*in clay none are*
in muddies sar	in clay nanar
in my deals are	en clainanar
in my ders	en clain
in model sar	in claynanar

Experimentally, the influence of context on listeners' ability to segment speech has been investigated by asking listeners to try to detect mispronunciations during the presentation of a spoken passage.[5] In the case of the segmentation issue, a key syllable like *go* is mispronounced *ko* in two different conditions, one in which this syllable appears as the second syllable in a bisyllabic word, as in *cargo,* the other in which the same syllable appears as a monosyllabic word, as in *car go.* The English language contains a host of phonological strings that can be alternatively represented by one word or two words (e.g., *quarter/back, snow/drift, home/made, fair/grounds, draw/back*), and a study of mispronunciations was carried out by Cole, Jakimik, and Cooper[7] to determine how listeners utilize contextual cues to guide their perception. In the task, listeners were asked to press a button as soon as a mispronunciation was detected, and it was reasoned that listeners should be faster at detecting a mispronunciation when it appeared as the second syllable of a bisyllabic word than as a monosyllable. In the current example, subjects should thus be faster at detecting the mispronunciation *carko* than *car ko* if the subjects utilize contextual cues to anticipate a one- versus two-word segmentation. In the case of the two-word segmentation, subjects would need to delay pressing the button until they realized that *ko* was intended to be *go* and not the first syllable of a *bona fide,* contextually appropriate multisyllabic word (such as *collide*).

In order to test the role of contextual information, a first experiment involved the use of pairs of passages, in which each pair member served to bias the listener in favor of a one- versus two-word segmentation of *car/go.* This biasing was attempted for the present example by presenting a pair of passages, with one passage describing a car that was about to be put onto a ferry and the other describing two dockworkers about to unload a shipment. Subjects' reaction time to detecting the mispronunciation was about 300 msec faster in the second passage, favoring the one-word segmentation, and suggesting that listeners indeed utilize the global context of a spoken passage to guide word segmentation. Since an identical representation of the key sentence was utilized in both passages, the present effect could be firmly attributable to the influence of prior context rather than to acoustical cues to word boundary location.

Additional experiments were conducted to examine more local contextual influences within a given sentence. In particular, we wanted to find out whether listeners utilize syntactic and/or semantic information provided just one word in advance of the key material in order to make a segmentation decision. In order to test this possibility, sentence pairs like the following were constructed:

The doctor said that nose*d*rops will help the cold.

The doctor said he knows *d*rops will help the cold.

In this pair, *drops* was mispronounced as *trops,* and, as in the preceding experiment, it was predicted that subjects would be faster at detecting the mispronunciation in the one-word segmentation (in this case *nosedrops*), provided listeners could utilize the contextual information supplied by the preceding word (*that*) to guide their segmentation. Listeners indeed showed significantly faster reaction times to detecting a mispronunciation in the one-word segmentation version, indicating their ability to make very fast use of contextual information provided by *that* versus *he.* In this case, the acoustical representation of the string beginning after *that* versus *he* was identical, so again the effect could not be attributed to acoustical cues to word boundary segmentation in the key region.

Identification

The problem of identifying words in fluent speech goes hand in hand with the problem of segmentation. As noted earlier, listeners are not very adept at correctly identifying words presented without their accompanying context, suggesting that context plays a role in our normal ability to identify words. A variety of experimental studies support this conclusion, and, in recent years, a considerable amount of research has been devoted to figuring out the detailed mental processes that mediate such influences.

At the most general level, the influence of context on word identification was demonstrated by Miller, Heise, and Lichten,[43] who showed that subjects were able to recognize words embedded in noise with greater accuracy when these words were presented in sentence contexts rather than in isolation. In a related study, Miller and Isard [44] presented in noise groups of word strings that either corresponded to normal English sentences, strings that were semantically anomalous but syntactically well formed, and strings that were syntactically as well as semantically anomalous. Listeners were able to correctly identify more words as a function of the degree to which the string corresponded to normal English, with word recognition being best for normal English sentences and worst for the strings that were both semantically and syntactically aberrant. Clearly, then, listeners do make use of higher-order grammatical context, relying on their implicit knowledge of linguistic rules, in guiding their recognition of words in noise-degraded speech.

As Cole and Jakimik [6] observe, the influence of context on word recognition is not limited to circumstances involving degraded speech. For example, Morton and Long [46] found that subjects reacted about 80 msec faster to detecting a target phoneme when it appeared in a word that was more highly predictable on the basis of preceding word context in clearly audible unambiguous sentences. In this phoneme-monitoring task,[16] subjects were faster, for example, at detecting the target phoneme (*b* in the string: *He sat reading his book/bill until it was time to go home for his tea.*) In an extension of this study, Foss and Blank [17] have shown that this effect is critically dependent on the influences of preceding context, since no effect is observed when the target phoneme is simply contained in a high- versus low-frequency word without any variation in the frequency of usage of the preceding word or of the transitional probability between the preceding and target word.

Aside from word identification, the influence of context has also been shown to affect listeners' perception of individual phonemes within a word. When a phoneme is replaced with a cough or other extraneous sound of about the same intensity, listeners report hearing the word intact and often fail to detect or mislocate the extraneous sound.[29, 58, 59, 64, 65] For the most part, it appears that the contextual influence that triggers this "phoneme restoration" effect is word-internal. For example, in Warren's original study,[64] the first *s* of *legislatures* was replaced by a cough or a tone in the sentence "The state governors met with their respective legislatures convening in the capital city." While the sentential context rendered the target word highly probable, the word *legislatures* is itself so highly distinctive from other English words on the basis of partial phonemic information that it seems likely that the restoration of the first *s* in this word can be largely attributable to the influence of lexical choice. As observed by Warren and Sherman,[66] this contextual influence can influence phonemic restoration even when it appears after the replaced phoneme, as in *deli–ery* versus *deli–eration,* for which listeners restored *v* and *b,* respectively.

In order to examine the influence of preceding word context on phonemic restorations, Samuel [58] presented sentence pairs like "The soldier's/pitcher's thoughts of the dangerous bat– made him very nervous" as well as sentence fragments containing just the portion up to and including the replaced phoneme after "bat." By having subjects also make judgments about sentences and fragments in which the key segment included extraneous noise that was superimposed on the target phoneme instead of replacing it, Samuel was able to include a signal-detectability analysis to factor out the extent to which listeners' restorations of phonemes represented an effect of perception versus response bias. In the case of sentence context, the subjects tended to restore phonemes that were appropriate to the sentence (for example, *soldier-battle* versus *pitcher-batter*), but the signal-detectability analysis revealed that the contextual influence operated primarily at the level of response bias rather than perception. That is, listeners are more likely to report words as being intact when they are predictable from the preceding context of the sentence than when they are not.

Other experiments by Samuel,[58, 59] utilizing the same signal detectability measures, have shown that the phonemic-restoration effect is also influenced by bottom-up acoustical factors. In particular, listeners were more likely to restore fricatives than vowels when the phonemes were replaced by white noise, whereas listeners were more likely to restore vowels than fricatives when the same phonemes were replaced by pure tones. This effect was attributable to variations in listeners' perception of restoration rather than response bias, unlike the effect noted earlier for sentence context. In the present case, the influence on perception is explicable in terms of the acoustic similarity of the target phoneme and the replacement sound, with the spectral compositions of fricatives/white noise and vowels/pure tones being more similar than those for the converse combinations of sounds. It thus appears that, in addition to using contextual influences on phoneme restoration, listeners also make use of acoustic similarity in guiding their perception of restoration. In this particular set of experiments, restoration was examined for isolated words, so the effect must be attributed to listeners' restoration of phonemes on the basis of word-internal context, with the likelihood of restoration influenced by whether or not the acoustic replacement is sufficiently close to the anticipated phoneme to confirm the listeners' expectations.

The argument for dual operation of acoustic-driven and knowledge-driven types of processing is also supported by evidence from listening for mispronunciations. In addition to the influences of higher-order context discussed earlier, listeners' ability to detect mispronunciations is influenced by the degree of acoustic similarity between the target and mispronounced phonemes, with a greater likelihood of detection and faster response times for acoustically more dissimilar target and error phonemes.[5, 7] Thus, under appropriate testing circumstances, both listening for mispronunciations and phoneme-restoration tasks reveal the joint operation of acoustic- and knowledge-driven information in speech recognition.

In order to examine the interplay between bottom-up and top-down processing in detail, Marslen-Wilson and his colleagues[37–42] have examined subjects' performance during the perceptual task of word-monitoring as well as in the more complex task of speech-shadowing, in which the subjects are asked to repeat utterances as they are being spoken in immediate word-by-word fashion. By asking subjects in a monitoring task to detect a word that either rhymes with or belongs to the same semantic category as a prespecified word, and by adding a variety of other conditions in a systematic fashion, Marslen-Wilson and Tyler[42] have been able to test whether listeners utilize phonological, syntactic, and semantic sources of information in an interactive, high-speed manner to constrain word recognition, or whether, instead, listeners utilize these sources in a more strictly serial fashion. The results of their studies support the notion that listeners bring to bear all possible sources of information, from phonological to discourse-level cues, as soon as these become available to constrain word choice.

On the basis of their findings and a consideration of related literature, Marslen-Wilson and Tyler propose a Cohort model of lexical access, in which bottom-up processing is given primary status in establishing a small set of candidate words, with subsequent interactive processes devoted to narrowing down the correct word choice. As the authors observe, upon hearing the first two phonemes of a word, a listener can normally constrain word choice to no more than approximately 30 candidates. On the other hand, prior context constrains word choice so severely only when words are highly predictable. A bottom-up procedure virtually insures that the correct word is among the list of candidates, whereas a procedure for lexical access that is driven firstly by a top-down process might propose candidates that do not include the correct word (see also Klatt,[26]). What chiefly distinguishes the Cohort model from other models of lexical access (such as the Logogen model[45]) is its more detailed specification of how the various sources of information from prior context can interact with the bottom-up processes to narrow down the range of candidate words and ultimately derive a single word choice. Yet even the Cohort model leaves unspecified a detailed representation of how the various interactions among sources of information operate in real-time, and a good deal of future work is needed to further define and test this and related models.[15]

Conclusion

Knowledge-driven processes play a significant role in both the segmentation and identification of words in speech perception. As Daniel Ling [35] has aptly put it, "There's more to hearing than meets the ear." Listeners utilize knowledge of lexical, syntactic, and semantic constraints of the language being spoken to guide the segmentation of speech into word-like units and to select among candidate word choices. But listeners do not neglect the acoustic data. Even in the case of phoneme restoration, we have seen that listeners are influenced by the acoustic similarity of the target phoneme and its replacement sound. For the most part, it appears that normal listening jointly engages acoustic-driven and knowledge-driven processes, and greater attention can now be directed at the issue of how these two types of process typically interact to yield comprehension.

Implications for Hearing-Impaired Listeners

From the foregoing discussion, it should be evident that the existing literature on the perception of fluent speech in listeners with normal hearing can, at best, provide only a handful of general guidelines relevant to the improvement of cochlear prostheses for the hearing-impaired. As for the hearing-impaired listeners' use of acoustic-driven information, the studies reviewed here suggest that the suprasegmental cue of F0 might be particularly helpful in providing such listeners with cues to a variety of higher-order speech properties, including word stress, syntactic structure, semantic interpretation, and nonlinguistic traits of the speaker. Since F0 is usually preserved to a relatively great extent in hearing-impaired listeners, it might be useful to include explicit training for such listeners, possibly in conjunction with visual feedback training of F0 in speech production,[23] to extract as much information as possible from this cue. Such training might be particularly beneficial in hearing-impaired children who are in the process of learning their native language.

A consideration of the literature on normal listening, combined with a regard for the special problems of the hearing-impaired, suggests that one potentially useful line of research might involve a detailed examination of the mental processes that accompany listening when the listener "misses" a word or phrase, or is unable to make a plausible guess at word choice, usually because of insufficient auditory information. The existing literature, while not addressing this problem directly, certainly suggests that the consequences of missing a word may be disastrous from the standpoint of lacking not only a representation of the missed word per se, but also potentially important contextual information that such a word might provide in aiding subsequent word choice. Since the phenomenon of missing a word probably occurs with relatively high frequency among hearing-impaired listeners, the problems associated with this sort of error in individual utterances might be quite severe and cascading in their effect. This phenomenon could be examined in normal listening by simply garbling or masking a critical word in selected sentences of a passage and observing the consequences for tasks that tap the listeners' ability to quickly recover from this experience. For the hearing-impaired, with whom this kind of experience is more frequent, it would be interesting to examine whether the strategies used to cope with the phenomenon are adaptive from the standpoint of overall comprehension and whether such strategies differ appreciably from those of normal listeners.

The idea of studying listener's performance after missing a word or an entire phrase may prove to be a useful complement to currently popular experimental methods that emphasize listening in a state of unusually high attentiveness. By the nature of the task demands, experiments that involve listening for mispronunciations, phoneme- or word-monitoring, speech-shadowing, and the like, place great demands on the listener to attend to the acoustic input, to a degree probably not very common in normal conversational settings.

Aside from these suggestions for research and training with hearing-impaired listeners, the evidence reviewed in this presentation leads to two observations about the development and testing of cochlear prostheses. The first and most obvious point involves acoustic-driven information, for which prostheses are most directly aimed. Any prosthesis that clarifies the suprasegmental aspects of speech is likely to produce an improvement in the listeners' ability to extract higher-order linguistic information from the speech wave and might also aid in the perception of speaker characteristics. Single-wire electrode prostheses that stimulate the auditory nerve fibers are capable of conveying information about the suprasegmentals,[14, 18] and, while such stimulation cannot render speech intelligible, it can provide information that is complementary to lipreading. The potential benefits of cochlear prostheses for the perception of suprasegmentals are underscored by the fact that lipreading or vibrotactile aids are generally inadequate as alternatives to residual hearing for perceiving these cues.[35, 56] Secondly, with respect to knowledge-driven information, it will be particularly interesting to compare listeners' use of knowledge-driven processes before and after a cochlear prosthesis has been in place for varying intervals of time, since it might be expected that the hearing-impaired listener (especially if prelingually impaired, who are currently not candidates for most cochlear prostheses) will eventually store up a larger (but nowhere near normal) repertoire of linguistic rules after the prosthesis has improved the acoustic-driven processes that allow normal listeners to naturally acquire an extensive set of linguistic rules at a very early age. The rudimentary nature of current prostheses would appear to render any such improvements negligible, but if future prostheses are capable of rendering speech intelligible, improvements in knowledge-driven processes might ensue. As Klatt,[26] Norman,[49] and others have observed, a great deal of so-called bottom-up lexical analysis from acoustic input probably makes use of extensive precompiled knowledge about the possible transitions between phonemes, phonological rules, and related information, avoiding the need for a large amount of on-line computation. This emphasis on precompilation has been a salient feature of some of the most successful attempts at machine recognition of speech (for a review, see Bisiani's article in this volume). According to Klatt,[26] human listeners also make extensive use of precompiled acoustic–lexical information. Over an extended period of time, a beneficial prosthesis of the future might permit the enlargement of this knowledge base in many hearing-impaired listeners. At present, however, there exists a considerable gap between this goal and the available technology.

Summary

The perception of fluent speech involves both acoustic-driven and knowledge-driven sources of information. Acoustic sources that directly convey information about higher-order linguistic characteristics include the suprasegmental aspects of speech, associated with the acoustic cues of fundamental frequency, duration, and intensity. From the standpoint of cochlear prostheses, interest in listeners' perception of these suprasegmentals is heightened by the fact that these properties are typically among the best preserved sources of speech information in the sensorineural hearing-impaired. Studies with normal listeners indicate that suprasegmentals provide cues to such linguistic factors as word stress, syntactic structure, and semantic interpretation. In addition, they supply information about many nonlinguistic characteristics of the speaker. Research on knowledge-driven processes indicates that normal listeners utilize knowledge of lexical, syntactic, and semantic constraints of the language to guide the segmentation of speech into word-like units and to select among candidate word choices. These findings are related to research with hearing-impaired listeners and prosthesis testing.

References

1. Apple, W., L. A. Streeter & R. M. Krauss. 1979. Pitch and speech rate. J. Personal. Soc. Psychol.
2. Boomer, D. S. & J. D. Laver. 1968. Slips of the tongue. Br. J. Disorders Commun. **3:** 1–12.
3. Boothroyd, A. 1976. Influence of residual hearing on speech perception and speech production by hearing-impaired children. The Clarke School for the Deaf, Sensory Aids Research Project, Report #26. Northampton, MA.
4. Boothroyd, A. 1978. Speech perception and sensorineural hearing loss. *In* Auditory Management of Hearing-Impaired Children. M. Ross and T. G. Giolas, Eds.: 117–144. University Park Press. Baltimore, MD.
5. Cole, R. A. 1973. Listening for mispronunciations: A measure of what we hear during speech. Percep. Psychophys. **13:** 153–156.
6. Cole, R. A. & J. Jakimik. 1980. A model of speech perception. *In* Perception and Production of Fluent Speech. R. A. Cole, Ed.: 133–163. Erlbaum. Hillsdale, NJ.
7. Cole, R. A., J. Jakimik & W. E. Cooper. 1980. Segmenting speech into words. J. Acoust. Soc. Am. **67:** 1323–1332.
8. Coleman, R. O. 1976. A comparison of the contributions of two voice quality characteristics to the perception of maleness and femaleness in the voice. J. Speech Hear. Res. **19:** 168–180.
9. Cooper, W. E. & J. Paccia-Cooper. 1980. Syntax and Speech. Harvard University Press. Cambridge, MA.
10. Cooper, W. E. & J. M. Sorensen. 1981. Fundamental Frequency in Sentence Production. Springer-Verlag. New York, NY.

11. DAMSTE, P. H. 1967. Voice change in adult women caused by virilizing agents. J. Speech Hear. Disord. **32:** 126–132.
12. DAVIS, H. & S. R. SILVERMAN. 1970. Hearing and Deafness. Holt, Rinehart, and Winston. New York, NY.
13. DE ROOIJ, J. J. 1979. Speech Punctuation: An Acoustic and Perceptual Study of Some Aspects of Speech Prosody in Dutch. Unpublished Ph.D. thesis.
14. EVANS, E. F. 1977. Disorders of hearing and language: Understanding, diagnosis, rehabilitation seminar report. *In* Recognition of Complex Acoustic Signals. T. H. Bullock. Ed.: 367–386. Berlin, Germany.
15. FORSTER, K. I. 1979. Levels of processing and the structure of the language processor. *In* Sentence Processing. W. E. Cooper and E. C. T. Walker, Eds.: 27–85. Erlbaum. Hillsdale, NJ.
16. FOSS, D. J. 1969. Decision processes during sentence comprehension: Effects of lexical item difficulty and position upon decision times. J. Verb. Learn. Verb. Behav. **8:** 457–462.
17. FOSS, D. J. & BLANK, M. A. 1980. Identifying the speech codes. Cognitive Psychol. **12:** 1–31.
18. FOURCIN, A. F., B. C. J. MOORE & E. E. DOUEK. 1977. Perception and presentation of artificial speech patterns. *In* Report of Medical Research Council Working Party on Artificial Stimulation.
19. FRY, B. D. 1955. Duration and intensity as physical correlates of linguistic stress. J. Acoust. Soc. Am. **27:** 765–768.
20. GROSJEAN, F., L. GROSJEAN & H. LANE. 1979. The patterns of silence: Performance structures in sentence production. Cognitive Psychol. **11:** 58–81.
21. HOLLIEN, H. & T. SHIPP. 1972. Speaking fundamental frequency and chronological age in males. J. Speech Hear. Res. **15:** 155–159.
22. HORII, Y. & W. J. RYAN. 1975. Fundamental frequency characteristics and perceived age of adult male speakers. J. Acoust. Soc. Am. **57:** S69 (abstr.).
23. HOUDE, R. A. Instantaneous visual feedback in speech training for the deaf. Paper presented at the Convention of American Speech and Hearing Association, October, 1973.
24. HUGGINS, A. W. F. 1972. Just-noticeable difference for segment duration in natural speech. J. Acoust. Soc. Am. **51:** 1270–1278.
25. KLATT, D. H. 1975. Vowel lengthening is syntactically determined in a connected discourse. J. Phonet. **3:** 129–140.
26. KLATT, D. H. 1980. Speech perception: A model of acoustic-phonetic analysis and lexical access. *In* Perception and Production of Fluent Speech. R. A. Cole, Ed.: 243–288. Erlbaum. Hillsdale, NJ.
27. KLATT, D. H. & W. E. COOPER. 1975. Perception of segment duration in sentence contexts. *In* Structure and Process in Speech Perception. A. Cohen and S. G. Nooteboom, Eds.: 69–89. Springer-Verlag. New York, NY.
28. LARKEY, L. 1980. The Role of Prosodic Information in Speech Perception. Unpublished Ph.D. thesis, University of Minnesota.
29. LAYTON, B. 1975. Differential effects of two nonspeech sounds on phonemic restoration. Bull. Psychonom. Soc. **6:** 487–490.
30. LEA, W. A. 1973. Segmental and suprasegmental influences on fundamental frequency contours. *In* Consonant Types and Tones. L. Hyman, Ed.: 15–70. University of Southern California Press. Los Angeles, CA.
31. LEA, W. A. 1980. Prosodic aids to speech recognition. *In* Trends in Speech Recognition. W. A. Lea, Ed. Prentice-Hall. Englewood Cliffs, NJ.
32. LEHISTE, I. 1977. Isochrony reconsidered. J. Phonet. **5:** 253–263.
33. LEHISTE, I., J. P. OLIVE & L. A. STREETER. 1976. Role of duration in disambiguating syntactically ambiguous sentences. J. Acoust. Soc. Am. **60:** 1199–1202.
34. LERMAN, J. W. 1969. Voice pitch of homosexuals. Folia Phoniatrica, **21:** 340–346.

35. LING, D. 1978. Auditory coding and recoding (an analysis of auditory training procedures for hearing-impaired children). *In* Auditory Management of Hearing-Impaired Children. M. Ross and T. G. Giolas, Eds.: 181–218. University Park Press. Baltimore, MD.
36. MAEDA, S. 1976. A Characterization of American English Intonation. Unpublished Ph.D. thesis, Massachusetts Institute of Technology.
37. MARSLEN-WILSON, W. D. 1973. Linguistic structure and speech shadowing at very short latencies. Nature **244:** 522–523.
38. MARSLEN-WILSON, W. D. 1975. Sentence perception as an interactive parallel process. Science **189:** 226–228.
39. MARSLEN-WILSON, W. D. Linguistic descriptions and psychological assumptions in the study of sentence perception. *In* New Approaches to the Study of Language. R. J. Wales and E. C. T. Walker, Eds. North-Holland. Amsterdam.
40. MARSLEN-WILSON, W. D., L. K. TYLER & M. SEIDENBERG. 1978. Sentence processing and the clause-boundary. *In* Studies in Sentence Perception. W. J. M. Levelt and G. B. Flores D'Arcais, Eds. Wiley. New York, NY.
41. MARSLEN-WILSON, W. D. & A. WELSH. 1978. Processing interactions and lexical access during word-recognition in continuous speech. Cognitive Psychol. **10:** 29–63.
42. MARSLEN-WILSON, W. D. & L. K. TYLER. 1980. The temporal structure of spoken language understanding. Cognition **8:** 1–71.
43. MILLER, G. A., G. HEISE & W. LICHTEN. 1951. The intelligibility of speech as a function of the context of the test materials. J. Exp. Psychol. **41:** 329–335.
44. MILLER, G. A. & S. ISARD. 1963. Some perceptual consequences of linguistic rules. J. Verb. Learning Verb. Behav. **2:** 217–228.
45. MORTON, J. 1970. A functional model for memory. *In* Models of Human Memory. D. A. Norman, Ed. Academic Press. New York, NY.
46. MORTON, J. & J. LONG. 1976. Effect of word transitional probability on phoneme identification. J. Verb. Learn. Verb. Behav. **15:** 43–51.
47. NOOTEBOOM, S. G. 1973. The perceptual reality of some prosodic durations. J. Phonet. **1:** 25–45.
48. NOOTEBOOM, S. G. & DOODEMAN, J. N. 1980. Production and perception of vowel length in spoken sentences. J. Acoust. Soc. Am. **67:** 276–287.
49. NORMAN, D. A. Copycat science or does the mind really work by table look-up? *In* Perception and Production of Fluent Speech. R. A. Cole, Ed.: 381-395. Erlbaum. Hillsdale, NJ.
50. O'SHAUGHNESSY, D. 1976. Modelling Fundamental Frequency, and Its Relationships to Syntax, Semantics, and Phonetics. Unpublished Ph.D. thesis, Massachusetts Institute of Technology.
51. OSHIKA, G. T., V. W. VUE, R. V. WEEKS, H. NEU & J. AURBACH. 1975. The role of phonological rules in speech understanding research. IEEE Trans. Acoust. Speech, Signal Processing **23:** 104–112.
52. PIERREHUMBERT, J. 1980. The Phonology and Phonetics of English Intonation. Unpublished Ph.D. thesis, Massachusetts Institute of Technology.
53. POLLACK, I. & J. M. PICKETT. 1963. Intelligibility of excerpts from conversational speech. Language and Speech **6:** 165–171.
54. REDDY, R. 1976. Speech recognition by machine: A review. Proc. IEEE **64:** 501–531.
55. REICH, S. S. 1980. Significance of pauses for speech perception. J. Psycholinguist. Res. **9:** 379–389.
56. RISBERG, A. 1974. The importance of prosodic speech elements for the lipreader. *In* Visual and Audiovisual Perception of Speech. H. B. Nielson and E. Kamp, Eds.: 153–164. Scandinavian Audiology, Suppl. 4. Almqvist & Wiksell. Stockholm.

57. RISBERG, A. 1976. Diagnostic rhyme test for speech audiometry with severely hard of hearing and profoundly deaf children. Speech Transmission Lab. Quart. Prog. Status Rep. **2–3:** 40–58.
58. SAMUEL, A. G. 1981. Phonemic restoration: Insights from a new methodology. J. Exp. Psychol. General **110**(4)**:** 474–494.
59. SAMUEL, A. G. 1981. The role of bottom-up confirmation in the phonemic restoration illusion. J. Exp. Psychol.: Human Percept. Perform. **7**(5)**:** 1124–1131.
60. STREETER, L. A. 1978. Acoustic determinants of phrase boundary perception. J. Acoust. Soc. Am. **64:** 1582–1592.
61. STUDDERT-KENNEDY, M. & K. HADDING-KOCH. 1973. Auditory and linguistic processes in the perception of intonation contours. Language and Speech **16:** 293–313.
62. VILLCHUR, E. 1978. Signal processing. *In* Auditory Management of Hearing-Impaired Children. M. Ross and T. G. Giolas, Eds.: 219–237. University Park Press. Baltimore, MD.
63. WALES, R. & H. TONER. 1979. Intonation and ambiguity. *In* Sentence Processing. W. E. Cooper and E. C. T. Walker, Eds.: 135–158. Erlbaum. Hillsdale, NJ.
64. WARREN, R. M. 1970. Perceptual restoration of missing speech sounds. Science **167:** 392–393.
65. WARREN, R. M. & C. OBUSEK. 1971. Speech perception and phonemic restorations. Percept. Psychophys. **9:** 358–363.
66. WARREN, R. M. & G. SHERMAN. 1974. Phonemic restorations based on subsequent context. Percept. Psychophys. **16:** 150–156.
67. TERRANGO, L. 1966. Pitch and duration characteristics of the oral reading of males on a masculinity-femininity dimension. J. Speech Hear. Res. **9:** 590–595.

ACOUSTIC CODING OF SPEECH AND NORMAL LIMITS ON TRANSFER OF INFORMATION: DISCUSSION PAPER

Paula Tallal

Department of Psychiatry
University of California, San Diego
La Jolla, California 92093

This first session has been devoted to a discussion of what is known concerning the acoustic coding of speech. Dr. Kenneth Stevens began by discussing the acoustic properties (noise, amplitude, pattern of spectral peaks, abrupt change in spectra) that characterize differences between various categories of speech sounds. He emphasized that of the acoustic properties that characterize these differences an underlying characteristic of speech is its temporal nature. That is, the acoustic waveform characterizing speech constantly changes over time. Thus, some of the critical distinctions between various categories of speech depend on distinctions occurring over a very brief segment of the acoustic spectra, whereas other acoustic cues are not quite so brief. One critical limit on the transfer of information from the periphery for central processing is rate. We have shown in subjects with developmental as well as acquired language disorders that patients with difficulty in processing rapidly changing acoustic information have specific difficulties in discriminating between speech sounds that are characterized by brief temporal cues.[1–3] These studies indicate that temporal constraints on processing can have a very direct effect on acoustic coding of speech.

Dr. Atal has emphasized the importance of determining at the perceptual level what we use in the speech code versus what we do not. He presented data that demonstrated that all aspects of the acoustic signal are not equally salient in speech perception. Certain aspects of the signal mask other aspects. Like Dr. Stevens, Dr. Atal emphasized the salience of temporal cues in the acoustic coding of speech and suggested that this salience should be taken into account in designing cochlear implants.

Dr. Studdert-Kennedy described research that demonstrates that what we perceive when we hear speech is not the actual sounds of the acoutic waveform, but an abstract code. So, at the neurologic level, it is likely that we perceive this abstract code rather than the initial sound that occurs at the periphery. However, as we all know, if the acoustic waveform is not transferred adequately from the periphery, then we are presumably unable to encode sound into this abstract form necessary for speech perception at the central level. Consequently, given that the acoustic waveform is initially transferred adequately, information pertaining to the acoustic coding of speech at the neurologic level is of importance for cochlear implant research. However, the acoustic characteristic of what must be transferred again becomes critical to speech perception. Dr. Studdert-Kennedy suggested that one of the most primary aspects of the acoustic waveform that must be captured in the acoustic signal is change over time. He suggests that this may be the single most important aspect of the signal and stated that the rate at which the signal changes, and thus must be encoded, is critical.

0077-8923/83/0405-0064 $01.75/0

There seems little doubt that the rate at which the acoustic waveform changes and needs to be encoded is a critical aspect of speech perception and one that should receive particular attention in the development of cochlear implants. In our own studies, we have been able to show in a group of children with acquired developmental language disorders that computer alteration of the rate of change of specific temporal characteristics of some speech sounds results in significant enhancement of speech perception by these children.[4] In these studies, the childern demonstrated difficulty in responding correctly to nonverbal tone stimuli presented rapidly in succession. In subsequent studies, it was demonstrated that a similar difficulty occurred in discriminating between speech syllables that were characterized by rapidly changing formant transitions. When the duration over which the formant transitions critical for characterizing these speech stimuli was synthetically extended, speech discrimination dramatically improved. These studies suggest that physiological limitations may be bypassed through the development of technological devices having the capability of altering those aspects of the acoustic waveform that are necessary for speech processing. In designing cochlear implant electrodes, it may be important to determine which aspects of the acoustic spectra are most salient, as suggested by Dr. Atal, and to attempt to enhance those aspects so that subjects have a maximum amount of the most important information being transferred for neural coding of speech.

References

1. Tallal, P. & M. Piercy. 1973. Developmental aphasia: Impaired rate of nonverbal processing as a function of sensory modality. Neuropsychologia **11:** 389–398.
2. Tallal, P. & M. Piercy. 1974. Developmental aphasia: Rate of auditory processing and selective impairment of consonant perception. Neuropsychologia **12:** 83–93.
3. Tallal, P. & F. Newcombe. 1976. Impairment of auditory perception and language comprehension in dysphasia. Brain and Language **5:** 13–24.
4. Tallal, P. & M. Piercy. 1975. Developmental aphasia: The perception of brief vowels and extended stop consonants. Neuropsychologia **13:** 67–74.

PART II. NORMAL CODING WITHIN THE AUDITORY SYSTEM

INTRODUCTION

Juergen Tonndorf

Department of Otolaryngology
College of Physicians & Surgeons
Columbia University
New York, New York 10032

The first session has dealt with the acoustic properties of speech sounds. Speech obviously is the most important and probably the most complex type of signal the auditory system is called on to handle. In this second session we must now turn our attention to the problem of sensorineural coding. In general, all external sensory inputs must be coded so as to generate neural signals, which the central nervous system can optimally transmit and process and from which it can ultimately extract maximal sensory information. In the normal ear, this coding takes place in the hair-cell/nerve-fiber junctions, where the incoming mechanoacoustic signals are transduced into neural signals.

In addition to this general sensorineural coding, there is a specific cochlear process—the systematic distribution of frequency to discrete hair-cell and nerve-fiber groups due to the traveling wave event, which occurs on a purely mechanical basis. Since in this respect the cochlea acts as a delay line, the spatial distribution is accompanied by a temporal delay of low frequencies relative to high frequencies that is also systematic and amounts maximally to 4 or 5 msec. The central reintegration of complex auditory signals must take into account these temporal differences between various frequency components. That is, there must be a permanent central program that systematically delays high frequencies to compensate for the peripheral low-frequency delay.

When the hair cells are missing, many of the essential details of the neural coding process are eliminated, including, of course, the spatial and temporal distribution of frequency. Electrical analogs of the acoustical waveform applied via cochlear prostheses elicit some neural responses to be sure, but the auditory centers are unable to extract much more than mere temporal information from them. Admittedly, the central nervous system possesses some plasticity, that is, it can adapt itself to some altered requirements, as evidenced by the success of nerve grafting. However, to let some peripheral motor nerve fibers acquire a new skill is a relatively simple task, especially when it does not involve the loss of the underlying coding process and the need to carry on operations with the aid of a greatly reduced process. It is very much doubted that the central auditory system can learn, even over the long run, to extract substantial sensory information from signals presented without proper coding. The sensory information provided by the reception of uncoded analog signals via a cochlear prosthesis, being largely limited to the time domain, clearly is not sufficient for the whole class of speech signals, but only for a relatively small fraction of them. According to Information Theory, the efficiency of a given transmission channel is not determined by the manner in which it handles selected signals, but by entire classes of them. Thus, the problem arises with respect to cochlear prostheses of how to develop a substitute external coding process. Since auditory coding may have some redundancy, one can hope that such a substitute can be simplified to some degree for the benefit of real-time processing.

Data required for these purposes cannot be obtained from simple trial and error methods, but only from systematic neurophysiological studies. We must recall that the present problem is primarily concerned with the manner in which acoustic properties of the auditory signals are being handled, not with their semantic content, which, from this standpoint, is a secondary problem. Therefore, meaningful experiments can be carried out in experimental animals.

SPATIOTEMPORAL RESPONSE PATTERNS IN POPULATIONS OF COCHLEAR NERVE FIBERS: SINGLE- AND TWO-TONE STUDIES [a]

D. O. Kim

Departments of Physiology and Biophysics,
Electrical Engineering, and Biomedical Engineering
Washington University
St. Louis, Missouri 63110

Introduction

A sound understanding of basic mechanisms underlying the transduction of acoustic signals into spike discharges of the population of cochlear nerve fibers distributed along the cochlear partition should be helpful in cochlear implant research. This paper reviews some of the salient features of cochlear mechanical and neural responses to single- and two-tone stimuli, especially as revealed by the method of cochlear nerve population recording, which illustrates spatiotemporal response patterns of the total length of the cochlear partition.

Tuning and Nonlinearity of Cochlear Response

Early mechanical experiments of Bekesy [2] and subsequent experiments [30] conducted until very recently have indicated that the mechanical response of each position of the cochlear partition is quite broadly tuned. Threshold excitation of a single cochlear nerve fiber, in contrast, shows a sharp tuning.[12] This apparent discrepancy has led Evans and Wilson [3] and other investigators to postulate a "second cochlear filter," which sharpens a broad mechanical tuning to produce a sharp neural tuning. On the other hand, Kim and Molnar [14] have cautioned that the apparent discrepancy between the mechanical and neural tuning should not be taken at face value because of physiological vulnerability and nonlinearity of cochlear partition motion.

Rhode [23] showed that tuning and nonlinearity of cochlear partition motion changed significantly after death of the experimental animal or after removal of the cochlear blood supply. Subsequent studies of LePage and Johnstone [19] also showed that nonlinearity of cochlear partition motion was physiologically vulnerable. Accumulating evidence from a number of neural [16, 18, 29] and otoacoustic [1, 5, 8, 17] studies have strengthened the conclusions that: (1) cochlear mechanical response is highly nonlinear in the normal cochlea; (2) cochlear partition motion is vulnerable to physiological disturbance of the cochlea; and (3) the cellular activity of the cochlear partition is bidirectionally coupled to the cochlear partition mechanics.

[a] This work was supported in part by Grant NS18426 from the National Institutes of Health.

0077–8923/83/0405–0068 $01.75/0 © 1983, NYAS

In recent cochlear mechanical experiments by Sellick *et al.*[27] and Khanna and Leonard,[11] utmost care was taken to minimize damage to cochlear mechanisms and to closely monitor the physiological state of the cochlea by measuring tone-pip thresholds for the cochlear nerve compound action potential (N_1). In these experiments, data obtained under an optimal physiological condition reveal much greater sensitivity and tuning of the cochlear mechanical response than that obtained under physiologically deteriorated conditions. FIGURE 1 shows a replot of the data of Sellick *et al.*, where the circles connected by a solid line represent an optimal mechanical tuning curve corresponding to 10Å-isodisplacement of a basal position of guinea pig basilar membrane, and the dashed line represents a typical tuning curve of a cochlear spiral ganglion neuron located in the similar basal region of guinea pig cochlea. The mechanical

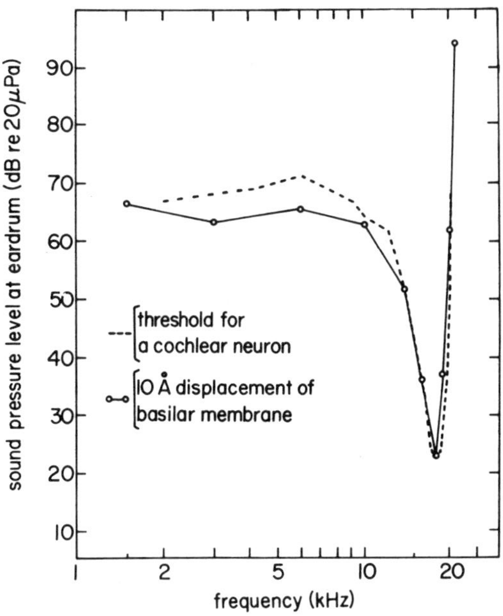

FIGURE 1. Tuning curves of the basilar membrane (*solid line*) and a cochlear neuron (*dashed line*) in a guinea pig. (From Neely and Kim,[21] where the original data of Sellick *et al.*[27] were replotted. Reprinted by permission.)

and neural tuning curves of FIGURE 1 are quite similar. The good agreement of the two curves in FIGURE 1 further suggests that a constant basilar membrane displacement of about 10Å (rather than a constant velocity of about 0.04 mm/sec, suggested by Sellick *et al.*) corresponds well to threshold excitation of a cochlear neuron.

Sharp tuning characteristics observed in suppression of otoacoustic emission signals by tonal stimuli[9, 31, 33] are consistent with the sharp tuning of basilar membrane motion shown in FIGURE 1.

FIGURE 2 shows recent results obtained from an active model for cochlear biomechanics developed by Neely and Kim.[21] The three curves represent tuning characteristics (in the form of 10Å-isodisplacement curves) of the basilar membrane under three different conditions of the model. Curve 1, which shows the highest sensitivity and the sharpest tuning among the three,

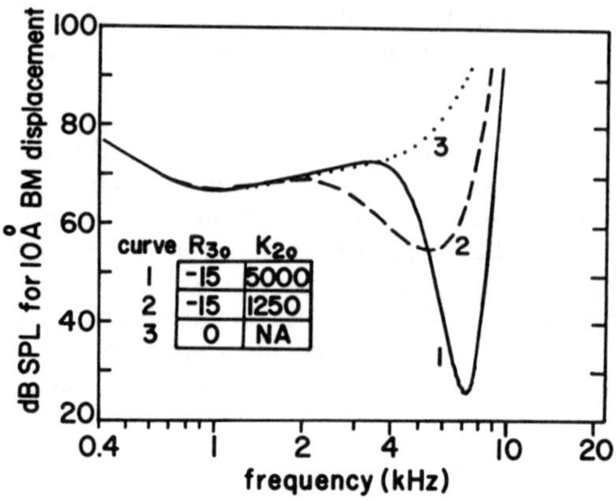

FIGURE 2. 10Å-isodisplacement tuning curves of a point on the basilar membrane (23% from the stapes) in an active cochlear model developed by Neely and Kim. The three curves represent responses of the model under three different conditions: curves 1 and 2 correspond to active conditions of the model indicated by the presence of a negative damping component R_{30} in the model; curve 3 corresponds to a passive condition of the model, where there are no negative damping components. (Adapted from Neely and Kim.[21])

corresponds to the most active condition of the model, where a large amount of mechanical energy is released from inside the cochlear partition into the surrounding fluid of the model. Curve 2, which shows a lower sensitivity and broader tuning, corresponds to a less active condition of the model, where a lesser amount of the internal energy is released. Curve 3, which shows the lowest sensitivity and the broadest tuning among the three, corresponds to a passive condition of the model, where the entire cochlear partition does not release any energy but always dissipates energy. These three curves of the model results are quite similar to the animal data of Sellick *et al.*[27] obtained under various physiological conditions of the cochlea, as just discussed.

RESPONSE TO SINGLE TONES

A useful method for investigating spike discharges of single cochlear nerve fibers to a periodic stimulus such as a single tone is to construct period histograms [24] and to analyze these histograms by the discrete Fourier transform to extract the average discharge rate, R_0, the amplitude, R_i and the phase, θ_i, of the i-th harmonic component of the period histogram as defined by Kim and Molnar.[15] FIGURE 3 illustrates an example of the response of a single cochlear nerve fiber to a single tone in the form of the period histogram on the left and the spectrum obtained by the discrete Fourier transform of the histogram on the right. The upper part of the spectrum corresponds to R_i in spikes/sec and the lower part corresponds to θ_i in radians for $i = 1, 2, \ldots, 6$. (The phase is not defined for $i = 0$, that is, the zero-frequency component.) The two dominant spectral components in this example are the average discharge rate component, R_0 (80 spikes/sec), and the fundamental frequency component, R_1 (60 spikes/sec). The fundamental component R_1 is a more sensitive measure of response than R_0 because R_1 conveys stimulus-dependent information even at very low levels of stimulus, where R_0 remains unchanged from the spontaneous rate (SR) of the nerve fiber.[15, 24]

By using this method of taking the period histogram and its Fourier transform of responses of each of more than 400 sequentially recorded single cochlear nerve fibers in an individual animal, it was possible to reconstruct spatiotemporal response patterns of the populations of cochlear neurons originating from various positions along the cochlear partition.[15, 22] FIGURE 4 shows such examples of spatial distributions of two measures of response amplitude, that is, R_0–SR and R_1 for single-tone stimuli of 1 kHz at 20, 45, and 75 dB sound pressure level (SPL) re 20 μPa. The left column of FIGURE 4 indicates that at 20 dB SPL only the fibers innervating a small region near the characteristic place of 1 kHz show increased average discharge rate over the fiber SR; at 45 dB a greater percentage of the neural population shows an increase in average rate; at 70 dB a bulk of the neural population, representing nearly 70% of the total length of the cochlear partition, shows average rate increase and, furthermore, the spatial distribution pattern at 70 dB is no longer a simple single-peaked pattern observed with the 20-dB stimulus. It should be noted that the 70 dB SPL is not a high stimulus level, but a moderate stimulus level comparable to a common conversational speech signal level.

As shown in the right column of FIGURE 4, spatial distributions of the fundamental Fourier component R_1 are consistent with the average-rate distributions, except that R_1 is a more sensitive and informative measure of response than R_0–SR. For example, the secondary peak located near the 7-kHz place is clearly detectable in the lower right two panels, whereas it is not detectable in the lower left two panels. Although the nature of this secondary peak and the cause for the complex spatial patterns at 70 dB SPL are not fully understood now, it is conjectured that these two phenomena have a common origin in standing-wave-like interactions between cochlear mechanical wave components propagating in the forward (apical) and backward (basal)

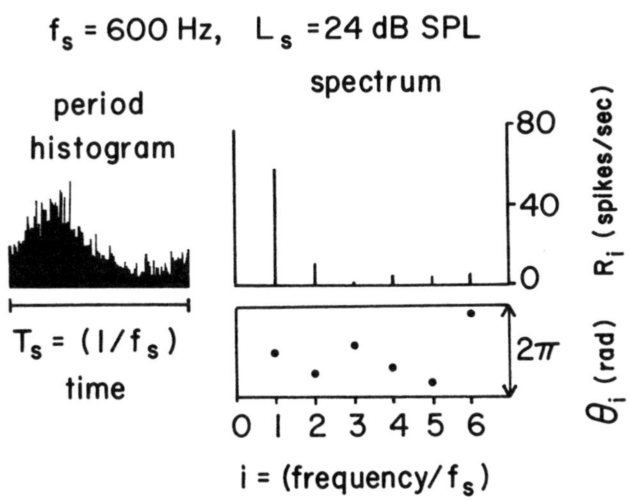

FIGURE 3. A period histogram and its spectrum (obtained by taking a discrete Fourier transform of the period histogram) for responses of a cat cochlear nerve fiber: characteristic frequency = 1050 Hz; spontaneous rate = 67 spikes/sec; sample time = 20 sec; bin width = 13 μsec. The stimulus was a single tone of 600 Hz, 24 dB re 20 μPa. The time origin of the period histogram corresponds to the negative-going zerocrossing of the voltage applied to the earphone.

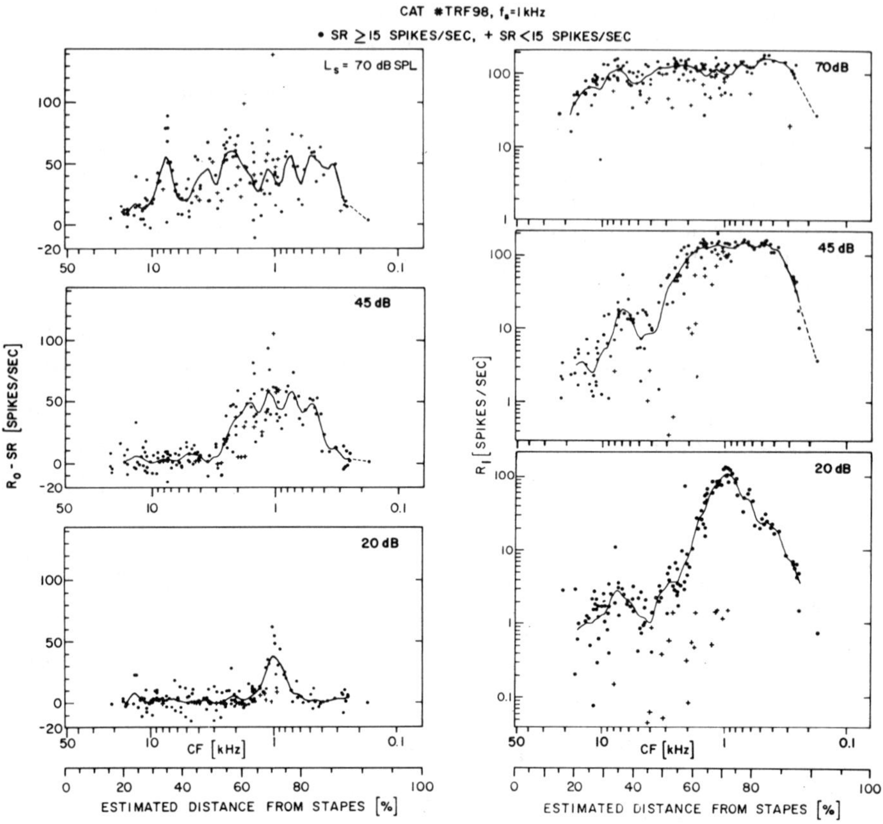

FIGURE. 4. Spatial profiles of two response measures, that is, (R_o–SR) and R_1, for a population of cochlear nerve fibers in one cat. R_o is the average discharge rate; R_1 is the amplitude of the Fourier transform of the period histogram at the fundamental frequency; both R_o and R_1 are in spikes/sec. The *dots* represent fibers with SR $\geqslant$ 15 spikes/sec and the *crosses* show fibers with lower SR. The continuous curve through the data points in each panel is a moving-window average based on the high-SR fibers only. The stimulus was a single tone of 1 kHz at 20, 45 and 70 dB re 20 μPa. (Adapted from Kim and Molnar.[15])

directions.[17] The backward propagation component is postulated to originate from an active energy source located in the cochlear partition which enhances mechanical response sensitivity by converting metabolic energy into mechanical energy.[10, 17, 21]

FIGURE 5 shows high-frequency (8-kHz) data reported by Evans [4] which were processed in the same way as those in the left column of FIGURE 4. The 8-kHz results in FIGURE 5 are qualitatively similar to the 1-kHz results in FIGURE 4, including the fact that the lowest stimulus level produces a simple single-peaked spatial response pattern, whereas the higher stimulus levels produce complex spatial response patterns. Differences between the results of FIGURES 4 and 5 include the fact that the 1-kHz tone, at 70 dB, excited a wide region of the cochlear partition spreading around the 1-kHz place toward both the apex and the base of the cochlea, whereas the 8-kHz tone, at 70 and 94 dB, excited the region spreading only toward the base from the 8-kHz place, thus maintaining a sharper apical slope of the excitation pattern at the 8-kHz place.

Response to Two Tones

The upper part of Figure 6 illustrates an example of a two-tone stimulus waveform and its spectrum, where we have $f_1 = 7f_0$, $f_2 = 9f_0$ and $f_0 = 300$ Hz. The lower part of Figure 6 illustrates five period histograms and their spectra representing responses to this stimulus recorded from five single cochlear nerve fibers innervating different positions along the cochlear partition in one cat. The response patterns of these cochlear nerve fibers to the same two-tone stimulus are strikingly different and demonstrate the prominent nonlinearity of cochlear mechanisms. The fiber with CF = 2700 Hz shows a response pattern most resembling the stimulus waveform; the spectrum for this fiber's response (second from the bottom) shows large primary frequency components, $f_1 = 7f_0$ and $f_2 = 9f_0$, besides other frequency components. However, the fiber with CF = 600 Hz responds as if the stimulus were a 600-Hz single tone rather than the 2100-Hz, 2700-Hz two-tone pair whose frequency difference, $(f_2–f_1)$, is 600 Hz. Likewise, the fiber with CF = 1160 Hz, which is near $(2f_1–f_2)$,

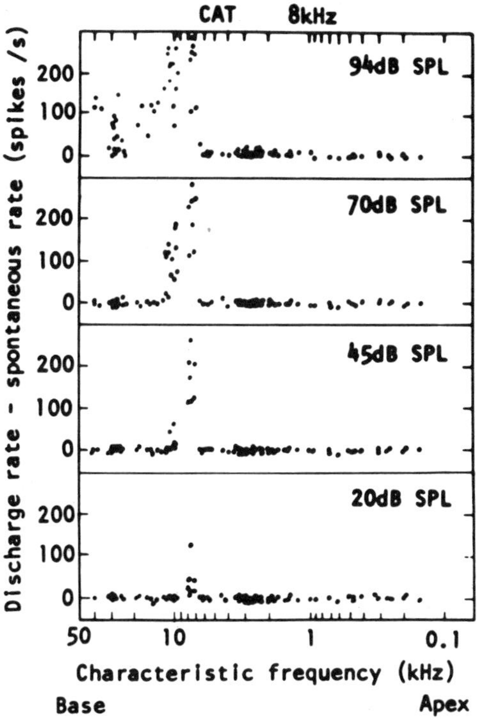

Figure 5. Spatial profiles of the response measure (R_o–SR) for a population of cochlear nerve fibers in one cat. The stimulus was a single tone of 8 kHz at 20, 45, 70 and 94 dB re 20 μPa. (From Evans.[4] Reprinted by permission.)

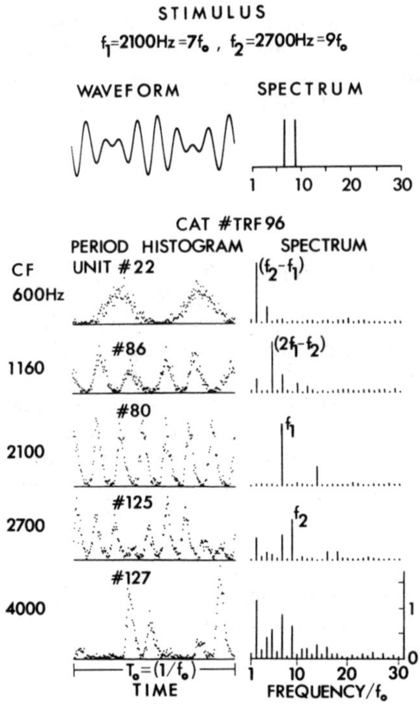

FIGURE 6. A two-tone stimulus waveform and five period histograms and their spectra. The period histograms represent responses of five single cochlear nerve fibers with different characteristic frequency (CF), as shown. (From Kim *et al.*[18] Reprinted by permission.)

shows a prominent ($2f_1$–f_2) distortion product in the response, as previously reported by Goldstein and Kiang.[6] The fiber with CF = 4000 Hz shows a response pattern that is grossly distorted from the stimulus waveform and contains a variety of distortion product components besides the primary components.

Spatial distributions of the amplitudes of the primary components $R(f_1)$ and $R(f_2)$ as well as the distortion product components $R(f_2-f_1)$ and $R(2f_1-f_2)$ have been investigated using the same cochlear nerve population method discussed earlier with the single-tone case. FIGURE 7 shows the amplitudes of these four components normalized by the fiber SR for a particular two-tone stimulus at eight stimulus levels ranging from 4 dB to 74 dB SPL. In FIGURE 7, the average curves are shown without the individual fiber data points for clarity of display. Spatial profiles of the response components are rather simple at very low stimulus levels, 4 to 24 dB SPL, where the primary (f_1 and f_2) components are dominant and the significant amplitudes of the distortion products are localized only in the region where the f_1 and f_2 components overlap. At and above 34 dB SPL, however, the spatial response profiles become increasingly more complex. In particular, each of the distortion products shows a peak of amplitude at the characteristic place of the distortion frequency as indicated by vertical arrows. These and related neural data [14, 17, 29] as well as results from nonlinear cochlear modeling studies [7, 13, 18] and studies of otoacoustic distortion products in the ear canal [17, 28, 34] support the following conclusions: (1) mechanical distortion product signals such as ($2f_1$–f_2) and

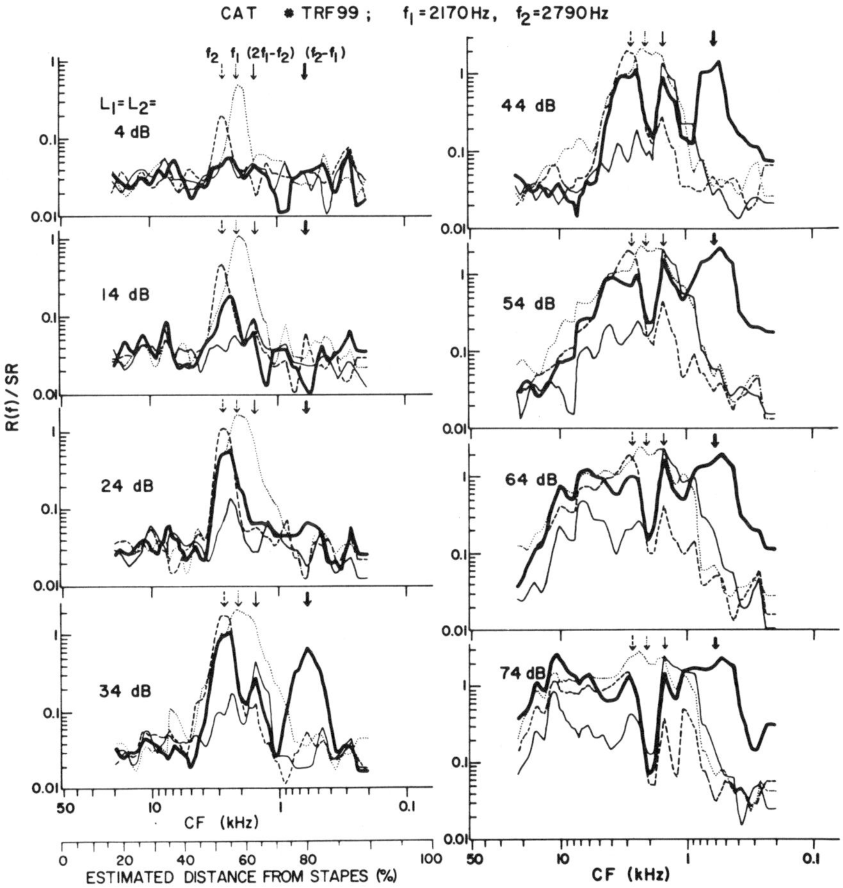

FIGURE 7. Spatial profiles of four response measures, $R(f_1)/SR$, $R(f_2)/SR$, $R(f_2-f_1)/SR$ and $R(2f_1-f_2)/SR$. $R(f_i)$ is the amplitude of the Fourier transform of the period histogram at the frequency value of f_i. These data are moving-window averages based on a population of cochlear nerve fibers in one cat. The stimulus was a two-tone pair, $f_1 = 2170$ Hz and $f_2 = 2790$ Hz, at eight levels ranging from 4 to 74 dB re 20 μPa. (From Kim *et al.*[18] Reprinted by permission.)

(f_2-f_1) are generated in the cochlear region, where the f_1 and f_2 components are both large; and (2) these distortion products mechanically propagate both toward the distortion frequency place and toward the stapes, through the middle ear and into the ear canal; and (3) the distortion product generation requires normal physiological processes, but not neural activity, in the cochlear sensory apparatus.

DISCUSSION

The biomechanical system of the cochlea, as we now understand it, is much more complicated than had been widely believed for decades on the basis of

Bekesy's[2] pioneering works conducted since the 1940s. Evidence currently available compels us to change our concept of the cochlear mechanical system drastically from a traditional passive and linear system to an active and nonlinear system which is significantly controlled by biological activities of the organ of Corti and the olivocochlear efferent neural system.[10, 17, 18, 20, 28]

The complex spatial response profiles of the cochlear neural population to single- and two-tone stimuli shown in FIGURES 4, 5, and 7 clearly demonstrate prominent nonlinear behavior which is present not only around the characteristic places of the stimulus frequencies, but also over most of the total length of the cochlear partition. Response profiles of the cochlear neural population of the cat for certain speech stimuli have been reported by Sachs and Young[25, 26] and Young and Sachs.[32] These neural population data obtained with speech stimuli are quite consistent with the single- and two-tone data discussed earlier in that the speech responses also show prominent nonlinear behavior widespread over most of the total length of the cochlear partition. It is remarkable that the Figures 3–5 and 7–9 of Young and Sachs[32] clearly show that at 50 to 80 dB SPL formant frequency components of the vowel stimulus excite a large proportion of cochlear neural population, not only those neurons tuned to the particular formant frequency, but also many other neurons spread over wide regions of the cochlear partition. The particular method of examining the "average localized synchronized rate" (ALSR) presented by Young and Sachs in their Figures 6, 10 and 11 has a potential danger of misleading an unsophisticated reader to think that responses to the formant frequency components are well localized spatially around the characteristic places of the formant frequencies. In fact, they are very broadly distributed.

A good design goal for an ideal cochlear prosthesis would be to stimulate the entire surviving cochlear neural population distributed along the cochlea such that the artificially excited neural response profiles closely resemble the normal response profiles such as those discussed in this paper. In this approach, it will be helpful to use an adequate model for biomechanics and the transduction process of the ear, which closely simulates normal response characteristics.

REFERENCES

1. ANDERSON, S. D. & D. T. KEMP. 1979. The evoked cochlear mechanical response in laboratory primates: A preliminary report. Arch. Otorhinolaryngol. **224:** 47–54.
2. BEKESY, G. VON. 1960. Experiments in Hearing. McGraw-Hill. New York, NY.
3. EVANS, E. F. & J. P. WILSON. 1975. Cochlear tuning properties: Concurrent basilar membrane and single nerve fiber measurements. Science **190:** 1218–1221.
4. EVANS, E. F. 1981. The dynamic range problem: Place and time coding at the level of cochlear nerve and nucleus. *In* Neuronal Mechanisms of Hearing. J. Syka and L. Aitkin, Eds.: 69–85. Plenum Press. New York, NY.
5. EVANS, E. F., J. P. WILSON & T. A. BORERWE. 1981. Animal models of tinnitus. *In* Tinnitus. Ciba Foundation Symposium **85:** 108–138. Pitman Books. London.
6. GOLDSTEIN, J. L. & N. Y.-S. KIANG. 1968. Neural correlates of the aural combination tone $2f_1–f_2$. Proc. IEEE **56:** 981–992.

7. HALL, J. L. 1974. Two-tone distortion products in a nonlinear model of the basilar membrane. J. Acoust. Soc. Am. **56:** 1818–1828.
8. KEMP, D. T. 1978. Stimulated acoustic emissions from within the human auditory system. J. Acoust. Soc. Am. **64:** 1386–1391.
9. KEMP, D. T. 1979. Evidence of mechanical nonlinearity and frequency selective wave amplification in the cochlea. Arch. Otorhinolaryngol. **224:** 37–45.
10. KEMP, D. T. 1980. Towards a model for the origin of cochlear echoes. Hearing Res. **2:** 533–548.
11. KHANNA, S. M. & D. G. B. LEONARD. 1982. Basilar membrane tuning in the cat cochlea. Science **215:** 305–306.
12. KIANG, N. Y. S., T. WANATABE, E. C. THOMAS & L. F. CLARK. 1965. Discharge patterns of single fibers in the cat's auditory nerve. Research Monograph **35:** MIT Press. Cambridge, MA.
13. KIM, D. O., C. E. MOLNAR & R. R. PFEIFFER. 1973. A system of nonlinear differential equations modeling basilar-membrane motion. J. Acoust. Soc. Am. **54:** 1517–1529.
14. KIM, D. O. & C. E. MOLNAR. 1975. Cochlear mechanics: Measurements and models. *In* The Nervous System. Vol. 3. Human Communication and Its Disorders. D. B. Tower, Ed.: 57–68. Raven Press. New York, NY.
15. KIM, D. O. & C. E. MOLNAR. 1979. A population study of cochlear nerve fibers: Comparison of the spatial distribution of average-rate and phase-locking measures of responses to single tones. J. Neurophysiol. **42:** 16–30.
16. KIM, D. O., J. H. SIEGEL & C. E. MOLNAR. 1979. Cochlear nonlinear phenomena in two-tone responses. Scand. Audiol. Suppl. **9:** 63–81.
17. KIM, D. O. 1980. Cochlear mechanics: Implications of electrophysiological and acoustical observations. Hearing Res. **2:** 297–317.
18. KIM, D. O., C. E. MOLNAR & J. W. MATTHEWS. 1980. Cochlear mechanics: Nonlinear behavior in two-tone responses as reflected in cochlear-nerve-fiber responses and in ear-canal sound pressure. J. Acoust. Soc. Am. **67:** 1704–1721.
19. LEPAGE, E. & B. JOHNSTONE. 1980. Nonlinear mechanical behaviour of the basilar membrane in the basal turn of the guinea pig cochlea. Hear. Res. **2:** 183–189.
20. MOUNTAIN, D. C. 1980. Changes in endolymphatic potential and crossed olivocochlear bundle stimulation alter cochlear mechanics. Science **210:** 71–72.
21. NEELY, S. T. & D. O. KIM. 1983. An active cochlear model shows sharp tuning and high sensitivity. Hearing Res. **9:** in press.
22. PFEIFFER, R. R. & D. O. KIM. 1975. Cochlear nerve fiber responses: Distribution along the cochlear partition. J. Acoust. Soc. Am. **58:** 867–869.
23. RHODE, W. S. 1973. An investigation of post-mortem cochlear mechanics using the Mössbauer effect. *In* Basic Mechanisms of Hearing. A. R. Møller, Ed.: 49–67. Academic Press. New York, NY.
24. ROSE, J. E., J. F. BRUGGE, D. J. ANDERSON & J. E. HIND. 1967. Phase-locked response to low-frequency tones in single auditory nerve fibers of the squirrel monkey. J. Neurophysiol. **30:** 769–793.
25. SACHS, M. B. & E. D. YOUNG. 1979. Encoding of steady-state vowels in the auditory nerve: Representation in terms of discharge rate. J. Acoust. Soc. Am. **66:** 470–479.
26. SACHS, M. B. & E. D. YOUNG. 1980. Effects of nonlinearities on speech encoding in the auditory nerve. J. Acoust. Soc. Am. **68:** 858–875.
27. SELLICK, P. M., R. PATUZZI & B. M. JOHNSTONE. 1982. Measurement of basilar membrane motion in the guinea pig using the Mössbauer technique. J. Acoust. Soc. Am. **72:** 131–141.

28. SIEGEL, J. H. & D. O. KIM. 1982. Efferent neural control of cochlear mechanics? Olivocochlear bundle stimulation affects cochlear biomechanical nonlinearity. Hearing Res. **6:** 171–182.
29. SIEGEL, J. H., D. O. KIM & C. E. MOLNAR. 1982. Effects of altering organ of Corti on cochlear distortion products f_2–f_1 and $2f_1$–f_2. J. Neurophysiol. **47:** 303–328.
30. WILSON, J. P. & J. R. JOHNSTONE. 1975. Basilar membrane and middle ear vibration in guinea pig measured by capacitive probe. J. Acoust. Soc. Am. **57:** 705–723.
31. WIT, H. P. & R. J. RITSMA. 1979. Stimulated acoustic emissions from the human ear. J. Acoust. Soc. Am. **66:** 911–913.
32. YOUNG, E. D. & M. B. SACHS. 1979. Representation of steady-state vowels in the temporal aspects of the discharge patterns of populations of auditory nerve fibers. J. Acoust. Soc. Am. **66:** 1381–1403.
33. ZUREK, P. M. 1981. Spontaneous narrowband acoustic signals emitted by human ears. J. Acoust. Soc. Am. **69:** 514–523.
34. ZUREK, P. M., W. W. CLARK & D. O. KIM. 1982. The behavior of acoustic distortion products in the ear canals of chinchillas with normal or damaged ears. J. Acoust. Soc. Am. **72:** 774–780.

ADAPTATION IN THE AUDITORY PERIPHERY[a]

R. L. Smith,[b] M. L. Brachman,[c] and D. A. Goodman[b]

[b] *Institute for Sensory Research*
Syracuse University
Syracuse, New York 13210

[c] *R. J. Brachman Associates*
Havertown, Pennsylvania 19083

Introduction

Adaptation of sensory receptors was defined by Adrian[1] in the following way: "The stimulus is represented as appearing suddenly and remaining at a constant value. The excitatory process in the receptor declines gradually, and as it declines the intervals between impulses in the sensory fibre become longer and longer." The purpose of this paper is to discuss the application of this description to the peripheral auditory system, especially the auditory nerve. The effects of adaptation on nonconstant (that is, dynamic) stimuli are reviewed and summarized. As is demonstrated, the results suggest that many of the effects of adaptation are relatively simple to describe and model and that adaptation has predictable influences on the responses to dynamic stimuli. Adaptation appears to have at least two effects of interest. First, it introduces spatiotemporal contrast since those fibers that were most recently stimulated are least responsive. Second, it can influence the operating range over which a fiber responds to changes in intensity. These considerations should be helpful in evaluating the need and manner in which to incorporate adaptation in an auditory prosthesis. Most of the data come from auditory neurons of anesthetized mongolian gerbils, and the assumption is made that similar results would be obtained in other mammalian species, including man.

As a first order of approximation it is assumed that adaptation can be described independently of other important properties of the auditory periphery, such as frequency selectivity and phase-locking to individual stimulus cycles. Consequently, the stimuli are defined in terms of their envelopes and applied in random phase, and responses are averaged over time intervals that span several stimulus cycles. The kinds of stimuli utilized are illustrated in FIGURE 1, which contains schematic representations of stimulus envelopes. These envelopes were chosen to represent simple kinds of dynamic stimuli for which changes in frequency content were small enough to be neglected. They are similar to the kinds of stimuli used by Delgutte[2] in his study of the responses of auditory nerve fibers to synthetic speech, a study that provides additional evidence and examples relevant to evaluating the importance of adaptation in the encoding of speech. In most cases the carrier was at the characteristic frequency (CF, the frequency of maximum sensitivity) of a unit, although

[a] This work was supported by Grant BNS81–04089 from the National Science Foundation and by Grants NS–00388 and NS–03950 from the National Institutes of Health.

0077–8923/83/0405–0079 $01.75/0 © 1983, NYAS

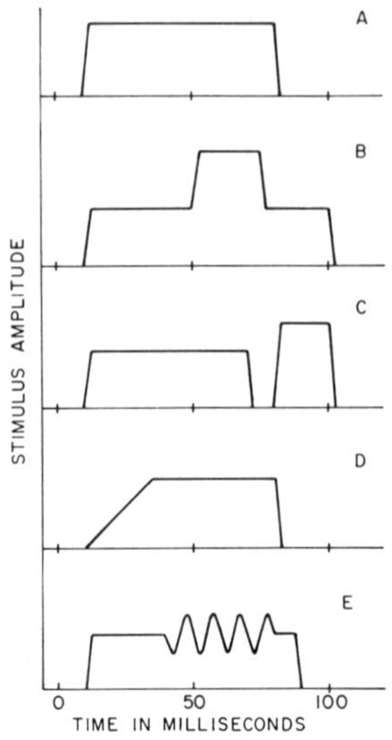

FIGURE 1. Schematic representations of the envelopes of some of the stimuli utilized in studying adaptation. **A:** Tone or noise burst of constant sound intensity. **B:** Background or adapting stimulus with an added test tone or increment in sound intensity. **C:** Test tone preceded by an adapting stimulus. **D:** Tone or noise burst with a long rise time. **E:** Tone burst whose amplitude is modulated by a sinusoid.

many of the experiments were also performed using wideband noise carriers. So far as has been determined, the results are independent of the frequency of the carrier.

RESPONSE TO CONSTANT INTENSITY

Strictly speaking, adaptation as defined above does not occur in the auditory system. This is because the "excitatory process in the receptor," that is, the receptor potential of an inner hair cell (IHC), does not "decline gradually" in response to a tone burst. Instead, it remains constant,[3, 4] as can be seen in FIGURE 2 and was shown previously for IHCs of the guinea pig.[5] This figure shows a typical plot of the change in intracellular voltage versus time in response to a high-frequency tone burst that lasted for about the duration of the response. Some cells in the gerbil departed from constancy

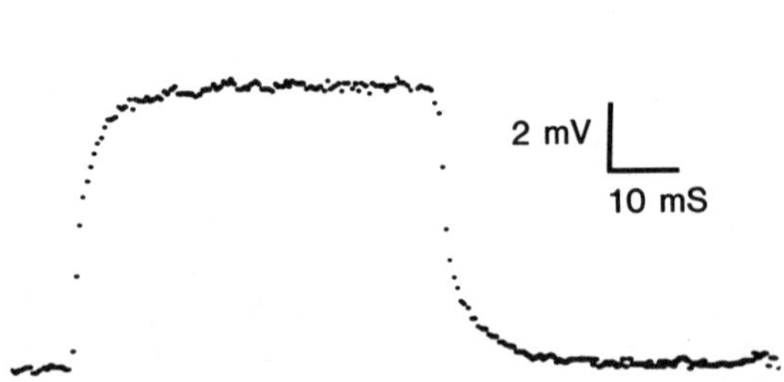

FIGURE 2. The DC receptor potential of an inner hair cell plotted versus time. The stimulus was a tone burst of 81 dB SPL at the characteristic frequency of the cell, 19 kHz. The depolarization lasted for the duration of the stimulus. Unit AN–49.

by exhibiting a slight increase over time, but a decay was never observed (unpublished results). Since the receptor potential is approximately constant, a single input–output or intensity function serves to describe the magnitude of the receptor potential as a function of sound intensity. A typical IHC intensity function is plotted in FIGURE 3. It can be seen that the receptor potential, plotted on a linear ordinate, is a monotonically increasing function of intensity level that does not reach saturation over the range of intensities shown,[3, 4] that is, at least 60 dB.

In contrast to IHCs, the responses of the next stage of processing, the auditory nerve fibers, decay with time during ongoing stimulation. This has also generally been called adaptation [6, 7] since it satisfies the second part of the foregoing definition. A typical response to a tone burst is shown by the poststimulus-time (PST) histogram in the left part of FIGURE 4C. The ordinate of the PST histogram effectively has units of spikes per second and

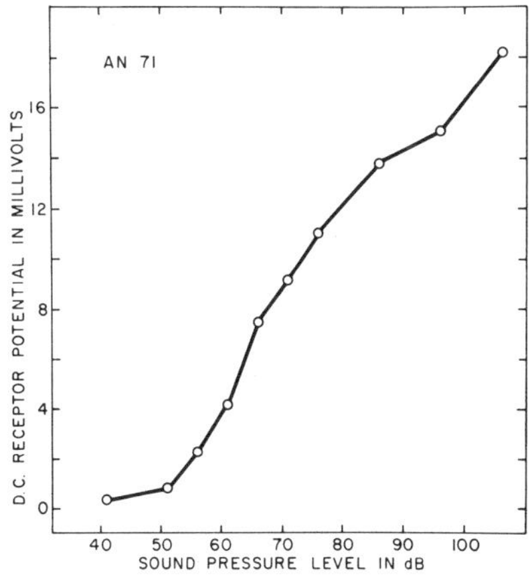

FIGURE 3. The magnitude of the DC receptor potential of an inner hair cell plotted versus sound-pressure level. The stimuli were tone bursts at the characteristic frequency of the cell, 16 kHz.

can be interpreted as the firing rate or as the probability of occurrence of a spike,[8, 9] and the abscissa is time in milliseconds. Histograms such as this can be approximated by the sum of two exponential decays, and a constant, leading to the suggestion that two adaptation phases exist—rapid adaptation with a time constant of several milliseconds, and short-term adaptation with a time constant of about 40 msec.[6, 7, 10, 11]

When the steady-state or adapted firing rate is plotted versus sound-intensity level, the rate generally increases monotonically over a range of about 30 dB and then approaches saturation. An example can be seen in the steady-state rate–intensity function of FIGURE 5A. The degree of saturation of the steady-state rate appears to be much greater than that observed in the receptor potential of IHCs (for example, that in FIGURE 3). This difference suggests that, in addition to decreasing the firing rate, adaptation may produce a decrease in overall operating range by changing the shape of the input–output characteristic. It should also be noted that some steady-state functions exhibit a decrease in slope, rather than full saturation, at high intensities.[12] However, their slopes still seem substantially smaller than that of the IHC function.[3]

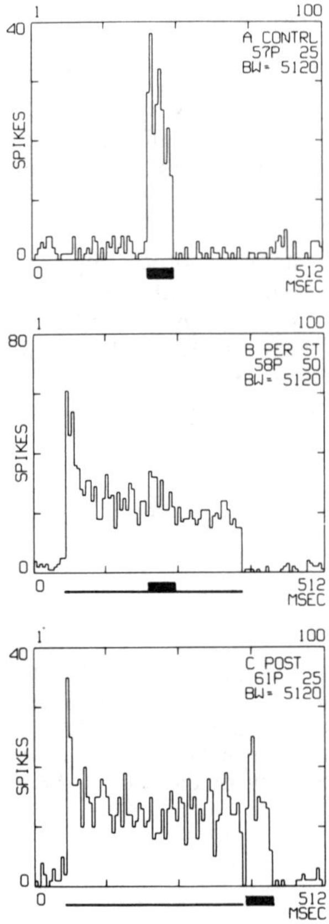

FIGURE 4. PST histograms showing typical auditory nerve responses for several stimulus paradigms. **A:** Short test tone applied alone. **B:** Test tone added to a background or adapting stimulus. **C:** Test tone applied after the adapting stimulus. (From Smith.[13] Reprinted by permission.)

If the shape of the rate–intensity function is influenced by adaptation, then the rate–intensity function measured at stimulus onset might be expected to have a different shape than the steady-state function. In contrast, both the onset and steady-state functions were shown [7, 13] to have the same shape provided that the onset firing rate is measured over a sufficiently long time interval, generally 10 msec or greater. This range of intervals was specifically chosen to emphasize the properties of short-term adaptation and to minimize the effects of rapid adaptation on the measurement. Typical data are shown in FIGURE 5A, where onset and steady-state firing rates are plotted versus sound-intensity level. Both sets of data were fitted by dashed curves with the same shape, suggesting that short-term adaptation does not alter the rate–intensity function or the operating range of a unit. In other words, as sound intensity is increased, the change in the onset response is proportional to the change in adapted response.

Partly on the basis of these results, it was hypothesized [7, 13, 14] that the invariant shape of the input–output characteristic resulted from a peripheral static nonlinearity that was followed by a short-term adaptation process that was inherently linear or additive, that is, obeyed the principle of superposition.

According to this model, a sudden increase or step in stimulus intensity produces an adapting response with an invariant shape when plotted as a function of time. The initial or onset magnitude of the response is determined from the static nonlinearity and equals the change in output of the nonlinearity produced by the given change in input. This two-stage model of adaptation is an oversimplified description of the actual system and some of its limitations and attempts at more complete modeling will be discussed later. Nevertheless, the model serves as a very useful way of characterizing many response properties related to short-term adaptation, and some examples of this will be discussed in the next section.

Effects of Short-Term Adaptation

Incremental Responses

The stimulus envelope shown in Figure 1B represents a paradigm where a test tone or increment in intensity is added to a background sound.[7, 13, 14] A typical PST histogram produced by this stimulus is shown in Figure 4B. To obtain the histogram, the test tone that produced the response in Figure 4A was added in the middle of a longer background sound. The background is seen to reduce both the total response and the incremental response, that is, the change in response produced by the increment. According to the model, the size of the incremental response should be a nonmonotonic function of intensity level. This is because as the background intensity is increased, the increment spans different regions on the S-shaped input nonlinearity. In addition, the superposition principle implies that the incremental response should be independent of the time delay and the amount of adaptation preceding the increment.

Typical incremental response functions are plotted in Figure 5B and show that these relationships are obeyed. The data were obtained by applying a 6-dB increment in intensity to a background tone at either the onset

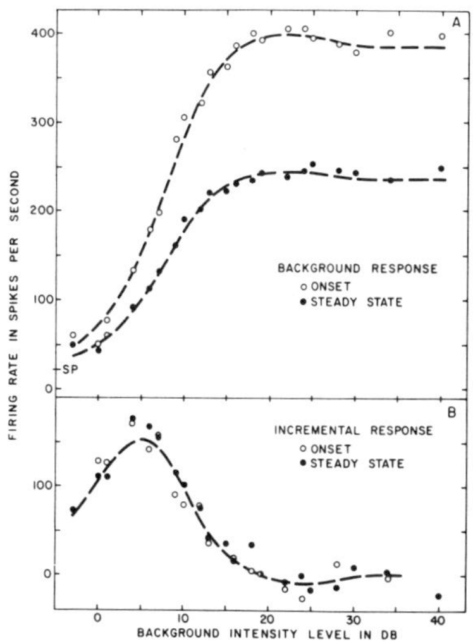

Figure 5. Responses of an auditory nerve fiber to a background tone with an added increment in sound intensity. **A:** Rate–intensity functions at the onset of the background and after the steady state had been reached. The *dashed curves* are proportional to one another after subtraction of the spontaneous rate (SP). **B:** The incremental response (the change in firing rate) produced by a 6-dB increment in sound intensity applied at background onset or after the steady state had been reached. The *dashed curve* is the theoretical incremental response function obtained from the rate–intensity function by computing the change in firing rate produced by the appropriate 6-dB change in intensity.[13, 17] Firing rates were measured over 40-msec-long time intervals. (From Smith.[13] Reprinted by permission.)

of the background, or after a time delay of 150 msec so that short-term adaptation was completed. At each background intensity level the onset and steady-state incremental responses can be seen to be equal. The dashed curve shows the nonmonotonic incremental response function predicted by the model, and the data lie close to the curve. At high intensities the incremental response decreases in spite of the fact that the increment in decibels is fixed so that the total energy added by the increment increases as the background intensity increases.

A related situation occurs when a test tone of fixed intensity is added to a background and the background intensity increased. If the test tone is sufficient to produce saturation, then according to the model the incremental response should equal that portion of the input nonlinearity that is not utilized by the background. Consequently, the sum of the incremental response and the response at background onset should be constant. As the background intensity increases, both the incremental response and the total response produced by the test tone should decrease monotonically. For this "physiological masking" paradigm, the data were also shown to be in quantitative agreement with the predictions of the model.[13]

Poststimulatory Effects

The principle of superposition can also be used to predict responses for the poststimulatory paradigm (FIGURE 1C). As can be seen in FIGURE 4C, the effect of prior stimulation is to reduce the response to the test tone. According to the model, the reduction should be by a constant number of spikes per second, independent of the intensity of the test tone. In addition, the amount of reduction should be proportional to the response to the adapting tone. Both of these effects were found to occur,[10, 13, 15–17] and an example of the former is shown in FIGURE 6. In FIGURE 6A the rate–intensity function

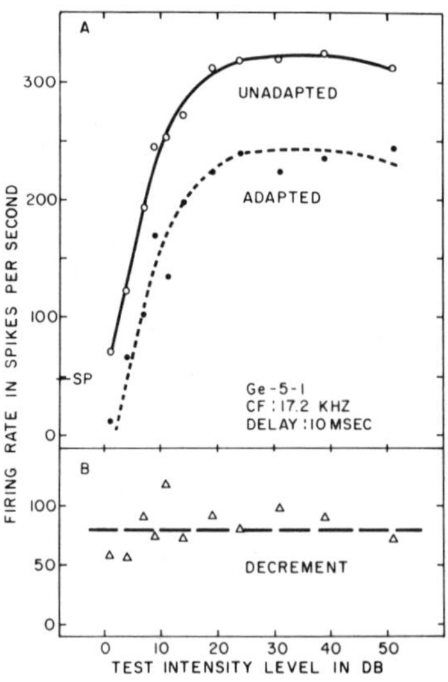

FIGURE 6. **A:** Rate–intensity functions for an auditory nerve fiber in response to a test tone in the presence (*solid circles*) and absence (*open circles*) of a prior adapting tone. There was a delay of 10 msec from the offset of the adapting tone to the onset of the test tone. **B:** Differences between the adapted and unadapted responses in **A** plotted versus the intensity level (re threshold) of the test tone. The *dashed line* was drawn through the median difference. (From Smith.[15] Reprinted by permission.)

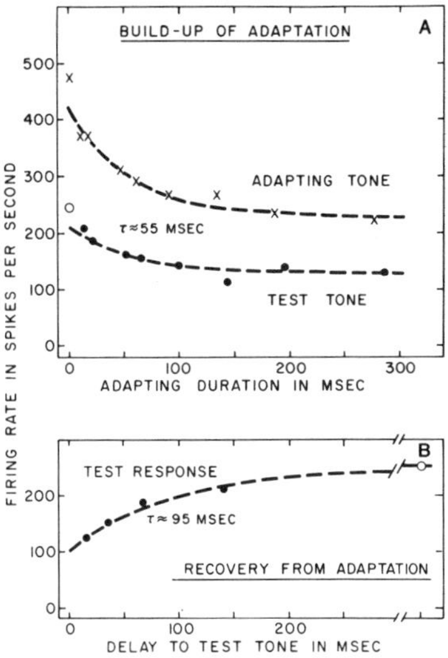

FIGURE 7. **A:** The *crosses* show the firing rate of an auditory nerve fiber during and at the end of an adapting tone having the duration indicated on the ordinate. The *solid circles* show the firing rate in response to a 40-msec-long test tone occurring 17 msec after the end of the adapting tone. The dashed curves are each the sum of a constant and an exponential term with a time constant of 55 msec. **B:** Firing rate in response to the test one in **A** as a function of the time delay from the end of the adapting tone to the start of the test tone. Adapting duration equals 202 msec. The *dashed line* is the sum of a constant and an exponential with a time constant of 95 msec. Unit Ge–16–4.

for a test tone is plotted in the presence and absence of a fixed adapting tone. The effect of adaptation is to produce a vertical shift of the rate–intensity function so that the dashed curve, which is a shifted and redrawn version of the solid curve, provides a reasonable fit to the data. Although this effect is unable to alter the operating range of a unit, it produces spatiotemporal gradients in response as a result of the past history of stimulation.[2, 15] The response to a stimulus depends upon both the excitation produced by the current stimulus and that produced by prior stimuli.

The duration of the adapting stimulus appears to have a simple relationship to the amount of poststimulatory adaptation.[10,15, 18] As is illustrated in FIGURE 7A, when the duration of an adapting stimulus increases, the decrement in the test response increases. However, the decrement does not depend on adapting duration per se, but rather on the amount of adaptation that occurs during the adapting exposure. Hence, once the response to the adapting stimulus has reached a steady state, further increases in duration do not affect the response to the test tone.

When the silent interval between the adapting and test tones is increased, the response to the test tone recovers along an exponential time course. However, the time constant of recovery is two or three times larger than that of short-term adaptation.[10, 13, 15, 18] An example is shown in FIGURE 7B for the same unit as in FIGURE 7A. This asymmetry is a departure from the superposition principle. It indicates that the buildup of adaptation and the recovery from adaptation involve separate system parameters, but the asymmetry does not otherwise alter the usefulness of the two-stage model.

Stimulus with a Long Rise Time

The foregoing results suggest that the same static nonlinearity produces saturation and limits firing rates for onset, steady-state, incremental, and poststimulatory responses. In terms of the model, the operating range is limited by the saturation of the input nonlinearity. Short-term adaptation does not alter this situation because it is located after the nonlinearity. Nevertheless, a more complex interaction occurs when a stimulus with a long rise time is applied, as in FIGURE 1D. By long is meant more than a few milliseconds and thus not negligible compared to the 40-msec time constant of short-term adaptation. Consequently, the input nonlinearity interacts with the time course of the input, effectively producing a time-dependent nonlinear effect.

To compute the response of the model, the rising portion of the stimulus can be viewed as producing a series of small steps or increments, each occurring on a progressively higher portion of the input nonlinearity. The magnitude of each step is proportional to the slope of the nonlinearity at the appropriate point and to the rate of change of the input. The output then equals the superposition or sum of the adapting responses to each small step.[19] For a given rise time, the rate at which the input nonlinearity is traversed depends upon the final intensity reached. The higher the overall intensity, the more decibels spanned per unit time during the rising portion. Because of the saturating shape of the input nonlinearity, as intensity is increased the effective rise time of its output will decrease. This results in a change in shape of the PST with intensity, as can be seen in the simulation of FIGURE 8. This figure shows model responses for four intensity levels, where the higher the intensity, the larger and earlier the maximum response. It should also be noted that the highest three intensities produce about the same steady-state response, while major differences occur near the onset. In particular the maximum response continues to grow with increasing intensity, even though the steady-state response has saturated. This occurs because the earlier the maximum occurs, the less the amount of adaptation at the time of the maximum. Hence, the model predicts that the interaction between adaptation, saturation, and the stimulus rise time will produce an increased operating range, if the latter is defined in terms of the maximum firing rate.

The PST histograms in FIGURE 9 illustrate that the predictions of the model are borne out.[19, 20] The right-hand column shows the responses to a stimulus with a short rise time for three intensity levels. Intensity increases in going from the top to the bottom of the figure, and both the onset and

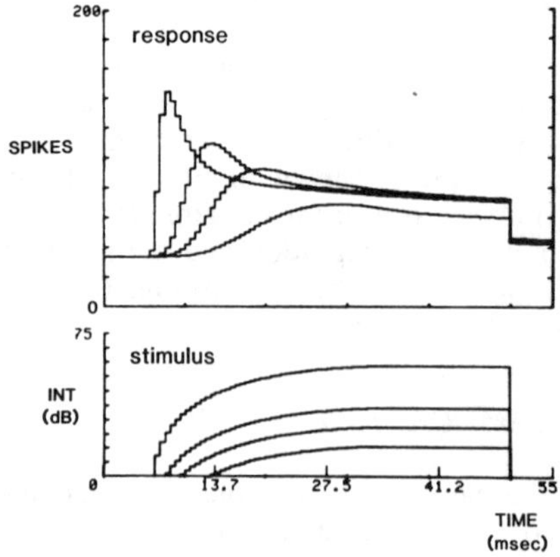

FIGURE 8. (*Top*) simulated responses (PST histograms) of the two-stage model to a stimulus with a long rise time at four intensity levels (see text). (*Bottom*) plot of logarithm of the envelope of each of the stimuli.

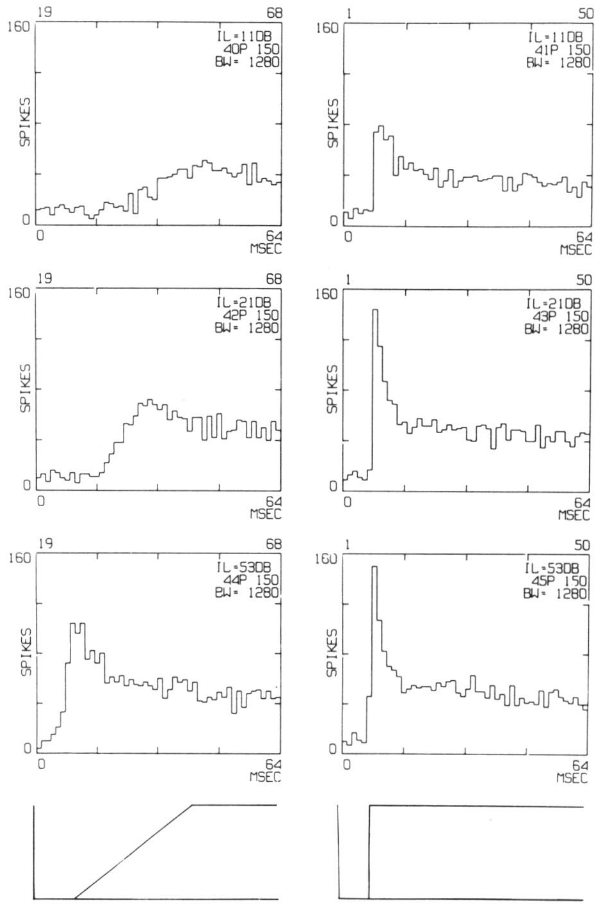

FIGURE 9. PST histograms for an auditory nerve fiber in response to stimuli with long (*left column*) and short (*right column*) rise times. Intensity level re threshold is indicated in the upper *right* corner of each histogram and increases from the top to the bottom of the figure. Stimuli were wideband noise bursts, but similar effects occur with tone bursts. Unit Ge–55–11.

steady-state responses can be seen to have reached saturation in the middle histogram. The responses to a stimulus with a 25-msec rise time are shown in the left-hand column for the same intensity levels as on the right. The histograms change shape in the predicted manner. Both the maximum and the steady-state rates are plotted versus intensity level in FIGURE 10, and it can be seen that the former continues to increase when the latter reaches saturation. The effects of rise time are of potential importance in the encoding and discrimination of speech sounds, although their interaction with background sounds must also be taken into account.[2, 21]

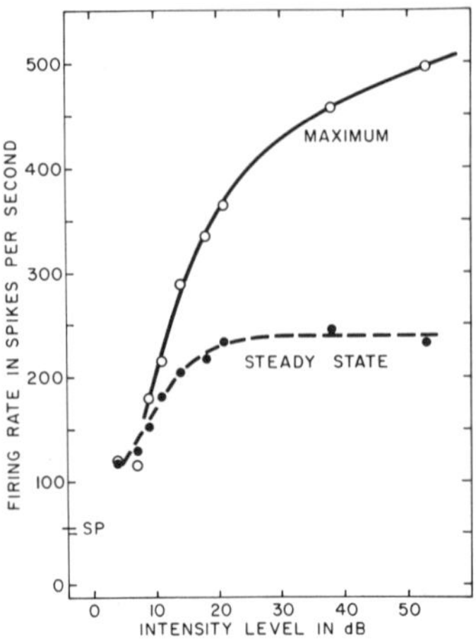

FIGURE 10. Rate–intensity functions for the unit in FIGURE 9. *Open circles* show the maximum firing rate in response to the stimulus with the long rise time, measured over a 5.12-msec interval. *Solid circles* show the steady-state rate in response to the stimulus with a short rise time.

RAPID ADAPTATION AND INCREASED OPERATING RANGE

The two-stage model just described provides a useful phenomenological description of short-term adaptation and its interaction with sound-intensity level. However, the onset function appears to differ in shape from the input–output function of inner hair cells. This suggests that additional transformations are occurring that are not incorporated in the model. In addition, the onset rate–intensity functions described earlier were measured using time intervals of 10 msec or more in order to emphasize the properties of short-term adaptation. Hence the possibility remained that rapid adaptation produced a change in the shape of the input-output characteristic that was overlooked by the measuring technique. In order to resolve the effects of rapid adaptation, onset firing rates were measured using small time intervals of 2 msec or less. The resulting rate–intensity functions differed systematically from the onset and steady-state functions described above.[19, 20, 22, 23] An example is shown in FIGURE 11, where FIGURE 11A is a steady-state rate–intensity function, and FIGURE 11B is the corresponding onset function measured with a small interval. It can be seen that this onset function, which is called the unadapted function, shows fewer effects of saturation and a larger operating range than does the steady-state function. Hence the unadapted function more closely resembles the input–output function of an inner hair cell than does the onset function measured with a larger time interval.[3, 23] It should also be noted that the unadapted shape resembles the maximum response function plotted in FIGURE 10. However, the latter was obtained using a much longer rise time as well as a larger measuring interval, and presumably is a different effect.[19, 20, 23]

The unadapted characteristic is present at stimulus onset, but its functional significance depends in part on whether it is also available, after adaptation has occurred, to respond to a sufficiently rapid change in intensity. To explore this possibility, responses were obtained for tones that were amplitude-modulated by sinusoids,[22–25] as in FIGURE 1E. Generally, modulation was applied after adaptation had occurred and response modulation was obtained by generating period histograms synchronized to the modulating waveform.[26] Results were typically as shown in the right-hand column of FIGURE 12, which contains two-cycle period histograms. Intensity increases in going from the top to the bottom figure and the amount of response modulation decreases. The decrease qualitatively resembles the corresponding decrease in incremental responses shown by the PST histograms on the left side of the figure. It should be noted that to obtain the particular data in FIGURE 12 the paradigm departed from that of FIGURE 1E. For purposes of illustration a 6-dB increment in intensity was applied simultaneously with the onset of modulation. Hence the PST and period histograms could be determined from the same data.

In general, response modulation is a nonmonotonic function of sound intensity resembling the incremental response function (for example, FIGURE 5B). However, unlike the latter, the response modulation function cannot be predicted from the steady–state rate–intensity function of a unit. The prediction generally has a maximum at too low an intensity and a narrower width than the actual function,[22–25, 27] as can be seen in FIGURE 11C. In contrast, when a prediction is made from the unadapted function, as in FIGURE 11D, a much better fit is obtained. Hence amplitude modulation appears to reflect the unadapted response characteristic and the latter appears to be available

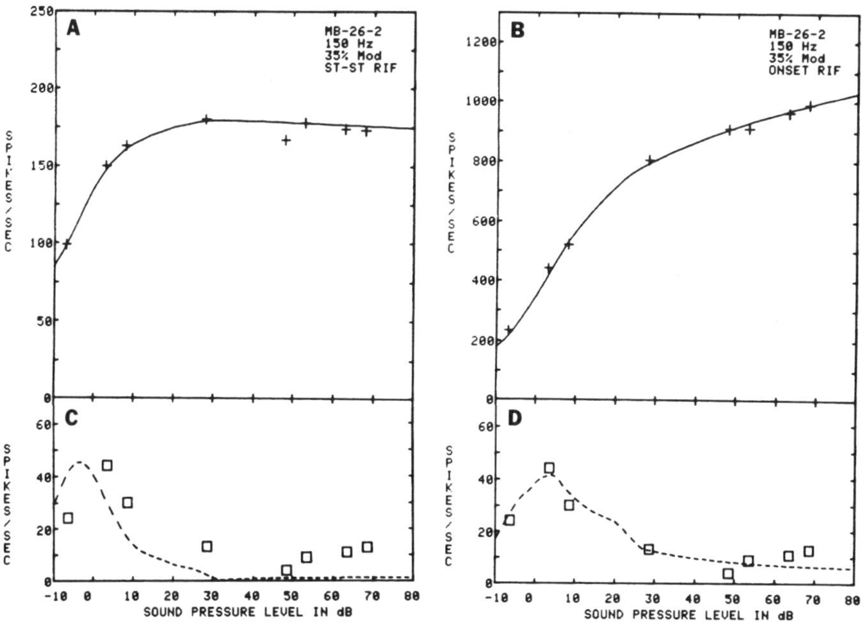

FIGURE 11. Rate–intensity functions and response modulation versus intensity for an auditory nerve fiber. **A:** Steady-state rate–intensity function for a tone burst. **B:** Unadapted rate–intensity function for the responses in **A**. The unadapted rate was the maximum firing rate at response onset, measured with a 0.64-msec time interval. **C:** *Open squares* represent the measured amplitudes of response modulation produced by 35% amplitude modulation with a 150-Hz sinusoid, plotted as a function of the average intensity. *Dashed curve* shows the predicted response modulation (see text) determined from the steady-state rate–intensity function. **D:** As in **C**, except that predictions are from the unadapted rate–intensity function. (From Brachman.[23] Reprinted by permission.)

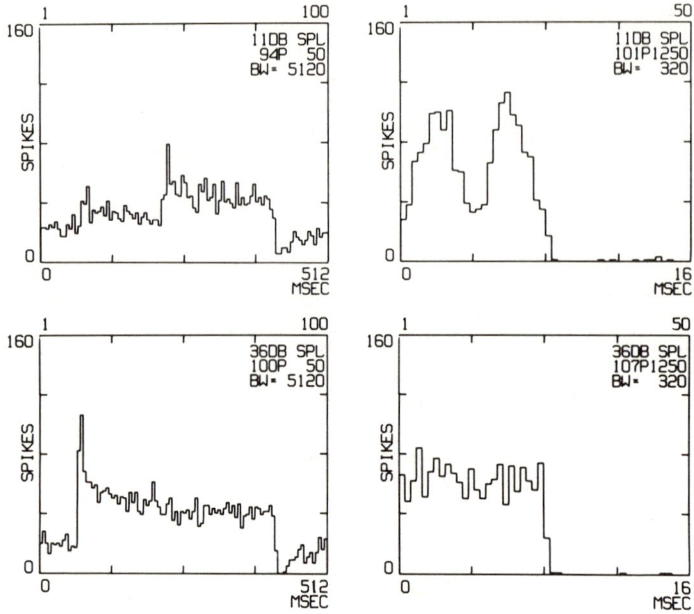

FIGURE 12. Response histograms for an auditory nerve fiber. The stimuli consisted of tone bursts with 6–dB increments in intensity added 150 msec after tone onset. The increments were amplitude-modulated by sinusoids with parameters as in FIGURE 11. The sound-pressure level of the tone increases by 25 dB in going from the *top* to the *bottom* row. The *left column* contains PST histograms synchronized to the onset of the tones, with a bin width of 5.12 msec. The *right column* contains two-cycle period histograms synchronized to the modulating waveform, with a bin width of 0.32 msec.

to respond to sufficiently rapid changes in intensity with an expanded operating range relative to the static function.

As was noted earlier, the shape of the unadapted rate–intensity function bears a suggestive resemblance to the input–output function of the IHC. In particular, both show fewer effects of saturation than does the steady-state rate–intensity function. This suggests that the unadapted function may be a more direct result of the receptor potential of the cell.[3, 23, 28] Rapid adaptation, possibly caused by decreases in synaptic transmission from hair cell to nerve fiber, may then reduce the operating range of the output. Furthermore, although the two-stage model just presented provides a useful description of many response properties, it does not produce the unadapted response or rapid adaptation. A more realistic model would seem to require an input nonlinearity whose shape matches the hair-cell function. This in turn would be modified by adaptation in order to produce the simpler situation. Such a model has been developed and is being tested.[23, 28] It successfully accounts for a large number of properties related to rapid and short-term adaptation, but its description and analysis are beyond the scope of the present paper.

Future Investigation and Some Speculations

On the basis of results reviewed herein it is evident that the properties of short-term adaptation are relatively simple to describe and model. Rapid adaptation introduces additional complexity, but can be described and accounted for. Both processes are bound to affect the responses of auditory nerve fibers to speech signals, with the magnitude of the effects dependent on the rapidity and strength of changes in intensity. Several studies incorporating effects of adaptation on responses to speech have appeared.[2, 21, 29] However, additional quantitative data and modeling seem required and important issues still remain to be resolved. For example, describing adaptation provides little direct insight into its importance in the perception of speech or into the relevant time scales of analysis. It is hoped that additional insights into these issues will result from the discussions and other papers in this symposium.

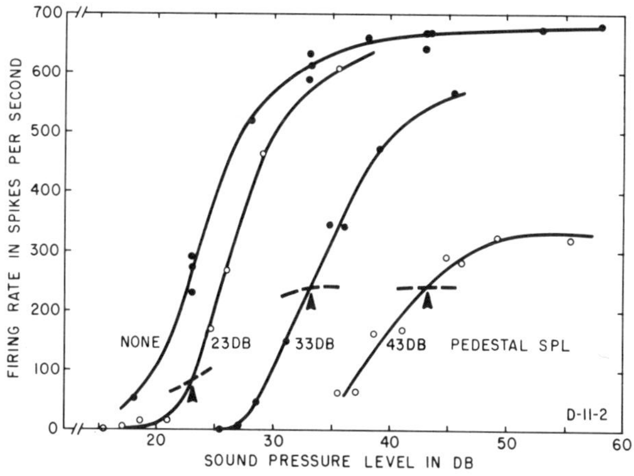

FIGURE 13. Rate–intensity functions for a cochlear-nucleus unit with increments and decrements in intensity applied as described in the text. (From Smith.[14] Reprinted by permission.)

Unresolved questions also concern whether and how adaptation is utilized in more central regions of the auditory nervous system and what time scales are utilized by cells in these regions. Although these issues have not been systematically studied, several results suggest that enhanced effects of adaptation may appear in some cells of the next stage of processing, the cochlear nucleus complex.[14, 26, 30–32] An example, is shown in FIGURE 13, which contains rate–intensity functions from a cell in the cochlear nucleus of a gerbil.[14] In response to tone bursts, the cell exhibited a primary-like PST histogram. The onset rate–intensity function (marked "none") and the steady-state rate–intensity function (dashed lines) increased monotonically and approached saturation within 30 dB of threshold, again similar to the auditory nerve response. However, when increments in intensity were applied after short-term adaptation was complete, substantial incremental responses were obtained in spite of the strong onset and steady-state saturation. In the figure each arrow points to a background or pedestal intensity, and the corresponding solid curve shows the total firing rate produced during the first 10 msec of an increment or decrement in intensity. Corresponding to each solid curve the ordinate gives the total intensity produced by the increment or decrement. Hence it appears that this cell exhibits a shift in its operating range and dynamic characteristic that significantly exceeds the range of dynamic effects observed in single units of the auditory nerve. Important issues for future investigation then involve determining the distribution and strength of these effects, the underlying mechanisms responsible for them, and, again, their importance in the perception of speech. It is possible for example, that an auditory prosthesis with adequate simulation of the adaptation seen in auditory nerve fibers is a prerequisite for enhanced adaptation in higher centers and that the latter is necessary for the meaningful encoding of speech.

One further speculation concerns the functional significance of the changes in operating range that appear to be occurring. The inner hair-cell response seems to have a large operating range but no contrast in time. The operating range is largely preserved in nerve-fiber responses, but only for dynamic stimulus components. Adaptation produces an increased temporal contrast but a smaller steady-state operating range. In higher centers the operating range for dynamic stimuli may be further extended, possibly through the interaction of converging inputs from lower centers, to equal or exceed that of hair cells. However, the operating range is now accompanied by a temporal contrast that was not originally present.

References

1. Adrian, E. D. 1928. The Basis of Sensation. Christophers. London.
2. Delgutte, B. 1980. Representation of speech-like sounds in the discharge patterns of auditory-nerve fibers. J. Acoust. Soc. Am. **68:** 843–857.
3. Goodman, D. A., R. L. Smith & S. C. Chamberlain. 1982. Intracellular and extracellular responses in the organ of Corti of the gerbil. Hearing Res. **7:** 161–179.
4. Goodman, D. A. & R. L. Smith. 1981. Cochlear inner hair cells: Intracellular responses and staining. Abstracts of the Fourth Midwinter Meeting, Association for Research in Otolaryngology: 7.
5. Russell, I. J. & P. J. Sellick. 1978. Intracellular studies of hair cells in the mammalian cochlea. J. Physiol. **284:** 261–290.
6. Kiang, N.Y.-S., T. Watanabe, E. C. Thomas & L. F. Clark. 1965. Discharge Patterns of Single Fibers in the Cat's Auditory Nerve. MIT Research Monograph No. 35, MIT Press. Cambridge, MA.
7. Smith, R. L. & J. J. Zwislocki. 1975. Short-term adaptation and incremental responses in single auditory-nerve fibers. Biol. Cyber. **17:** 169–182.
8. Gerstein, G. L. & N. Y.-S. Kiang. 1960. An approach to quantitative analysis of electrophysiological data from single neurons. Biophys. J. **1:** 15–28.
9. Moore, G. P., D. H. Perkel & J. P. Segundo. 1966. Statistical analysis and functional interpretation of neuronal spike data. Annu. Rev. Physiol. **28:** 493–523.
10. Harris, D. M. & P. J. Dallos. 1979. Forward masking of auditory nerve fiber responses. J. Neurophysiol. **42:** 1083–1107.
11. Yates, G. K. & D. Robertson. 1980. Very rapid adaptation in auditory ganglion cells. *In* Psychophysical, Physiological, and Behavioural Studies in

Hearing. G. van den Brink and F. A. Bilsen, Eds.: 200–205. Delft University Press. The Netherlands.
12. SACHS, M. B. & P. J. ABBAS. 1974. Rate versus level functions for auditory-nerve fibers in the cat: Tone burst stimuli. J. Acoust. Soc. Am. **56:** 1835–1847.
13. SMITH, R. L. 1979. Adaptation, saturation, and physiological masking in single auditory-nerve fibers. J. Acoust. Soc. Am. **65:** 166–178.
14. SMITH, R. L. 1973. Short-term Adaptation and Incremental Responses in Single Auditory-Nerve Fibers. Ph.D. dissertation and Special Report LSC-S-11, Institute for Sensory Research, Syracuse University. Syracuse, NY.
15. SMITH, R. L. 1977. Short-term adaptation in single auditory-nerve fibers: Some poststimulatory effects. J. Neurophysiol. **40:** 1098–1112.
16. SMITH, R. L. 1976. Eighth nerve responses and permanent sensorineural hearing loss. *In* Effects of Noise on Hearing. D. Henderson, R. P. Hamernik, and D. S. Dosanjh, Eds.: 225–244. Raven Press. New York, NY.
17. ABBAS, P. J. 1979. Effects of stimulus frequency on adaptation in auditory-nerve fibers. J. Acoust. Soc. Am. **65:** 162–165.
18. HARRIS, D. M. 1977. Forward Masking and Recovery from Short-Term Adaptation in Single Auditory-Nerve Fibers. Ph.D. dissertation, Northwestern University, Evanston, IL.
19. SMITH, R. L. & M. L. BRACHMAN. 1980. Dynamic response of single auditory-nerve fibers: Some effects of intensity and time. *In* Psychophysical, Physiological, and Behavioural Studies in Hearing.[11]: 312–319.
20. SMITH, R. L. & M. L. BRACHMAN. 1980. Operating range and maximum response of single auditory-nerve fibers. Brain Res. **184:** 499–505.
21. YOUNG, E. D., M. B. SACHS & H. F. VOIGT. 1981. Wider dynamic range during stimulus onset transient: Effects on the representation of steady-state vowels in cat auditory nerve discharge rate profiles. Abstracts of the Fourth Midwinter Meeting, Association for Research in Otolaryngology.: 9.
22. BRACHMAN, M. L. & R. L. SMITH. 1979. Dynamic versus static characteristics of single auditory-nerve fibers. Soc. Neurosci. Abs. **5:** 16.
23. BRACHMAN, M. L. 1980. Dynamic Response Characteristics of Single Auditory-Nerve Fibers. Ph.D. dissertation and Special Report ISR-S-19, Institute for Sensory Research. Syracuse University, Syracuse, NY.
24. SMITH, R. L. & M. L. BRACHMAN. 1977. Response of auditory-nerve fibers to sinusoidal amplitude modulation. J. Acoust. Soc. Am. **65:** S83(A).
25. SMITH, R. L. & M. L. BRACHMAN. 1980. Response modulation of auditory-nerve fibers by AM stimuli: Effects of average intensity. Hearing Res. **2:** 123–133.
26. MØLLER, A. R. 1974. Responses of units in the cochlear nucleus to sinusoidally amplitude-modulated tones. Exp. Neurol. **45:** 104–117.
27. YATES, G. K. 1982. Auditory nerve response to amplitude modulated tones: Modulation frequency effects. Abstracts of the Fifth Midwinter Meeting, Association for Research in Otolaryngology.: 32.
28. SMITH, R. L. & M. L. BRACHMAN. 1982. Adaptation in auditory-nerve fibers: A revised model. Biol. Cyber. **44:** 107–120.
29. KIANG, N.Y.-S., D. K. EDDINGTON & B. DELGUTTE. 1979. Fundamental consideration in designing auditory implants. Acta Otolaryngol. **87:** 204–218.
30. EVANS, E. F. & A. R. PALMER. 1975. Response of units in the cochlear nerve and nucleus of the cat to signals in the presence of bandstop noise. J. Physiol. **252:** 60–62P.
31. SMITH, R. L. & J. J. ZWISLOCKI. 1971. Response of some neurons of the cochlear nucleus to tone-intensity increments. J. Acoust. Soc. Am. **50:** 1520–1525.
32. GIBSON, D. J. & E. D. YOUNG. 1982. Adaptation in the dorsal cochlear nucleus of the cat. Abstracts of the Fifth Midwinter Meeting, Association for Research in Otolaryngology. :30.

SPEECH ENCODING IN THE AUDITORY NERVE: IMPLICATIONS FOR COCHLEAR IMPLANTS[a]

Murray B. Sachs, Eric D. Young, and Michael I. Miller

Department of Biomedical Engineering
The Johns Hopkins University School of Medicine
Baltimore, Maryland 21205

INTRODUCTION

Discussions of stimulus encoding for cochlear prostheses have focused on replacement of peripheral auditory processing by at least a crude simulation of the function of the normal system.[1,2] The ultimate goal of the prosthesis is to provide the central nervous system with information adequate for the perception of speech. An understanding of the normal encoding of speech in the auditory nerve is therefore fundamental to the development of a simulation-type prosthesis or even to the evaluation of the potential for success of such devices. In this paper we shall review some recent studies of speech encoding in the auditory nerve. In particular, we shall consider representations of speech spectra in terms of average discharge rates of fiber responses and in terms of temporal (phase-locked) properties of the discharge patterns. As we will emphasize, we cannot at this point rule out either representation as the one actually used by the normal auditory system. We will, however, discuss the relationship of both average rate and temporal encoding to stimulation strategies for cochlear implants.

ENCODING IN TERMS OF AVERAGE DISCHARGE RATE AND BASILAR MEMBRANE PLACE

One simple notion of the encoding of speech is that peaks in the acoustic spectrum (such as formant peaks) of the speech sound would result in peaks in the discharge rate in the population of auditory nerve fibers at places along the basilar membrane where characteristic frequencies correspond with the formant frequencies. We refer to this as the "rate–place" scheme. An example of how this scheme would work for vowels is shown in FIGURE 1. At the top we show the spectrum of a synthesized steady-state vowel /ɛ/ whose first three formant frequencies are 512, 1792, and 2432 Hz. The center plot shows tuning curves from three auditory nerve fibers in one cat.[b] The characteristic frequencies (CFs) of these fibers are near the formant frequencies of the vowel. Because the vowel has more energy in the vicinity of its CFs,

[a] This work was supported by a grant from the National Institute for Neurological and Communicative Disorders and Stroke. E. D. Young is supported by a Research Career Development Award from the National Institutes of Health, and M. I. Miller is supported by the Whiting School of Engineering and the School of Medicine of the Johns Hopkins University.

[b] Tuning curves from the Eaton-Peabody Laboratory.

0077-8923/83/0405-0094 $01.75/0 © 1983, NYAS

these units should begin to respond to the vowel at lower sound levels than units with CFs between the formants and should respond at higher discharge rates, at least at moderate vowel levels. The bottom plot shows a rate–place profile for a population of auditory nerve fibers recorded in one cat when the /ɛ/ was presented at 38 dB SPL. Discharge rate is normalized in this figure

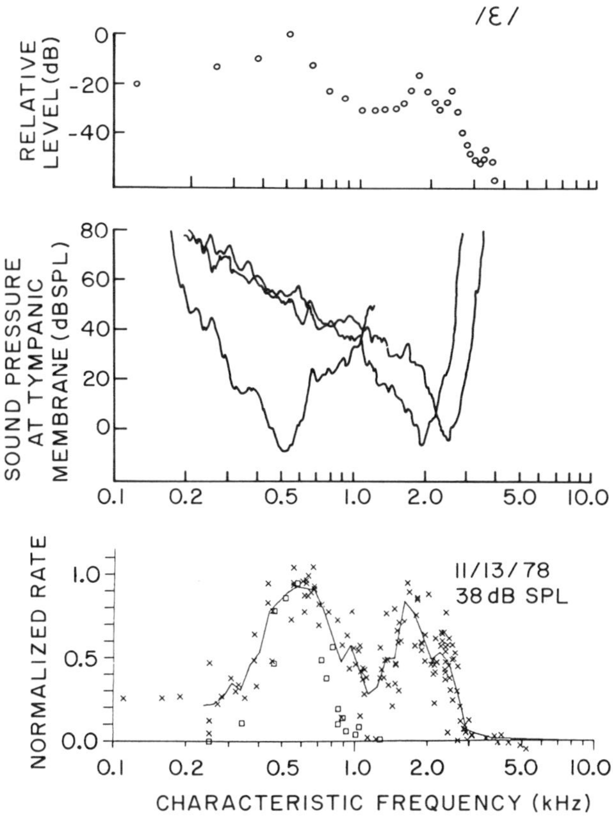

FIGURE 1. (*Top*) amplitude spectrum of /ɛ/. (*Middle*) tuning curves (from Eaton-Peabody Laboratory) from three auditory nerve fibers whose characteristic frequencies are close to the formant frequencies of /ɛ/. (*Bottom*) plot of normalized rate versus characteristic frequency for units studied on 11/13/78 with /ɛ/ at 38 dB SPL as the stimulus. Each point is rate of one unit plotted at the unit's CF. Normalized rate is rate to the vowel minus spontaneous rate (R_s in FIG. 2A and B) divided by saturation rate (R_m in FIG. 2A and B) minus spontaneous rate. Units with spontaneous rate less than 1/sec plotted with squares; other units with Xs. Line is average rate of units with spontaneous rate greater than 1/sec, computed using a sliding triangular window with a base 0.25 octave wide; the centers of adjacent windows were 0.125 octaves apart. (From Sachs and Young.[42] Reprinted by permission.)

so that each fiber's rate increase to the vowel is plotted as a fraction of its maximal rate increase. There is some evidence that auditory nerve fibers with very low spontaneous rates form a separate population;[3, 4] for this reason data from fibers with spontaneous rates less than 1/sec are plotted with open square symbols and data from higher spontaneous units are plotted with Xs. The average curve was computed from the high spontaneous rate population only. In this case, this rate profile shows peaks at CFs corresponding to the first three vowel formants, as required by the rate–place scheme.

As sound level is increased, however, the representation of the stimulus spectrum in terms of such rate profiles degenerates. The principal cause of this degeneration is the limited dynamic range of auditory nerve fibers,[5–7] which is illustrated by the rate versus level functions in FIGURES 2A and 2B. The effect of this saturation on rate profiles as sound level increases is illustrated in FIGURE 2C for the vowel /ϵ/ and in FIGURE 2D for the vowel /a/. For /ϵ/ at about 58 dB SPL the response rate of fibers with CFs near the formants (arrows) saturates and the continued increase of discharge rates of fibers with CFs between the formants causes the rate profiles to flatten out. The behavior of rate profiles of responses to /a/ shown in FIGURE 2D is similar.

Notice that for both vowels shown in FIGURE 2 the rate profiles saturate at values of normalized rate less than 1.0 in the frequency range above the first formant; that is, fibers with CFs in the vicinity of the second and third formants do not reach rates as high as their maximal rate even at high stimulus levels. In the vicinity of the first formant, however, the profiles saturate at normalized rates near 1.0. The behavior of units with CFs above the first formant has been explained as resulting from the phenomenon of two-tone rate suppression.[8, 9]

The loss of formant peaks in rate profiles such as those in FIGURE 2 occurs at sound levels within the conversational range. This could be a serious problem for a theory of vowel perception based on rate and place, since speech intelligibility is stable at levels well beyond those where the formant peaks are lost in rate profiles. Representation of vowels based on average discharge rate cannot be ruled out by the data of FIGURE 2 alone, however, because of a number of uncertainties:

1. Vowels could be discriminated on the basis of the gross shape of their rate profiles, even in the absence of formant peaks. The shape of the rate profiles for different vowels is slightly different even at high levels. In FIGURE 2, for example, the 77-dB profile for responses to /a/ falls off more rapidly at high frequencies than does the 78-dB profile for /ϵ/. The difference in shape for vowels like /ϵ/ and /I/ is relatively small,[8] however, and it is not clear that all the vowel distinctions could be supported by this mechanism. As we have pointed out previously,[8] two-tone suppression is crucial in maintaining these differences in gross shape. It is this apparent suppression that keep fibers with CFs above the first formant from reaching their full saturation rates as stimulus level increases.

2. Auditory nerve fibers of low spontaneous rate have higher thresholds[3] and wider dynamic ranges[10] than do the higher spontaneous rate fibers from which the rate profiles of FIGURE 2 were computed. Thus, formant-related peaks might be observed in rate profiles for this population at levels above those at which the high spontaneous rate population has saturated. Rate profiles for the low spontaneous rate fibers from the same population as those in FIGURE 2C are shown in FIGURE 3. Although the data are sparse, there are clearly formant-

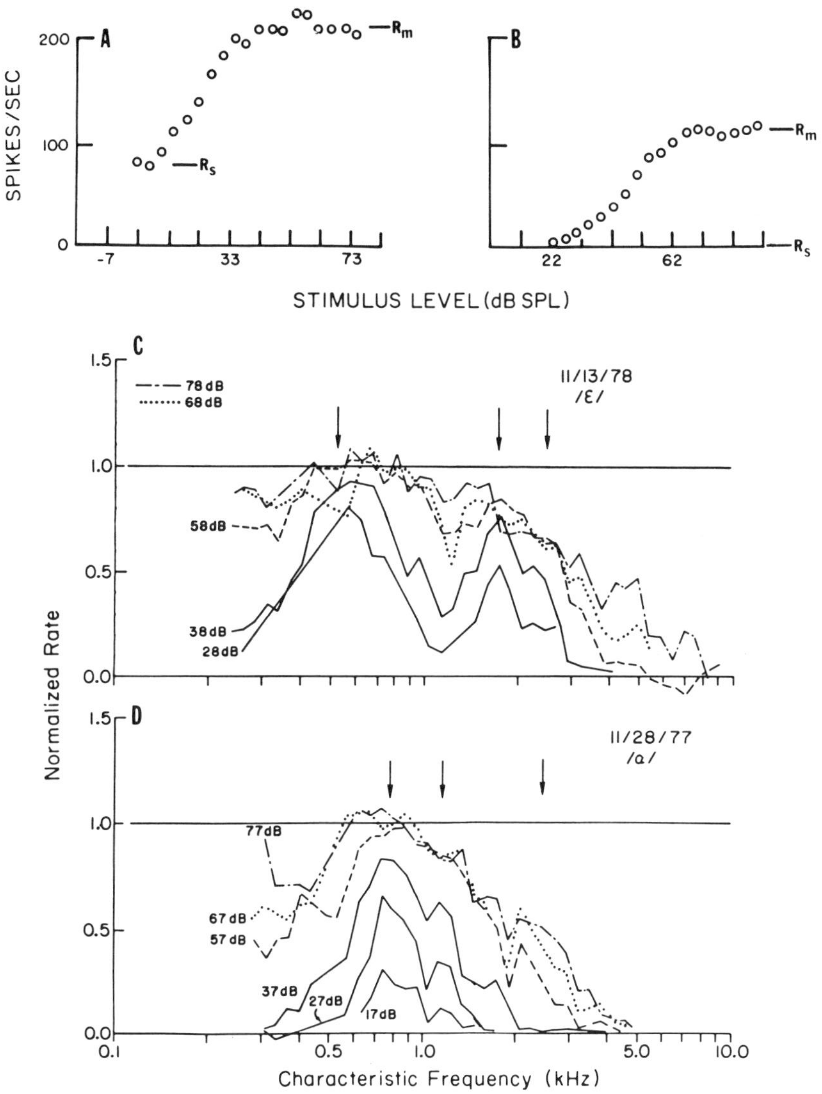

FIGURE 2. (**A** and **B**) discharge rate versus stimulus level for two auditory nerve fibers. (**C** and **D**) average rate profiles for /ɛ/ and /a/, respectively, for several vowel levels. Average curves computed as in FIGURE 1. *Arrows* show formant frequencies. (From Young and Sachs.[15] Reprinted by permission.)

related peaks in these profiles at 78 dB. Low spontaneous rate units show the effects of two-tone suppression more strongly than do high spontaneous rate units [8, 10]; because they are strongly suppressed, the response rate of fibers near the second formant and therefore the second formant peak in the 78-dB rate profile in FIGURE 3 is quite small. It is doubtful that this peak would remain at a 20-dB higher level, where vowels are still easily discriminable.

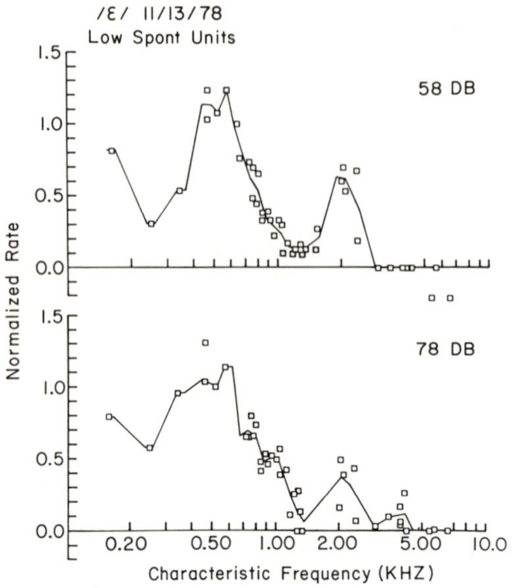

FIGURE 3. Normalized rate versus CF for low spontaneous rate units (less than 1/sec) studied on 11/13/78 with /ɛ/ as stimulus. (From Sachs and Young.[8] Reprinted by permission.)

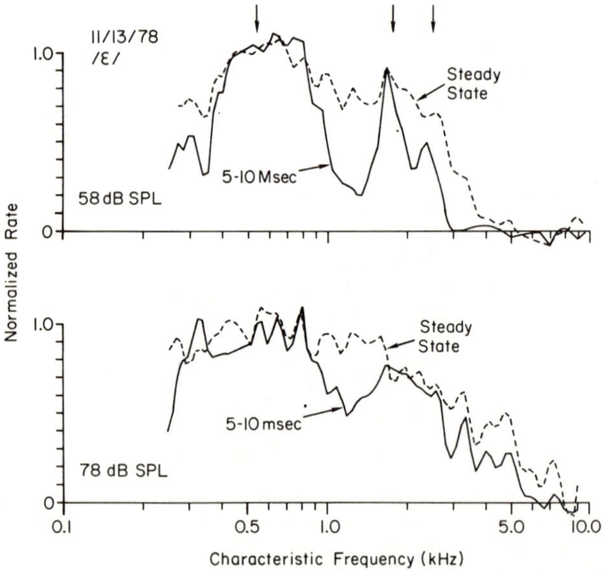

FIGURE 4. Normalized rate versus CF for steady state and onset of /ɛ/ stimulus. Steady-state rates (*dashed lines*) were averaged over last 380 msec of 400-msec stimulus bursts. *Solid curves* show rates averaged over interval from 5 to 10 msec after onset of stimulus burst. Computation of average curves as in FIGURE 1 except that the centers of adjacent windows used to average rates across units were 0.0063 octaves apart in this figure only. *Arrows* show formant frequencies.

3. Effects of the external ear canal resonances [11] and middle ear muscles [12–14] which are not present in our anesthetized preparation have been considered in detail previously.[15] The effects expected appear to be small.

4. The role of the efferent olivocochlear system in encoding at high stimulus levels is unknown. Electrical stimulation of the crossed olivocochlear bundle (COCB) leads to a rightward shift along the abscissa of rate versus level functions for CF tones. This shift corresponds roughly to an attenuation of the acoustic signal and cannot amount to more than 20 dB.[16] These shifts have the effect of moving the dynamic part of the rate function to higher stimulus levels and could preserve formant peaks in rate profiles at higher levels than those shown in FIGURE 2. The efferent system is unlikely to be active in an anesthetized preparation like ours.

5. The rate profiles shown in FIGURE 1 were computed over the last 380 msec of a 400-msec stimulus burst. That is, they represent "steady-state" discharge rates. Smith and his associates [17] have shown that the dynamic range of auditory nerve fiber rate response is considerably larger when rate is measured over short (5 msec) intervals near stimulus onset than when measured over longer intervals. They have suggested that this increased dynamic range could be important in representing speech stimuli; obviously, it could increase the range of stimulus levels over which a rate–place profile could represent the formant structure of a vowel. We have carried out rate analyses using only those spikes occurring in the interval from 5 to 10 msec after stimulus onset. FIGURE 4 shows examples of this analysis for the vowel /ϵ/ from the same data shown in FIGURE 2. The curves marked steady-state are the same as the ones shown in FIGURE 2; they show rate computed over the last 380 msec of 400-msec stimulus bursts. At 58 dB SPL there is a broad peak at the first formant and a small peak in the region of the second and third formants; there are no formant-related peaks at 78 dB. The profiles for rate during the 5–10-msec interval (solid lines) do show formant-related peaks even at 78 dB SPL, and at 58 dB the peaks are better differentiated than those in the steady-state profiles. Thus, the range over which rate profiles show formant-related peaks is greater if we limit rate computation to the onset of the stimulus.

We have extended our investigations of the role of low spontaneous rate fibers and extended dynamic range at stimulus onset in a series of experiments in which vowels were presented in background noise. FIGURE 5 shows an example in which the vowel /ϵ/ was presented at a level of 88 dB SPL in background noise at a signal-to-noise ratio of +9 dB.[c] At this signal-to-noise ratio vowels are easily discriminated from one another; [18] for /ϵ/ second formant frequency shifts of about 100 Hz can be discriminated by untrained human observers.[19] In FIGURE 5 we have plotted rate change versus CF for a population of fibers from one cat. Rate change is the difference between total rate to the vowel plus noise and total rate during the 400-msec interval before each vowel presentation (that is, when the background noise was on alone). The first three formant frequencies are indicated by arrows in both sets of plots. For both steady-state and onset profiles, rate increases were observed for fibers with CFs less than about 0.7 kHz. For higher CFs, rate actually decreased when the vowel was turned on in the presence of noise; that is, at

[c] Signal-to-noise ratio is defined as the ratio (dB) of signal energy to noise power in the frequency band from 0 to 3000 Hz.

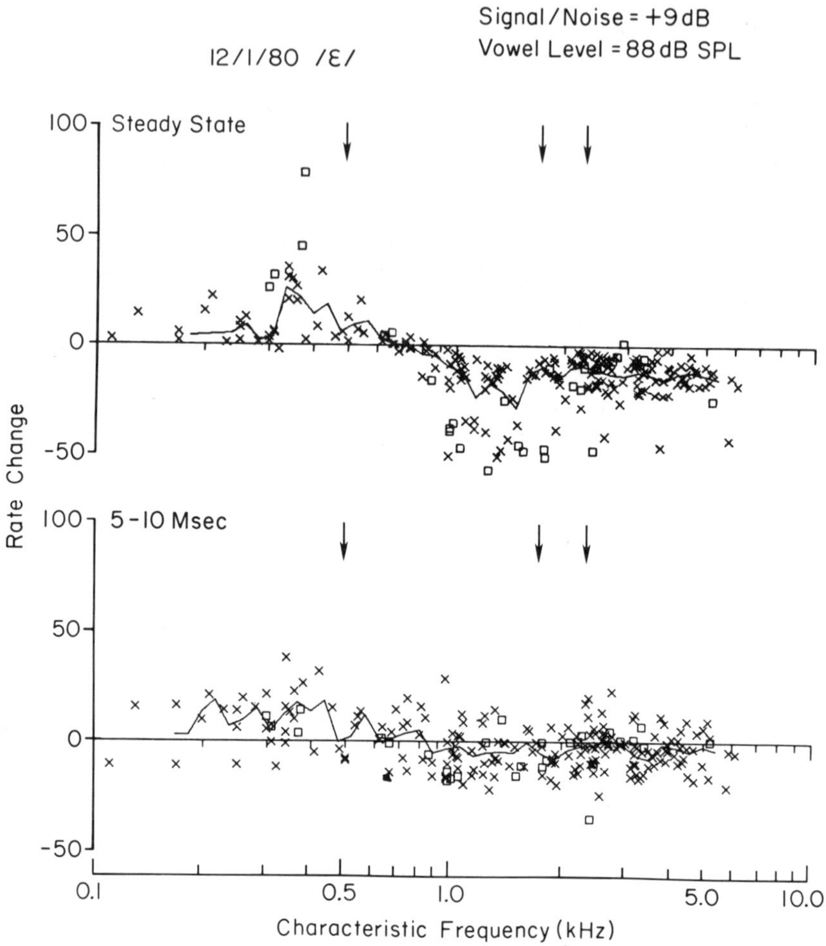

FIGURE 5. Rate change versus CF for units studied on 12/1/80 with /ɛ/ as stimulus in background noise at a signal-to-noise ratio (ratio of signal power to noise power in the frequency band from 0 to 3000 Hz) of +9 dB. Rate change is rate to the stimulus in noise minus rate to the noise alone. *Top* shows steady-state rates; *bottom* shows rates measured from 5 to 10 msec after stimulus onset. *Arrows* show formant frequencies.

these CFs responses to noise were apparently suppressed by the addition of the vowel stimulus. There is, however, little obvious structure related to the second formant frequency. Yet as stated earlier, a second formant frequency shift of about 100 Hz can be discriminated in this signal and noise situation. The lack of any clear second formant structure here is seen in both steady-state and onset profiles. Notice, furthermore, that the low spontaneous rate fibers (square symbols) show greater suppression of their noise-evoked rate than the average of the rates of the high spontaneous rate fibers (solid line). The general behavior of the sparse population of low spontaneous rate fibers makes it unlikely that they would encode second formant frequency in this situation. When interpreting these noise results, however, we must carefully consider the role that the efferent system might play. Dewson[18] has shown that monkeys whose efferent pathway has been cut do not discriminate noise-masked vowels as well as do intact monkeys. It is possible that the efferents could operate to preserve rate profiles in background noise.

Encoding in Terms of Temporal Properties and Basilar Membrane Place

An alternative to rate–place profiles for the representation of the spectral features of speech can be found in the temporal patterns of responses of auditory nerve fibers. We shall see that this representation is stable with changes in stimulus level and in the presence of background noise. For single tones or multicomponent stimuli, there is considerable information about the spectral content of the stimulus in the "phase-locked" structure of auditory nerve discharge patterns.[20] The instantaneous rate (or probability of discharge) of auditory nerve fibers responding to stimuli with frequencies below about 6 kHz is modulated by a rectified version of the stimulus waveform, as modified by cochlear filtering and nonlinearities.[20–22] Thus if an auditory nerve fiber is responding to a 1-kHz tone, there will be alternate 0.5-msec periods of increased and decreased probability of discharge which will be phase-locked to the stimulus; as a consequence, the fiber will tend to discharge at intervals of about 1 msec and multiples of 1 msec (since the fiber will not fire on every cycle of the stimulus). This temporal response can be analyzed by several means: *post-stimulus time (PST) histograms,* which estimate discharge probability or instantaneous rate as a function of time over some interval after stimulus onset; *period histograms,* which estimate probability of discharge as a function of time through one cycle of a periodic stimulus and can be thought of as PST histograms folded at the period of the stimulus; and *interspike interval histograms.* FIGURE 6 shows examples of period and interval histograms of three fibers in response to a steady–state vowel. This vowel is a perfectly periodic /a/ with fundamental frequency equal to 128 Hz. One period of the /a/ is shown at the top of column A. The six prominent peaks in the waveform reflect the fact that the first formant dominates the temporal pattern because it has considerably more energy than any other components. Because the stimulus is periodic it contains energy only at the harmonics of its fundamental frequency (128 Hz). In this case, the first formant is at 768 Hz, which is equal to the sixth harmonic of the fundamental vowel frequency; hence there are six cycles of the first formant in one period of the vowel. The second formant is at 1152 Hz (ninth harmonic of the fundamental); the third formant is at 2432 (nineteenth harmonic). Column A shows period histograms of responses to /a/ of the three fibers; the abscissa of these histograms is one fundamental period of the vowel. Column B shows the amplitude spectrum of the discrete Fourier transform of the period histograms. Column C shows interval histograms constructed from the same data as the corresponding period histograms. Column D shows the amplitude spectrum of the discrete Fourier transform of the interval histogram next to it. Because the stimulus has energy only at harmonics of its 128-Hz fundamental, we have labeled the abscissas of the Fourier transforms in

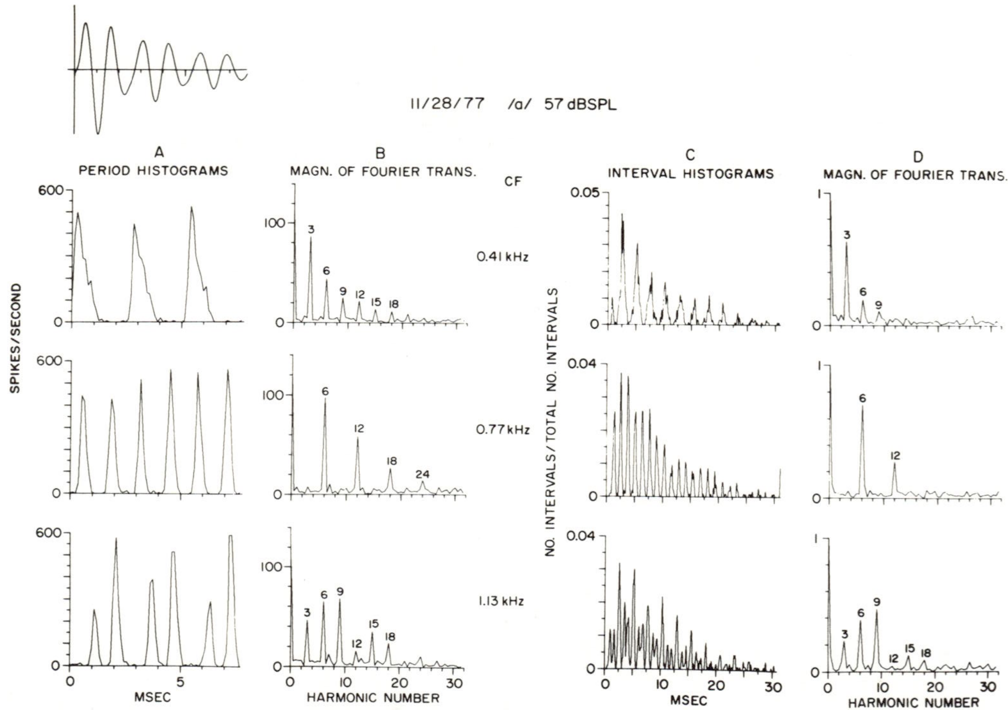

FIGURE 6. Period histograms (**A**), magnitude of Fourier transforms of period histograms (**B**), interval histograms (**C**), and magnitude of Fourier transform of interval histograms (**D**) for single fibers studied on 11/28/77 using /a/ as the stimulus. CFs of units are shown between **B** and **C**. The period histograms show estimates of instantaneous discharge rate as a function of time through one cycle of the vowel; they were computed with 64 bins per cycle. One pitch period of the vowel is shown at the top of column **A** with the same time scale as the period histograms. Interval histograms are estimates of the probability of various intervals in a long record of responses. The ordinate gives the number of intervals in a 122-μsec bin divided by the total number of spikes in the record. The maximal interval plotted is 31.25 msec. The height of the bin farthest to the right gives the relative number of intervals longer than 31.25 msec. (From Sachs and Young.[42] Reprinted by permission.)

this plot as harmonic number. The data in FIGURE 6 illustrate some of the most commonly observed patterns of response to vowels; they also serve to illustrate our method of analysis of the temporal patterns of these responses.

The top two units in FIGURE 6 are cases in which one frequency component dominates the response. The top unit responded to the vowel with three phases of increased discharge rate of approximately equal amplitude, indicating that the unit responded principally to the third harmonic of the vowel. The frequency of the third harmonic (384 Hz) is near this unit's CF. Similarly, the second unit has a CF near the sixth harmonic (first formant) of the vowel and its response is dominated by the sixth harmonic. Responses so dominated by one component are most often seen in units whose CFs are near a formant frequency. The Fourier transforms of these two period histograms (Column B) have a large component at the frequency of the dominant harmonic. Notice that they also have significant energy at integer multiples of the dominant harmonic, most likely a result of "rectifier distortion." [23] The third histogram in FIGURE 6 illustrates a case in which more than one stimulus component contributes significantly to the response. The Fourier transform shows almost equal components at the ninth and sixth harmonics. Some of the remaining significant components (the third, twelfth, fifteenth, and eighteenth harmonics) can be interpreted as rectifier distortion products arising from the responses to the sixth and ninth harmonic stimulus components. The spectra of the transforms of the interval histograms are quite similar to those of the period histograms. In particular, the same components dominate both transforms, and other components, either stimulus-related or rectifier distortion, are present. The close relation between the spectral composition of the period and interval histograms has been considered theoretically.[24] Fourier transforms of PST histograms for vowels also show structure similar to those for period and interval histograms.[25]

The magnitudes of the components in the Fourier transforms of period, interval or PST histograms provide a good measure of the temporal response strength of auditory nerve fibers to the corresponding frequency components of the stimulus. Adequate account must be taken of rectifier distortion products and combination tones. FIGURE 7 shows how the responses at three harmonics of the stimulus were distributed in a population of auditory nerve fibers for the vowel /ɛ/. The temporal responses were computed from the same data as the rate profiles in FIGURE 2C. The spectrum of /ɛ/ is shown in FIGURE 1A. Its first formant is the fourth harmonic of the fundamental frequency (512 Hz) and its second formant is the fourteenth harmonic (1792 Hz). Each column in FIGURE 7 shows the distribution of temporal response to one of three harmonics, the fourth (first formant) in the left column, the tenth in the center column, and the fourteenth (second formant) in the right column. Each row shows the responses to the three harmonics at one of three different sound levels (38, 58 or 78 dB SPL, indicated at right). The plots in FIGURE 7 were constructed in the same fashion as the rate profile in FIGURE 1C; there is one point for each unit which shows the amplitude of the fourth, tenth, or fourteenth harmonic in the Fourier transform of the unit's period histogram (the ordinate is normalized by dividing by the average discharge rate [23]) plotted against the unit's CF (abscissa). The arrow in each graph points to the CF, which is equal to the frequency of the harmonic plotted in that graph; this will be referred to later as the "place" of that harmonic.

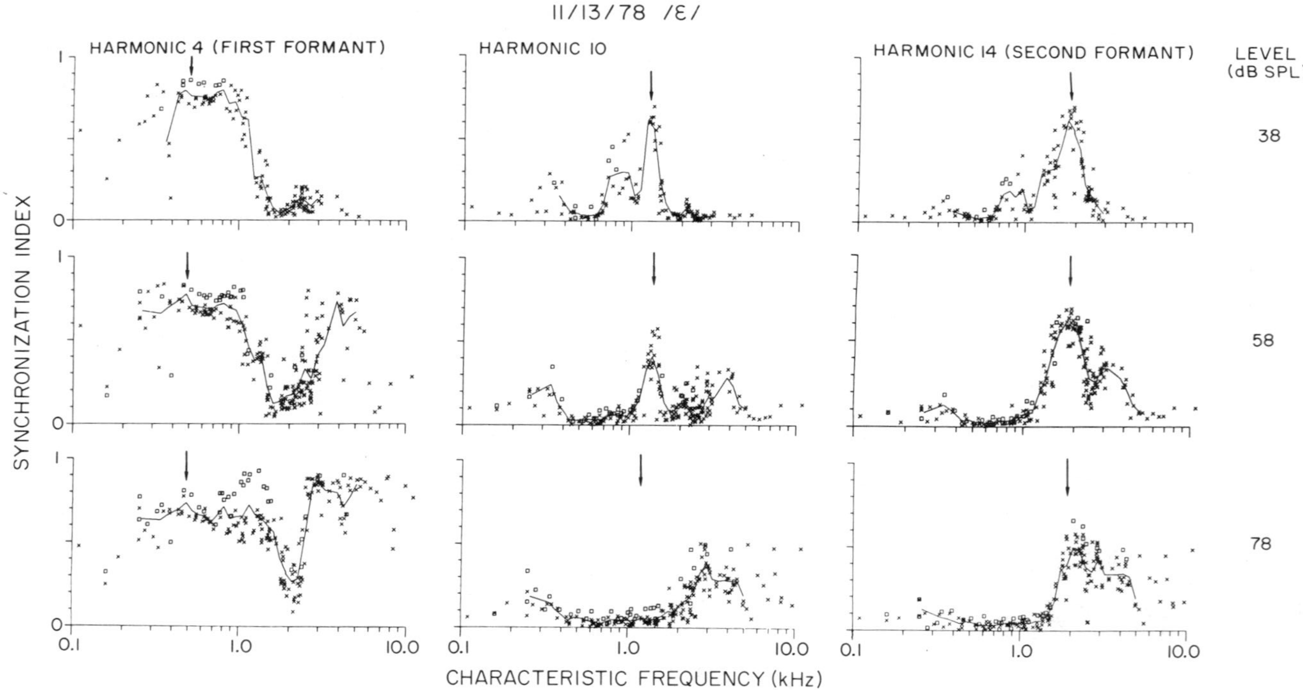

FIGURE 7. Distribution of synchronization as a function of CF for units studied on 11/13/78 with /ɛ/ as the stimulus. Each plot shows distribution of synchronization to one harmonic of the /ɛ/. The calculations are based on period histograms with 64 bins. Synchronization is the amplitude of the harmonic in a unit's period histogram, divided by average discharge rate. Distributions are shown for the fourth, tenth and fourteenth harmonics at 38, 58, and 78 db SPL. *Arrows* point to the CF, which is equal to the frequency of the harmonic (that is, place of the harmonic). Each point is derived from response of one unit. Symbols and lines are as in FIGURE 1.

The temporal response distributions in FIGURE 7 have been chosen to illustrate the behavior of responses to all stimulus harmonics. At the lowest stimulus level (38 dB, top row) the response to each harmonic is maximum in the vicinity of its place; that is, the largest amount of response to each harmonic is found among fibers whose CFs are approximately equal to the frequency of the harmonic. The strongest responses are seen at the formant frequencies, in this case the fourth and fourteenth harmonics; the first formant response is particularly strong and widespread. As stimulus level is increased, the response to the first formant spreads over a wide range of CFs; at 78 dB, almost the entire population of fibers is responding to the first formant. Response to the second formant near its place stays roughly constant from 38 to 58 dB, although some changes in its distribution occur. At 78 dB, the response to the second formant is reduced slightly near its place, but significant response to this harmonic remains.

In contrast to the behavior of the formant harmonics, the response to the tenth harmonic near its place decreases monotonically as sound level is increased until at 78 dB there is no sign of the peak that was observed at 38 dB. Instead, units with CFs near the tenth harmonic's place are responding to the fourth harmonic, the first formant. This behavior is similar to the behavior of two-tone synchrony suppression, which has been previously described in detail.[21, 22, 24, 27–29] The behavior observed for the tenth harmonic in FIGURE 7 is typical of nonformant harmonics in our data. Although there is no response to the tenth harmonic near its place at 78 dB, there is significant response to this harmonic at CFs between about 2.5 and 5.0 kHz. Notice that this is the frequency region in which units are responding strongly to both the fourth and fourteenth harmonics and the distribution of the tenth harmonic has roughly the same shape as the distribution of the fourteenth harmonic. As we have discussed in detail previously, this is the behavior expected of a rectifier distortion product.[23]

The fact that the formant harmonics dominate the patterns of temporal response of auditory nerve fibers suggests that a good idea of the spectrum of a vowel stimulus could be gained by comparing the amount of temporal response at various harmonics of the stimulus. Examination of the top line in FIGURE 7 suggests that it is appropriate to look for response to each harmonic in a restricted region centered around that harmonic's place in the population, because when a response occurs to a particular harmonic, it will be maximal at this place. Using a restricted region centered on a harmonic's place has the added advantage that it discriminates against responses that are rectifier distortion products.[23] The average temporal contours shown in FIGURE 8 were motivated by these considerations. The points in FIGURE 8 show the average value of temporal response in distributions like those of FIGURE 7 (except not normalized, but expressed as discharge rate) for each harmonic (ignore the lines for now); the average was computed only over fibers whose CFs were within 0.5 octave of the frequency of the harmonic. Thus these curves show the average temporal response to each harmonic among fibers with CFs within 0.5 octave of the harmonic's place. For convenience we will refer to these temporal response contours as ALSR (average localized synchronized rate) curves. The points at the first three formant frequencies harmonics (fourth, fourteenth, and nineteenth) have been plotted with solid circles. Notice that the ALSR is always largest at the first formant. At

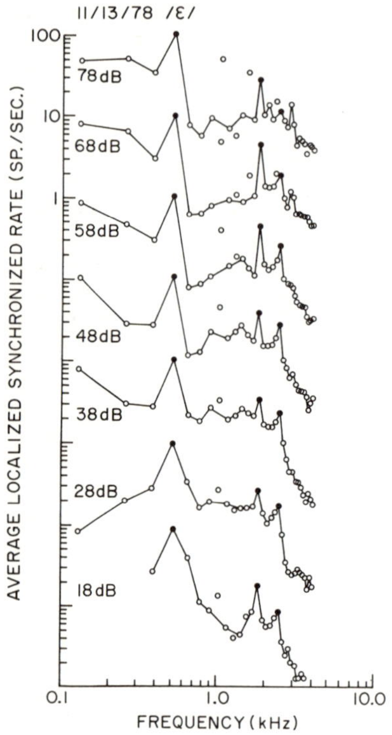

FIGURE 8. The points show the average localized synchronized rate averaged over all fibers within 0.5 octave of each harmonic for the /ɛ/ at all levels used in experiment on 11/13/78. There is one point for each harmonic up to the thirty-second. Points corresponding to formant frequencies are plotted with *solid circles.* Ordinate is scaled logarithmically. Plots are shifted vertically from one another by one order of magnitude for clarity. Ordinate scale refers to 78-dB data only. Maximal response in each plot is about 100 spikes/sec. The lines are drawn through all points except those corresponding to the second and third harmonics and the sum and difference tones of the first two formants. See rules given in text. (From Young and Sachs.[23] Reprinted by permission.)

lower sound levels the profile of the ALSR is a good reflection of the spectrum of the /ɛ/ (FIGURE 1A), with local maxima at the first three formant frequencies. The only serious deviation is the slightly elevated response at the second harmonic of the first formant (harmonic 8). At higher levels the first and second formants continue to stand out; the salience of the third formant is reduced, as response to it is suppressed. Responses to the second and third harmonics of the first formant (eighth and twelfth harmonics) grow considerably at higher levels until they are larger than the second formant response at the highest level. Except for these two distortions products related to the first formant, however, all response components between the first and second formants are suppressed at higher levels.

The lines drawn through some of the points in FIGURE 8 are meant to show the extent to which the ALSR resembles the stimulus spectrum if presumed distortion components are ignored. The lines are drawn through all the points, except those at the second and third harmonics of the first two formants and the first sum and difference tone of the first two formants.[23] The similarity of these plots to the spectrum of the stimulus (FIGURE 1C) is clear. Notice particularly that changes in stimulus level over a 50–60 dB range do not greatly alter the qualitative aspects of these plots; they continue to reflect the first two formants of the stimulus. This stability is in marked contrast to the behavior of response profiles based on discharge rate alone (FIGURES 2C and 2D) where saturation and suppression limit the representation of the formants at higher levels.

The importance of two-tone synchrony suppression in the ALSR plots of FIGURE 8 is shown in FIGURE 9. Average localized synchronized rates (with distortion products removed) have been reproduced from FIGURE 8 for the 38-, 58-, and 78-dB SPL cases. The average response to the first formant stays approximately constant as level increases. The response to the second formant is somewhat suppressed at the highest level. However, responses to harmonics between the first and second formants are also suppressed and it is the suppression of these harmonics that allows the maintenance of a local maximum of response at the second formant frequency.

The temporal response profiles (ALSR) shown in FIGURES 8 and 9 were derived from period histograms for perfectly periodic stimuli. It is natural to question whether a temporal representation can be used to encode the spectrum of an aperiodic speech signal. We have previously shown that the spectra of synthetic whispered vowels, produced by exciting a model of the vocal tract with noise, are well represented by such a temporal place mechanism.[30] Such stimuli are totally aperiodic. In the case of these aperiodic stimuli, temporal response profiles were generated from Fourier transforms of interval histograms rather than period histograms.

FIGURE 10 shows that a temporal place mechanism can also represent the time-varying spectra of stop consonants. The left column of FIGURE 10 shows the spectra of 20-msec segments of the syllables /da/ (top) and /ba/ (bottom). These segments occurred 20 msec after stimulus onset, during the formant transition of the stop consonant. The arrows indicate the instantaneous formant positions. The second and third formants for /ba/ are lower than those of /da/ at this time during the transition, reflecting the rising second and third formants of /ba/ and falling second and third formants of /da/. The right column shows the corresponding ALSR plots for a population of 277 auditory nerve fibers. These ALSRs were derived from PST histograms computed over the same 20-msec interval of the stimulus as the spectra at left. The instantaneous spectral differences between /ba/ and /da/ are clearly reflected in these ALSR plots. Indeed, we have shown pre-

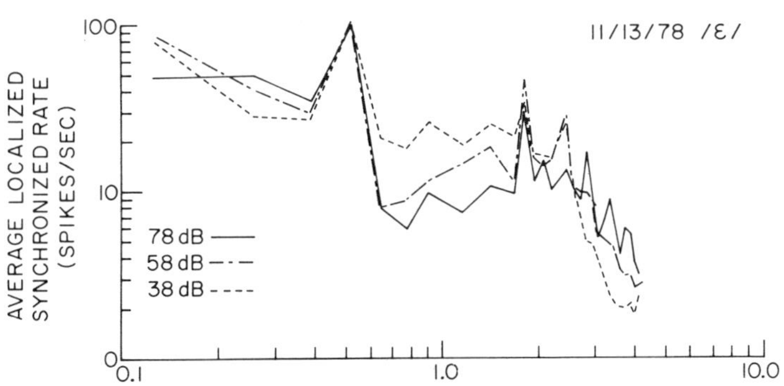

FIGURE 9. Average localized synchronized rate profiles, with distortion points eliminated, for /ɛ/ at 38, 58, and 78 dB (taken from FIG. 8). Plots are superimposed for comparison.

viously[25] that such a temporal–place representation can closely follow the spectral changes in a stop consonant throughout the duration of the formant transitions.

Finally, we have recently shown that a temporal–place representation does not suffer the same degradation with noise background as does the rate–place profile.[19] At all noise levels where second formant discriminations can be made there is a clear representation of the second formant in the ALSR.

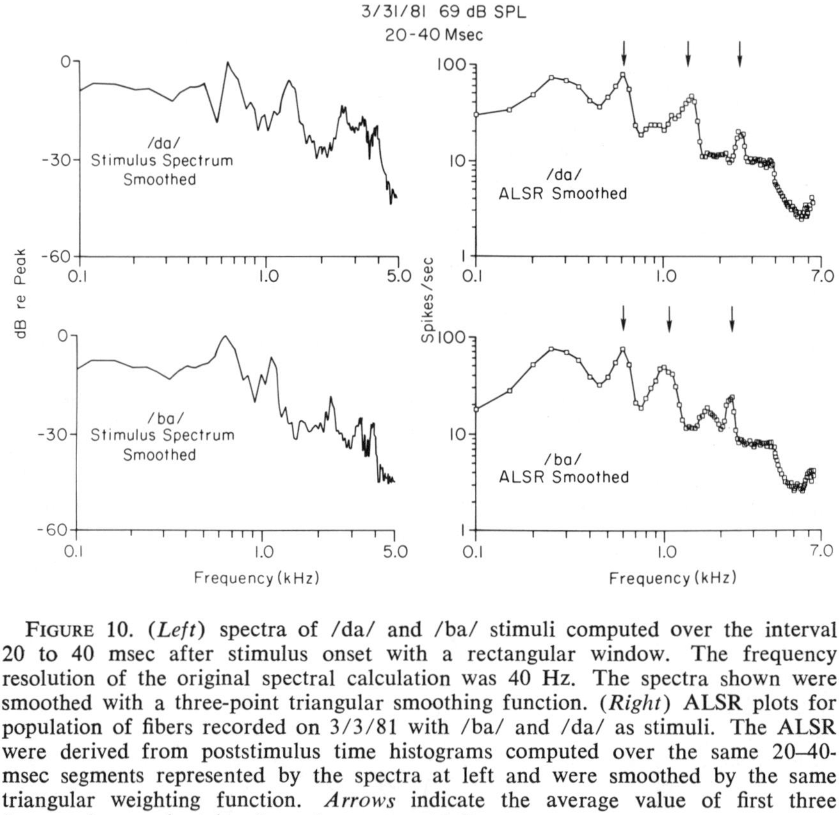

FIGURE 10. (*Left*) spectra of /da/ and /ba/ stimuli computed over the interval 20 to 40 msec after stimulus onset with a rectangular window. The frequency resolution of the original spectral calculation was 40 Hz. The spectra shown were smoothed with a three-point triangular smoothing function. (*Right*) ALSR plots for population of fibers recorded on 3/3/81 with /ba/ and /da/ as stimuli. The ALSR were derived from poststimulus time histograms computed over the same 20–40-msec segments represented by the spectra at left and were smoothed by the same triangular weighting function. *Arrows* indicate the average value of first three formant frequencies taken from the spectra at left.

IMPLICATIONS OF NORMAL CODING FOR COCHLEAR IMPLANT CODING

We have discussed two representations for speech in the normal discharge patterns of auditory nerve fibers. It is important to emphasize here that both of these representations reflect place in the population of auditory nerve fibers (that is, basilar membrane place or equivalently, characteristic frequency). The profiles in FIGURES 1–5 plot average rate versus place (characteristic frequency). In the ALSR plots of FIGURES 8–10, response to a given component is given by the responses phase-locked to that component averaged only over those fibers with CFs (that is, place) appropriate to that component. Thus, any cochlear implant coding scheme which is designed as even a crude simulation of these two normal representations must preserve some basilar membrane place information. That is, simulation of the normal patterns in terms of either average rate or temporal response requires a multichannel device. We shall return to this point when we discuss the temporal code in more detail below.

The rate–place representation is quite unstable as signal level changes, either for vowels presented in silence or in background noise (FIGS. 2 and 5). As vowel level increases, formant-related peaks disappear, largely because of rate saturation effects, which limit the dynamic ranges of the auditory nerve fibers. In noise backgrounds, the noise itself causes the population of fibers to saturate.

The problem of limited dynamic range is even more severe for electrical stimulation. For example, Kiang and Moxon [31] have shown that a sinusoidal current stimulus at a level of less than 4 dB above threshold can produce a discharge rate greater than the saturation rate of a fiber to acoustic stimuli. More indirect evidence of limited dynamic range comes from studies of brainstem potentials evoked by electrical stimulation of the cochlea. These potentials can saturate at current levels less than 10 dB above threshold for bipolar stimulation.[32] Psychophysical studies in subjects with implants indicate that the range of current levels between threshold and stimuli that are uncomfortably loud is between 4 and 30 dB.[33] This narrow dynamic range seems to make some sort of dynamic range adjustment (that is, an automatic gain control) an essential feature of the ultimate auditory prosthesis.

The sound level of normal speech varies in a number of ways, all of which must be accounted for by an implant encoding scheme if the implant is to operate within its dynamic range. Normal speech is easily perceived over a range of overall sound levels of at least threshold to 100 dB SPL,[34] and the overall level changes with speaker, range, and environment. Such slow changes in the overall level of speech might be compensated for by a variety of automatic gain control schemes.[35] More rapid changes in level occur during the course of normal speech even though overall average level remains constant. Consonant portions of syllables are much less intense than vowel portions. The vowel to consonant ratio can be greater than +20 dB.[36] Thus, without some dynamic compression scheme, it is likely that either the consonants would be below implant threshold or the vowels would fall into the saturation range of the responses to electrical stimulation. It is possible that such long-term changes in overall speech level or short-term consonant-to-vowel changes can be handled by a single channel compression system.

It may not be necessary to maintain the formant-related peaks in a rate–place profile for a speech stimulus. As pointed out earlier, vowels could be discriminated on the basis of the gross shape of the rate-place profile and it could be that an array of a relatively small number of electrodes could be used to represent this gross spectral shape. However, the differences between gross shapes of profiles illustrated in FIGURE 2 are maintained by two-tone suppression, which counteracts the fibers' limited dynamic range by preventing fibers with CFs above the first formant from attaining their full saturation rates. In order to maintain discriminable differences in gross shapes of profiles in the face of much smaller electrical stimulation dynamic range, some form of interchannel two-tone suppression would have to be employed in the implant encoding scheme.

The temporal–place representation of speech does not suffer the same instabilities with stimulus level or background noise as does the place–rate representation. A temporal–place code does, however, pose some serious questions in terms of the development of a cochlear prosthesis. For example, in order for a temporal code to represent a 1.5-kHz stimulus component (that is, a component in the range of second formant frequencies), auditory nerve fibers must be phase-locked to this component. Furthermore, the central nervous system must be able to extract frequency information from the phase-locked spike trains. Under acoustic stimulation the auditory nerve fibers discharge at rates generally less than 300 spikes per second in the steady state [3, 6] and thus do not fire a spike in every cycle of a 1.5-kHz stimulus. This is essential since synaptic transmission is rarely maintained at rates above 200/sec. Thus, if the central nervous system uses phase-locked activity in extracting stimulus spectrum information, it must sum the activity over a number of fibers. Because spike trains of different auditory nerve fibers appear to be statistically independent of one another,[37] a central neuron could operate on a "summed" input process which has one or more spikes per stimulus cycle without any of its synapses operating at rates in excess of 2–300 per second.

Let us consider the implications of these ideas for implant coding. Consider the encoding of a second formant frequency in the temporal patterns of electrically stimulated auditory nerve fibers. Moxon [31] has shown that there is phase-locked information in the electrically driven firing patterns of auditory nerve fibers from which the central nervous system might be able to extract frequency information. There are, however, important differences between these electrically driven patterns and the normal acoustically evoked patterns. First, the spike rates are considerably higher for the electrically driven activity than for acoustic driving. Thus, because of the very limited dynamic range for electrical stimulation, it is likely that a sinusoidal electric stimulus at 1.5 kHz applied above threshold will drive auditory nerve fibers at rates far above those normally encountered. Second, the period histograms of individual fibers exhibit narrower peaks for electrical stimulation than for acoustic stimulation and sometimes show multiple peaks not present for acoustic stimulation. This difference may result from the fact that at the high rates elicited by electrical stimulation, the refractory properties of the neurons determine the temporal distributions of spikes, whereas at the lower rates for natural stimulation the properties of hair-cell transduction and synaptic transmission dominate. Third, the relative phase of responses across fibers of different CFs does not, for single electrode stimulation, match the wide spread of phase for acoustic stimulation. Finally, and this is a matter of speculation, it is not clear whether different auditory nerve fibers are independent under electrical stimulation.

Thus, in the presence of sinusoidal electrical stimulation the synapses in the cochlear nucleus which must relay or process phase-locked information from the auditory nerve are likely to be presented with highly unnatural inputs. These inputs will be coming at rates which are too high and with temporal distributions different from those seen for acoustic stimulation. It is also possible that central neurons will not be receiving the independent inputs they might need in order to effectively sum inputs. In light of these constraints, it is not entirely surprising that subjects with implants do not make pitch discriminations for tonal electrical stimulation at frequencies above 400–500 Hz.[38–40] It may be very relevant in this context that Merzenich *et al.*,[40] in experiments with electrical stimulation of cat cochlea, found "phase-locking" in the inferior colliculus at frequencies below about 700 Hz but not above.

This discussion points up two issues that need to be addressed before serious thought can be given to an implant based on temporal coding of spectral information. First, it is important to determine what is the upper bound on auditory nerve spike rates at which cells in the cochlear nuclei are capable of processing their inputs from the periphery. Put another way, we need to know how response properties of cochlear nucleus cells are affected by the abnormally high rates elicited by electrical stimulation of the cochlea. Second, the possibility of generating more-normal temporal patterns in the auditory nerve with electrical stimulation should be pursued. A simple auditory nerve fiber model whose output is a simulated spike train could be used to drive each electrode. Such a model could generate normal temporal patterns (that is, normal rates and statistical properties). It is unlikely, however, that it would produce independent discharge patterns in different fibers.

Our discussion thus far has attempted to relate our results to coding in multichannel implants. We will close with a brief, perhaps obvious, comment about single-channel electrodes. FIGURE 6 shows that the temporal waveform of a vowel (or any stimulus for that matter) is dominated by the frequency component with the largest energy. FIGURE 7 shows that, except in the vicinity of the other formants, the first formant dominates the response of the population of auditory nerve fibers. It is only the nonlinear, place-dependent filtering of the cochlea that preserves any responses to these higher components. Without this filtering we would presumably see only responses to the dominant component throughout the population. A single-channel system cannot reproduce this filtering and one would thus expect that such a system could provide information relevant only to the dominant spectral component (formant) and to the fundamental frequency of speech.

REFERENCES

1. KIANG, N. Y. S., D. K. EDDINGTON & B. DELGUTTE. 1979. Fundamental considerations in designing auditory implants. Acta Otolaryngol. **87:** 204–218.
2. MERZENICH, M. M. & M. WHITE. 1980. Coding considerations in design of cochlear prostheses. Ann. Otol. Rhinol. Laryngol. **89:** 84–87.
3. LIBERMAN, M. C. 1978. Auditory-nerve response from cats raised in a low-noise chamber. J. Acoust. Soc. Am. **63:** 442–455.
4. KIM, D. O. & C. E. MOLNAR. 1979. A population study of cochlear nerve fibers: Comparison of spatial distributions of average-rate and phase-locking measures of responses to single tones. J. Neurophysiol. **42:** 16–30.
5. KIANG, N. Y. S., T. WATANABE, E. C. THOMAS & L. F. CLARK. 1965. Discharge Patterns of Single Fibers in the Cat's Auditory Nerve. MIT Press. Cambridge, MA.
6. SACHS, M. B. & P. J. ABBAS. 1974. Rate versus level functions for auditory-nerve fibers in cats: Tone-burst stimuli. J. Acoust. Soc. Am. **56:** 1835–1847.

7. Evans, E. F. 1978. Place and time coding of frequency in the peripheral auditory system: Some physiological pros and cons. Audiology **17:** 369–420.
8. Sachs, M. B. & E. D. Young. 1979. Encoding of steady-state vowels in the auditory nerve: Representation in terms of discharge rate. J. Acoust. Soc. Am. **66:** 470–479.
9. Sachs, M. B. & N. Y. S. Kiang. 1968. Two-tone inhibition in auditory-nerve fibers. J. Acoust. Soc. Am. **43:** 1120–1128.
10. Schalk, T. B. & M. B. Sachs. 1979. Nonlinearities in auditory-nerve fiber responses to bandlimited noise. J. Acoust. Soc. Am. **67:** 903–913.
11. Wiener, F. M. & D. A. Ross. 1946. The pressure distribution in the auditory canal in a progressive sound field. J. Acoust. Soc. Am. **18:** 401–408.
12. Wever, E. G. & J. A. Vernon. 1955. The effects of the tympanic muscle reflexes upon sound. Acta Otolaryngol. **45:** 433–439.
13. Borg, E. 1978. A quantitative study of the effect of the acoustic reflex on sound transmission through the middle ear of man. Acta Otolaryngol **66:** 461–472.
14. Borg, E. & J. Zakrisson. 1973. Stapedius reflex and speech features. J. Acoust. Soc. Am. **54:** 525–527.
15. Young, E. D. & M. B. Sachs. 1981. Processing of speech in the peripheral auditory system. *In* The Cognitive Representation of Speech. T. Myers, J. Laver, and J. Anderson, Eds. North Holland Publishing Co. Amsterdam.
16. Wiederhold, M. L. 1970. Variations in the effects of electric stimulation of the crossed olivocochlear bundle on cat single auditory-nerve fiber responses to tone bursts. J. Acoust. Soc. Am. **48:** 966–977.
17. Smith, R. L. & M. L. Brachman. 1980. Dynamic responses of single auditory-nerve fibres: Some effects of intensity and time. *In* Psychophysical, Physiological and Behavioral Studies in Hearing. G. van den Brink and F. A. Bilsen, Eds. Delft University Press. Delft, the Netherlands.
18. Dewson, J. H. 1968. Efferent oliovocochlear bundle: Some relationships to stimulus discrimination in noise. J. Neurophysiol. **31:** 122–130.
19. Sachs, M. B., H. F. Voigt & E. D. Young. 1982. Representation of vowel spectra in the auditory nerve in the presence of masking noise. In preparation.
20. Rose, J. E., J. F. Brugge, D. J. Anderson & J. E. Hind. 1967. Phase-locked response to low frequency tones in single auditory nerve fibers of the squirrel monkey. J. Neurophysiol. **30:** 769–793.
21. Hind, J. E., D. J. Anderson, J. F. Brugge & J. E. Rose. 1967. Coding of information pertaining to paired low-frequency tones in single auditory-nerve fibers of the squirrel monkey. J. Neurophysiol. **30:** 794–816.
22. Brugge, J. F., D. J. Anderson, J. E. Hind & J. E. Rose. 1969. Time structure of discharges in single auditory-nerve fibers of the squirrel monkey in response to complex periodic sounds. J. Neurophysiol. **32:** 386–401.
23. Young, E. D. & M. B. Sachs. 1979. Representation of steady-state vowels in the temporal aspects of the discharge patterns of populations of auditory-nerve fibers. J. Acoust. Soc. Am. **66:** 1381–1403.
24. Johnson, D. H. 1974. The Response of Single Auditory-Nerve Fibers in the Cat to Single Tones: Synchrony and Average Discharge Rate. Thesis, Massachusetts Institute of Technology, Cambridge, MA.
25. Miller, M. I. & M. B. Sachs. 1981. Temporal representation of CV syllables in populations of auditory-nerve fibers, J. Acoust. Soc. Am. **70:** S9.
26. Rose, J. E., L. M. Kitzes, M. M. Gibson & J. E. Hind. 1974. Observations on phase-sensitive neurons of anteroventral cochlear nucleus of the cat: Nonlinearity of cochlear output. J. Neurophysiol. **37:** 218–253.
27. Arthur, R. M. 1976. Harmonic analysis of two-tone discharge patterns in cochlear nerve fibers. Biol. Cybernetics **22:** 21–31.
28. Kim, D. O., J. H. Siegal & C. E. Molnar. 1978. Cochlear nonlinear effects in two-tone responses. Scand. Audiol. (Suppl. **9**): 63–82.

29. Reale, R. A. & C. D. Geisler. 1980. Auditory-nerve fiber encoding of two-tone approximations to steady-state vowels. J. Acoust. Soc. Am. **67:** 891–902.
30. Voigt, H. F., M. B. Sachs & E. D. Young. 1982. Representation of whispered vowels in discharge patterns of auditory-nerve fibers. Hearing Res. **8:** in press.
31. Kiang, N. Y. S. & E. C. Moxon. 1972. Physiological considerations in the artificial stimulation of the inner ear. Ann. Otol. Rhinol. Laryngol. **81:** 714–730.
32. Merzenich, M. M. & M. White. 1977. Cochlear implant—the interface problem. *In* Functional Electrical Stimulation. F. T. Hambrecht & J. B. Reswick, Eds.: 321–340. Marcel Dekker. New York, NY.
33. Eddington, D. K., W. H. Dobelle, D. E. Brackmann, M. G. Mladejovsky & J. L. Parkin. 1978. Auditory prostheses research with multiple channel intracochlear stimulation in man. Ann. Otol. Rhinol. Laryngol. **87** (Suppl. 53): 1–39.
34. Pollack, I. & J. M. Pickett. 1958. Masking of speech by noise at high sound levels. J. Acoust. Soc. Am. **30:** 127–130.
35. Braida, L. D., N. I. Durlach, R. P. Lippmann, B. L. Hicks, W. M. Rabinowitz & C. M. Reed. 1979. Hearing Aids—A Review of Past Research on Linear Amplification, Amplitude Compression and Frequency Lowering. ASHA Monographs No. 19. American Speech, Language, Hearing Association. Rockville, MD.
36. House, A., C. Williams, M. Hecker & K. Kryter. 1965. Articulation testing methods: Consonantal differentiation with a closed response set. J. Acoust. Soc. Am. **37:** 158–166.
37. Johnson, D. H. & N. Y. S. Kiang. 1976. Analysis of discharges recorded simultaneously from pairs of auditory nerve fibers. Biophys. J. **16:** 719–734.
38. Eddington, D. K. 1980. Speech discrimination in deaf subjects with cochlear implants. J. Acoust. Soc. Am. **68:** 885–891.
39. Simmons, F. B., R. L. White, M. G. Walker & R. G. Mathews. 1981. Pitch correlates of direct auditory nerve stimulation. Ann. Otol. Rhinol. Laryngol. **90** (Suppl. 82): 15–18.
40. Merzenich, M. M., R. P. Michelson, R. C. Petit, R. A. Schindler & M. Reid. 1973. Neural encoding of sound sensation evoked by electrical stimulation of the acoustic nerve. Ann. Otol. Rhinol. Laryngol. **82:** 486–503.
41. Moxon, E. C. 1971. Neural and Mechanical Responses to Electrical Stimulation of the Cat's Inner Ear. Doctoral dissertation, Massachusetts Institute of Technology, Cambridge, MA.
42. Sachs, M. B. & E. D. Young. 1980. Effects of nonlinearities on speech encoding in the auditory nerve. J. Acoust. Soc. Am. **68:** 858–875.

THE IMPACT OF AUDITORY NERVE EXPERIMENTS ON COCHLEAR IMPLANT DESIGN [a]

N. Y. S. Kiang,[b] E. M. Keithley,[c] and M. C. Liberman [d]

[b] *Department of Electrical Engineering and Computer Sciences and*
[b, c] *Research Laboratory of Electronics*
Massachusetts Institute of Technology
Cambridge, Massachusetts 02139

[b, d] *Department of Physiology*
Harvard Medical School
Boston, Massachusetts 02115

[b] *Neurology Service*
Massachusetts General Hospital
Boston, Massachusetts 02114

[b, c, d] *Eaton-Peabody Laboratory of Auditory Physiology*
Massachusetts Eye and Ear Infirmary
Boston, Massachusetts 02114

As data accumulate on cochlear-implant patients, it seems difficult to deny that the goal of having profoundly deaf people understand free-running speech has still not been reached. In recent years, knowledge of how speech stimuli are encoded in the auditory nerve has advanced significantly. Thus, it may be useful to examine what is known, what is still unknown, and what can be implemented.

Functional Organization of the Auditory Nerve

First, we shall summarize the present view of the functional organization of the mammalian auditory nerve. The afferent components of the auditory nerve are the central processes of spiral ganglion cells.[e] The ganglion cells are of two types. Bipolar type I cells have myelinated peripheral processes that end on inner hair cells and thick (>3 μm) myelinated central processes that end on cochlear nucleus neurons. The type II cells have unmyelinated peripheral processes that end on outer hair cells.[1, 2] Little is known about the central processes of the type II neurons except that they are thin (<0.5 μm), apparently unmyelinated, and enter the cochlear nucleus.

Since there are approximately twenty times as many type I cells as type II cells, the bulk of the auditory nerve is made up of the central axons of

[a] This work was supported by Grants 1 RO1 NS 18339, 5 PO1 NS 13126, and 1 T32 NS 07047 from the U.S. Public Health Service.

[b] Address for correspondence: N.Y.S. Kiang, Eaton-Peabody Laboratory of Auditory Physiology, 243 Charles Street, Boston, Massachusetts 02114.

[e] In addition to the afferent neurons, which take a fairly direct course through the nerve trunk, there are also fine fibers that wander about in the nerve, seemingly associated with blood vessels. The latter are assumed to be autonomic in origin, but have never been traced to their cell bodies.

0077–8923/83/0405–0114 $01.75/0 © 1983, NYAS

neurons innervating inner hair cells. In the cat, where careful counts have been made, each inner hair cell receives approximately 20 endings, presumably all from type I cells.[1, 3] Thus, there is roughly one type II neuron per inner hair cell. These observations suggest a modular organization of afferent neurons as depicted in FIGURE 1. The number of such modules is obviously the number of inner hair cells: approximately 2500 in cats and 3500 in humans (in both cases there are about 100 inner hair cells per millimeter of cochlear length).[f] The functional significance of such a modular organization will depend upon how the central projections are distributed in the cochlear nucleus, but the orderly arrangement of modules along the cochlear spiral is undoubtedly the basis for tonotopic organization at higher levels of the system.

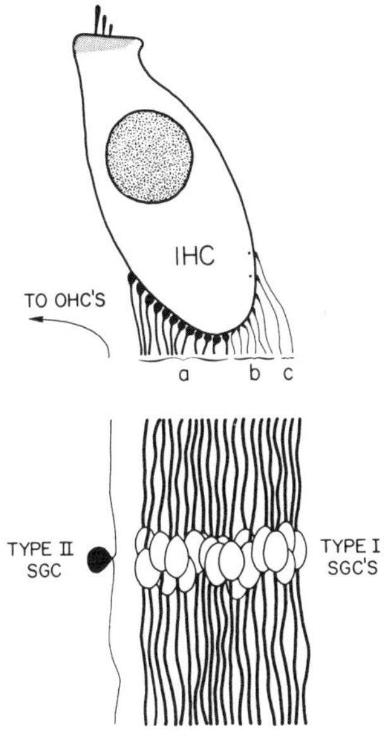

FIGURE 1. Stylized representation of afferent components in the auditory nerve based on studies on cats. IHC = inner hair cells; OHC = outer hair cells; and SGC = spiral ganglion cells. The three types of unmyelinated terminals (labeled a, b, and c) represent the high, medium, and low spontaneous-rate units (respectively) as described in the text.

The present view of the afferent innervation is further complicated by the finding[4] that three types of single units are distinguishable in the nerve on the basis of spontaneous-discharge rate and thresholds to tones (FIG. 2). Recently, intracellular marking techniques have been used to demonstrate that all three types of units correspond to type I neurons and innervate only inner hair cells.[5] Neurons with high spontaneous-discharge rates have low thresholds for acoustic stimuli and give rise to large, mitochondrion-rich endings on inner hair cells. Neurons with medium or low spontaneous-discharge rates have intermediate or high thresholds, respectively, and give rise to small, mitochondrion-poor endings also on inner hair cells. The neurons with the lowest spontaneous-

[f] Both the ratio of type I to type II ganglion cells and the ratio of type I cells to inner hair cells may differ for different species. For example, there are fewer type I ganglion cells per inner hair cell in humans than in cats.

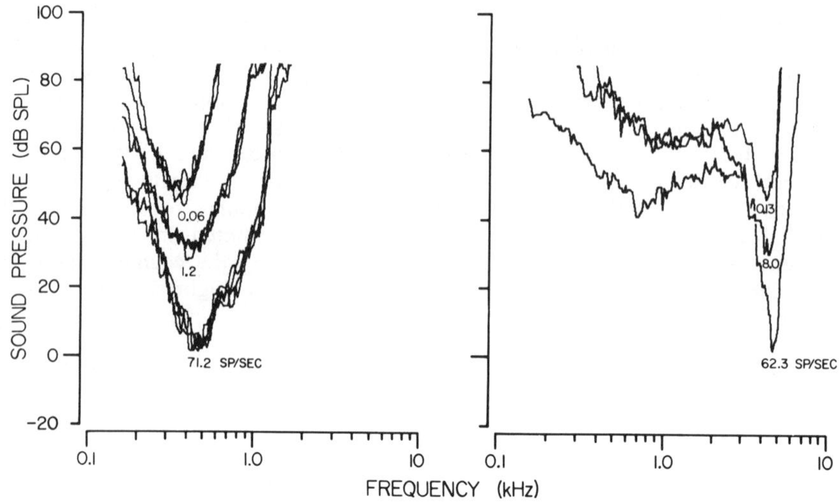

FIGURE 2. Tuning curves from six auditory nerve fibers, each from a different animal. (*Left*) tuning curves from three low-frequency units. Several tuning curves from each unit are shown to indicate reproducibility of the curves. The number under each set of curves gives the spontaneous-discharge rate of the fiber (in spikes per second). (*Right*) tuning curves from three fibers of higher characteristic frequency, again with the spontaneous-discharge rates indicated. All six fibers were injected with horseradish peroxidase during recording. After appropriate processing, the labeled fibers were traced to their terminations under inner hair cells.

discharge rates may be associated with specialized synaptic structures at the hair cell and may be contacted by especially large numbers of efferent fibers in the region underneath the inner hair cells.[3, 6] At present, the only demonstrated morphologic differences among type I neurons are in the unmyelinated segments within the organ of Corti. Differences in the morphology of the myelinated peripheral processes, cell bodies, or central projections have yet to be established.

Little, if anything, is known about the activity of the thin unmyelinated fibers innervating the outer hair cells. In recent experiments, we have detected long-latency responses to electric shocks delivered at the cochlea (FIG. 3). These extracellularly recorded responses are of very small amplitude and appear to be "all-or-none." When sound is presented, the background electric noise in the recordings increases. Thus, it has been impossible to determine how acoustic stimuli affect the responses. It may be relevant for cochlear prosthesis work that the thresholds for these long-latency responses to 0.1-msec electric shocks are always much higher than those for short-latency responses (FIG. 4). Preliminary data suggest that there are no systematic differences in thresholds to shocks for the different classes of short-latency units. If the long-latency responses are indeed the action potentials of the thin central axons of type II spiral ganglion cells, then under some circumstances, electrical stimulation in the cochlea could activate only the myelinated fibers innervating inner hair cells. It may be that most cochlear-implant patients adjust the gain controls so that only the type I neurons would be stimulated, since the range from threshold to discomfort for electrical stimulation is narrow.[7]

Speech-Coding Experiments on the Auditory Nerve

Thus far, all of the data on single-unit responses to speech sounds are consistent with results obtained using simpler sounds.[8] Descriptive properties (such as adaptation, synchrony, saturation, and nonlinear interactive effects of multiple stimuli) that were derived from work with clicks, tones, and noise are also useful in characterizing responses to speech. Although a formalized quantitative theory for simple stimuli has not yet been constructed to account for all of the known data from the nerve, such a theory might also prove adequate to account for responses to speech. A tenable hypothesis at present is that by knowing the tuning curve (which would characterize both the frequency selectivity and the absolute threshold), one could predict the responses to all acoustic stimuli, including speech, because all other response properties are related to the tuning curve.

Most descriptions of speech coding in the auditory nerve have concentrated on single units that have relatively low thresholds and intermediate or high spontaneous activity. There is a practical difficulty in finding sufficient numbers of units with high thresholds and low spontaneous activity, since they constitute only 10% of the recordable units, even when electric shocks are used as search stimuli.[4] When there have been attempts to address the issue of how low spontaneous-discharge rate units respond to complex stimuli, the samples obtained have been small.[9]

There is an increasingly detailed body of data for responses of the high and medium spontaneous-discharge rate units to various speech sounds.[10–13] The synthetic stimuli alone now include vowels,[14, 15] voiceless fricatives,

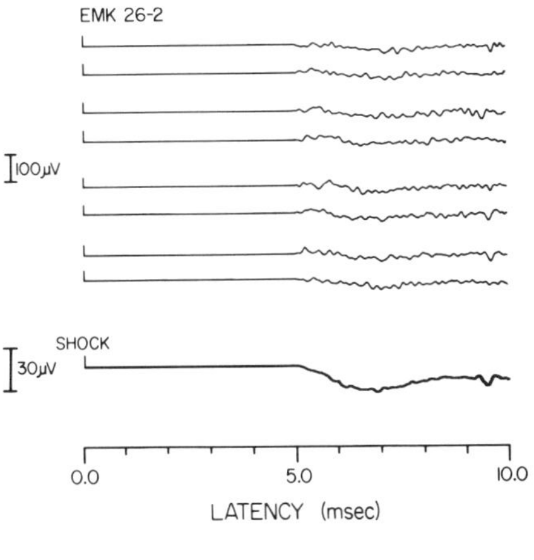

Figure 3. One long-latency unit response to electric shocks recorded from the auditory nerve in the internal auditory meatus. Eight successive traces are shown at the top, each trace starting with the delivery of a shock. The lowest trace (at a higher amplification) shows an average of 16 consecutive traces. Shocks were generated by delivering 10/sec, 1.0-mA pulses of 0.1-msec duration to a platinum wire in the scala tympani of the basal turn with a return electrode inserted into a hole drilled in the apical part of the cochlear capsule. The first 5 msec of each trace are blanked to remove the large stimulus artifact and gross potentials. Upward deflections in the traces represent negativity at the platinum-plated indium recording electrode relative to the headholder.

dynamically changing sounds,[16, 17] whispered vowels,[9] and vowels in noise.[16, 18] The results of these studies suggest that, even if one considers only the most sensitive units, there may be sufficient cues to discriminate speech sounds that are psychophysically distinguishable. In most cases multiple cues are available.

Under some conditions, such as high-intensity speech, high background noise level, or chopped speech, the usual multiplicity of cues may be reduced. Consider, for example, the problem posed by the saturation in average discharge rates of single fibers as steady-state vowel stimuli reach high levels.[14, 15] The available evidence on anesthetized animals indicates that,

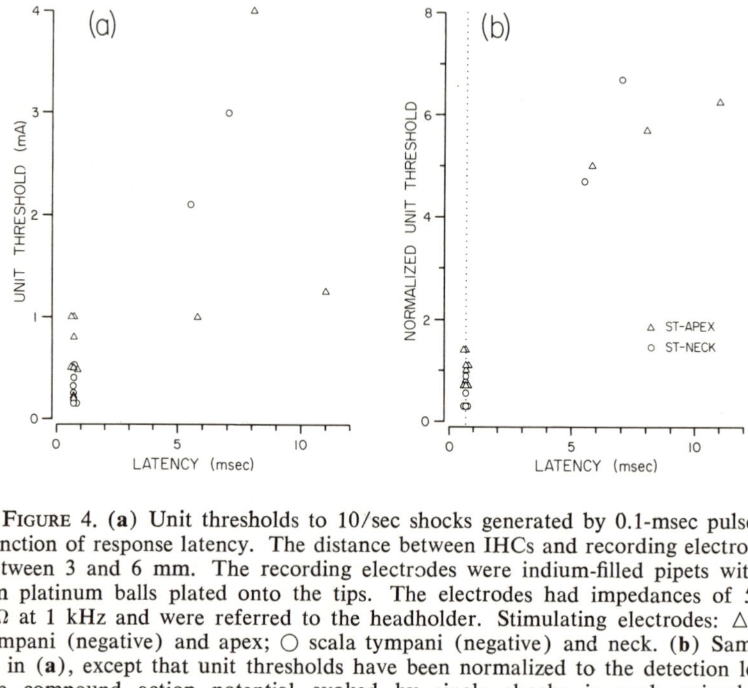

FIGURE 4. (**a**) Unit thresholds to 10/sec shocks generated by 0.1-msec pulses as a function of response latency. The distance between IHCs and recording electrode was between 3 and 6 mm. The recording electrodes were indium-filled pipets with 5–8-μm platinum balls plated onto the tips. The electrodes had impedances of 50–150 KΩ at 1 kHz and were referred to the headholder. Stimulating electrodes: △, scala tympani (negative) and apex; ○ scala tympani (negative) and neck. (**b**) Same data as in (**a**), except that unit thresholds have been normalized to the detection level of the compound action potential evoked by single shocks in each animal. This potential is recorded with a gross electrode in the internal auditory meatus (referred to headholder). Its latency (*dotted line*) is constant across animals and is virtually identical to that seen for the single units with short-latency responses to shocks.

even allowing for the presence of high-threshold units, the average rate cues should become less effective at high intensities, simply because most fibers are firing maximally to many of the vowel stimuli. There are, however, other cues that remain distinctive for different vowels even at high intensities, for example, the synchrony of activity to selected frequency components of the stimuli. In unanesthetized animals the possible effects of efferent activity (either via activation of the olivocochlear bundle or contraction of the middle-ear muscles) must also be considered. Although the role of those active processes in normal speech perception is unclear, all the known effects seem to be suppression of activity or a decrease in sensitivity. Middle-ear muscle activity may serve to keep acoustic signals within some maximally effective intensity range. Similarly, individual olivocochlear fibers may act as gain controls for small local regions in the cochlea. (The heavy efferent innervation of the small terminal segments under inner hair cells [6] may be important in this context.) Whether the spatial patterning of such efferent activity will prove to be significant in processing speech sounds remains to be seen. However, there are suggestions that the apparatus for such subtle effects is present, since there is topographic specificity in the cochlear projections of efferent fibers from brainstem nuclei.[19]

Relation of Auditory Nerve Data to Cochlear Implants

It is obvious that there is no immediate hope of generating a completely normal pattern of activity in the nerve by electrical stimulation. For example, the activity of the unmyelinated fiber system can hardly be imitated if it remains unknown. Moreover, there is no practical way to stimulate type I neurons so that the three classes will be activated differently. Thus, at present, one can provide only a crude and distorted version of the richly detailed information in normal auditory nerve activity.

The main issue in implant design is how to provide cues that can be used easily by the central processor. Given the great flexibility of the central nervous system, one could conceivably argue that as long as the information is present in some form, the central processor might learn to use whatever cues exist. For example, single-channel implants have been of some use even when the coding schemes are decidedly unnatural.[20, 21] However, there are some costs attached to the use of inappropriate codes. If the central processor has to work very hard to make discriminations, it will take longer and be more susceptible to mistakes under adverse conditions. This may be why some subjects can perform well on word discrimination or even recognition tasks given sufficient time or repeated presentations but fail to decipher speech at normal conversational rates. The erratic performance of even the best subjects [22] suggests that high levels of concentration are required to decode the signals. The best results are apparently achieved when the postlingual hearing losses develop slowly. Presumably, this situation provides a long period of adjustment to stimuli that are being degraded gradually. Indeed, the cues available to many profoundly deaf patients might be very similar to those obtainable with certain single-channel devices.

Given these considerations, it makes sense to code the information in the most natural way possible, so that the central processor will not be unnecessarily taxed. In head-to-head comparison testing, multiple-channel stimulation gives better results than single-channel stimulation for postlingually deaf subjects,[7] presumably because spatial cues for spectral frequency are present in the former case. Also critical for good results are the dynamic properties of the channels.[22] This is consistent with speech-coding experiments which indicate that dynamic properties of nerve responses can contain important cues for many speech sounds.

One can readily appreciate many of the observations made on patients with multiple-channel implants by drawing an analogy in which recognizing words in conversation is likened to recognizing books in a library. Perfect vision enables us to read the titles, thus unambiguously identifying each volume.

However, in a very familiar library, one can identify many volumes using cues such as color, height, thickness, or location (context). If two books of similar appearance are interchanged, one would find the error by reading the titles. However, if one can only make out the gross appearance of the volumes, one might recognize books in their usual locations (interchanging two similar books from different sections would cause confusion). Under these circumstances, learning could presumably lead to great improvements in performance. One might expect the role of learning to be greatest in children and that more latitude might be permitted in designing implants for young prelingually deaf subjects (because of the greater flexibility of the central processor in such brains).

The observations on postlingually deaf patients are consistent with a view that the closer one approaches the normal representation of neural activity, the better the performance. The use of multiple, frequency-selective channels with proper adaptation times, individually adjustable gains, and an overall volume control are all important in attempting to mimic the natural condition. However, many other factors will influence the ultimate usefulness of any implant, including the condition of the nerve, the location of the electrodes, the stimulus waveforms, the coding schemes for intensity and frequency, as well as the needs, motivation, age and teachability of the patients, the state of the central nervous system, the language of most familiarity, and the time course of hearing loss. A major problem for cochlear implant design is the interactive nature of many of these important variables: changing any of these factors can interact with any of the others. In such a complicated situation, it seems advisable to adopt well-controlled ways of testing performance, keeping track of empirical data, and assessing the significance of the results.

References

1. Spoendlin, H. 1973. The innervation of the cochlear receptor. *In* Basic Mechanisms of Hearing. A. R. Møller, Ed., Academic Press. New York, NY.
2. Kiang, N. Y. S., J. M. Rho, C. C. Norhtrop, M. C. Liberman & D. K. Ryugo. 1982. Hair cell innervation by spiral ganglion cells in adult cats. Science **217:** 175–177.
3. Liberman, M. C. 1980. Morphological differences among radial afferent fibers in the cat cochlea: An electron-microscopic study of serial sections. Hearing Res. **3:** 45–63.
4. Liberman, M. C. 1978. Auditory-nerve response from cats raised in a low-noise chamber. J. Acoust. Soc. Am. **63**(2): 442–455.
5. Liberman, M. C. 1982. Single neuron labeling in the cat auditory nerve. Science **216:** 1239–1241.
6. Liberman, M. C. 1980. Efferent synapses in the inner hair cell area of the cat cochlea: An electron microscopic study of serial sections. Hearing Res. **3:** 189–204.
7. Eddington, D. K. 1980. Speech discrimination in deaf subjects with cochlear implants. J. Acoust. Soc. Am. **68**(3): 885–891.
8. Kiang, N. Y. S. 1980. Processing of speech by the auditory system. J. Acoust. Soc. Am. **68**(3): 830–836.
9. Voight, H. F., M. B. Sachs & E. D. Young. 1981. Representation of whispered vowels in the temporal patterns of auditory-nerve fiber discharges. J. Acoust. Soc. Am. **69:** S53 (A).

10. KIANG, N. Y. S. & E. C. MOXON. 1972. Physiological considerations in artificial stimulation of the inner ear. Ann. Otol. Rhinol. Laryngol. **81**(5): 714–730.
11. KIANG, N. Y. S. & E. C. MOXON. 1974. Tails of tuning curves of auditory-nerve fibers. J. Acoust. Soc. Am. **55**(3): 620–630.
12. HASHIMOTO, T., Y. KATAYAMA, K. MURATA & I. TANIGUCHI. 1973. Auditory nerve response to speech sounds. Proc. Japan Acad. **49:**(7): 559–563.
13. HASHIMOTO, T., Y. KATAYAMA, K. MURATA & I. TANIGUCHI. 1975. Pitch synchronous response of cat cochlear nerve fibers tot speech sounds. Jap. J. Physiol. **25:** 633–644.
14. SACHS, M. B. & E. D. YOUNG. 1979. Encoding of steady-state vowels in the auditory-nerve: Representation in terms of discharge rate. J. Acoust. Soc. Am. **66:** 470–479.
15. YOUNG, E. D. & M. B. SACHS. 1979. Representation of steady-state vowels in the temporal aspects of the discharge patterns of populations of auditory-nerve fibers. J. Acoust. Soc. Am. **66:** 1381–1403.
16. DELGUTTE, B. 1981. Representation of speech-like sounds in the discharge patterns of auditory-nerve fibers. Doctoral thesis, Dept. of Electrical Engineering and Computer Science, Massachusetts Institute of Technology.
17. DELGUTTE, B. 1980. Representation of speech-like sounds in the discharge patterns of auditory-nerve fibers. J. Acoust. Soc. Am. **68**(3): 843–857.
18. VOIGHT, H. F., M. B. SACHS & E. D. YOUNG. 1981. Effects of masking noise on the representation of vowel spectra in the auditory nerve. *In* Neuronal Mechanisms of Hearing. J. Syka and L. Aitkin, Eds.: 113–118. Plenum Press. New York, NY.
19. GUINAN, J. J., JR. & W. B. WARR. 1980. Efferent innervation of the organ of Corti: Asymmetrical topographic projections. Soc. Neurosci. **6:** 544.
20. BILGER, R. C. 1977. Evaluation of subjects presently fitted with implanted auditory prostheses. Ann. Otol. Rhinol. Laryngol. Suppl. **38:** 1–176.
21. HOCHMAIR-DESOYER, I. J., E. S. HOCHMAIR, R. E. FISCHER & K. BURIAN. 1980. Cochlear prostheses in use: Recent speech comprehension results. Arch. Otorhinolaryngol. **229:** 81–89.
22. EDDINGTON, D. K. Personal communication.

Part III. Electrical Stimulation of the Auditory System

INTRODUCTION

Gerald E. Loeb

Laboratory of Neural Control
National Institute of Neurological and Communicative Disorders and Stroke
National Institutes of Health
Bethesda, Maryland 20205

Like any other electrically excitable cells, the nerve fibers of the auditory nerve can be stimulated to generate propagated action potentials by electrical currents of the proper amplitude and spatial distribution. It is now clear that the central nervous system interprets these artificial activations as if they were generated by sound energy acting via the normal transduction mechanisms of the hair cells; that is, the elicited activity is perceived as sound.

Of course, the details of the spatiotemporal activation pattern so achieved are unlikely to be similar to anything ever experienced by a normal hearing individual. Thus, it has not been surprising that the percepts reported by auditory prosthesis patients are complex and difficult to describe. Fortunately, the sensory nervous system has a remarkable ability to extract meaningful information from noisy or distorted inputs. Thus it is that with even the crudest of techniques, patients have reported sensations that scale pitch and loudness in the appropriate directions with changes in amplitude, frequency, and place of electrical stimulation.

But the information-handling requirements for the real-time perception of intelligible speech are very much harder to satisfy than those for performing these psychophysical discriminations (and are covered in detail elsewhere in this volume). It is generally conceded that they can be met only by a significant number (perhaps four to twelve) of parallel and reasonably independent channels. Channel separation for electrical stimuli can be achieved only by spatially separating the current fluxes in the vicinity of the target neural elements. In the contributions that follow, my coworkers and I outline the theoretical factors that influence neuronal activation and Black and coworkers present some of the empirical findings that have led many investigators to concentrate on bipolar and pseudobipolar electrode configurations.

The use of small, intense, highly localized current sources has brought the design of intracochlear prostheses to the cutting edge of electrochemical research. Much of the controversy regarding stimulation-induced damage, as discussed by Clopton and his coworkers, revolves around the classes of electrochemical reactions which transfer electrical currents from the motion of electrons in wires to the motion of ions in solutions, presented here by Brummer *et al.* As we attempt to crowd larger numbers of channels into closer spacings, these problems must be resolved or we shall have to settle for performance that is less than optimal.

Finally, we should keep in mind that the auditory system is unique in its abilities to extract information from temporal as opposed to spatial patterns. Speech perception from both normal and prosthetic hearing depends on preserving at least some of both aspects of an input signal. My coworkers and I as well as Clopton *et al.* discuss the temporal factors influencing the recruitment of neurons by electrical waveforms of differing durations and shapes. The psychophysical effects of these variables are just beginning to be explored (see elsewhere this volume) and have yet to be systematically exploited to improve the performance of auditory prostheses.

BIOPHYSICAL CONSIDERATIONS IN ELECTRICAL STIMULATION OF THE AUDITORY NERVOUS SYSTEM[a]

Gerald E. Loeb,[b] Mark W. White,[c] and William M. Jenkins[c]

Laboratory of Neural Control
National Institute of Neurological and Communicative Disorders and Stroke
Bethesda, Maryland 20205

[c] *Coleman Laboratory*
Department of Otolaryngology
University of California School of Medicine
San Francisco, California 94143

A considerable body of both theoretical and experimental data exists regarding the electrical activation of nervous tissue. Over the past decade, the increasing use of this technique as both a quantitative research tool and a prosthetic approach to restoration of function has spurred attempts to develop general descriptions of the relevant physical processes so that models and experimental results pertaining to widely different circumstances could be compared. The emerging picture has generally been that of an orderly, well-behaved system in good agreement with the properties of the Hodgkin–Huxley model of the excitable nerve membrane.[1] However, a rather large number of variables must be accurately specified to obtain useful predictions from such models, and the relevant data are frequently either unavailable or impractical to obtain for the complicated circumstances pertaining to many clinical devices. Therefore, it is important to develop an efficient set of empirical descriptors of each system which can be used to relate clinical and animal experiments to each other and to the operating curves of such models.

It is not our purpose to present a detailed model of the electrical activation of the auditory nerve. Too little is known about the electrical and physical properties of this system and too many technical variations of prosthetic electrodes and waveforms have been employed for this to be either feasible or useful (see the review by Eddington [2]). Rather, we here point out at least the general effects of the relevant factors and suggest some simplifying assumptions and insights that appear to account for most clinical results and that might guide future development. There appears to be a general consensus that the scala tympani affords the best-distributed access to the auditory nerve. Therefore, we have limited the ranges of many variables to those found in this setting to try to draw as many hard conclusions as possible, at the expense of generalizability to other situations.

There are four general considerations in the electrical activation of neural tissue. First, the electrically excitable target elements must be defined and

[a] This work was supported by Grant NS–11804 and Contract NS–0–2337 from the National Institutes of Health, and by Hearing Research, Inc.

[b] Address for correspondence: Dr. Gerald E. Loeb, National Institutes of Health, Bldg. 36, Rm. 5A29, 9000 Rockville Pike, Bethesda, Maryland 20205

0077–8923/83/0405–0123 $01.75/0 © 1983, NYAS

their physical dimensions and structural details described sufficiently to make reasonable guesses about their electrical cable properties.[1] Second, the stimulating electrical waveforms and physical arrangement of the electrodes must be specified so that the resultant electrical fields may be calculated. Third, special circumstances in the transmission medium, usually assumed to be a homogeneous volume conductor, must be noted and their effects on the fields experienced by the target elements estimated. Finally, and this is potentially quite important in an auditory prosthesis, the investigator must consider secondary factors such as the response of higher-order neurons to the fine spatiotemporal details of the resultant first-order recruitment.

The Target

From the time that electrical stimulation was first employed in neurophysiology, it was noted that there were systematic differences in the responsiveness of neural elements, depending on their size, shape, and composition.

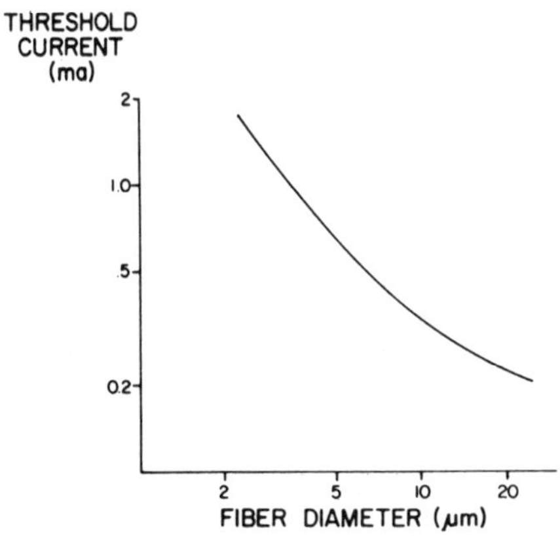

FIGURE 1. Theoretical relationship between the threshold current of a 100-μsec duration monopolar cathodal pulse delivered 1 mm above a node of Ranvier and the diameter of the myelinated nerve fiber. (From McNeal[4] [based on the Frankenhaeuser and Huxley[1] model of the electrical cable properties of such fibers]. Reprinted by permission.)

From such experiments, two properties emerged that continue to be used to categorize their sensitivity: threshold and chronaxie.[3] To a first approximation, threshold can be related both theoretically and empirically to the physical dimensions of the target structure, and chronaxie (defined later) to the electrical properties of its membranes.

Threshold

All other things being equal, large-diameter fibers have a lower action-potential *threshold* than do small diameter fibers, and large-diameter cell bodies have lower thresholds than small ones, for extracellularly applied electrical currents. For nerve fibers, a fairly good theoretical understanding of the size effect is possible and is in good agreement with empirical results.[4] The relationship for myelinated fibers is shown in FIGURE 1. The fiber diameter of the human auditory nerve myelinated fibers falls generally in the midportion of this curve (3–10 μm),[5] where the threshold current is nearly a linear inverse of the fiber diameter. Unmyelinated fibers have very high thresholds, and any unmyelinated portion of the spiral ganglion cell's apical dendrite that might survive in a deaf cochlea is unlikely to be the site of spike initiation, even if it lies closer to the stimulating electrode than do the other parts of the cell. Similarly, the small-diameter myelinated and unmyelinated fibers present in the nerve probably do not contribute to the percepts of auditory prosthesis patients unless they are being stimulated at levels far above the large-fiber threshold, and thus far above perceptual threshold. However, if there has been a selective and nearly complete loss of the large-diameter fibers, the psychophysical threshold may be sufficiently elevated that modest increments in stimulation current over this will, in fact, recruit small fibers whose normal perceptual roles are not understood.

The effect of the cell body is very much harder to model accurately. The depolarization of a neuron to the point of threshold requires a fairly extended spatial distribution of current flow through elongated processes attached to the cell body; a spherical cell body without processes is virtually inexcitable extracellularly.[6] The fact that the spiral ganglion cell is a moderately sized and spindle-shaped (20×30 μm) bipolar cell with its own myelin sheath suggests that its presence does little to alter the electrical excitability of the overall structure.

Chronaxie

Chronaxie is the classical measure of the responsiveness of the target neuron to temporal as opposed to spatial features of the electrical stimulation field. Operationally, it is determined by the threshold duration of a monopolar, monophasic electrical stimulation pulse whose current amplitude is twice that of the minimum activating current needed by an infinite duration pulse.[3] The standard linear plot of threshold current strength (y-axis) versus stimulus duration (x-axis) for single monophasic square pulses has a hyperbolic shape from which a horizontal asymptote is readily estimated (FIG. 2). Only a few points on the curve are needed to obtain a fairly reliable interpolation of the pulse duration at twice this level. This time relates both theoretically and empirically to the time constant of the target cell membrane, which is the product of the membrane capacitance and resistance per unit area. Conceptually, it can be appreciated as the degree to which the capacitance in the cell membrane slows its ability to follow a quickly changing applied extracellular field.

The chronaxies of myelinated nerve fibers are generally independent of their diameter. Most measurements cluster around 100 μsec, with a range of 20 to 200 μsec, in agreement with models of such fibers. This probably relates to the relatively low membrane capacitance imparted by the myelin sheath, and is in reasonable agreement with estimates of the membrane time constant made from intracellular recordings (time constant should be about 1.4 times chronaxie). The chronaxie of unmyelinated nerve fibers and cell bodies is generally much larger, on the order of 500–6000 μsec. This is probably related to the much larger amount of exposed, high-capacitance membrane. However, the effect of cell bodies is impossible to separate from their attached processes, which may be myelinated (output axons) or unmyelinated, but made of membranes whose electrical properties are not directly measurable (dendrites). In such complex geometries, the chronaxie actually observed depends complexly on the orientation of the target neuron to the stimulating electric field and the actual site of spike initiation (see Ranck[6] for a review of preceding points).

In the case of the auditory nerve, the presence of myelin over all three structures—apical dendrite, soma, and output axon—suggests that the chronaxies should be relatively short.[7] In preparing this discussion, we discovered that no estimate of chronaxie using the classical paradigm seems to have been made for auditory nerve fibers activated via intracochlear electrodes. This is presumably because of the recent emphasis on biphasic waveforms for safety, bipolar electrodes for selectivity, and continuous frequency trains for psychophysical relevance. We, therefore, undertook a simple experiment to relate the classical measurement to the more commonly used waveforms.

A pair of closely spaced microelectrodes was passed dorsoventrally and caudorostrally along the parasagittal plane through the cochlear nucleus of an anesthetized cat. Acoustic stimuli were used to map the structure, identifying the responses typical of the dorsal and ventral cochlear nuclei and, in particular, the low-frequency, large spherical cell region lying deep in the anteroventral cochlear nucleus (see FIGURE 4 and related text in the section THE EFFECTS). The latter cells have been described as "primary-like" in that they appear to follow one-for-one the action potentials of their input auditory nerve fibers.[8] The round window of the ipsilateral cochlea was then exposed, opened,

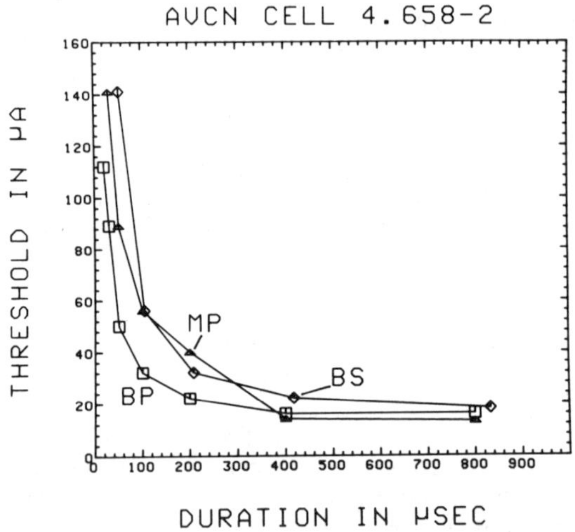

FIGURE 2. Classical strength/duration curve for a presumed "primary-like" large spherical cell recorded in the anteroventral cochlear nucleus of an acutely neomycin-deafened cat. Curve MP indicates monopolar, monophasic cathodal stimulation (single pulses at 8 pps) from a scala tympani electrode; BP indicates bipolar, monophasic cathodal stimulation from the electrode used for MP referenced to another similar contact located 0.7 mm more basal along the basilar membrane; BS indicates bipolar, biphasic stimulation using a continuous sinusoidal waveform whose half-cycle duration is plotted on the x-axis.

TABLE 1

RESPONSE PROPERTIES OF AVCN CELLS TO INTRACOCHLEAR ELECTRICAL STIMULATION

Cell No.	Depth in Track (μm)	Threshold—100 μsec Cathodal (μA)	Chronaxie—Cathodal (μsec)
1	4155	100	380
2	4175	112	650
3	4313	89	200
4	4658	56	310
5	4122	126	850

and 0.1 cc of 5% neomycin infused over a 20-min period, without losing the stereotaxic orientation of the skull. This treatment has been shown to lead to an immediate destruction of the mechanosensitivity of the hair cells, leaving the spiral ganglion cells and their apical dendrites at least temporarily intact and excitable.[9] An appropriately scaled-down version of the human scala tympani electrode array was then introduced through the round window opening so that its four longitudinally spaced electrodes were positioned about halfway around the first turn and lying up against the organ of Corti. The microelectrode pair was reintroduced along approximately the same track originally mapped, and single units encountered at various depths were characterized by their responsiveness to various locations, orientations, and waveforms of electrical stimulation in the scala tympani. Lesions were made at the ends of the tracks to verify histologically the location of the recorded units.

Chronaxie was estimated for five cells which were located in the large spherical cell region of the anteroventral cochlear nucleus. They were distributed over a range of 200 to 850 μsec (mean 478 μsec) (TABLE 1). Theshold currents varied by a factor of two, presumably as a result of different distances between the origination point of each cell's input from the basilar membrane and the distance to the nearest available stimulation electrode. However, it is not clear from this small sample size whether the large range of chronaxies may represent some heterogeneously distributed property of the spiral ganglion cells, possibly correlated with their thresholds.

One cell (FIG. 2) was tested for the effects of pulse duration with both monopolar (MP) and longitudinal bipolar (BP; 0.7-mm separation) cathodal pulses (AC coupled to minimize damage but with a time constant of 100 msec to approximate the classical monophasic condition). Monopolar chronaxie of 310 μsec was reduced to about 100 μsec bipolar. This same cell was also tested with continuous sinusoids (BS; same bipolar pair) in which the pulse duration was taken to be the duration of each half-cycle. "Chronaxie" estimated in this manner was 200 μsec. This cell had the lowest threshold of any tested, suggesting that its input came from a region of the basilar membrane closest to a stimulating electrode, and thus most likely to represent the threshold phenomena reported psychophysically by patients [10] or found behaviorally in monkeys.[11]

Monopolarly measured classical chronaxies thus appear to be distinctly longer for these cells than for other myelinated axons, where theory and intra-

and extracellular measurements all converge around 50–150 μsec. The values reported here are typical of those of grey-matter chronaxies, which have been presumed to result from the complex product of unmyelinated soma/dendrite components and myelinated axons. However, the architecture of the heavily myelinated spiral ganglion cells is clearly not like that of most CNS nuclei. If unmyelinated membrane capacitance is not a factor, then it seems likely that the increased time constant of the cells implicit in this measurement comes from higher than usual resistivity, perhaps from an unusually thick or resistive myelination or smaller nodes of Ranvier. This may have implications for the interaction of multiple stimuli that are close to each other in time and space, since the residual intracellular effects of one subliminal stimulus may persist considerably beyond its actual current duration. Attempts to estimate these neuronal time constants using bipolar and/or biphasic stimuli appear to underestimate them by a considerable factor.

Efficiency

One reason for measuring strength/duration relationships is that it provides useful information regarding the optimal design of stimulation equipment. The critical variable in the damage of tissue and electrodes by electrolytic reactions is the charge density per phase, expressed in microcoulombs per real square centimeter of exposed metal ("real" refers to accessible surface area including roughening effects). The actual limit depends complexly on the composition of the metal, its electrical history, and the composition of the electrolyte, particularly including trace additives of proteins and amino acids.[12, 13] For platinum alloy electrodes, the safe limit below which electrolytic reactions are entirely avoided is likely to be around several hundred $\mu C/cm^2$. Translated to cochlear electrode dimensions, this is several $\mu C/mm^2$. A disk electrode 0.3 mm in diameter has about 0.1 mm^2 area (using geometric rather than real area for simplicity), so the maximum charge per pulse should be kept to considerably less than 1 μC, or 1 mA $\times$ 1 msec. For single-pulse stimuli, the product of the threshold current amplitude and the pulse duration can be used as a measure of the stimulus efficiency. In this experiment, it is interesting to note that this threshold charge is slowly but steadily decreasing for progressively narrower pulses, even those requiring very high current levels (FIG. 3). For pulses longer than chronaxie, efficiency becomes rapidly poorer. Of course, it may be impractical to build stimulation circuits capable of the high driving voltages and fast slewing rates that are needed for very short pulses.

It should be noted that this fast-pulse efficacy does not hold for continuous waveforms, such as the bipolar sinusoid, whose effects are plotted in FIGURE 3 (curve BS frequency scale is plotted at x-axis positions where pulse duration and half-cycle time are approximately equal). This probably pertains also to symmetrical biphasic pulses, since the efficiency reversal probably occurs at the point at which the electrical response of the voltage-dependent gates in the neuron membrane cannot keep up with rapidly reversing fields. This effect is distinct from and in addition to the time constants inherent in the axon membranes, which affect monophasic and biphasic pulses equally. Stimulation at frequencies in excess of about 5 kHz occurs primarily by successive

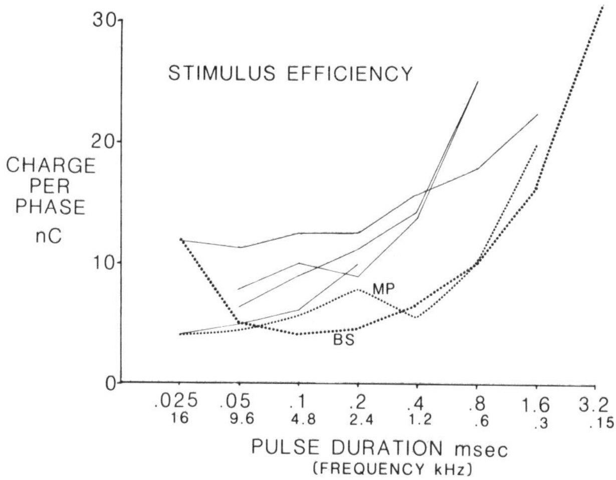

FIGURE 3. The charge per phase (area of the waveform) is plotted for intracochlear activation of five different AVCN cells at threshold amplitude for various pulse durations. Curves marked MP and BS are from same cell as in FIGURE 2; the frequency of the sinusoidal stimulus for curve BS is plotted at the single pulse duration corresponding closest to a half-cycle duration. The four unmarked fine lines represent four other cells activated by monopolar, monophasic cathodal pulses delivered through the scala tympani electrode with the lowest threshold for the unit (which was the apical-most electrode for all five units shown here).

summation of only partially rectified membrane currents from each successive stimulus cycle, resulting in progressive loss of efficiency. The actual current level required to reach threshold for the 16-kHz point shown in curve BS of FIGURE 3 was 560μA, far off the scale of FIG. 2, despite the more similar chronaxies of these curves.

THE STIMULI

The sequence of events by which an applied electrical signal gives rise to a conducted action potential involves a series of electrical processes, some of which are best characterized by their voltages and others by their current, but all of which are related by Ohm's law:

If a voltage is applied between two electrodes (one of which may be a remotely located common or reference electrode), a current will flow whose amplitude depends inversely on the vector sum of three impedances: the resistance of the saline solution between the two electrodes and the impedance of the metal/electrolyte interface of each electrode. At the frequencies and dimensions of cochlear prostheses, the latter two are by far the larger and dominant factor. Once there is current flow through the medium, it gives rise to changes in the relative potentials at various locations in the extracellular fluids. The distribution of such potentials can be determined from a knowledge of the possibly heterogeneous impedances of the medium (discussed later). This, in turn, gives rise to fluxes of current into and out of nerve membranes which span these voltage gradients. This process depends on the orientation of these membranes with respect to the fields and their intrinsic time constants, as discussed earlier. Finally, these transmembrane currents produce changes in the normal resting potential which the cells maintain between the inside and the outside. When any local area of membrane becomes depolarized by about 20 mV from its usual resting potential of about 80 mV (inside negative), this initiates a series of rapid changes in the conductance of that patch of the membrane to sodium and potassium ions. This gives rise to the neural action currents which propagate the local depolarization rapidly throughout the neuron as an action potential.

Waveform

In the final analysis, the variable that gives the investigator the best control over the situation is the waveform of the current that flows through the electrodes. Normally, this is controlled by a constant-current stimulator. However, several circumstances may cause the stimulus generation apparatus to have control of voltage only. Telemetry devices relying on simple inductive coupling of an amplitude-modulated carrier provide essentially only voltage control of their outputs. More sophisticated metering of current or charge requires much more sophisticated circuitry.[14] If several sets of electrodes are connected in parallel, even a current-regulated circuit cannot guarantee any particular distribution of current through any particular electrode. If the impedance of each electrode were constant and known, then the current distribution could be calculated from Ohm's law. However, metal/electrolyte interfaces are complex impedances whose resistive and capacitive terms are nonlinear, time-dependent functions of frequency, current density, polarization voltage, and total charge flow. The most obvious nonlinearity occurs when the voltage drop across the junction passes the 1–2 VDC required to drive the electrolysis reactions of water. In a typical intracochlear electrode with a nominal impedance of 10 kilohms at 1 kHz, this potential would be reached (assuming linear behavior) with 100 μA of current, right in the middle of the operating range of most such devices. Thus, whenever possible, current should be controlled or at least monitored.

For continuous waveforms such as sinusoids, the stimulus is obviously biphasic. However, when pulses are employed, the question arises as to whether a monophasic pulse of anodal current (electrode-positive) or cathodal current (electrode-negative) should be used, or whether the stimulus will be a biphasic pulse, in which case there arises the question of which phase will be first and whether they will be symmetrical in shape. It is now generally recognized that the stimulation should cause equal and opposite amounts of charge to flow in each phase of the biphasic waveform so that no net DC current results.[15] This minimizes the various electrolytic reactions of both the medium (saline solution) and the electrodes (usually oxidizable metals), which otherwise give rise to products that are highly damaging to both the tissue and the electrodes themselves. It seems reasonable that initially cathodal pulses will have somewhat lower thresholds since this current tends to depolarize the portions of the cell membrane that are closest to the electrode, where the current density is highest. However, the effect depends complexly on the target geometry, the distances involved, the position of the other electrode of a bipolar pair, and the pulse durations and their symmetry. In the human cochlea, the activation threshold is unlikely to be more than a factor of two higher for anode-first pulse pairs, although there may be considerable differences in the fine details of the spatial and temporal distribution of fibers actually producing action potentials. In our study in cats of monopolar, monophasic 100 μsec pulses, anodal thresholds averaged twice cathodal thresholds, probably a worst-case situation.

Geometry

The most significant variable in the *selective* activation of subpopulations of neurons, such as desired for multichannel prostheses, is the physical arrangement of the stimulating electrodes with respect to the target fibers. The current density in a volume-conducting medium is highest at the surface of the current sources and sinks (electrodes), and drops off rapidly in the intervening fluid. For monopolar electrodes (large remote reference sink), threshold current has been found to vary almost linearly with distance over the range of 100 to 1000 μm.[6] Depending on fiber or cell diameter, the threshold current for a 200-μsec duration cathodal pulse tends to be 5–20 μA at 100-μm distance; and 50–200 μA at 1000-μm distance. This is in general agreement with both the thresholds and the limited dynamic ranges reported for intracochlear monopolar electrodes.[10] Once the current density in the modiolus reaches threshold, virtually all remaining auditory nerve fibers will be activated, regardless of their distance from the electrode.[16] The best selectivity and largest dynamic range will be achieved when the electrode is closest to the target subpopulation, since this maximizes the relative distance to the remainder of the population. The loss of apical dendrites has a pronounced effect on the excitability of spiral ganglion cells, primarily because it removes their closest excitable membrane from the immediate vicinity of a scala tympani electrode.[17] This will affect selectivity as well as threshold, no matter what design of intracochlear electrode is chosen.

The use of bipolar electrodes is often advocated to improve the selectivity by confining the spread of current to a limited volume of fluid "between the two electrodes." Of course, current flow in a volume conductor is not like sparks across an air gap. The degree to which current flow can be controlled depends on the actual spacing between the electrodes; the degree to which an advantage is so obtained depends on the relative spacing to the target subpopulation. If the electrodes are too far apart, they act simply as two local monopolar electrodes which happen to be out of phase. If the targets are too far away, the high-current density gradient in the immediate vicinity of the pair is of no use, as the neurons are actually being activated by the much more homogeneous current densities obtaining at that distance.

The electrical field gradients surrounding monopole and dipole antennas are mathematically well defined and well understood by radio engineers. The field strength around a monopole varies inversely with distance ($1/r$) and around a dipole with distance squared ($1/r^2$). While the situation is more complex in biological preparations, some useful general rules arise. To a first approximation, the optimal spacing between the bipolar elements should be of the same order as the distance to the presumed target elements. In this range, the function of threshold versus distance approaches distance squared, significantly improving selectivity over the linear function for monopolar stimulus spread. Since the object of electrical stimulation is to generate longitudinal gradients along elongated neural elements, the orientation should be parallel to the fibers, further enhancing the selectivity.[17] Again, the closer the target, the better the selectivity.

Occasionally it is stated that electrode surface areas must be kept small to improve selectivity or reduce shunting in bipolar pairs. The former consideration applies only when the effective diameter of the exposed electrode disc begins to approach the distance between the electrode and the target, since the current from the perimeter areas then has less selective effect on the targets closest to the center. The latter consideration applies only when the resistance of the intervening saline medium in a bipolar pair is equal to or greater than the metal/electrolyte contact impedance; otherwise current density is uniform over the surface of each contact so that their shape has no effect on shunting. For the frequencies and surface geometries available to cochlear prostheses, this condition simply never arises, and the current is always distributed almost uniformly rather than selectively concentrated at adjacent edges. Bipolar electrode contacts should therefore be as large as the distance between them permits, stopping only when danger of physical shorting arises. This decreases their impedance, which lowers the necessary driving voltages, linearizes their behavior, reduces the danger of elctrolytic reactions, and reduces the shunting effects of any small electrical leaks along leads and connectors.[18]

The Medium

The bony spiral lamina and soft tissue membranes of the cochlea can be expected to cause electrical currents to flow differently than they would in perilymph alone, which is electrically similar to normal saline solution, that is, a homogeneous, isotropic volume conductor with a specific resistivity of 65 ohm-cm. On the other hand, these boundaries are electrically unlike simple plastic tubes. While the different conductivities of membranes, scar tissue, axon bundles, and bone have been much studied in isolation, the most salient point to keep in mind is that they are all only moderately less conductive than saline solution, a fairly poor conductor. Even bone requires for its metabolic sustenance an intricate system of blood vessels and cytoplasmic channels which are fluid-filled and contribute to its conductivity. Probably no element present in either the normal or the pathologic cochlea has a conductivity more than an order of magnitude poorer than that of saline solution or perilymph, and probably all are isotropic within a factor of two.[19] In particular, scar tissue is likely to have no more than two or three times the resistivity of perilymph, which is consistent with the relatively unchanged electrode impedances, psychophysical thresholds, and percepts obtained during the first few weeks of implant function when such encapsulation is developing (unpublished results from two most recent patients implanted at UCSF with 16-contact electrode arrays fabricated in the Coleman Laboratory). Larger fluctuations in electrode impedances measured at low current densities have been noted both *in vitro* and *in vivo*. These have been ascribed to contamination of metal surfaces by silicone oil, oxide build-up, and other debris which are removed by current flow at normal levels of use.[20]

In volume-conducting situations, such inhomogeneities have surprisingly little effect on the distribution of current density, particularly when compared with the large, predictable effects of physical distance from a bipolar electrode. Several attempts have been made to measure the actual distribution of fields inside the cochlea during intracochlear stimulation by using the inactive electrodes either as probes or distributed common electrodes.[21, 22] So far this has not been particularly useful, stemming from limitations of technique and interpretability. In fact, the best detector of current distribution in the cochlea still appears to be the array of nerve fibers themselves, whose output may be inferred, albeit indirectly, by carefully designed psychophysical studies. This is particularly the case in elucidating complex interactions such as those between adjacent electrodes.

The Effects

The spatiotemporal patterns of activity resulting from electrical activation of any ensemble of nerve fibers will be quite unlike their normal physiological activation patterns. In some systems, the effect of stimulation is more or less in proportion to the total amount of activity elicited without regard to such details. In the auditory nervous system, there is reason to believe that the central processor is exquisitely sensitive to the details, perhaps even to the active exclusion of "noise-like" patterns lacking spatial or temporal detail.

We have already addressed the limitations in spatial selectivity encountered by various electrode configurations. The enhanced detection of spatial gradients and a concomitant insensitivity to poorly differentiated activity levels is a common second-order property in neural perceptual systems. It is usually accomplished by sets of concentrically arranged inhibitory fields surrounding the excitatory field of a given second-order neuron. Such inhibitory action has been noted in the dorsal cochlear nucleus,[23] and might be expected to limit the sensitivity of these neurons to poorly localized electrical stimulation of the first-order neurons.

AVCN versus DCN

FIGURE 4 shows the distribution of thresholds to electrical stimulation as a function of the depth in the cochlear nuclei at which each unit was encountered in our experiment. This is superimposed on the frequency mapping of this depth axis by the acoustically tuned penetration made prior to acute neomycin treatment. The tracks pass through two tonotopically organized structures which presumably correspond to first the dorsal (DCN) and then anteroventral (AVCN) cochlear nuclei. A poorly responsive region presumably devoid of large cells was noted in the second area (broken hatched line), and was followed by large, sharply tuned, strictly excitatory responses typical of the large spherical cells of the AVCN. The estimated location of the four stimulating electrodes (based on insertion depth) is shown translated into best frequency position (right side ordinate) on the basilar membrane, with A for apical-most and B for basal-most contact. The capital letters refer to the thresholds for evoking single unit action potentials with a latency of 0.9–1.4 msec for a 100-μsec duration monopolar, monophasic search stimulus at the electrode that gave the lowest threshold. The lowercase letters indicate responses at latencies of 1.5–4.0 msec, which were possibly polysynaptic. Capital letters in parentheses refer to thresholds for evoking short-latency field potentials which were clearly not unitary and presumed to be from terminal arborizations of primary afferents. It is noteworthy that DCN units required stimulation currents an order of magnitude greater than AVCN units, even though this region appeared to be receiving low-threshold afferent input and was equally sensitive to acoustic stimuli. This suggests that the normal inhibitory mechanisms of the DCN may virtually eliminate it from contributing to the perceptual effects of intracochlear prostheses, which would then have to be conveyed to higher centers via the AVCN relay.

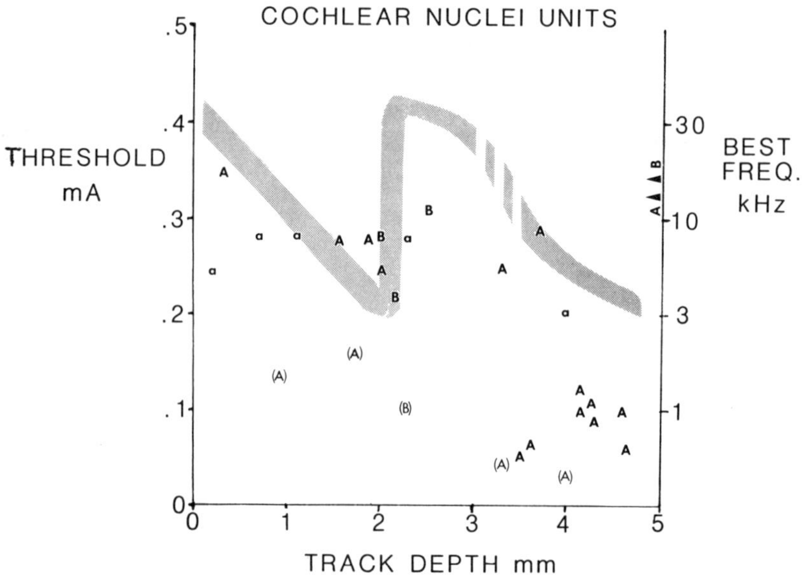

FIGURE 4. Intracochlear stimulation thresholds for all cells encountered in three double-microelectrode penetrations plotted against depth along the track (zero is just touching the dorsal cochlear nucleus; parasagittal tracks are oriented dorsocaudal to ventrorostral at approximately 30° from horizontal stereotaxic coordinates). The *shaded line* indicates the acoustical tuning curves (right ordinate) of cells encountered in a prior penetration along the same axis before acute neomycin deafening. See text for explanation of symbols.

Phase-Locking

Temporal effects are particularly interesting since the normal mechanisms for the interpretation of speech sounds almost certainly rely at least partly on the unique "phase-locking" of afferent activity to stimulus frequencies far above the physiological limit of one-to-one frequency following.[24] We have recently demonstrated that electrical stimuli cause a very similar, perhaps even enhanced, phase-locking effect over the relevant sinusoidal frequencies up to at least 3.2 kHz.[25] This leads to a paradox in the apparent insensitivity of prosthesis patients to frequency modulation beyond about 300 Hz, which is the subject of a theoretical treatment published elsewhere.[26] Despite the lack of a clear psychophysical pitch correlate of periodicity, such temporal effects may well be responsible for the rather complex sounds that auditory prosthesis patients describe even for the best localized stimuli that can be delivered. Temporal effects probably also relate to the empirical observation that pulse amplitude and duration cannot be traded arbitrarily to achieve similar quality percepts at threshold or at any constant loudness level. Even when equal numbers of neurons are activated, there will be considerably more temporal dispersion in the firing resulting from a long, low-amplitude pulse than from a short, high-level pulse. When complex waveforms such as the polyharmonic spectra of speech are applied directly to multiple intracochlear electrodes, the psychophysical effects are far beyond prediction by even the most sophisticated theories. Thus, it is likely that the continued development of auditory prostheses and speech processors for the encoding of electrical stimuli will have to proceed largely on empirical grounds, with electrophysiological theory able to provide general guidance on electrode design and placement and, perhaps, some *post hoc* rationalization of the results.

Acknowledgments

These experiments were performed in the Coleman Laboratory with the advice and assistance of Dr. Michael M. Merzenich, Director. We thank Dr. F. T. Hambrecht for his comments on the manuscript.

References

1. Frankenhauser, B. & A. F. Huxley. 1964. The action potential in the myelinated nerve fibre of xenopus laevis as computed on the basis of voltage clamp data. J. Physiol (Lond.) **171:** 302–315.
2. Eddington, D. K. 1980. Speech discrimination in deaf subjects with cochlear implants. J. Acoust. Soc. Am. **68:** 885–891.
3. Erlanger, J. & H. S. Gasser. 1937. Electrical Signs of Nervous Activity. University of Pennsylvania Press. Philadelphia, PA.
4. McNeal, D. R. 1976. Analysis of a model for excitation of myelinated nerve. IEEE Trans. Biomed. Eng. **23:** 329–337.
5. Rasmussen, A. T. 1940. Studies of the VIIIth cranial nerve of man. Laryngoscope **50:** 67–83.
6. Ranck, J. 1975. Which elements are excited in electrical stimulation of mammalian central nervous system? A review. Brain Res. **98:** 417–440.
7. Thomsen, E. 1967. The ultra structure of the spiral ganglion in the guinea pig. Acta Otolaryng. Suppl. **224:** 442–448.
8. Pfeiffer, R. R. 1966. Classification of response patterns of spike discharges for units in the cochlear nucleus: Tone-burst stimulation. Exp. Brain Res. **1:** 220–235.
9. Leake-Jones, P. A., M. C. Vivion, B. F. O'Reilly & M. M. Merzenich. Deaf animal models for studies of a multichannel cochlear prosthesis. Hearing Res. In press.
10. Eddington, D. K., W. H. Dobelle, M. G. Mladejovsky, D. E. Brackmann & J. L. Parkin. 1978. Auditory prostheses research with multiple channel intracochlear stimulation in man. Ann. Otol. Rhinol. Laryngol. **87**(53): 5–38.

11. PFINGST, B. E., F. A. SPELMAN & D. SUTTON. 1980. Operating ranges for cochlear implants. Ann. Otol. Rhinol. Laryngol. **89**(66): 1–4.

12. MCHARDY, J., L. S. ROBBLEE, J. M. MARSTON & S. B. BRUMMER. 1980. Electrical stimulation with Pt electrodes: IV. Factors affecting Pt dissolution in inorganic saline. Biomaterials **1:** 129–134.

13. ROBBLEE, L. S., J. MCHARDY, J. M. MARSTON & S. B. BRUMMER. 1980. Electrical stimulation with Pt electrodes: V. The effect of protein on Pt dissolution. Biomaterials **1:** 135–142.

14. SOMA, M. 1980. Design and fabrication of an implantable multichannel neural stimulator. Tech. Report No. G908–1, Integrated Circuits Lab., Department of Electrical Engineering, Stanford University. Stanford, CA.

15. PUDENZ, R. H., W. F. AGNEW, T. G. YUEN & L. A. BULLARA. 1977. Electrical stimulation of brain: Light and electron miscroscopy studies. *In* Functional Electrical Stimulation. F. T. Hambrecht and J. B. Reswick, Eds.: 437–458. Marcel Dekker. New York, NY.

16. WHITE, M. W., M. M. MERZENICH & M. C. VIVION. 1980. A non-invasive recording technique for evaluating electrode and nerve function in cochleas implanted with a multichannel electrode array. *In* Advances in Prosthetic Devices for the Deaf: A Technical Workshop. D. L. McPherson, Ed. The National Technical Institute for the Deaf, Rochester Institute of Technology. Rochester, NY.

17. MERZENICH, M. M., C. L. BYERS, M. WHITE & M. C. VIVION. 1980. Cochlear implant prostheses: Strategies and progress. Ann. Biomed. Eng. **8:** 361–368.

18. LOEB, G. E., J. MCHARDY, E. M. KELLIHER & S. B. BRUMMER. 1982. Neural prosthetics. *In* Biocompatibility in Clinical Practice, Vol. 2. D. F. Williams, Ed.: 123–149. CRC Press. Boca Raton, FL.

19. SCHWAN, S. P. & C. F. KAY. 1956. Specific resistance of body tissues. Circulation Res. **4:** 664.

20. LOEB, G. E., C. L. BYERS, S. J. REBSCHER, D. E. CASEY, M. M. FONG, R. A. SCHINDLER, R. F. GRAY & M. M. MERZENICH. The design and fabrication of an experimental cochlear prosthesis. Med. Biol. Eng. Comput. In press.

21. SPELMAN, F. A., B. M. CLOPTON, B. E. PFINGST & J. M. MILLER. 1980. Design of the cochlear prosthesis: Effects of the flow of current in the implanted ear. Ann. Otol. Rhinol. Laryngol. **89**(66): 8–10.

22. BLACK, R. C., G. M. CLARK & J. F. PATRICK. 1981. Current distribution measurements within the human cochlea. IEEE Trans. Biomed. Eng. **28:** 721–725.

23. EVANS, E. F. & P. G. NELSON. 1973. The responses of single neurones in the cochlear nucleus of the cat as a function of their location and the anaesthetic state. Exp. Brain Res. **17:** 402–427.

24. SACHS, M. B. & E. D. YOUNG. 1980. Effects of non-linearities on speech encoding in the auditory nerve. J. Acoust. Soc. Am. **68:** 858–875.

25. WHITE, M. W., M. M. MERZENICH & G. E. LOEB. Electrical stimulation of the eighth nerve in cat: Temporal properties of unit responses in the large spherical cell region of the AVCN. In preparation.

26. LOEB, G. E., M. W. WHITE & M. M. MERZENICH. Spatial cross-correlation: A proposed mechanism for acoustic pitch perception. Bio. Cybernetics. Submitted for publication.

CURRENT DISTRIBUTIONS IN COCHLEAR STIMULATION [a]

R. C. Black, G. M. Clark, Y. C. Tong, and J. F. Patrick

Department of Otolaryngology
University of Melbourne
Victoria 3052, Australia

INTRODUCTION

The success of a multiple-channel cochlear implant depends, in part, on localizing the electrical current to discrete groups of auditory nerve fibers. A number of studies are described that were performed to investigate this issue. First, a three-dimensional resistance model of the normal cat cochlea was developed to examine general properties of electrically stimulating the cochlea. The distribution of the excited nerve fibers for monopolar and bipolar stimulation of the cat scala tympani were then determined. In addition certain measurements of the current distribution within the human cochlea for a pseudobipolar electrode array were performed. Finally, measurements were made in saline-solution-filled tube models of current distributions for bipolar and pseudobipolar stimulation, with both single-electrode and coincident multi-electrode stimulation.

RESISTANCE MODEL OF THE NORMAL COCHLEA

The spread of current in the cochlea was initially studied [1] with reference to a three-dimensional resistance model (FIG. 1). The cross-sectional resistances lying between the scala vestibuli, scala media, scala tympani, spiral ligament, and body were obtained by averaging and scaling the values of resistances cited in the literature for the guinea pig cochlea,[2, 3] and the longitudinal resistances were calculated from values for the resistivity of perilymph [4] and from measurements of the cross-sectional areas of the scalas. The resistance values for the spiral ligament were from Strelioff.[5]

The distribution of voltages along the scalae, the current through the the unmyelinated nerve dendrites in the organ of Corti (current through R3), and also the current through the auditory nerve to ground (current through R6) were calculated for a number of different positions of the stimulating electrodes. The results for stimulation between the scale tympani and the body are shown in FIGURE 2.

It can be seen that scalar voltage distributions do not necessarily reflect the current distributions at sites where the nerve fibers are going to be excited by the scala tympani electrodes. Thus, the length constant for the organ of Corti current was a third the length constant for the scalar voltages, while the length constant for the current flowing through the auditory nerve to ground was more than twice as large as that of the scalar voltage.

[a] This work was supported in part by the National Hospital and Medical Research Council of Australia and by the Channel 10 Deafness Appeal.

0077-8923/83/0405-0137 $01.75/0 © 1983, NYAS

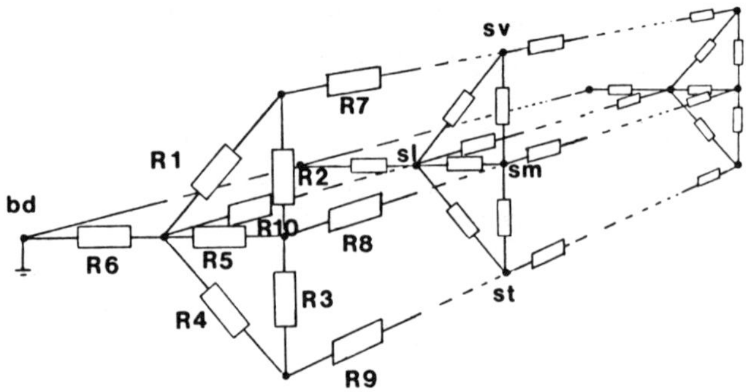

FIGURE 1. Resistance model for calculation of current distributions within the organ of Corti (R3), the cochlear grounding resistances containing the auditory nerve (R6), and the scala tympani (R9) resulting from electrical stimulation of the scala tympani. The model consists of 16 identical sections with stimulation occurring in the central section. There are five model nodes: sv, scala vestibuli; sm, scala media; st, scala tympani; sl, spiral ligament; bd, body.

CURRENT DISTRIBUTIONS IN THE CAT COCHLEA

In view of these model results it is clear that to assess different stimulus electrode configurations it is important to measure the current distribution in the direct vicinity of the nerve fibers. This can be done by a method in which the propagation of the current in the cochlea is measured by recording inferior colliculus cell thresholds to electrical stimulation.[6] The site of stimulation in the cochlea and distance from the stimulating electrode can be determined by recording the characteristic frequencies of the cells to sounds pre-

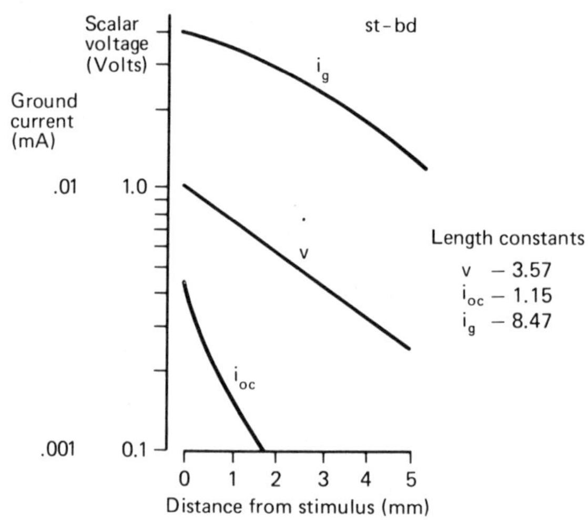

FIGURE 2. Scala tympani voltage (v), organ of Corti current (i_{oc}), and cochlear ground current (i_g) for monopolar stimulation of scala tympani (st-bd).

sented to the unoperated ear. Using this technique, thresholds were measured for monopolar and bipolar stimulation of the scale tympani, and for stimulation between the scala tympani and scala vestibuli. The stimulus electrodes were made of insulated fine wires with the ends exposed and fitting freely into the scala. It can be seen (FIG. 3) that for these fine-wire electrodes, the spread of the stimulus current was much less for bipolar than monopolar stimulation. In fact the length constant for bipolar stimulation was 2–4 mm, and for monopolar stimulation 8–16 mm.

These results emphasize the advantages of bipolar over monopolar stimulation for multiple-channel implants.

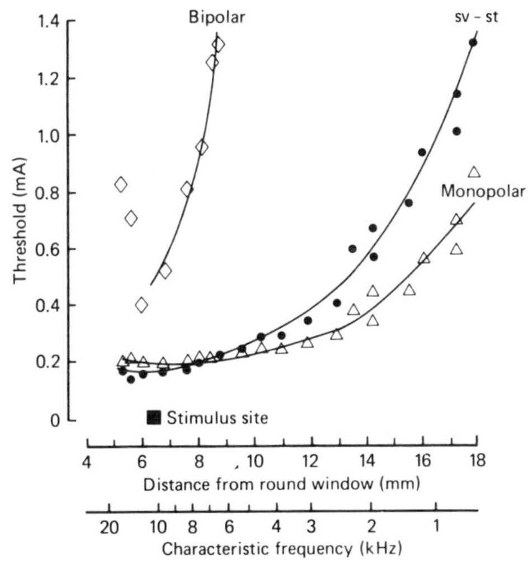

FIGURE 3. The threshold of single inferior colliculus units to electrical stimulation from fine-wire electrodes situated 6–7 mm from the round window, plotted as a function of the characteristic frequency of the units and their computed distances from the round window. Results due to both monopolar (△) and bipolar (◇) stimulation of the scala tympani are shown together with results from stimulation of the scala tympani relative to a reference electrode in scala vestibuli (●). The approximate position of the stimulus site is shown by the position of ■.

CURRENT DISTRIBUTION IN THE HUMAN COCHLEA

Following these experimental studies on cats' cochleas, it was considered most important to also make measurements of the current distribution in the human cochlea insofar as this was possible, to assist in the interpretation of our later psychophysical findings. In this case a pseudobipolar electrode was used, in which stimulation was referenced to the ten ground electrodes that were shorted together to form a common ground (FIG. 4). The electrode array was inserted just prior to the cochlear implant procedure, and was similar to the implanted electrode. Although it was not possible to measure the actual current in the cochlea itself, measurements could be made of the current in the ground lines of electrodes C1–C9, when stimulating the active electrodes A1, 2, 3 and 4 with 500-μA current pulses.[7]

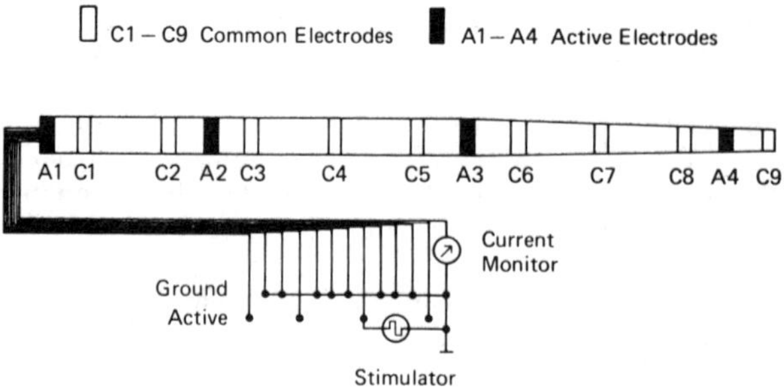

FIGURE 4. Pseudobipolar electrode array for measurement of ground-line current within the human cochlea. Ground electrodes were separated by 1.5 mm and were 0.3 mm wide. Array diameter was 0.4 mm at the tip and 0.6 mm at position of A3.

Ground currents measured in this way in one of the patients are shown in FIGURE 5. In general, these currents exhibited a significant propagation along the length of the array, and were generally nonmonotonically distributed with distance from the stimulation electrode. For example, when electrode A4 was stimulated, the current in an adjacent group electrode C8 was the same as that in the most distant electrode C1, while C7, which lay between C1 and C8, carried considerably less current. For stimulation of A3, the current in the adjacent ground electrode C6 was less than in the most distant electrode C1.

Similar patterns of ground current distribution and nonmotonicity are also seen when the same electrode was placed in a large beaker filled with saline solution and in a saline-solution-filled tube 5 mm in diameter (FIG. 6). There-

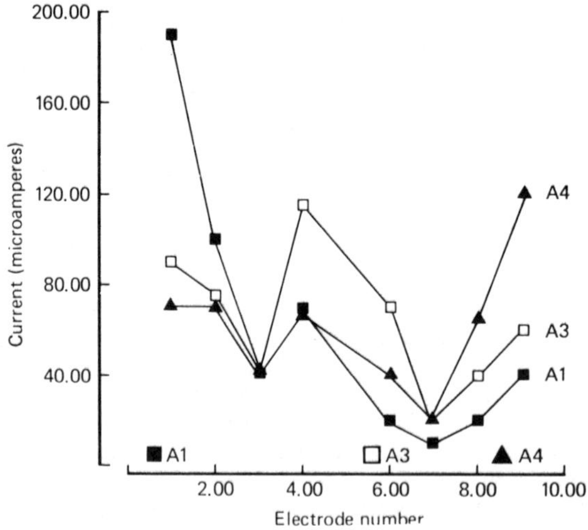

FIGURE 5. Ground-line current measurements made in a single patient for stimulation of A1, A3 and A4 with 500-μA current pulses.

fore, in these cases the ground currents appeared to be determined by properties of the electrode itself rather than by those of the surrounding environments. It was thought that the impedances of the ground electrodes themselves were substantially greater than the impedance of the fluid paths between the active and ground electrodes, in which case the total impedance from an active electrode to any ground electrode would be approximately equal. This would result in wide distribution of the ground current. Furthermore, if there were substantial random differences in impedances of the ground electrodes due to manufacture, nonmonotonicity of the ground current magnitudes with distance from the stimulus electrode would be expected.

Later measurements made in the 5-mm tube (which served as a good model for the distribution of ground currents in the cochlea) showed that the impedances of the ground electrodes were of the order of 1 kΩ and quite

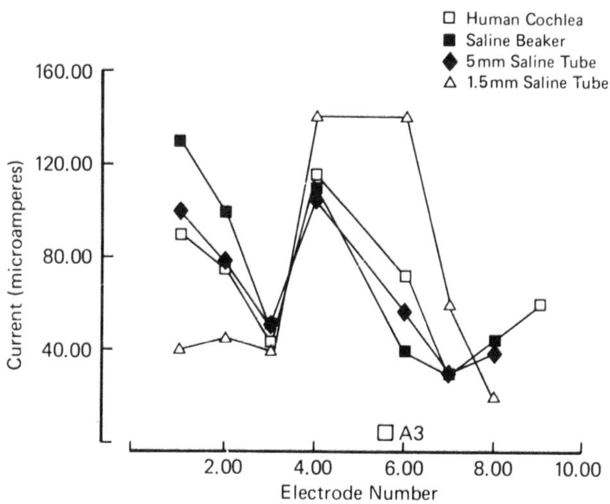

FIGURE 6. Ground current distributions for stimulation with electrode A3 in the human cochlea, a saline-solution-filled beaker, and saline-solution-filled tubes of diameters of 5 mm and 1.5 mm.

variable, while the fluid impedances were approximately 30Ω/mm, thus indicating these hypotheses to be correct. Furthermore, in the tube 1.5 mm in diameter, in which the fluid impedances were 330 Ω/mm, the ground currents were much more localized to the stimulus site and monotonic.

The ground currents in the cochlea for stimulation of A1 were quite well localized because the electrode design meant that electrodes C1–C5 had larger surface areas than C6–C9 but also because manufacturing variations led to significant impedance increases from C1–C3.

These findings are interesting for a number of reasons. First, we know from psychophysical results with the implant electrode that stimulation of separate populations of auditory nerve fibers was possible with the pseudobipolar electrode.[8] Although the ground current distribution was widespread,

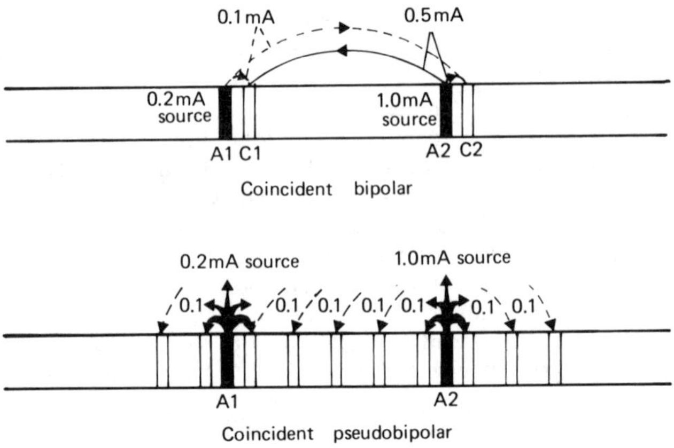

FIGURE 7. Ground current diagram for coincident stimulation with bipolar and pseudobipolar electrodes.

local excitation was nevertheless possible because the total current density in the region of the active electrode was much greater than elsewhere. Second, the results indicate that if we are to use coincident stimulation, the high ground electrode impedance will result in interaction of the stimulus currents. This will, however, be less for pseudobipolar stimulation than for bipolar stimulation (FIG. 7). In the case of coincident bipolar stimulation, ground currents have been measured to be approximately equal. Therefore, coincident stimulation of 0.2 mA from active electrode A1 and 1.0 mA from active electrode A2 means that the excitation at A1 will be due largely to the ground current from electrode A2, but will be less in the case of pseudobipolar stimulation where the currents in the ground electrodes are widely distributed over a large number of ground electrodes and therefore smaller.

SALINE-SOLUTION-FILLED TUBE MODELS OF CURRENT DISTRIBUTIONS FOR SINGLE- AND SIMULTANEOUS MULTIPLE-ELECTRODE STIMULATION

The current distribution around bipolar and pseudobipolar electrodes in a 5-mm (diameter) tube filled with saline solution were also calculated from voltage measurements recorded in the saline solution. While these results cannot be extrapolated quantitatively to the situation of cochlear stimulation, qualitative insight is obtained.

The radial and longitudinal current components for pseudobipolar stimulation using only four ground electrodes are shown in FIGURE 8. The measurements were made 0.5 mm from the array surface. It can be seen that the longitudinal current changes direction, as would be expected over the active electrode, and as is also evident over the right ground electrode, which returned a disproportionately large amount of current. In addition to the radial current maximum situated over the active electrode, radial sink currents are observed over each common electrode. If there is a large number of ground electrodes, these radial currents will not be excitatory since they decrease in proportion to the number of ground electrodes.

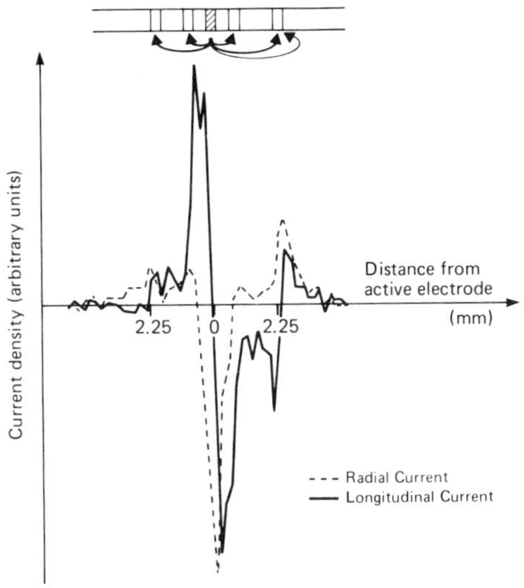

FIGURE 8. Radial and longitudinal current distributions for a pseudobipolar electrode of only four ground electrodes.

The total current distributions for bipolar stimulation and pseudobipolar stimulation with an electrode containing ten ground electrodes were also measured (FIG. 9), and it can be noted that over a 6–10-dB dynamic range, which is the normal operating range of the cochlear implant with this electrode type, the current distributions were similar. The total current distribution for coincident stimulation of two active electrodes was also measured for this array (FIG. 10). Cancellation of the current between the two stimulus maxima

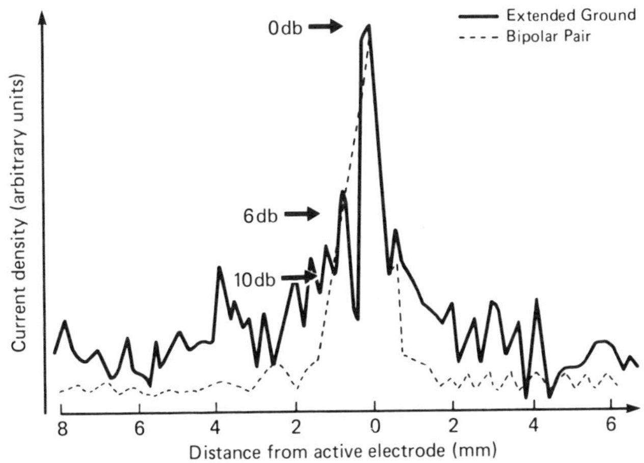

FIGURE 9. The total current distribution for bipolar and pseudobipolar stimulation with an electrode containing ten ground electrodes.

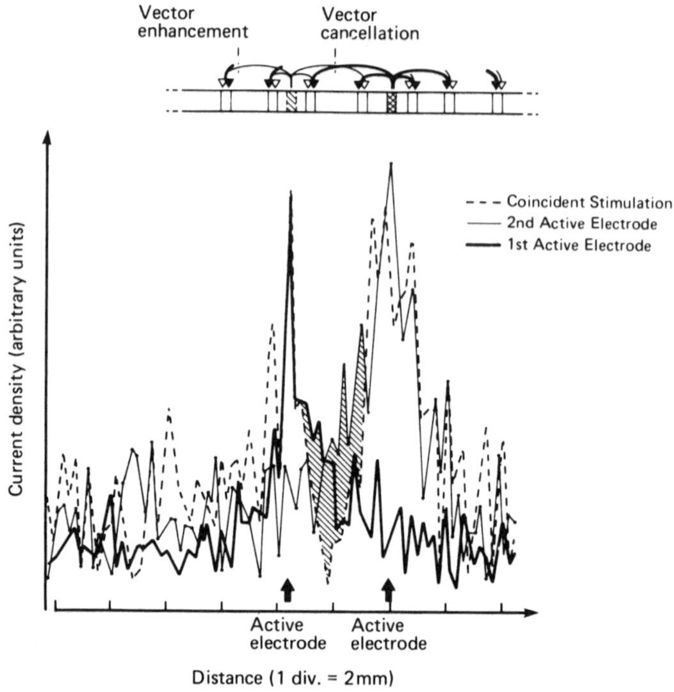

FIGURE 10. The total current distribution around a pseudobipolar electrode for coincident stimulation of two electrodes with equal currents.

occurred, with some summation at the outside edges, resulting in increased stimulus separation. This result is presumed to arise mainly from the ground current moving in opposite directions between the active electrodes, and in the same direction outside this region. These effects will, however, be less significant for unequal currents because cancellation will then be incomplete. The findings should also largely be true for bipolar stimulation.

SUMMARY

Animal experimental studies have shown length constants of 2–4 mm for bipolar and 8–16 mm for monopolar stimulations. Studies in models using saline-solution-filled tubes have allowed us to examine the radial and longitudinal current distribution for pseudobipolar stimulation and have demonstrated that current localization is the same for bipolar and pseudobipolar stimulation over a 6–10-dB operating range. With coincident pseudobipolar multiple-channel stimulation there was suppression of the current between the stimulus maxima and enhancement at the edges leading to less stimulus interaction. Experiments performed with a pseudobipolar electrode implanted into the human cochlea showed that there was significant spread of current along the ground electrode because the electrode ground impedance was significantly greater than the cochlear tissue impedances. Because this leads to less current returned at each ground electrode, the pseudobipolar array will result in less interaction for coincident stimulation.

ACKNOWLEDGMENTS

We wish to acknowledge the surgical assistance of Dr. Q. Bailey, Dr. B. Pyman and Dr. R. Webb, the assistance of the theatre staff of The Royal Victorian Eye and Ear Hospital, and the technical assistance of Mr. L. Cole and Mr. G. Cook.

REFERENCES

1. BLACK, R. C. & G. M. CLARK. 1980. Differential electrical stimulation of the auditory nerve. J. Acoust. Soc. Am. **67**(3): 868–874.
2. JOHNSTONE, B. M., J. R. JOHNSTONE & I. O. PUGSLEY. 1966. Membrane resistance in endolymphatic walls of the first turn of the guinea pig cochlea. J. Acoust. Soc. Am. **40:** 1398–1404.
3. HONRUBIA, V., D. STRELIOFF & S. T. SITKO. 1976. Physiological basis of cochlear transduction and sensitivity. Ann. Otol. **85:** 697–710.
4. BEKESY, G. 1951. Patterns of electrical resistance in the cochlea. J. Acoust. Soc. Am. **23:** 18–28.
5. STRELIOFF, D. 1973. A computer simulation of the generation and distribution of cochlear potentials. J. Acoust. Soc. Am. **54:** 620–629.
6. MERZENICH, M. M. 1974. Studies on electrical stimulation of the auditory nerve in animals and man: Cochlear implants. *In* The Nervous System, Vol. 3: Human Communication and its Disorders. Raven Press. New York, NY.
7. TONG, Y. C., R. C. BLACK, G. M. CLARK, I. C. FORSTER, J. B. MILLAR, B. J. O'LOUGHLIN & J. F. PATRICK. 1979. A preliminary report on a multiple-channel cochlear implant operation. J. Laryngol. Otol. **93:** 679–695.
8. BLACK, R. C., G. M. CLARK & J. F. PATRICK. 1981. Current distribution measurements within the human cochlea. IEEE Trans. Biomed. Eng. **28:** 721–725.

NEURAL ENCODING OF ELECTRICAL SIGNALS [a]

Ben M. Clopton,[b] Francis A. Spelman, Itzhak Glass,
Bryan E. Pfingst, Josef M. Miller, Peter D. Lawrence,[c]
and Douglas P. Dean [c]

Department of Otolaryngology
Regional Primate Research Center, and
Center for Bioengineering
University of Washington
Seattle, Washington 98195

[c] *Department of Electrical Engineering*
University of British Columbia
Vancouver, British Columbia, Canada

Research on the cochlear prosthesis is increasingly concerned with the nature of sounds that we encounter and how we might encode them for introduction through a cochlear prosthesis. As we progressively define the physiological and technical limitations on extracting, transforming, and introducing information from these sounds in electrical form, the rules relating the electrical waveforms used to drive a prosthesis and afferent neural activity become a central concern to prosthesis operation. These rules act at the interface between local electrical events and the response of neural membranes, giving rise to questions about stimulus encoding as well as the central processing leading to perception and responses.

This is a selective review of published and ongoing research on some topics especially relevant to the encoding of signals presented through a cochlear prosthesis. Its purpose is to summarize in an organized manner information that we view as important for understanding and optimizing prosthesis operation. Data from our laboratories on animal and mathematical models form much of the matrix for the discussion that follows.

OVERVIEW

An organized approach to information transfer from a stimulus voltage waveform to behavioral responses might be represented as a collection of input–output relationships, some as familiar and accessible as the transfer function for a stimulator, and others as complicated and undefined as "central processing." The stimulus waveform is usually a voltage waveform which is the result of sound transformation and processing that is termed "encoding." An effective, practical specification of the stimulus waveform (or in the case of multichannel stimulation, waveforms) is the goal of research on encoding. To be precise, representing this waveform as a voltage is somewhat inappro-

[a] This work was supported by Grants NS 13056 and RR 00166 from the National Institutes of Health and by Grant A 9341 from the Natural Sciences and Engineering Research Council of Canada.

[b] Address for correspondence: Dr. Ben M. Clopton, Department of Otolaryngology RL–30, University of Washington, Seattle, Washington 98195.

0077–8923/83/0405–0146 $01.75/0 © 1983, NYAS

priate since the stimulus parameter most directly related to neural excitation is current (or its integral, charge). Use of a constant-current stimulator whose output current proportionately reflects a stimulus voltage waveform makes this distinction unnecessary, and the impedance of the electrode–tissue interface is removed as a determinant of stimulation effectiveness. The electrode–tissue interface remains, however, as an important site of physical and chemical events that influence the limits of safe stimulation due to the possibility of electrode and tissue damage.

Tissue properties determine the spread of electrical current to the sites of neural excitation. Multiple-current pathways, each characterized by a specific complex impedance, result in unique electrical conditions which affect each neural element. Current spread through the tissues thus determines the spatial pattern of excitation within the neural population. Any distortion of the amplitude-phase characteristics of the stimulus waveform as it is distributed through the tissue will change the temporal structure of the stimulus reaching each neural element.

Current and voltage values in the vicinity of each neural element result in transmembrane voltage differences which are integrated within the neuron to produce a temporal pattern of spike activity traveling toward the cochlear nuclei in the auditory portion of the eighth nerve. The spatial and temporal pattern of this spike activity across the neural population constitutes the information available to the implant patient. Most aspects of central processing under these atypical conditions of stimulation are not understood.

The discussion that follows deals with the major transforms between the stimulus waveform and central processing. These include electrode and tissue properties, transformation of the electrical stimulus to spike activity, and some initial observations on the properties of central processing.

Electrode Properties and Tissue Damage

The primary function of electrodes in a cochlear prosthesis is to allow the production of current densities at sites of neural excitation sufficient to cause neural responses. The determinants of their success are placements relative to neural elements, sizes, service life, and the absence of associated tissue damage or adverse reactions. An absolute limit on stimulus encoding is the charge density at which hydrogen is evolved at the surface of the electrode. This has been estimated at 300 $\mu C/cm^2$ per phase for platinum electrodes in simulated cerebrospinal fluid at 37° C.[1] This limit holds for the real surface area, which invariably exceeds the geometric surface area.[2] In our laboratory, spheres flamed at the ends of 1-mil platinum–iridium wires show real surface areas of approximately 0.001 cm^2 or greater. The gassing limit estimated for this surface area is 6.7 μA rms with 10-Hz stimulation increasing at 6 dB/octave with frequency.[3]

While gassing is an obvious condition to be avoided, stimulation mediated by ionic surrents induced through metal electrodes can have damaging effects on tissues that are presently evident only by their pathologic effect on the surrounding tissues. A recent study[4] of cochlear damage in the guinea pig with scanning electron microscopy found damage after only 3 hours of stimulation at 1 kHz with charge densities as low as 70 $\mu C/cm^2$ per phase. This damage was restricted to the immediate vicinity of the stimulating electrode.

More prolonged stimulation in cats [5] indicates that as little as 40 μC/cm^2 per phase produces histopathologic changes. These observations provide specific frequency and intensity boundaries within which stimulus waveforms might prudently be restrained until more extensive histopathologic observations are available.

Other constraints on waveform parameters must be considered in light of the prevalence of osteogenesis observed in implanted cochleas.[6, 7] It is at present uncertain to what extent bone growth results from tissue damage produced at the time of implantation, tissue reaction from prolonged exposure to implant materials, chemical events at the electrode–tissue interface, or from the electrical currents themselves. Direct-current stimulation, already excluded because of gassing considerations, is known to stimulate bone growth at extremely low current densities,[8] and 60-Hz stimulation has been reported [9] to induce osteogenesis at a charge density of only 1.13 μC/cm^2 per phase. In light of these considerations, stimulus encoding must be accomplished within frequency–intensity limits that at best are mildly, and at worst severely, restrictive.

Tissue Properties and Current Spread in the Cochlea

The electrical architecture of the cochlea has been studied primarily to explain the nature of cochlear potentials and their role in sound transduction. While impedances between the major labyrinthine compartments have been measured,[10, 11] the electrical microstructure governing the current distribution from scalar electrodes is not well defined. Measurement of electrical impedances in the cochlea requires separate stimulation and voltage-sensing electrodes in order to exclude the impedances of the stimulating electrodes. We have implanted pairs of stimulating and sensing electrodes in guinea pigs and some monkeys to measure tissue impedances within the scala tympani and between it and other sites, such as the modiolus and cochlear nuclei. Using both sinusoids and synthesized wideband waveforms, we have observed that tissues of the cochlea and its surroundings are essentially resistive and linear in their current-spread properties.[12, 13] This characterization of the electrical properties may have to be modified as the microstructure is resolved, but it is most accurate presently to consider extracellular current as undergoing an attenuation specific for a pathway to a neural element with little phase shift. Thus, charge and voltage fluctuations at individual neural elements are likely to be highly reflective of waveforms measured in tissue near the stimulating electrode.

A path of relatively low resistance appears to exist between the basal scala tympani and the modiolus, approximately 3 kΩ in the guinea pig. The resistance of the scalar fluids over the 4–5-mm extent of an implant is less than 3 kΩ.[13] Currents introduced between bipolar electrodes thus are shunted to some extent within the fluids of the scala, but significant currents flow in the loop including the modiolus. When currents are manipulated within these pathways by stimulating between the various possible pairs for electrodes at the apical, basal, and modiolar sites, changes in the threshold for evoking tract responses at the brachium of the inferior colliculus are observed. Response thresholds vary most directly with currents flowing in the pathways exiting the scala, especially the basal–modiolar pathway.[14] This indicates that the neural elements being stimulated lie outside the fluid compartment of the scala. Placing bipolar stimulating electrodes nearer the eighth nerve as it approaches the cochlear nuclei or near the nuclei themselves does not result in thresholds as low as with scalar placements,[15] so current spread to the cochlear nuclei is not likely to mediate neural excitation with scalar stimulation. The somas and axons of the cells of the spiral ganglion are implicated.

These observations suggest that a path of low electrical resistance may exist across the bone of the spiral lamina, that is, between the scala tympani and cells of the spiral ganglion. The resistance of this pathway (a few kΩ) stands in contrast to the resistance observed to bound the scala media. These consist of 13 kΩ for the stria vascularis, 24 kΩ for the basilar membrane, and the extreme 40 kΩ for Reissner's membrane.

In summary, there appears to be little distortion of stimulus waveforms due to tissue properties intervening between the electrodes and the sites of neural excitation, but many of the details of current distribution have yet to be worked out. This will require finer electrode placements, a determination of the electrical properties of cochlear structures in greater detail, and possibly the aid of field models based on such information. It is especially important that changes in electrical properties of tissues with pathology and ossification be characterized in order to better understand prosthesis operation in the pathologic ear.

Neural Membranes

In the absence of hair cells, the responses of neural membranes to transmembrane voltage differences induced by electrical stimulation are responsible for transduction. Our observations suggest that many features of CNS physiological responses and behavior with electrical stimulation are probably determined by events at neural membranes. This is illustrated by considering threshold functions in relation to stimulus frequency and intensity. Figure 1 shows threshold functions for three representative single units in the ventral cochlear nucleus from a sample of about 100 that we have studied so far. Units do, indeed, have tuning curves with electrical stimuli. Their greatest sensitivity invariably lies near 100 Hz, and while the sharpness of tuning is significantly less than that of acoustically stimulated units, it is present.

This selectivity for lower-stimulus frequencies is evident in field and tract potentials also. Figure 2 shows threshold functions for field potentials in the anteroventral cochlear nucleus and for tract potentials in the brachium of the inferior colliculus. Both curves were collected using single cycles of sinusoids to minimize the considerable electrical artifact associated with stimulation, but the frequency selectivity for both response relationships is evident and comparable. The stimulus artifact prevented collection of responses at the brachium below 250 Hz, but later, improved artifact suppression allowed a relatively complete response curve at the anteroventral cochlear nucleus.

These data implicate events at the site of spike initiation for imposing a characteristic frequency bias to responses at the primary and secondary levels of brainstem auditory levels with electrical stimulation. In the context of previous work on the responses of neural membranes to electrical stimuli, these results are not surprising. Guttman and Hachmeister[16] have observed

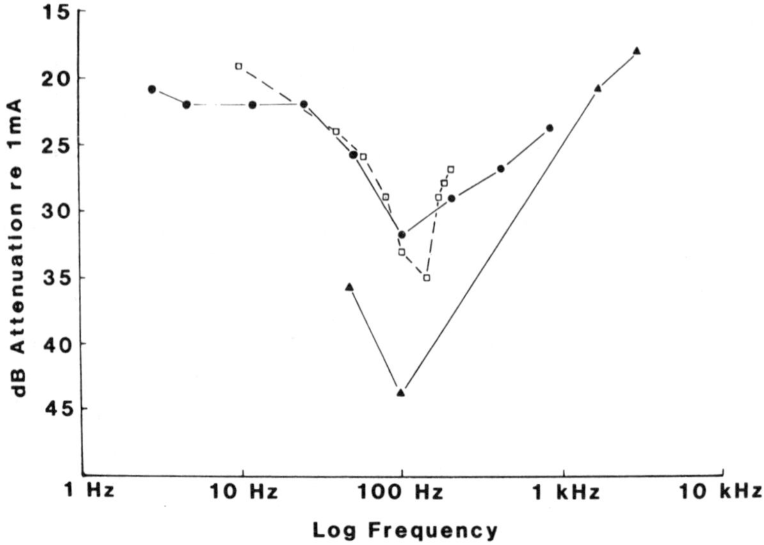

FIGURE 1. Threshold tuning curves of three units in the ventral cochlear nucleus of guinea pig for sinusoidal electrical stimulation through electrodes in the scala tympani. These units are representative of about 100 sampled to date. Stimulation was bipolar between electrodes separated by about 1 mm along the axis of the scala. Single units were isolated with glass microelectrodes introduced vertically into the cochlear nuclei near the entry of the eighth nerve. Threshold criterion was a 10% increase in spike rate over the spontaneous rate.

similar tuning curves for electrical stimulation in squid giant axon. These curves were noticeably affected by experimental variables, such as calcium concentration in the surrounding medium and temperature, but their similarity to our data from the mammalian cochlea is quite reasonable, considering the differences in species, temperature, and other variables. We have observed with middle-ear stimulation that changes in the calcium concentration of fluids bathing the perilymphatic spaces change thresholds for brachial responses above 500 Hz, which is in agreement with the invertebrate work.[17]

Neural membranes have, of course, been intensely studied. In order to compare our results with this line of research and to explore more analytic approaches to the problem of electrical transduction, we have employed a computer implementation of the Frankenhaeuser–Huxley model of the toad nodal membrane.[18, 19] FIGURE 3 shows threshold values for the nerve simulation at 33°, 35°, and 37° C. It must be noted that this model was derived from experimental observations on *Xenopus laevis* (toad), is designed to simulate responses at one node of a myelinated axon, and was extrapolated significantly beyond the temperature range for the original data base. Stimulation through electrodes in the cochlea involves unknown combinations of multiple nodal, somatic, and dendritic membranes. In spite of these qualifications, the nodal model produced tuning curves similar to those from the cochlea except for a higher "best frequency". We are examining the correspondence between the conditions under which the physiological data are collected and the assumptions of the membrane simulation. While such modeling cannot replace physiological observations, it can help us to better place responses to electrical stimuli in a well-established body of knowledge and guide our studies of neural responses to electrical stimulation.

Behavioral Thresholds

Behavioral threshold relationships are available for both human patients and animals performing in psychophysical tasks. Figure 4 displays threshold curves for two monkeys obtained with the reaction-time task.[6] These animals had different survival rates for their populations of spiral ganglion cells. One demonstrated excellent sensitivity and a typical threshold curve for an animal having minimal cell loss. The other shows threshold elevation primarily for

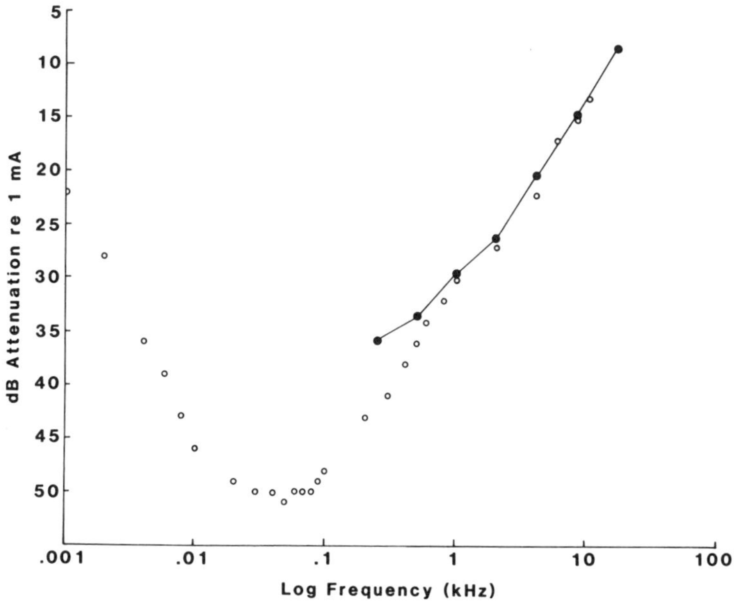

Figure 2. Threshold tuning curves for tract responses at the brachium of the inferior collicuius (*solid circles*) and field potentials in anteroventral cochlear nucleus (*open circles*) in the guinea pig. Stimuli were single cycles of sinusoids delivered to bipolar electrodes on the medial surface of the middle ear (brachial responses) and to a monopolar, saline-agar glass microelectrode resting on the spiral lamina of the first turn in scala tympani with excess perilymph removed (cochlear nucleus). All responses were "waveform-averaged" for 25 to 50 stimulus presentations, and the minimum stimulus intensity for appearance of the response was determined manually using visual criteria for the averaged waveform, a determination that was replicable to within 1 to 2 dB. Lower frequencies were associated with electrical artifacts, which prevented reliable threshold determinations for brachial responses, but improved artifact suppression allowed a complete curve for the field potentials. The brachial curve is the average of responses for five guinea pigs. The curve from the cochlear nucleus is from one animal in which the temperature of the opened cochlea was 32° C.

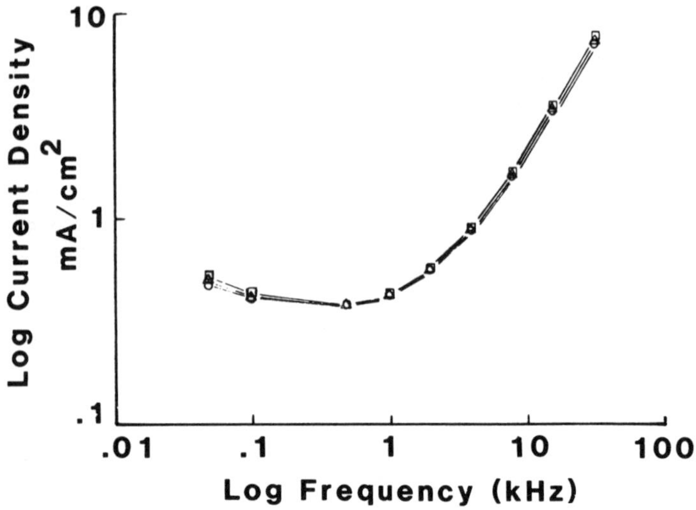

FIGURE 3. Threshold curves for a single-spike response to a single cycle of a sinusoid for a computer simulation of the Frankenhaeuser-Huxley approximation of the nodal membrane of *Xenopus laevis* (African clawed toad).[18, 19] The model was extrapolated to three temperatures near mammalian values: 33° (*circles*), 35° (*triangles*), and 37° C (*squares*). These curves were generated in an initial attempt to compare membrane properties to observed responses from cochlear stimulation. The stimulation was implemented on a PDP 11/23 processor.

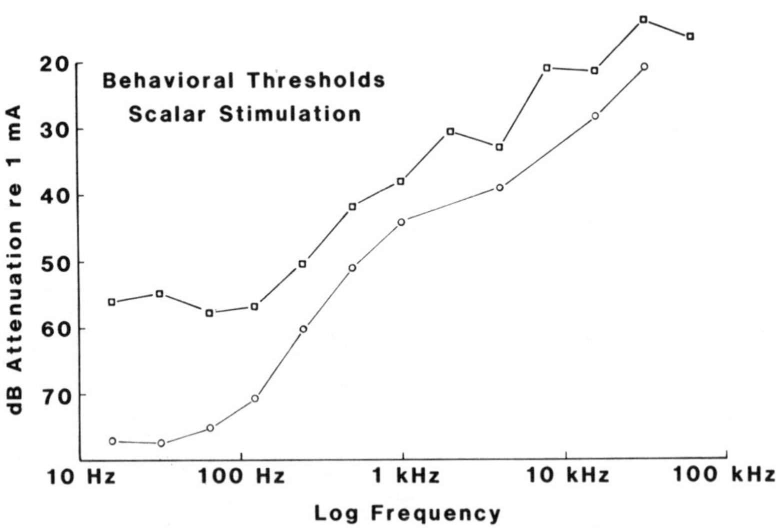

FIGURE 4. Behavioral thresholds for two monkeys performing in a reaction-time task. Stimulation was through a scalar implant using gated sinusoids and bipolar stimulation. The electrodes were separated by approximately 3 mm in both cases. The cochleas differed in histopathology, the more sensitive animal having a greater complement of spiral ganglion cells (see Pfingst and Sutton[6] for details).

low frequencies. These data are comparable to threshold contours observed in some human implant patients.[20, 21] The overall shape and minima of the curves are reminiscent of the neurophysiological and model data described with differences. The minimum threshold range for both curves is rather

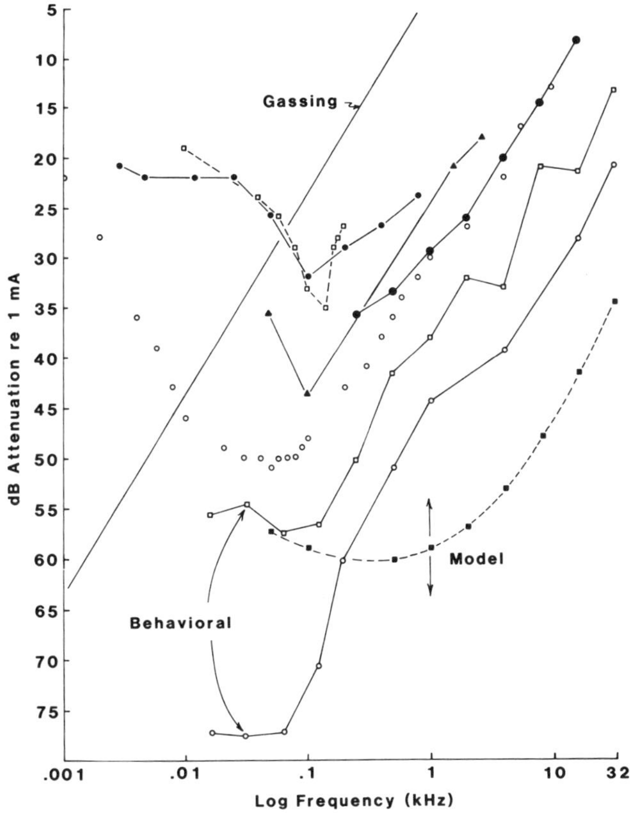

FIGURE 5. Composite graph for all threshold functions discussed to aid comparison. The results from simulation of the toad nodal membrane have been included for 37° C using an arbitrary shift in ordinate values. Gassing limits for a platinum electrode having a real surface area of 0.001 cm^2 are shown to indicate the most conservative upper limit on stimulus intensity. The more sensitive behavioral curve appears to have a range of enhanced sensitivity at low frequencies, but the similarity of all threshold curves is notable, considering the differences in species, stimulation waveforms (single versus multiple cycles of sinusoids), electrode types and placements, histopathology of the cochleas, and other differences.

broad. The slope of the high-frequency limb for the lower curve has a distinct inflection at about 1 kHz with slope differences on either side. Finally, the lower behavioral curve falls significantly below the neurophysiological curves.

In order to facilitate comparisons, the data mentioned to this point have been combined in FIGURE 5. The gassing limits for platinum electrode limits appropriate to our scalar implants have been included. The curve for the Frankenhaeuser–Huxley simulation is shown using an arbitrary ordinate shift. The divergence of the behavioral data for the more sensitive animal is greatest at the low frequencies, but the overall similarities between the general shapes of the curves are apparent. While significant differences need to be resolved between the neurophysiological, the model, and the behavioral thresholds, we submit that the continued investigation of the roles played by peripheral membrane responses is clearly justified by these data.

Temporal Responses

Thresholds provide a convenient basis for the comparisons just discussed, but the introduction of temporally patterned responding in afferent nerve fibers is even more pertinent to stimulus encoding than the limits of responding. We have observed unit responses at the ventral cochlear nucleus to waveforms consisting of sinusoids and the combination of two or five sinusoids.[22] These results again demonstrate response features for electrically evoked neural activity that appears attributable to a nonlinear transform at neural membranes. Figure 6 illustrates that responses of units in the guinea pig cochlear nucleus are quite synchronous to low-frequency electrical sinusoids. Additive combinations of two or five sinusoids evoke spikes primarily near their largest peaks so that the envelope of the stimulus waveform dominates the temporal

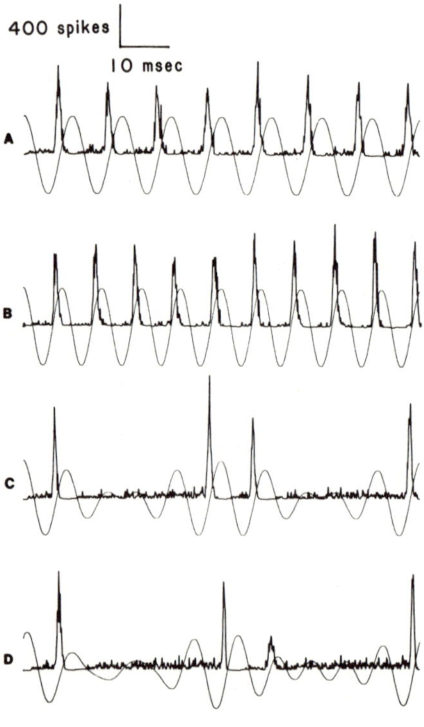

Figure 6. Response histograms for single-unit responses to bipolar stimulation in the scala tympani of guinea pigs. Waveforms consisted of sinusoids (**A** = 97.7 Hz, **B** = 122.1 Hz) or additive combinations of equal-amplitude sinusoids (**C** = 97.7 + 122.1 Hz, **D** = 85.4 + 97.7 + 109.9 + 122.1 + 134.3 Hz). Waveforms are shown as *thin lines.* Each histogram represents 1000 repetitions of the waveform segment shown at an intensity corresponding to 3 dB above the threshold for the waveform in **A.** In contrast to the synchronous responses to every cycle of the individual sinusoids, only the largest peaks of the more complex waveforms evoked spikes. This form of responding held with increased stimulus intensity and after application of neomycin sulfate to destroy structures on the basilar membrane. Neomycin treatment resulted in higher thresholds and narrower peaks in the histogram.

records of the responses. Increases in stimulus intensity do not appear to overcome this pattern of responses. The mechanism for this type of response is probably an alternate depolarization and hyperpolarization of the neural membrane by the stimulating waveform. These low-frequency displacements from the resting potential are opposed by membrane accommodation processes that tend to restore the resting transmembrane voltage. Only stimulus peaks of sufficient size cause threshold to be exceeded and a spike to occur. The result is a rectifier-like nonlinearity which prevents the peak-to-peak periodicities for the frequencies in a narrow-band waveform whose amplitude varies from being faithfully transformed to neural spike patterns. Instead, the higher peaks associated with the period of the envelope of the waveform appear in the response record. A greater knowledge of this process might allow us to effect a more efficient transfer of information from waveform to neural activity, but at present we should be cautious about how we encode speech information for introduction through a cochlear prosthesis. Synchronous neural responding to low-frequency sinusoids does not imply that we can induce temporal patterns in neural firing with low-frequency, narrow-band-filtered speech components that match the frequencies of the speech. The pattern of neural firing will reflect not the frequencies of the speech component that we tried to select with the filter, but the generally lower-frequency envelope waveform determined by the shape of the narrow-band filter that we use and the speech waveform we feed into it. The results demonstrate that the vagaries of membrane responses and neural integration must be dealt with in order to optimally encode stimulus information.

Just as temporal locking has been demonstrated to occur to acoustic stimuli in afferent fibers for sound intensities below thresholds estimated from rate measures,[23] it is possible that temporal features enhance the detection of low-intensity electrical stimuli. For example, a candidate for the augmentation of low-frequency sensitivity is the extraction of temporal information from a population of responding afferent fibers. Using a process such as autocorrelation for the fiber's activity in the afferent array with spontaneous background responding, it is plausible that behavioral detection of electrical sinusoids could occur at levels significantly below those at which our neural measures were affected. In line with this speculation, we have conducted some preliminary behavioral tests designed to reveal any influence of temporal-pattern detection on behavioral thresholds.[24] One group of tests was aimed at removing some of the periodicity from low-frequency sinusoids to determine whether thresholds were raised. FIGURE 7 illustrates that frequency modulation of a low-frequency sinusoid in an attempt to disperse peak-to-peak periodicities did not result in a shift in behavioral threshold. In addition, amplitude modulation of a 4-kHz sinusoid to introduce periodicities at high frequencies through the temporal mechanism that we have just discussed failed to lower the threshold. Thus, we have not yet found support for an explanation, such as a temporal-pattern detector, that might account for the great sensitivity to low electrical frequencies observed for some animals. There are clearly more questions to be explored, but it is becoming easier to ask these questions, if not to answer them.

SUMMARY AND CONCLUSIONS

The transforms discussed are schematically summarized in FIGURE 8. Except for "central processing," the properties of each input–output relationship can be described, some quite accurately and others to at least a first order. Properties from the encoded voltage waveform through the electrode–tissue interface have primarily technical problems associated with them, although the tissue interface itself offers significant opportunity for study. Tissue properties affecting current spread are not yet defined in sufficient detail to allow confidence in designing optimal prosthetic arrangements. The transform from extracellular electrical events to spike activity at neural elements seems to impress very characteristic features on threshold and temporal-pattern observations that we have made. We believe that this step in the stimulus–response pathway deserves continuing attention to allow us to understand and utilize its features most effectively for prosthesis operation. Finally, it is the ability of central processes to interpret these strange signals that we introduce that determines the success of our efforts. Behavioral observations in patients and in animal models must provide the means for understanding this most complex set of problems.

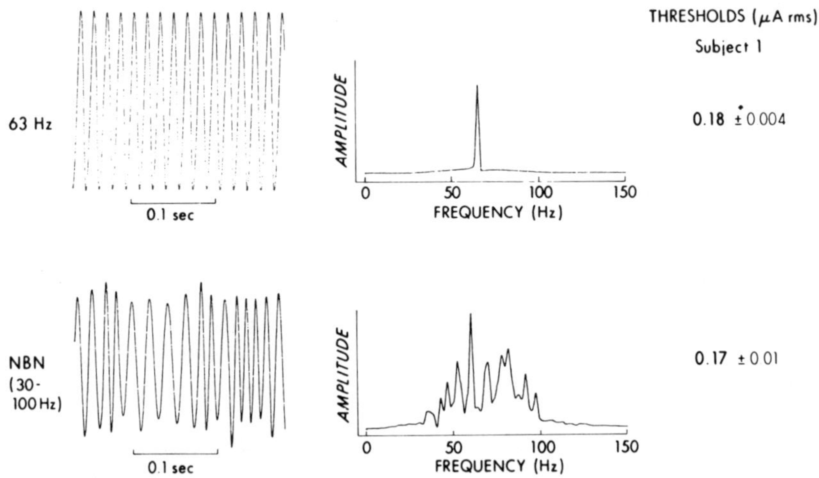

FIGURE 7. Behavioral thresholds for two low-frequency waveforms differing in the uniformity of peak-to-peak intervals. No significant changes in threshold were observed for this experiment designed to determine whether detection of a temporal pattern in afferent spike activity was responsible for enhanced behavioral sensitivity to low-frequency electrical waveforms. The sinusoid (63 Hz) and a semirandomly frequency-modulated sinusoid or narrow-band noise (NBN) centered at 63 Hz were associated with insignificantly different thresholds. In a similar experiment, no difference was observed in thresholds for a 4-kHz sinusoid and the same sinusoid with 50% amplitude modulation at 100 Hz designed to induce low-frequency synchrony in responses to high-frequency stimuli. These observations represent some initial attempts to define contributions of central processing to behavioral thresholds.

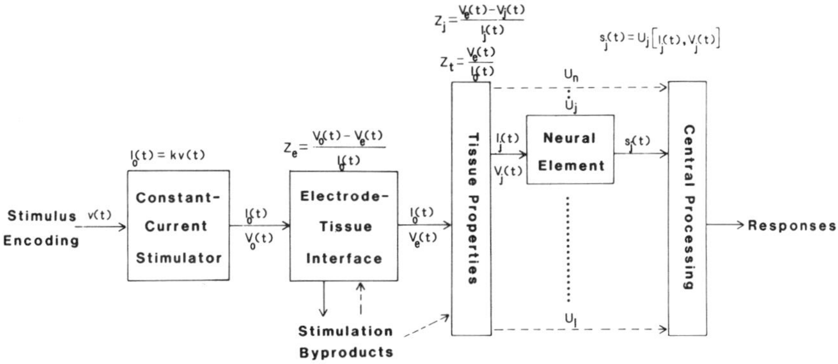

FIGURE 8. Schematic diagram of the transforms discussed in this paper. Values from the encoded stimulus voltage waveform v(t) to the neural element are complex electrically. Complex impedances characterize the electrode–tissue interface and total tissue and single neural element pathways. The constant-current stimulator obviates consideration of the tissue–interface impedance, except for the limits imposed by damage. Tissue properties determining current flow appear to be linear and resistive for first approximations. The transform at the neural element results in a point process representing spike occurrences in afferent fibers. When threshold functions are considered, the transform at the neural element is the primary determinant of the outcome. Nonlinearities at this step also shape responses to temporal aspects of stimulation waveforms. $I_o(t)$, $V_o(t)$ = current and voltage at stimulator output; $V_e(t)$ = voltage in tissue near electrode; Z_e, Z_t, Z_j = impedances for electrode, total tissue, and jth element pathway; $I_j(t)$, $V_j(t)$ = current and voltage at jth neural element; $s_j(t)$ = point process representing spike occurrences of jth element.

ACKNOWLEDGMENT

Parts of the data in this study were processed on the Prophet Network.

REFERENCES

1. BRUMMER, S. B. & M. J. TURNER. 1977. Electrical stimulation with Pt electrodes: II. Estimation of maximum surface redox (theoretical non-gassing) limits. IEEE Trans. Biomed. Eng., BME-**24:** 440–443.
2. BRUMMER, S. B. & M. J. TURNER. 1977. Electrical stimulation with Pt electrodes: I. A method for determination of "real" electrode areas. IEEE Trans. Biomed. Eng., BME-**24:** 436–439.
3. SPELMAN, F. A., B. PFINGST, W. POWERS, J. MILLER, M. HASSUL & B. CLOPTON. 1979. Biophysics of the implanted ear: Electrical parameters. *In* Advances in Prosthetic Devices for the Deaf. D. L. McPherson, Ed.: 312–323. National Technical Institute for the Deaf. Rochester, NY.
4. DUCKERT, L. G. & J. M. MILLER. 1982. Acute morphological changes in guinea pig cochlea following electrical stimulation: A preliminary scanning electron microscope study. Ann. Otol. Rhinol. Laryngol. **91:** 33–40.
5. WALSH, S. M., P. A. LEAKE-JONES, L. VUREK & M. M. MERZENICH. 1980. Effects of chronic electrical stimulation of auditory nerve in the cat. Abstracts of the Midwinter Meeting of the Association for Research in Otolaryngology.

6. Pfingst, B. E. & D. Sutton. Relation of cochlear implant function to histopathology in monkeys. This volume.
7. Johnsson, L. G., W. F. House & F. H. Linthicum. 1979. Bilateral cochlea implants: Histological findings in a pair of temporal bones. Laryngoscope **89:** 759–762.
8. Marino, A. A., J. M. Cullen, R. O. Becker & E. Fukuda. 1981. Electret-induced bone formation in rats. *In* IEEE 1980 Frontiers in Health Care. D. A. Cohen, Ed.: 220. IEEE Press. New York, NY.
9. Hassler, C. R., E. F. Rybicki, R. B. Diegle & L. C. Clark. 1977. Studies of enhanced bone healing via electrical stimuli. Clin. Orthop. **124:** 9.
10. Johnstone, B. M., J. R. Johnstone & I. D. Pugsley. 1966. Membrane resistance in endolymphatic walls of the first turn of the guinea pig cochlea. J. Acoust. Soc. Am. **40:** 1398–1404.
11. Honrubia, V., D. Strelioff & S. Sitko. 1976. Electroanatomy of the cochlea: Its role in cochlear potential measurements. *In* Electrocochleography. R. J. Ruben, C. Elberling & G. Salomon, Eds.: 23–29. University Park Press. Baltimore, MD.
12. Spelman, F. A., B. M. Clopton, B. E. Pfingst & J. M. Miller. 1980. Design of the cochlear prosthesis: Effects of the flow of current in the implanted ear. Ann. Otol. Rhinol. Laryngol. **89** (Suppl. 66): 8–10.
13. Spelman, F. A., B. M. Clopton & B. E. Pfingst. 1982. Tissue impedance and current flow in the implanted ear: Implications for the cochlear prosthesis. Ann. Otol. Rhinol. Laryngol. **91** (Suppl. 98): 3–8.
14. Clopton, B. M. & F. A. Spelman. 1982. Neural mechanisms relevant to the design of an auditory prosthesis: Location and electrical characteristics. Ann. Otol. Rhinol. Laryngol. **91** (Suppl. 98): 9–14.
15. Clopton, B. M., F. A. Spelman & J. M. Miller. 1980. Estimates of essential neural elements for stimulation through a cochlear prosthesis. Ann. Otol. Rhinol. Laryngol. **89** (Suppl. 89): 5–7.
16. Guttman, R. & L. Hachmeister. 1971. Effect of calcium, temperature, and polarizing currents upon alternating current excitation of space-clamped squid axons. J. Gen. Physiol. **58:** 304–321.
17. Clopton, B. M. & M. M. Bosma. 1982. Effectiveness of middle-ear electrical stimulation for activating central auditory pathways. Ann. Otol. Rhinol. Laryngol. **91:** 285–291.
18. Frankenhaeuser, B. & A. F. Huxley. 1964. The action potential in the myelinated nerve fibre of *Xenopus laevis* as computed on the basis of voltage clamp data. J. Physiol. **171:** 302–315.
19. Butikafer, R. & P. D. Lawrence. 1978. Electrocutaneous nerve stimulation: I. Model and experiment. IEEE Trans. Biomed. Eng., BME-**25:** 526–531.
20. Simmons, F. B. 1966. Electrical stimulation of the auditory nerve in man. Arch. Otolaryngol. **84:** 2–54.
21. Eddington, D. K., W. H. Dobelle, D. E. Brackmann, M. G. Mladejovsky & J. L. Parkin. 1978. Auditory prostheses research with multiple channel intracochlear stimulation in man. Ann. Otol. Rhinol. Laryngol. **87** (Suppl 53): 1–39.
22. Clopton, B. M. & I. Glass. 1982. Unit responses at cochlear nucleus to electrical stimuli presented through a cochlear prosthesis. Abstracts of the Midwinter Meeting of the Association for Research in Otolaryngology: 7.
23. Johnson, D. H. 1980. The relationship between spike rate and synchrony in responses of auditory-nerve fibers to single tones. J. Acoust. Soc. Am. **68:** 1115–1122.
24. Pfingst, B. E. & B. M. Clopton. 1982. Detection of complex electrical stimuli. Abstracts of the Midwinter Meeting of the Association for Research in Otolaryngology: 51.

CRITERIA FOR SELECTING ELECTRODES FOR ELECTRICAL STIMULATION: THEORETICAL AND PRACTICAL CONSIDERATIONS

S. B. Brummer and L. S. Robblee

EIC Laboratories, Inc.
Newton, Massachusetts 02158

F. T. Hambrecht

National Institute of Neurological and
Communicative Disorders and Stroke
National Institutes of Health
Bethesda, Maryland 20014

Toxicity of Electrochemical Reactions Associated with Neural Stimulating Electrodes

It is well known that unidirectional stimulus currents through metallic electrodes can result in severe pH shifts in the tissue around the electrodes. These shifts are a result of faradaic (oxidation–reduction) reactions. The use of biphasic stimulus waveforms with zero net charge flow, or "balanced" waveforms as they are often called, does not guarantee that toxic electrochemical reaction products will not be generated and will not leave the surface of the electrodes.

Besides being concerned with local pH shifts, which can cause irreversible changes in tissue proteins, one also has to be wary of metallic dissolution products, gross hydrogen and oxygen gas bubbles, and oxidized organic and inorganic species. Some of the metallic ions, such as cobalt, silver, lead and mercury, are notoriously toxic to neural tissue. The toxicity of platinum is suspected, but has not been conclusively proven. In 1965, Rosenberg [1] noted the inhibition of cell division in bacteria by electrolysis products from a platinum electrode. Subsequent testing of platinum compounds on human tissue culture cells led to the development of new antitumor drugs. One of these, *cis*-platinum, has been reported to be ototoxic,[50] and audiologic monitoring is recommended for all patients on the drug. This report did not include histologic evaluation of the effects on the eighth nerve fibers. Agnew *et al.*[51] evaluated the effects of platinum salts injected into cortical tissue at concentrations equivalent to the levels calculated in tissue from platinum electrode corrosion studies as the result of high-intensity electrical stimulation. Compared with saline control injections, the platinum salts produced significant histologic reactions, including lethal effects on surrounding neurons. The histologic effects resembled in many, but not all, respects the damage seen from high-intensity stimulation through platinum electrodes. For these reasons, as well as to minimize corrosive loss of the platinum electrode, it behooves us to utilize stimulus values that minimize electrode dissolution.

The generation of oxygen or hydrogen is potentially toxic because of both the tissue pH shifts that can accompany the reactions and the tissue-disrup-

0077–8923/83/0405–0159 $01.75/0 © 1983, NYAS

tive effects of gross gas bubbles. However, if the rate of generation is low enough for normal tissue solubility and diffusion to carry the substances, in dissolved form, away from the electrodes, these substances should not be toxic.

Also to be avoided are oxidized inorganic species, such as some of the oxidation products of chlorine, which are strong oxidizing agents. Fortunately, the charge density levels at which they are formed during stimulation through platinum electrodes appear to be high.[33]

The auditory prosthesis is one of the more rapidly developing applications of neural tissue stimulation by means of chronically implanted electrodes. This paper surveys the present state of the electrode–tissue interface. It focuses on electrochemical considerations and how they affect the choice of electrode materials.

Physiological Considerations

The precise mechanisms by which neurons respond to electrical stimulation remain in doubt despite an abundance of phenomenological data on the subject. The difficulty in interpreting these data can be appreciated by considering the idealized case of a single cell that lies in the current path between two electrodes, and thus experiences an electric field. The minimum current needed to trigger an action potential (the "threshold current") will depend both on the electric field vector and on the nature and position of the cell. The field vector at a given point will be a function of electrode geometry and polarity and of electrolyte resistivity. The response will depend on the cell type (myelinated or nonmyelinated), the portion of the cell that experiences the field (dendrite, cell body, or axon), the cell size and conduction velocity, and its orientation with respect to the electric field (for a review, see Ranck [2]).

The interior of a nerve cell is normally maintained at a potential about 75 mV negative to the exterior. An applied field in the opposite direction will tend to depolarize the membrane and trigger an action potential; the associated current flowing through the membrane in the depolarized region is said to be "cathodal." "Anodal" current, on the other hand, will tend to hyperpolarize the membrane and hence inhibit an action potential. (The terms "anodal" and "cathodal" are only indirectly related to the terms "anodic" and "cathodic," which designate the polarity of charge transfer reactions at electrodes [3]. Direct control of anodal or cathodal currents would require that one electrode be placed inside the cell, but this is not usually practical. Instead, a form of indirect control is achieved by manipulating the electric field outside the cell. Thus, there will be points on the cell surface where the external field tends to depolarize the membrane and initiate an action potential. By the same token, there will be points on the surface where the external field will tend to hyperpolarize the membrane and inhibit an action potential. If the degree of hyperpolarization is too great, an action potential generated at the site of depolarization may not be propagated through the hyperpolarized region. This phenomenon may explain why cells near an electrode are often not stimulated, while more distant cells are.[4, 5] Stimulating currents that are at or near threshold are less likely to produce the extreme hyperpolarization effects encountered with higher currents.

In the more complex *in vivo* situation, where electrodes are implanted in or on tissue surfaces, all of the foregoing relationships prevail, but superimposed on them are unknown variables due to the heterogeneity of the tissue. A variety of cell types is present, and different portions of various cells will be in the area of the electric field. Numerous structures and matrices of different ionic composition and resistivities intervene between an electrode and the cells to be stimulated. It is difficult to determine which cells will be stimulated or what a threshold current will be. Consequently, it is usually necessary to employ higher currents than might be used in the ideal case because of the complicated geometry present in the tissue. For cortical electrodes applied to the pial surface, the higher current needed to elicit a response from cells within the cortex may be delivered through electrodes with a high-enough surface area so that the current and charge densities will be at an electrochemically "safe" level, as we shall discuss later. If electrodes are placed within the cortical tissue in close proximity to the cells that are to be stimulated, then smaller currents are adequate,[6] but the small electrode size can mean that current and charge densities are very large.

TABLE 1

EXAMPLES OF CHARGE DENSITIES EMPLOYED IN STIMULATION OF CEREBRAL CORTICAL NEURONS

Electrode Surface Area (cm^2 geometric)	Charge Density ($\mu C/cm^2$ geometric)	Investigator
10^{-2}	30–300	Pudenz *et al.*[10]
$1.3 \cdot 10^{-3}$	600	Marks [11]
$0.5–2 \cdot 10^{-3}$	25–4000	Pollen *et al.*[12]
$0.3–1.6 \cdot 10^{-3}$	100–1800	Doty *et al.*[13]
$1.7 \cdot 10^{-6}$	200–2000	Stoney *et al.*[6]
$0.5 \cdot 10^{-6}$	4000–10,000	Schmidt and McIntosh [14]

APPLICATIONS OF AND REQUIREMENTS FOR ELECTRICAL STIMULATION

Typical charge densities employed in a number of applications, taken from our recent publication [9] are summarized in TABLE 1. We should make it clear that, following the pioneering work of Lilly,[20] the pulse waveforms are always carefully charge-balanced and that the charge densities shown are calculated per half-phase.

The relative importance of a given electrode characteristic varies from one application to another. The stimulation of muscle fibers places a premium on mechanical flexibility, and electrodes of stainless steel are often used for this application.[15] By contrast, cortical stimulation with cortical surface electrodes demands little mechanical strength and pure platinum electrodes are commonly used.[10] Charge densities in this application also tend to be moderate, and Ta/Ta_2O_5 capacitor electrodes have been used successfully.[16–18]

Intracortical stimulation with semimicroelectrodes requires a material which has sufficient mechanical strength to pierce the cortical surface, and yet can support charge densities up to an order of magnitude larger than those required from surface electrodes.[17] An alloy of Pt and Ir was used for these electrodes,[17] but we have seen that traces of Pt and Ir dissolve with typical stimulation regimes.[19] Perhaps the most demanding application of all involves microelectrode stimulation with electrodes the size of single neurons. Stoney *et al.*[6] injected 0.2 msec pulses of 2–20 μA using a glass-insulated W microelectrode that had an exposed surface area of about 1.7×10^{-6} cm^2 (geometric) The charge density for the largest pulse was thus over 2000 μC$\cdot$cm^{-2} geometric. Schmidt and McIntosh[14] have injected similar pulses with even smaller electrodes ($\leq 0.5 \times 10^{-6}$ cm^2 geometric), giving rise to charge densities of up to 10^4 μC$\cdot$cm^{-2} geometric. With metal electrodes, all but a small fraction of this charge must flow through irreversible faradaic reactions, which is not acceptable. As we shall discuss, our most recent work (on Ir for example) is directed at investigation of electrode materials that might be capable of delivering the charge required for intracortical stimulation via *reversible* faradaic reactions.

Electrochemical Considerations

The flow of electric current between an electronic conductor (the metal electrode) and an ionic conductor (the biological medium) requires some type of process at the interface to mediate the change in charge carriers. The nature of processes that may occur at the metal–solution interface can be visualized in terms of a simple "double-layer" model. According to this model, there is generally a net electrostatic charge on the metal surface (governed in a complex manner by the chemistry of the system[21]) and this charge attracts an excess of oppositely charged ions in the solution. To a first approximation, the ions can be assumed to occupy a plane parallel to the electrode, known as the outer Helmholtz plane, or OHP. A layer of oriented water molecules adsorbed on the metal surface acts as a dielectric between the two charged layers and the whole system acts like a parallel plate condenser. An increment of anodic charge, dQ, will make the metal surface more positive, while an equal and opposite change will occur in the ionic charge of the OHP. In the process, the electrode potential, and hence the voltage across the double layer, will rise by an increment dV. (Similarly, the flow of cathodic charge would make the surface less positive, and thus lower the electrode potential). A parameter known as the double-layer capacitance, C_{dl}, is defined by the relationship, $C_{dl} = dQ/dV$. The value of C_{dl} is remarkably large (10–20 μF$\cdot$cm^{-2}) by normal capacitor standards because the dielectric layer is only 1 water molecule thick. However, useful charge injection is typically limited to a few μC$\cdot$cm^{-2} before the equivalent of dielectric breakdown occurs and faradaic reactions begin. Faradaic reactions involve electron transfer across the interface and result in the formation of new chemical species.

The foregoing remarks draw attention to the central importance of electrode surface area in discussions of electrode processes. The *real* area of an electrode is generally larger than the geometric area because (except for a liquid electrode like Hg) the surface is never perfectly smooth. The ratio of real to geometric surface area is referred to as the "roughness factor." For example, a bright mirror-like Pt surface will generally have a roughness factor of 1.3 to 1.4. We must always carefully distinguish between the real and the geometric area. We have described a technique for measuring the real surface areas of smooth Pt electrodes under stimulation conditions.[22]

The scope of possible charge injection processes during electrical stimulation has been analyzed earlier [22, 23] and touched upon by other authors.[24, 25] For the purposes of the present discussion, the processes may be divided into two groups—"reversible" and "irreversible." We define a reversible charge injection process as one that introduces no new species into solution. Reversible charge injection is possible either by a capacitive process (such as double-layer charging) or by *faradaic reactions involving species that remain bound to the electrode surface.* Charge injection by any other faradaic reaction will be at least partially irreversible because some of the products will escape from the electrode surface. Irreversible charge injection can thus lead to cumulative chemical changes that may be harmful to biological tissue. Examples of irreversible reactions include water electrolysis to H_2 or O_2, saline oxidation, metal dissolution, and the oxidation of organic molecules. Examples of reversible faradaic reactions are the oxide formation and H-atom plating reactions that occur on Pt and other noble metals [23] and the proton transfer and valence transitions that occur within a *multilayer* oxide film such as that which can be produced on Ir, Ru and Rh under certain conditions.[26–28]

The individual contributions of the foregoing reactions to charge injection during electrical stimulation will depend strongly on the potentials traversed by the electrode. Thermodynamically, a reaction can proceed anodically only if the electrode reaches potentials more positive than E_0, the "reversible potential" for that reaction. Conversely, the reaction can proceed cathodically only if the electrode potential is less positive than E_0. The values of E_0 for various relevant reactions were listed earlier.[9] However, thermodynamic conditions alone are not sufficient to determine whether or how fast a given reaction will occur. Platinum is a good "electrocatalyst" for many reactions but, even on Pt, organic oxidation reactions (such as glucose oxidation) are very slow—particularly in chloride solution.[29, 30] The contribution of such reactions to charge injection during electrical stimulation is thus likely to be small.

The types of charge injection processes that can occur during a stimulation pulse are illustrated for Pt in FIGURE 1. The data were obtained by applying a single biphasic pulse pair to a Pt bead electrode in 1*N* $HClO_4$ solution and recording the transient response of the electrode potential. Similar results are obtained in neutral saline solution, but the different processes are less clearly resolved. FIGURE 1A shows the potential transient produced by an anodic-first (AF) pulse of $\pm 500\ \mu C \cdot cm^{-2}$, $\pm 32\ mA \cdot cm^{-2}$. FIGURE 1B shows the potential transient produced by a cathodic-first (CF) pulse of the same magnitude. The curves have been divided into a number of regions, according to the main processes that are involved in charge injection. Referring to FIGURE 1A, anodic charge injection begins by capacitive charging of the double layer (DL). After the injection of about 5 $\mu C \cdot cm^{-2}$, oxide formation (OF) becomes the dominant process. Oxygen evolution (O_2E) becomes important when about 300 $\mu C \cdot cm^{-2}$ have been injected and the transient curve begins to level off. Upon reversal of the current, the curve first exhibits an "IR" drop, reflecting the contribution of ohmic losses to the measured potential. Again, a small region of double-layer charging is observed, and then a large region in which Pt oxide (formed in the anodic pulse) is reduced (OR). Once the oxide is totally reduced (after the cathodic injection of about 300 $\mu C \cdot cm^{-2}$), further cathodic charge drives the potential down below its starting point into the region where H-atom plating (HP) occurs. The charge consumed in this region is a measure of the charge "lost" to irreversible reactions (mainly O_2 evolution) in the anodic half of the pulse. A number of other reactions may also occur during the biphasic pulse (for example, Pt dissolution or O_2 reduction), but their contribution is too small to show up in this fast potential transient.

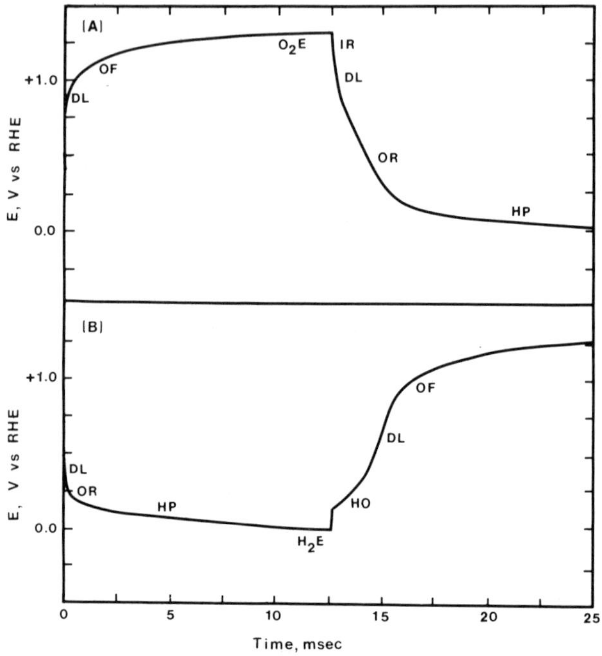

FIGURE 1. (**A**) Potential transient during anodic-first biphasic pulsing at $\pm$ 500 $\mu C \cdot cm^{-2}$. (**B**) Potential transient during cathodic-first biphasic pulsing at $\pm$ 500 $\mu C \cdot cm^{-2}$.

The response of the electrode potential to a cathodic-first pulse (FIG. 1B) has many features in common with the anodic-first transient. Thus, there are regions of double-layer charging and an "IR drop" at the point of current reversal. On the cathodic half of the pulse, double-layer charging is followed by oxide reduction, H-atom plating, and then H_2 evolution. On the anodic half of the pulse, the monolayer of H-atoms is first reoxidized (HO), and then double-layer charging and oxide formation occur. Charge that was "lost" to the irreversible process of H_2 evolution in the cathodic half of the pulse is made up by extra Pt-oxide formation and eventually by some O_2 evolution. Consideration of these potential transients indicates that *the charge limits before H_2 or O_2 evolution would be extended if it were possible to inject more charge via surface reactions.*

In both AF and CF transients, the onset of an irreversible faradaic reaction (O_2 or H_2 evolution) is accompanied by a tendency for the potential to level off, that is, become independent of charge. It has been suggested that the appearance of a region where potential becomes independent of charge can be used as an *in vivo* criterion for irreversible charge injection.[31] It is certainly true that such an "ohmic" response would signal irreversible charge injection and should, therefore, be avoided. However, the absence of "ohmic" regions in the potential transient is not sufficient to ensure reversible charge injection. For example, O_2 evolution begins before the anodic transient levels off (FIG. 1A) and several minor reactions (metal dissolution, for example) may occur without any discernible effect on the transient. Bergveld's criterion [31] is thus likely to overestimate the limits for reversible charge injection. The correct approach is to establish the reversible limits directly, by microscopic examination of the electrodes and by analysis of the fluid medium for the products of faradaic reactions.

With these concepts in mind, we now briefly summarize results for the most widely used noble metal electrode, Pt. Platinum is too soft to be used in its pure form as a penetrating cortical microelectrode. Furthermore, it dissolves slightly under stimulation conditions. Preliminary data for Ir, a very hard and corrosion-resistant metal, are also presented. They suggest that it may be the ideal, all-purpose noble metal electrode for stimulation. An alternative concept, the use of dielectric film capacitor electrodes, is illustrated with data on Ta/Ta_2O_5, the most developed material in the class.

PLATINUM: THE NOBLE METAL OF CHOICE

Platinum is the noble metal of choice of most workers. We have reported on it previously.[9, 22, 23, 32-36] Here, we only summarize our final conclusions.

- Water electrolysis begins after 300 $\mu C \cdot cm^{-2}$ real/half phase,[22, 32] but actual gas bubbling does not occur below 400 $\mu C \cdot cm^{-2}$ real/half phase.

- Saline oxidation was not detected.[35]

- Metal dissolution is only a minor charge admittance process in inorganic saline solution.[33, 35, 37] In the presence of protein, which inhibits dissolution,[34] Pt dissolution is even more minor, constituting often only a few parts per million of the applied current. Dissolved Pt is toxic, however,[43, 50, 51] and it does appear to be an inevitable consequence of use of the metal in stimulation regimes.[34]

- To minimize Pt dissolution in applications that must use large charge densities (≥ 400 $\mu C \cdot cm^{-2}$ real), we suggest the following waveforms:

1. For monopolar stimulation with charge-balanced biphasic pulses:

   Symmetrical[a] AF pulses—short duration ($\lesssim 1$ msec).
   Symmetrical CF pulses—long duration ($\gtrsim 4$ msec).
   Asymmetrical AF or CF pulses—first half-pulse of short duration; second half longer than first.

[a] Symmetrical refers to biphasic stimuli in which the magnitude of the current density in the first pulse of the biphasic pair is the same as in the second pulse. This is not true for asymmetrical charge-balanced biphasic pulses.

2. For bipolar stimulation with charge-balanced biphasic pulses:

   Asymmetrical AF or CF pulses—first half-pulse of short duration; second half longer than first.

Monophasic capacitively coupled pulses might be considered to be electrically equivalent to an asymmetrical biphasic pulse pair, in which case a short-current pulse (either polarity) followed by a long capacitive discharge might produce the same effect on dissolution as a long applied current pulse in the second half of a biphasic pulse pair.

Activated Iridium: A Noble Metal for the Future

It is clear that alternatives to Pt are needed since both its electrochemical and mechanical properties are not adequate, especially for very small ($<10^{-4}$ cm^2) electrodes). Pure Ir is a hard metal, and its mechanical properties are such that it can meet physical requirements for an intracortical electrode of small size and great strength.[38] Iridium also has electrochemical properties favorable for projected use as an intracortical electrode. When appropriately treated, that is, "activated," it can store large amounts of coulombic charge in the form of reversible surface oxides.[39–41] This should enhance the limits of reversible charge injection. Moreover, it has excellent resistance to corrosive attack by chloride ions, as evidenced by its use as a dimensionally stable anode for Cl_2 evolution.[42]

Ir may be activated by repetitive cycling of the potential between 0 and 1.5V versus RHE in 0.1–1.0M H_2SO_4 [26, 27, 39–41] and in buffered saline solution at pH 7.[7, 8] This treatment results in a progressive development of three, large current peaks in the oxide region above 0.4V versus RHE. These current peaks are due to highly reversible proton transfer reactions and valence transitions within the oxide layer.[26, 41] Because of these reactions, the charge capacity of activated Ir, in the potential range 0.4–1.5 V versus RHE, may be up to 100 times greater than that of untreated Ir.

Preliminary data with activated Ir show great promise.[7, 8] We find that Ir can be readily activated at pH 7 and that it remains activated throughout 7 days of biphasic pulsing in protein-containing saline solution with 800 $\mu C \cdot cm^{-2}$ at 800 $mA \cdot cm^{-2}$. Metal dissolution under these conditions is very small: With AF pulses, the dissolution rate is 0.0 ± 0.1 $ng \cdot C^{-1}$; with CF pulses, it is only 0.8–1.0 $ng \cdot C^{-1}$. In contrast, Pt shows 6–7 $ng \cdot C^{-1}$ and Pt:30% Ir, 1–10 $ng \cdot C^{-1}$ Pt and 0.1–6 $ng \cdot C^{-1}$ Ir at the same current and charge densities. Furthermore, activation of the Ir surface extends the useful charge-injection limits before gassing for anodic pulses by a factor of 10 compared with untreated Ir or Pt:30% Ir. Gassing limits for activated Ir are as high as 40 $mC \cdot cm^{-2}$.

Research on activated Ir is continuing apace. It appears to be an excellent charge-injection electrode.

Nonfaradaic (Capacitor) Electrodes

The idea behind capacitor stimulation electrodes is to introduce a dielectric at the electrode–solution interface that will withstand substantial voltages without leakage, and hence allow charge flow without the risk of faradaic reactions.[16, 44] An early attempt to apply this principle was made by Mauro,[45] who employed Teflon®-insulated wire. The low dielectric constant of Teflon ($\epsilon \sim 2$) and the substantial thickness needed to ensure freedom from pinholes resulted in a very small capacitance in a rather large volume.

A more practical approach is to exploit the type of metal/oxide combination used in electrolytic capacitors. The need for corrosion-resistance as well as a high-quality dielectric film pointed towards anodized Ta as a material of choice. Schaldach[46] demonstrated the feasibility of using anodized Ta for electrical stimulation, but the capacitance of his wire electrode was relatively small. Guyton and Hambrecht[16, 44] improved upon Schaldach's electrode by taking advantage of technology developed in the capacitor industry. Their electrode was made by anodizing a porous disc of sintered Ta powder. This resulted in an electrode having an effective surface area many times greater than the geometric area of 0.8 mm^2 so that stimulation charge densities of up to 250 μC/cm^2 (geometric) could be applied successfully. The feasibility of using sintered Ta powder for electrodes smaller than those of Guyton and Hambrecht (geometric area $\sim$0.16 mm^2) has been demonstrated in our laboratory at EIC and by others at Giner, Inc.[47] using two different methods for applying the Ta powder in small quantity. A volumetric charge-storage capability comparable to that of Ta powder has also been obtained by electrolytic etching of Ta wire. We favor this method because it does not require high-temperature fabrication techniques. Also, the method is applicable to the fabrication of very small electrodes.

Our data were summarized in a recent publication.[48] Fine Ta wire (0.25-mm diameter) was etched electrolytically in methanolic NH_4Br containing 1.5 wt% H_2O. Conical tips with a length of $\sim$0.5 mm and shaft diameters ranging from 0.10–0.16 mm were produced. Electrodes were anodized to 10 volts (versus saturated calomel electrode [SCE]) in 0.1 vol % H_3PO_4. The capacitance values normalized to geometric area of etched electrodes ranged from 0.13–0.33 $\mu F \cdot mm^{-2}$. Comparisons of these values to the capacitance of "smooth" Ta anodized to 10 volts (0.011 $\mu F \cdot mm^{-2}$) indicated that the degree of surface enhancement, or etch ratio, was 12–30. The surface roughness was confirmed by scanning electron microscopy studies, which revealed an intricate array of irregularly shaped surface projections about 1–2 μm wide.

The etched electrodes were capable of delivering 0.06–0.1 μC of charge with 0.1-msec pulses at a pulse repetition rate of 400 Hz when operated at 50% of the anodization voltage. This quantity of charge corresponded to volumetric charge densities of 20–30 $\mu C \cdot mm^{-3}$ and area charge densities of 0.55–0.88 $\mu C \cdot mm^{-2}$. Charge storage was proportionately higher at higher fractional values of the formation voltage. Leakage currents at 5 V were $\sim$2 nA. Neither long-term passive storage (1500 hr) nor extended pulsing time (18 hr) had a deleterious effect on electrode performance.

We estimate that this technology is capable of yielding conical electrodes 0.1 mm in diameter with 0.2-mm tip which can deliver $>$0.02 μC in 0.1 msec at 80% of the formation voltage, which is usually 5 V versus SCE.

Further improvement is required to obtain electrodes an order of magnitude smaller. One approach we have been following[49] is to use Ti/TiO_2. Titanium is biocompatible as the result of the TiO_2 film on its surface. TiO_2 is insulating and has a dielectric constant of 110–117 in the rutile modification as compared with 25 for Ta_2O_5. Thus, for a given metal roughness and oxide thickness, we would obtain four times the capacity of Ta/Ta_2O_5. The two problems we have had to date have been to obtain sufficient roughening of Ti by etching and to minimize the leakage currents, which are higher than those of Ta/Ta_2O_5.

An even more exciting possibility that we are exploring is to use the ferroelectric $BaTiO_3$.[49] This material has a dielectric constant in excess of 1000.

Summary

Smaller, more charge-intensive electrodes are needed for "safe" stimulation of the nervous system. In this paper we review critical concepts and the state of the art in electrodes. Control of charge density and charge balance are essential to avoid tissue electrolysis. Chemical criteria for "safe" stimulation are reviewed ("safe" is equated with "chemically reversible"). An example of a safe, but generally impractical, charge-injection process is double-layer charging. The limit here is the onset of irreversible faradaic processes. More charge can be safely injected with so-called "capacitor" electrodes, such as porous intermixtures of Ta/Ta_2O_5. $BaTiO_3$ has excellent dielectric properties and may provide a new generation of capacitor electrodes. Faradaic charge injection is usually partially irreversible since some of the products escape into the solution. With Pt, up to 400 $\mu c/cm^2$ real area can be absorbed by faradaic reactions of surface-adsorbed species, but a small part is lost due to metal dissolution. The surface of "activated" Ir is covered with a multilayer hydrated oxide. Charge injection occurs via rapid valence change within this oxide. Little or no metal dissolution is observed, and gassing limits are not exceeded even under stringent conditions.

References

1. Rosenberg, B., L. VanCamp & T. Drigas. 1965. Inhibition of cell division in *Escherichia coli* by electrolysis products from a platinum electrode. Nature **205:** 698.
2. Ranck, J. B., Jr. 1975. Which elements are excited in electrical stimulation of mammalian central nervous system? Brain Res. **98:** 417.
3. Giese, A. C. 1962. Cell Physiology. Saunders. Philadelphia and London.
4. Katz, B. & R. Miledi. 1965. Propagation of electrical activity in motor nerve terminals. Proc. Roy. Soc. Biol. **161:** 453.
5. Johannson, G. G. 1969. Electrical stimulation of a human ventrolateral-subventro-lateral thalamic target area. II. Combination of different durations of single pulses with peak current just adequate to evoke clinical responses. Acta Physiol. Scand. **72:** 446.
6. Stoney, S. D., Jr., W. D. Thompson & H. Asanuma. 1968. Excitation of pyramidal tract cells by intracortical microstimulation: Effective extent of stimulation current. J. Neurophysiol. **31:** 659.
7. Brummer, S. B., L. S. Robblee & J. L. Lefko. 1981. Evaluation of electrode materials and their electrochemical reactions. 7th, 8th and 9th Quarterly Progress Reports, NINCDS Contract No. N01–NS–9–2315.
8. Robblee, L. S., J. L. Lefko & S. B. Brummer. Activated iridium, an electrode suitable for reversible charge injection into saline solutions. J. Electrochem. Soc. Accepted for publication.

9. LOEB, G. E., J. MCHARDY, E. M. KELLIHER & S. B. BRUMMER. 1982. Neural prostheses. *In* Biocompatibility in Clinical Practice, vol. II. David F. Williams, Ed.: 123–149. CRC Press, Boca Raton, FL.
10. PUDENZ, R. H., W. F. AGNEW & L. A. BULLARA. 1977. Effects of electrical stimulation of brain. Brain Behav. Evol. **14:** 103.
11. MARKS, W. B. 1977. Polarization changes of simulated cortical neurons caused by electrical stimulation at the cortical surfaces. *In* Functional Electrical Stimulation. F. T. Hambrecht and J. B. Reswick, Eds.: 413. Marcel Dekker. New York, NY.
12. POLLEN, D. A., B. W. ANDREWS & J. C. LEVEY. 1977. Electrical stimulation of the visual cortex in man and cat. *In* Functional Electrical Stimulation.[11]: 277.
13. DOTY, R. W., J. R. BARTLETT & W. H. OVERMAN, JR. 1977. Quarterly Progress Report No. 28, April 1–June 30, Visual Prosthesis Contract NIH–70–2279, NINCDS, National Institutes of Health.
14. SCHMIDT, E. & J. MCINTOSH. 1979. Exp. Neurol. **63:** 485.
15. PECKHAM, P. H. & J. T. MORTIMER. 1977. Restoration of hand function in the quadriplegic through electrical stimulation. *In* Functional Electrical Stimulation.[11]: 83.
16. GUYTON, D. L. & F. T. HAMBRECHT. 1974. Theory and design of capacitor electrodes for chronic stimulation. Med. Biol. Eng. **7:** 613.
17. BARTLETT, J. R., R. W. DOTY, B. B. LEE, N. NEGRAO & W. H. OVERMAN. 1977. Deleterious effects of prolonged electrical stimulation of striate cortex in macaques. Brain Behav. Evol. **14:** 46.
18. BERNSTEIN, J. J., J. L. HENCH, P. F. JOHNSON, W. W. DAWSON & G. HUNTER. 1977. Electrical stimulation of the cortex with Ta_2O_5 capacitive electrodes. *In* Functional Electrical Stimulation.[11]: 465.
19. BRUMMER, S. B., L. S. ROBBLEE & J. L. LEFKO. 1981. Evaluation of electrode materials and their electrochemical reactions. 9th Quarterly Progress Report, NINCDS Contract No. N01–NS–9–2315.
20. LILLY, J. C. 1961. *In* Electrical Stimulation of the Brain. D. E. Sheer, Ed.: 60–64. Texas University Press. Dallas, TX.
21. PARSONS, R. 1954. Equilibrium properties of electrified interface. *In* Modern Aspects of Electrochemistry. vol. 1. J. O'M. Bockris, Ed.: 103. Butterworths, London; reprinted 1968 by Plenum Press, New York, NY.
22. BRUMMER, S. B. & M. J. TURNER. 1977. Electrical stimulation with Pt electrodes: I. A method for determination of "real" electrode areas. IEEE Trans-Biomed. Eng. BME-24: 436.
23. BRUMMER, S. B. & M. J. TURNER. 1977. Electrochemical considerations for safe electrical stimulation of the nervous system with platinum electrodes. IEEE Trans. Biomed. Eng. BME-**24:** 59.
24. DYMOND, A. M. 1976. Characteristics of the metal-tissue interface of stimulation electrodes. IEEE Trans. Biomed. Eng. BME-**23:** 274.
25. ZEUTHEN, T. 1978. Potentials and small-signal impedance of platinum microelectrodes *in vivo* and *in vitro*. Med. Biol. Eng. Comp. **16:** 489.
26. RAND, D. A. J. & R. WOODS. 1974. Cyclic voltammetric studies on iridium electrodes in sulphuric acid solutions. Nature of oxygen layer and metal dissolution. Electroanal. Chem. Interfac. Electrochem. **55:** 375.
27. RAND, D. A. J., R. WOODS & D. MICHELL. 1977. Electrochemical and physicochemical studies of oxygen layers on iridium and ruthenium electrodes. *In* Electrode Materials and Processes for Energy Conversion and Storage. J. D. E. McIntyre, S. Srinivasan & F. G. Will, Eds.: 217. The Electrochemical Society. Princeton, NJ.

28. BURKE, L. D. & E. J. M. O'SULLIVAN. 1978. Enhanced oxide growth at a rhodium surface in base under potential cycling conditions. J. Electroanal. Chem. **93:** 11.

29. MARINCIC, L., J. S. SOELDNER, C. K. COLTON, J. GINER & S. MORRIS. 1979. Electrochemical glucose oxidations on a platinized Pt electrode in Krebs-Ringer solution. I. Potentiometric studies. J. Electrochem. Soc. **126:** 43.

30. BREITER, M. W. 1964. Voltammetric study of the inhibition of methanol oxidation on platinum by chloride ion in acid solution. Electrochim. Acta **9:** 827.

31. BERGVELD, P. 1976. Simple test for electrophysiologically tolerable parameters of artificial stimulation. Med. Biol. Eng. **14:** 497.

32. BRUMMER, S. B. & M. J. TURNER. 1977. Electrical stimulation with Pt electrodes: II. Estimation of maximum surface redox (theoretical non-gassing) limits. IEEE Trans. Biomed. Eng. BME-**24:** 440.

33. BRUMMER, S. B., J. MCHARDY & M. J. TURNER. 1977. Electrical stimulation with Pt electrodes: III. Trace analysis for dissolved platinum and other dissolved electrochemical products. Brain Behav. Evolution **14:** 10.

34. ROBBLEE, L. S., J. MCHARDY, J. M. MARSTON & S. B. BRUMMER. 1980. Electrical stimulation with Pt electrodes. V. The effect of protein on Pt dissolution. Biomaterials **1:** 135.

35. MCHARDY, J., L. S. ROBBLEE, J. M. MARSTON & S. B. BRUMMER. 1980. Electrical stimulation with Pt electrodes. IV. Factors influencing Pt dissolution in inorganic saline. Biomaterials **1:** 129.

36. ROBBLEE, L. S., J. L. LEFKO, J. MCHARDY & S. B. BRUMMER. 1982. Electrical stimulation with Pt electrodes, Part VI. The control of metal dissolution. Biomaterials. Submitted for publication.

37. JOHNSON, P. F. & L. L. HENCH. 1977. An *in vitro* analysis of metal electrodes for use in the neural environment. Brain Behav. Evol. **14:** 23.

38. SALCMAN, M. & M. J. BAK. 1976. A new chronic recording intracortical microelectrode. Med. Biol. Eng. **14:** 42.

39. BREITER, M. W. 1967. Mechanism of the formation and reduction of the oxygen layer on Ir in sulphuric acid solution. Z. Phys. Chem. N. F. **52:** 1.

40. OTTEN, J. M. & W. VISSCHER. 1974. The anodic behavior of iridium. II. The oxygen coverage. Electroanal. Chem. Interfac. Electrochem. **55:** 13.

41. ZERBINO, J. O., N. R. DETACCONI & A. J. ARVIA. 1978. The activation and deactivation of iridium electrodes in acid electrolytes. J. Electrochem. Soc. **125:** 1266.

42. ARIKADO, T., C. IWAKURA & H. TAMURA. 1978. Some oxide catalysts for the anodic evolution of chlorine: Reaction mechanism and catalytic activity. Electrochim. Acta **23:** 9.

43. MELIUS, P. & M. E. FRIEDMAN. 1977. Complexes of platinum with polypeptides and proteins. Inorganic Perspectives in Biology & Medicine **1:** 1.

44. GUYTON, D. L. & F. T. HAMBRECHT. 1973. Capacitor electrode stimulates nerve or muscle without oxidation-reduction reactions. Science **181:** 74.

45. MAURO, A. 1960. Science **132:** 356.

46. SCHALDACH, M. 1971. Trans. Am. Soc. Artif. Int. Organs. **17:** 29.

47. —— 1978–1980. Giner, Inc. Development of improved capacitor stimulating electrodes. Quarterly Progress Reports No. 1–7, NINCDS Contract No. N01–NS–8–2300.

48. ROBBLEE, L. S., E. M. KELLIHER, M. E. LANGMUIR, H. VARTANIAN & J. MCHARDY. 1983. Preparation of semi-micro capacitor stimulation electrodes by electrolytic etching of tantalum wire. J. Biomed. Biomat. Res. Accepted for publication.

49. —— 1980–1982. EIC Laboratories, Inc. Development of improved capacitor stimulating electrodes. Quarterly Progress Reports No. 1–4, NINCDS Contract No. N01–NS–8–2356.

50. HELSON, L., E. OKONKWO, L. ANTON & E. CVITKOVIC. 1978. cis-Platinum ototoxicity. Clin. Toxicology **13:** 469.

51. AGNEW, W. F., T. G. H. YUEN & R. H. PUDENZ. 1977. Neuropathological effects of intracerebral platinum salt injections. J. Neuropath. Exp. Neurol. **36:** 533.

Part IV. Electrode Fabrication Techniques

INTRODUCTION

F. Terry Hambrecht

Neural Prosthesis Program
National Institute of Neurological and Communicative Disorders and Stroke
National Institutes of Health
Bethesda, Maryland 20205

Crucial to the development of truly useful cochlear implants is the development of safe, effective electrode arrays which serve as interfaces between auditory nerve fibers and implantable electrical stimulators. The choice of materials for the arrays is dictated by many factors including biocompatibility, mechanical characteristics, electrical properties, stability during long-term exposure to saline environments, and electrochemical behavior during high-charge-density stimulation. The materials that are available were generally developed for other applications and usually are not optimal for use in clinical implants. The choice of electrode contact size must be a compromise between using small electrode surface areas for selectivity of stimulation and using large surface areas to minimize potentially toxic electrochemical reactions. The electrode contact positions in the array will affect the place pitch characteristics of the array. It is generally felt that if a cochlear prosthesis is to be useful as an aid for understanding speech, it should be designed so that most of its contacts are in positions in the cochlea that are innervated by nerve fibers with characteristic frequencies in the same range as human speech. Some electrode arrays have also been designed so that the electrode contacts will be in optimal positions to stimulate the auditory nerve fibers with minimal shunting of the stimulus current through the extracellular fluid. Considerable ingenuity has been demonstrated in the mechanical engineering aspects of electrode arrays to assure the final desired electrode positions while maintaining a flexible array which can be inserted with minimal trauma to cochlear tissues.

The development of electrode arrays, especially multichannel cochlear arrays, is still in its infancy. New materials are being designed specifically for neural prostheses and will be incorporated with new fabrication techniques in future implants. The papers in this section give examples of the present state of the art.

DESIGN AND FABRICATION OF MULTIWIRE SCALA TYMPANI ELECTRODES [a]

Ingeborg J. Hochmair-Desoyer,[b] Erwin S. Hochmair,[b] and K. Burian [c]

[b] *Department of Electrical Engineering*
Technical University of Vienna
A-1040 Vienna, Austria

[c] *Second ENT Department*
University of Vienna
A-1090 Vienna, Austria

INTRODUCTION

A suitable stimulation electrode is a crucial part of an auditory prosthesis for the deaf. A number of different sites for the placement of such electrodes have been suggested and are being investigated. At present, the optimum site for electrode placement is still being discussd. As yet no results have been found that could scientifically demonstrate an advantage of multichannel stimulation versus single-channel stimulation. It will take some time and more experience with both types of systems before this question can be answered.

This report deals with multichannel electrodes that are designed to be inserted into the scala tympani via the round window. Other sites for multichannel electrodes that have been tried or are being used, as well as other approaches into the cochlea, will not be discussed.

The majority of researchers working on multichannel implants prefer the access into the scala tympani via the round window. The main reason for this is the short duration and comparatively small risk of the implant surgery required as compared to methods in which wires are put into the cochlea or close to it from outside its outer wall.

The requirements that a suitable scala tympani electrode must fulfill are similar to the requirements for electrodes of other neuroprostheses. They have to achieve an unknown degree of neuronal selectivity. This task involves adequate geometry of the electrode body and the stimulating areas and the possibility of sufficiently atraumatic placement in close-enough proximity to the excitable structures. If the number of channels exceeds ten and the spacing between electrode contacts has to be less than 1 mm, then thin- or thick-film techniques seem to offer an especially adequate tool for the realization of multichannel stimulation electrodes. Investigators at a number of centers have worked or are working on the design of thin-film electrodes for cochlear prostheses.

Several problems have to be overcome before it will be possible to use modern thin-film techniques for the realization of scala tympani electrodes [1] and to be able to eventually benefit from their lower production costs.

[a] This work was supported by the Austrian Science Research Fund.

0077–8923/83/0405–0173 $01.75/0

The contemporary multichannel scala tympani electrode that can be used for chronic stimulation as part of a cochlear prosthesis is a molded multiwire electrode.

Geometry of the Electrode

The flexible four-channel electrode that is currently used in one version of our cochlear prosthesis (the other version comprises a pair of electrodes that are placed external to the cochlea) is made of eight Teflon®-insulated 90% platinum–10% iridium wires embedded in a body from silicone elastomer. Each wire ends up in a ball within a diameter of 0.35 mm. The balls protrude just very slightly from the carrier. The diameter of the resulting bare areas is 0.25 mm, and the exposed geometric area amounts to approximately 0.06 $mm.^2$ The electrode body is of circular cross section tapering towards the tip. The contact balls are arranged in two rows on opposite sides of the electrode body. The four channels are formed by bipolar pairs of contacts. The distance between contacts forming one channel (Fig. 1) is a compromise between good channel separation and low thresholds. The contacts are arranged in two rows on opposite sides of the electrode body because the electric field should have an azimuthal component in order to reliably reach excitable nerve structures situated within the bony spiral lamina and/or in the spiral ganglion. This field component also guarantees that nerve structures can be excited at acceptable values even if the electrode should twist during insertion. Experience gathered thus far (in X-ray photographs taken postoperatively) shows that unintended twisting of the electrode almost never occurs. Different arrangements of the contacts within the electrode body have been employed in the 13 patients who received intracochlear electrodes. Not only was the distance between contacts varied, but also different connection schemes were tried: Besides a bipolar arrangement of contacts, a field configuration was tried in which every other contact was interconnected, thus forming a "common, intracochlear distributed ground" (see the legend to Figure 1). Unipolar stimulation against a remote ground was also used.

In patients who received an implant that allowed switching between the bipolar and the common-ground configuration just described, it was found that

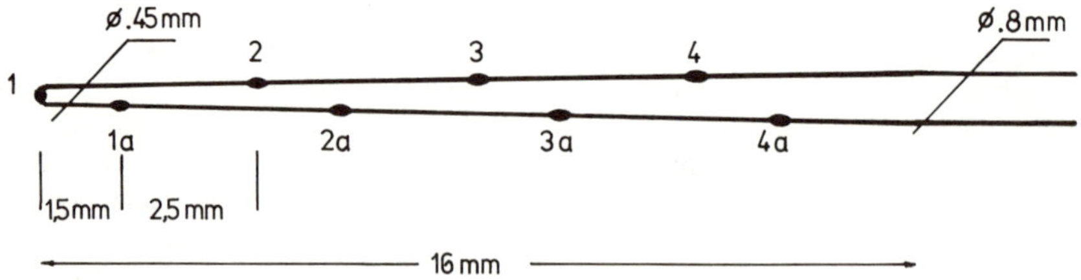

Figure 1. Geometry of the four-channel scala tympani electrode that is currently used. For bipolar stimulation, contacts 1 and 1a, 2 and 2a, 3 and 3a, and 4 and 4a form bipolar pairs. For the "common distributed intracochlear ground" configuration, contacts 1a, 2a, 3a and 4a are interconnected. For unipolar stimulation, contacts 1a, 2a, 3a and 4a are missing, and the remote-ground electrode is fixed to the implanted electronic circuitry.

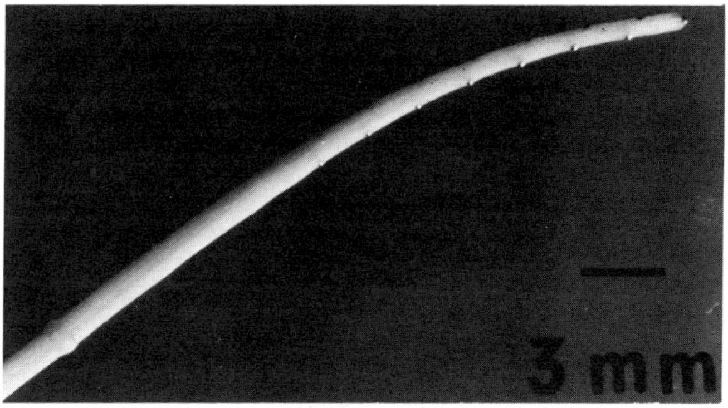

FIGURE 2. Eight-channel version of the molded multiwire electrode.

the threshold in terms of current is a little lower at all frequencies for the common-ground configuration than for the bipolar configuration. The electrical dynamic range is larger in the bipolar configuration. Unipolar stimulation of an electrode contact against a remote ground (for example, on the implanted receiver circuitry itself) results in considerably reduced thresholds as compared with those of the two other configurations. In the small number of patients with whom we could do this, we have not found significant differences in speech-understanding results among the three field configurations (using single-channel stimulation of the best-suited channel).

Six-, eight- (FIG. 2), and twelve-channel versions of this electrode have been constructed.

MECHANICAL PROPERTIES

A scala tympani electrode has to have a geometric shape and mechanical properties that enable the surgeon to place contacts as close to excitable nerve structures as possible and avoid insults to the basilar partition or to the bony spiral lamina.

Currently, two basic mechanical designs exist for molded scala tympani electrodes: First, there are coiled electrodes, the shape of which matches the coiled structure of the human cochlea.[2] These are temporarily straightened before insertion and regain their coiled shape, for which they have a memory, upon insertion. Second, there are straight electrodes, which are very flexible and acquire their adequately coiled shape during insertion.[3, 4] One advantage of a straight electrode is that, in case this becomes necessary, it can be pulled out of the cochlea again (see later). Even if an implantable disconnect system is used, the electrode might have to be pulled out if the disconnect system fails, if the connections between electrode wires and disconnect system fail, or if the electrode wires themselves break.

A straight scala tympani electrode has to be circular in cross section. If it is not, but, for example, resembles the cross section of the scala tympani, it would always tend to bend in such a way that the longer axis of the elliptic cross section (for example) would be parallel with the axis of the cochlea.

Thus, damage to the basilar partition would be very likely. A straight electrode also must not contain any stiff, springy wires, for if it did, atraumatic insertion would not be possible because the electrode would scrape along the outer wall of the cochlea. A straight electrode has to be extremely soft and nonelastic to keep the coiled shape that it acquires during insertion (FIG. 3). If at the tip there is a slight bend in the desired direction, two things are ascertained: (1) The tip does not get "hung up" when it first touches the outer wall of the cochlea after entering straight through the round window and the first part of the basal turn. (2) The bend of the tip also predetermines the direction in which the main body of the electrode bends with respect to the circumferential position of the two contact-rows.

FABRICATION

As opposed to other designs made for insertion into the cochlea, the fabrication of the electrode described in this paper is relatively easy, does not require an unacceptable investment of time, and, in addition, results in electrodes with good reproducibility with respect to geometry and location of electrode contacts within the electrode body.

The most important features of the fabrication process are (1) that the thin wires are knurled and (2) that a guide wire is used. With pacemaker electrodes, the electrode cables are tightly wound around a central wire which is removed afterwards. The electrodes thus are provided with good flexing properties and can also stand stress and movements. A scala tympani electrode, once implanted, does not move inside the cochlea, and if the leads to the implanted circuitry are properly placed and fixed to the bone at several locations, they too do not move extensively. The most critical phase for the wires inside a cochlear implant is the implant surgery. Knurling of the thin platinum–iridium wires guarantees that no extensive stress will be exerted on these wires. The knurled wires with a diameter of 25 μm almost do not contribute to the mechanical properties of the electrode. Since this is the case, they can be distributed at random within the cross section of the electrode (FIG. 4). They need not be within a central canal or tied together as a central wire bundle. The mechanical properties of the electrode are almost entirely determined by the mechanical properties of the one guide wire that is positioned in the center of the electrode body. A small contribution is added by the electrode body itself.

An injection molding technique is used. During this process the contacts are held in place inside the mold by vacuum suction.

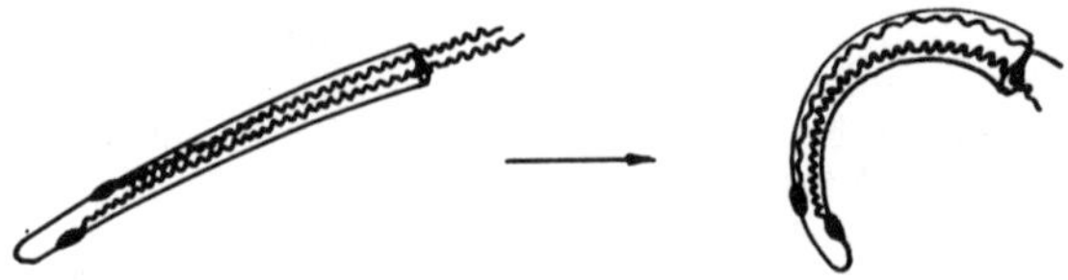

FIGURE 3. Wrinkling of the platinum–iridium wires.

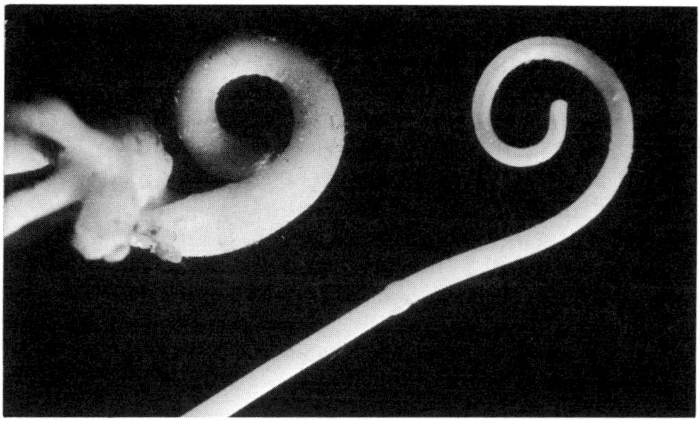

FIGURE 4. Cast of human scala tympani compared with electrode.

EXTENSION OF THE STIMULATING ELECTRIC FIELD

The electric field excited by a dipole source is well known. The other possible electrode configurations are either a special case (unipolar configuration) or a superposition of dipole fields (common-ground configuration). Nevertheless, it is of interest to *measure* the actual fields in order to determine the influence of the electrode body and the influence of the other channels, which, although not excited, *may* lead to slight aberrations of the dipole field.

During the measurements the electrode was driven via the same type of AM receiver that is used in the actual implant. The residual interchannel coupling for two-channel combinations is about −18 dB (less than 5%), and in most cases it is considerably less than that.[5] In either case, this coupling is too small to show up in the plots of the electric field that follow.

The measurement of the electric field strength was performed by a variation of the well-known electrolytic-trough method. The magnitude of the radial, azimuthal, and longitudinal electric field strength ($|E_r|$, $|E_a|$, and $|E_z|$, respectively) was measured in the plane indicated in FIGURE 5. The field was sensed by a small two-contact probe (contact distance: 0.5 mm) which was moved within the plane shown in FIGURE 5 along the z-direction (in parallel with the axis of the electrode).

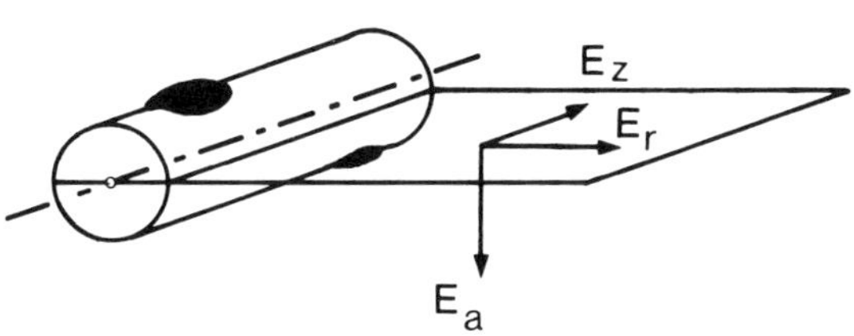

FIGURE 5. Orientation of longitudinal (E_z), radial (E_r), and azimuthal (E_a) components of the electric field. To the *left,* part of the electrode containing two contact balls is shown.

The cochlea is not a homogenous, isotropic medium. Nevertheless, it may be instructive as a first approximation to compare the various field configurations *in vitro*.

Since the output impedance of the receiver is comparatively low (in the order of the electrode impedance), the electrode current is larger in the unipolar and common-ground configurations than in the bipolar configuration by a factor of 1.6 and 1.4, respectively. These factors have to be taken into account and compensated for when using the plots shown here for comparing the electric field strength for the different configurations in the case of an electrode driven by a current source.

FIGURE 6 shows, as a typical example, the radial-field component for three different distances from the electrode axis for a bipolar configuration. In this and in the following figures the magnitude of the particular component of the electric field is plotted versus the distance along the z-direction. Points of polarity changes of the electric field can easily be recognized by the magnitude rapidly approaching zero.

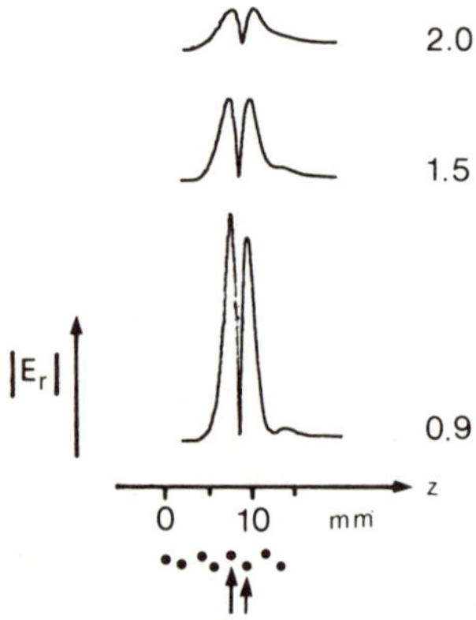

FIGURE 6. Radial-field component in the bipolar configuration for three different distances from the axis of the electrode. These distances are indicated in millimeters to the right of the plots. In this figure and in the following ones, the dots indicate the positions of the electrode contacts along the z-direction. This distance is also indicated in millimeters. The *arrows* indicate the active electrodes.

The extension of the stimulating electric field for different configurations is shown in FIGURES 7 through 10. The plots have been made using a constant AC voltage. If one wants to compare different field configurations at the same loudness, presumably the peak values of the electric-field strength should be normalized to the same level. At the distance of 1.5 mm from the electrode axis (FIG. 7) $|E_z|$ is confined most in the bipolar configuration, whereas $|E_r|$ (FIG. 8) is narrower in the unipolar configuration. In the common-ground configuration the side lobe, although -13 dB down, might influence the percept at louder sensation levels.

In case capacitively coupled monophasic pulses are used, only one polarity (the cathodic part) of the field of the bipolar electrode will stimulate, which makes both the bipolar and the common-ground field configuration narrower than the unipolar field configuration.

$|E_a|$ is compared for the unipolar and the bipolar case only (FIGS. 9 and 10). Especially at larger distances there is no significant difference between the two configurations. $|E_a|$, as defined in FIGURE 5, falls off with distance, of course, more rapidly than r^{-2} for both configurations.

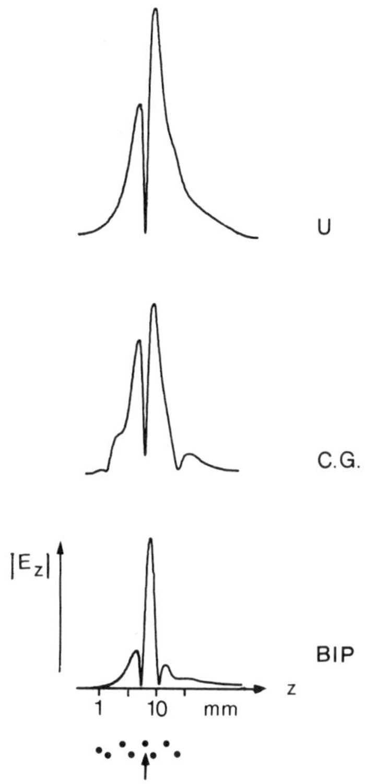

FIGURE 7. Comparison of axial component E_z of the electric field for the following field configurations (from top to bottom): unipolar (U), common-ground (C.G.), and bipolar (BIP). The active electrode(s) are the ones indicated by the *arrow* (U and C.G.) and the next one to the *lower right* (BIP). In the common-ground configuration, the four lower electrode contacts are interconnected to form the common ground. The distance from the electrode axis is 1.5 mm.

A measure for the channel separation can be obtained by the determination of the overlapping area of two such plots, whereby one is shifted by the interchannel distance of 4 mm. It cannot be said that a particular configura-

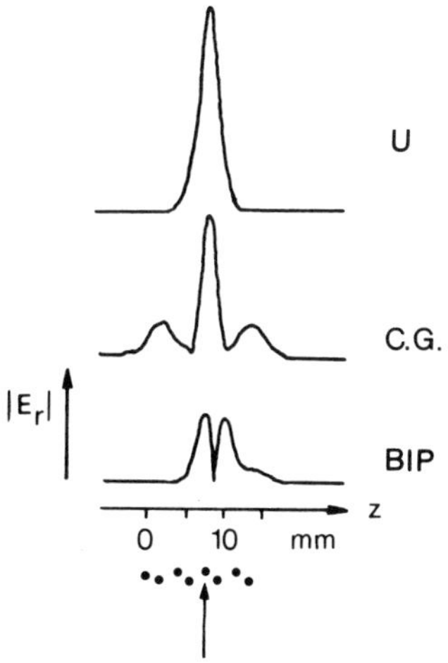

FIGURE 8. Comparison of the radial component E_r of the following electric-field configurations: unipolar (U), common-ground (C.G.), and bipolar (BIP). The vertical scale differs from that of FIGURE 7 by a factor of 2.5. The distance from the electrode axis is 1.5 mm.

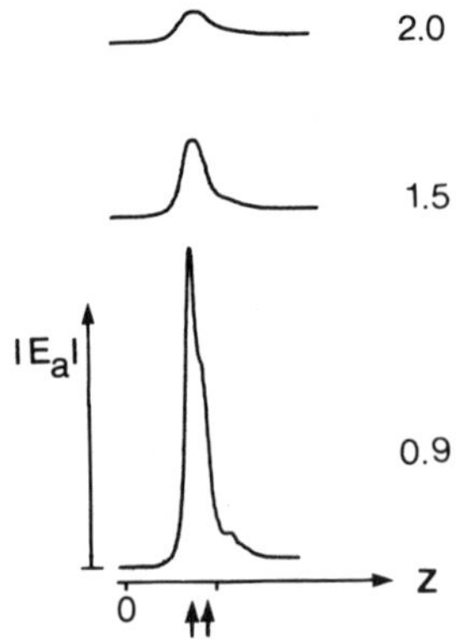

FIGURE 9. Azimuthal component of the electric field for the bipolar configuration measured at three different distances (0.9, 1.5, and 2.0 mm) from the axis of the electrode. The position of the active electrode pair along the z-axis is indicated by *arrows.*

tion shows a considerably better channel separation than another one. The channel separation achieved in a particular configuration depends, among other factors, on the field component parallel to the nerve fibers and on the dynamic range.

Since a nerve fiber is mainly excited by longitudinal fields, the component relevant for the electric stimulation of the auditory nerve depends on the orientation of the fibers. Stimulation by radial and/or azimuthal components seems to be more likely than by the longitudinal component.

At this time it is difficult to correlate these field configurations with results of psychoelectric measurements. Nevertheless some general remarks can be made. It is possible to obtain an estimate for the distance from the electrode to excitable nerve structures by comparing unipolar and bipolar thresholds. Since, except for aberrations of the near field, the electric field strength in the unipolar case falls off with distance r from the electrode axis by r^{-2}, and in the bipolar case by r^{-3}, differences in thresholds expressed as the stimulation

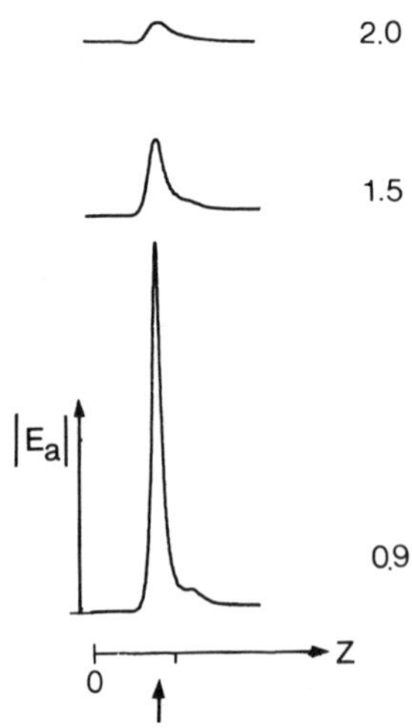

FIGURE 10. Azimuthal component E_a of the electric field for the unipolar configuration measured at three different distances (0.9, 1.5, and 2.0 mm) from the axis of the electrode. The position of the active electrode along the z-axis is indicated by an *arrow*.

current necessary for threshold sensation will occur for distances to nerve fibers greater than the width of the bipolar pair.

A different, although somewhat indirect, method to determine this distance is to correlate results of masking experiments to the extension of the electric field in z-direction.

Experience with Patients

So far thirteen deaf patients have received an intracochlear six, eight-, or four-channel electrode. The electrodes could be inserted for between 14 and 25 mm. Results on speech understanding and on psychophysical performance can be found in Hochmair-Desoyer *et al.*[6, 7]

Several conclusions regarding the electrode can be drawn from the experience with patients:

1. With the exception of two patients, both of whom had trauma to the head, it is practically impossible to evoke percepts other than auditory ones through electrical stimulation. This holds true for the entire dynamic range up to occasionally used amplitudes that are above the "uncomfortable listening level," for the whole frequency range from 50 Hz to 3.5 kHz that is normally used, and also for any higher frequency that has occasionally been used. If there is any connection between insertion damage and side effects of stimulation, this experience would suggest that no extensive damage did occur during insertion.
2. In all of our patients who use their sound processor, we see permanent improvement in performance. This is true for results on psychophysical tests as well as for communication abilities. No patient's performance has reached its "saturation" point yet. In none of the patients has any deterioration occurred that could be a sign of a "physiological failure" of a cochlear prosthesis. (The term "physiological failure" was used by skeptics who also suggested that the performance of a cochlear prosthesis could deteriorate with time due to a continuous degeneration of excitable nervous structures until electric stimulation stops causing sound sensations at all.) Thus far we have seen no such effect. If there was a substantial change in subjective loudness that could be evoked at a certain stimulus amplitude, this could be traced to a degraded electronic component or to an electrode that slipped out of the cochlea. In the majority of patients, threshold as well as suprathreshold loudness estimates versus stimulus amplitude stay constant over long periods of time.[8]

The Possibility of Revision Surgery

So far, one revision operation has been performed in a patient who had had a cochlear implant for 20 months. The scala tympani electrode was taken out and a new electrode of the same design was easily inserted. The new system works well again. None of the results of psychophysical or speech-understanding measurements after reimplantation had gotten worse; indeed, most of them had improved, such as the understanding of words and sentences without the additional help of lipreading.[8] This demonstrates that: (1) there is no extensive formation of new bone caused by either the initial insertion or by chronic electrical stimulation (as verified during revision surgery) and (2) the reinsertion of an electrode caused no further damage of a kind that would have manifested itself in the psychophysical or speech-understanding results.

The explanted electrode was carefully inspected for signs of electrolysis, increased roughness of contacts, or changes in color or anything else. No changes could be found through either light microscopy or scanning electron microscopy.[8] Other techniques will be used to try to study the material composition at the surface of the electrode.

References

1. White, R. L., L. A. Roberts, N. E. Cotter & O.-H. Kwon. 1983. Thin-film cochlear electrodes. This volume.
2. Merzenich, M. M., D. N. Schindler & M. W. White. 1974. Feasibility of multichannel scala tympani stimulation. Laryngoscope **LXXXIV:** 1887–1893.
3. Clark, G. M., J. F. Patrick & Q. Bailey. 1979. A cochlear implant round window electrode array. J. Laryngol. Otol. **93:** 107–109.
4. Hochmair-Desoyer, I. J. & E. S. Hochmair. 1980. An eight-channel scala tympani electrode for auditory prostheses. IEEE Trans. Biomed. Eng. BME-**27:** 44–50.
5. Hochmair, E. S. & I. J. Hochmair-Desoyer. 1983. Percepts elicited by different speech-coding strategies. This volume.
6. Hochmair-Desoyer, I. J., E. S. Hochmair & K. Burian. 1981. Four years of experience with cochlear prostheses: A review. Med. Progr. Technol. **8:** 107–119.
7. Hochmair-Desoyer, I. J., E. S. Hochmair, K. Burian & H. K. Stiglbrunner. 1983. Percepts from the Vienna cochlear implant. This volume.
8. Hochmair-Desoyer, I. J., K. Burian & E. S. Hochmair. 1983. Reimplantation of a molded scala tympani electrode. Psychophysical and speech understanding results. In preparation.

THIN-FILM ELECTRODE FABRICATION TECHNIQUES [a]

Robert L. White, Lester A. Roberts, Neil E. Cotter,
and Oh-Hyun Kwon

Department of Electrical Engineering
Stanford University
Stanford, California 94305

INTRODUCTION

It has been recognized for a number of years that the very high dimensional control characteristic of photolithographic technology makes it an attractive technique for the fabrication of the small multielectrode stimulation arrays required for complex neural prostheses such as the cochlear prosthesis. The dimensional resolution of planar photolithography is, in fact, considerably higher than is required by current cochlear prosthesis designs; alone of current electrode fabrication technologies, planar photolithography is extensible to further generations of prostheses, where denser arrays of smaller electrodes will allow more sophisticated and finer-scale control of neural stimulation patterns.

The minimum size of current cochlear stimulation electrodes is determined by the requirement that each electrode individually be capable of producing an auditory perception above threshold and, ideally, extending to maximum comfortable loudness. This requirement translates roughly into the requirement that the stimulation electrode be capable of delivering approximately 100 nanocoulombs of charge per phase of a charge-balanced stimulus, pulsatile or sinusoidal. On the other hand, the charge delivered per unit area per phase, or the current delivered per unit area per phase, are both limited by the ability of the metal to deliver charge without electrolysis and the ability of the neural tissue to accept such charge and current without irreversible damage. These two constraints differ. Careful electrochemical studies of platinum and iridium as biostimulation electrodes [1,2] set the electrolytic limit at something like 300 μC/phase per cm^2. The thresholds for (long-term) tissue damage are not yet as clearly established, but appear to be on the order of 100 μC/phase per cm^2 or perhaps less.[3] To keep charge and current densities within acceptable limits, the electrode area must therefore be on the order of 10^{-3} cm^2 or approximately 300 μm $\times$ 300 μm. For photolithographic fabrication, 10-μm resolution is easy to obtain, 5-μm resolution is routinely achieved in production circumstances, and that of 1 μm is achievable using advanced but presently available technology. The dimensional control capability of photolithographic fabrication, then, is one or two orders of magnitude better than is currently required, so simply attaining the required geometric configuration is not now and has not for some time been the limiting difficulty in fabricating viable long-term implantable stimulation electrode arrays.

[a] This work was supported by Contracts NO1–NS–2366 and NO1–NS–2336 from the National Institutes of Health, Bethesda, Maryland.

0077–8923/83/0405–0183 $01.75/0 © 1983, NYAS

The limiting technological difficulties in fabricating thin-film neurostimulation arrays have been:

(1) preservation of insulation integrity over distances of tens of micrometers with insulation thicknesses of a few micrometers;
(2) preventing delamination of the several layers characteristic of thin-film electrodes;
(3) building sufficient metal mass into the stimulation electrode area to give adequate lifetime protection against electrolysis; and
(4) achieving satisfactory lead attachment: making the transition from the thin-film world to the "wires and plugs" world.

In this paper, we will describe how these problems have been attacked and mostly overcome in the fabrication of two kinds of cochlear prosthesis electrodes, a rigid modiolar electrode designed for insertion into the eighth nerve in the modiolus as it exits the cochlea, and a flexible electrode for insertion into the scala tympani.

The Tantalum-on-Sapphire Rigid Electrode

Since the Stanford cochlear prosthesis project has mostly focused on modiolar implants, the first type of electrodes to be fabricated by thin-film techniques were rigid electrodes for modiolar insertion. Early versions used silicon, molybdenum, or tungsten for substrates, gold or platinum as the conductor metal, and SiO_2 (glass) as the insulation material.[4,5] Except for the platinum conductor metal, all these materials proved inadequate for their purposes. SiO_2 in thin films does not survive long-time soaking in a saline solution; silicon as a substrate is too brittle; molybdenum and tungsten offer problems associated with supporting an adequate and durable insulation layer between substrate and conductor; and gold is subject to an unacceptable level of electrolysis.

Our present design, which we feel has solved most of the foregoing problems, utilizes a single-crystal sapphire substrate, tantalum conductors to which platinum stimulation pads are alloyed, and insulation that consists of successive layers of Ta_2O_5, Si_3N_4, SiO_2, and Parylene. Since a fairly complete description of these electrodes is already in the literature,[6] we will only describe highlights here.

A drawing of the tantalum-on-sapphire electrode is given in Figure 1, and a photograph of such an electrode is shown in Figure 2. The single-crystal sapphire gives a tough, intrinsically insulating substrate. Tantalum metal bonds firmly to the Al_2O_3 substrate, probably through the formation of an intermediate oxide, so delamination at that level is not a problem. More important, the tantalum conductors can be anodized to produce a first layer of insulation, which is a native oxide tightly bound to the metal, allowing no penetration of fluids between conductor and insulation, as is inevitably the case for insulation systems involving metals wrapped with polymers. A second insulation layer is formed of silicon nitride, Si_3N_4, which is highly ion-impervious. The Si_3N_4 coat provides a polarization-insensitive insulation layer, provides mechanical protection to the Ta_2O_5, and reduces the capacitive coupling of the conductor to the surrounding environment which the thin Ta_2O_5 would otherwise allow. For further protection, overlayers of SiO_2 and

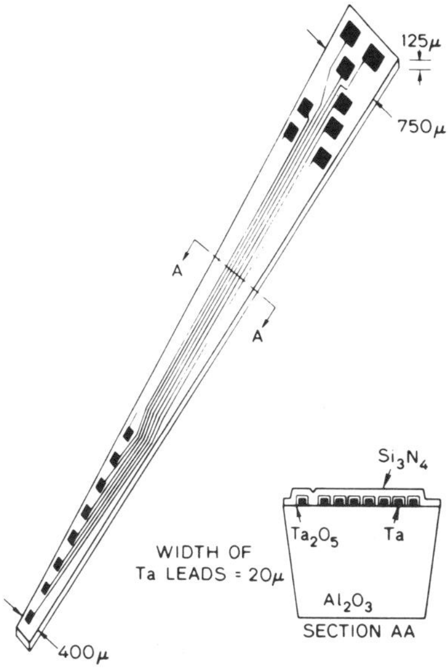

FIGURE 1. Eight-channel tantalum-on-sapphire multielectrode array. The total length of the array is 1.25 cm. The area of each stimulation site is 4×10^{-4} cm^2.

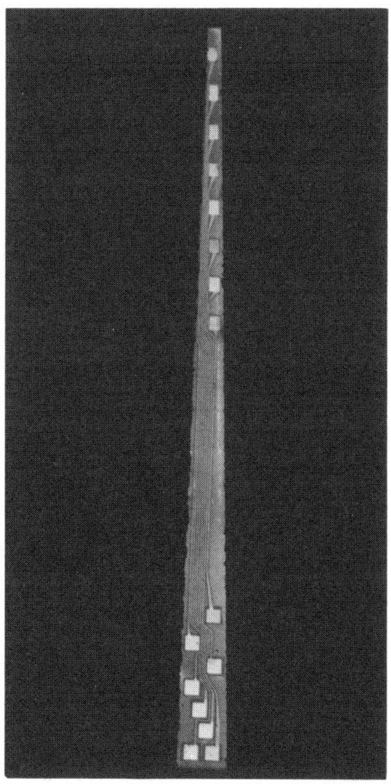

FIGURE 2. Photomicrograph of eight-channel tantalum-on-sapphire rigid microelectrode array.

Parylene are added. FIGURE 3 shows the multilayer insulation. The Parylene plays a significant role in providing mechanical strength to the welded joint between the tantalum lead wires and the thin-film electrode. At the stimulation sites, the tantalum is overcoated with platinum, which is then interdiffused with the tantalum to prevent delamination of the platinum from the tantalum. The principal failure modes of thin-film electrodes have, we think, been successfully countered in this structure; only long-term tests, now under way, will confirm this hope.

It is perhaps worthy of mention that the tantalum-on-sapphire construction may be particularly adaptable to extension to much more dense arrays. The achievement of truly multiple fine-scale arrays requires the development of on-electrode multiplexing; one simply cannot tolerate a hundred or so lead wires to a small electrode. Silicon-on-sapphire active circuits are already in commercial use; if adequate passivation techniques can be developed, active tantalum-on-sapphire multiple electrodes are feasible.

FLEXIBLE SCALA TYMPANI ELECTRODES

The earliest attempts to fabricate thin-film electrodes centered on flexible scala tympani electrodes. Pioneering efforts in this direction were made by Sonn [7] and Clark and Hallworth [8] in particular. The principal difficulty encountered by these scientists, as well as by others attempting to fabricate polymer–metal–polymer electrodes, was that of delamination. The preferred metals, platinum and iridium, are chemically very inert, as are the acceptable biocompatible polymers, such as Teflon® or Mylar® or Parylene® or Kapton®. These materials therefore do not bond readily to other materials, much less to one another, so structures fabricated of layers of such materials tend to come apart when soaked, particularly when subject also to electrical challenge. A second class of fabrication problems arose from the difficulty of cutting small holes in the polymer in the right places to expose stimulation and lead contact pads. The very property of chemical inertness that made the polymers biocompatible made them resistant to the chemical etching characteristic of photolithographic technology, and even resistant to the plasma etching of more recent dry-chemistry photolithography.

We believe we have solved these problems using a family of new materials and techniques. Much of this has been reported previously,[9] so we will again

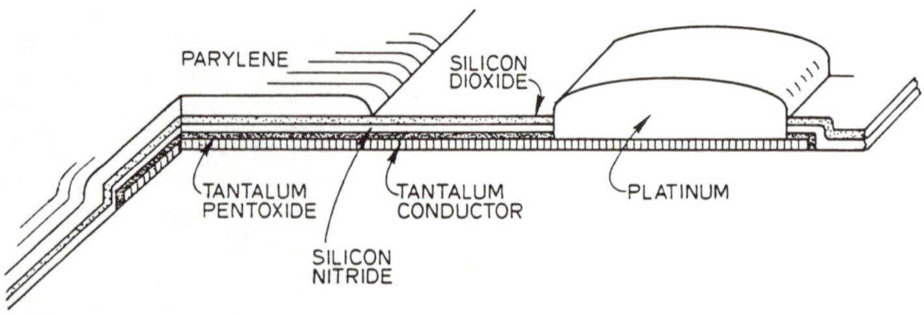

FIGURE 3. Schematic cross-section of tantalum-on-sapphire electrode array, showing insulation layers.

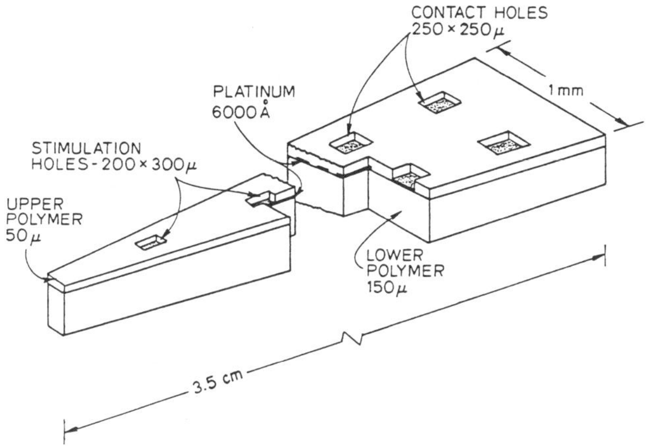

FIGURE 4. Schematic drawing of polyimide–metal–polyimide scala tympani electrode.

give a summary description here. A drawing of our thin-film flexible electrode is given in FIGURE 4. A key element is the use of a liquid polymer, a polyimide, which cures in two stages. After the first cure, the material is solid, but chemically active enough to be susceptible to chemical etching; the appropriate "windows" can be cut in the structure at this stage. After the second stage of curing, the polymer becomes inert biocompatible Kapton®. There still remains the problem of obtaining a good bond between the noble metals, platinum or iridium, and the cured polymer. This problem has been attacked, and, we believe, solved, by the use of a thin intermediate layer of tantalum or titanium. The surface of the polymer substrate is activated by a hydroxide pretreatment and neutralization followed by a plasma etch and surface activation. A few hundred angstroms of tantalum or titanium are then deposited. (Our first successful bonding used tantalum, but we have found titanium to yield even better adhesion characteristics.) Next, platinum is deposited, either by sputtering or by electron beam evaporation. Once the platinum has been patterned using photomask and back-sputtering techniques, the upper layer of the polymer–metal–polymer sandwich is spun on, and subjected to the first stage of the curing technique. The appropriate access holes are then cut through the upper polymers. FIGURE 5 shows a photomicrograph of one of the stimulation sites. Note that a tab of polymer centered in the stimulation pad helps to provide mechanical containment of the stimulation site. The polymer is then given its final cure to produce the inert final compound. FIGURE 6 shows a thin-film scala tympani electrode before lead attachment.

The stimulation and lead attachment pads are thickened through the electrodeposition of platinum on the stimulation site to increase electrode lifetime against electrolysis and on the lead attachment end to provide increased bonding metal. The electrodeposition of platinum on platinum has proven to be a nontrivial procedure, presumably because of the thin layer of platinum oxide formed on the base platinum layer during its exposure to

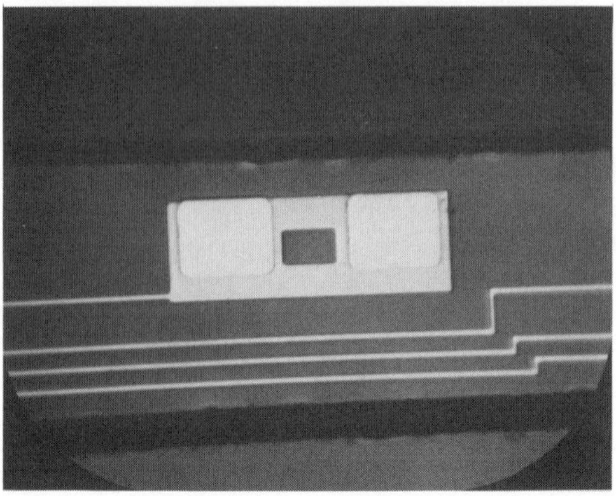

FIGURE 5. Photomicrograph of stimulation electrode of thin-film scala tympani electrode array.

air, and to other process steps. It has proved possible to obtain bright platinum electrodeposits after a chemical cleaning of the surface (or reducing the oxide) followed by a high current "strike." Some problems remain, however, related to a build-up of tensile stress in the platinum as the plated layer thickens. Such stress may cause the plated region to peel and curl; interestingly enough, the break for the peel comes between the plated platinum and the vacuum-deposited platinum, not between the platinum and the polymer. A combination of improved surface treatment of the vacuum-deposited platinum and a different plating solution seems to have solved this problem; again life tests will establish the completeness of the cure.

Lead attachment is currently made using a solder reflow technique. Welding does not work satisfactorily in this case because of the high melting temperatures of the two metals (platinum–iridium leads, platinum pads) and because of the tendency of the polymer to soften and deform at the pad

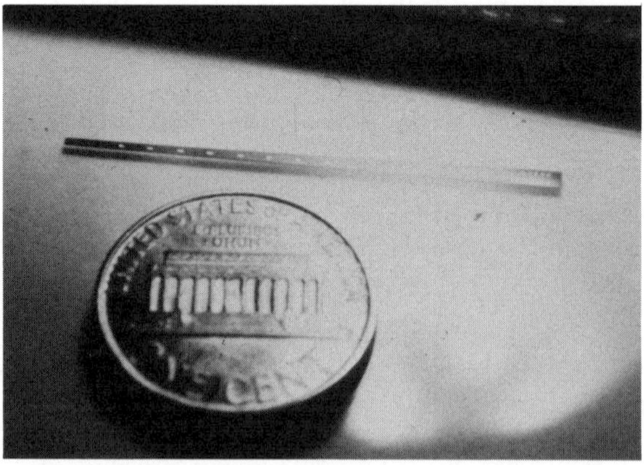

FIGURE 6. Photograph of thin-film scala tympani electrode.

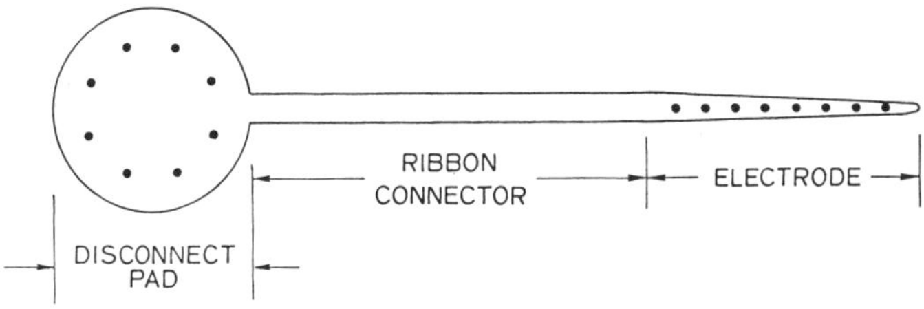

FIGURE 7. Drawing of integrated thin-film electrode-conductor ribbon–disconnect structure.

during welding. After lead attachment, the lead attachment region is again coated with liquid polyimide and cured. The insulation coating bonds to both the electrode structure and to the Teflon insulation on the lead wires.

A more satisfactory solution to the lead attachment problem is to eliminate lead wires entirely and to make the lead structure, a conductor ribbon, a direct extension of the electrode itself. Such an integrated electrode-lead ribbon–disconnect structure is drawn in FIGURE 7. The round disconnect pad is designed to mate with the feedthroughs on the round implantable stimulation electronic units. We are just beginning to fabricate such integrated structures and to explore the practicality of a gasketed disconnect structure using the thin-film contact pads.

The thin-film polymer–platinum–polymer electrode is very much smaller dimensionally than the scala tympani into which it is to be inserted. We found, however, two problems associated with the actual implantation of these electrodes. The first is that the polyimide tended to be attracted to and stick to the inner wall of the scala tympani, reducing to an unsatisfactory degree the distance into the cochlea it was possible to implant the electrode (we would like at least 2 cm of insertion). The second is that the narrow edge of the electrode frequently damaged the basilar membrane during insertion. As the electrode penetrated the climbing spiral of the cochlea, its upper edge was pressed against the basilar membrane, and the thin, relatively hard edge of the electrode cut the basilar membrane near its outer edge. A solution to these problems has been to back the thin-film electrode with a thin Silastic® mold, as shown in FIGURE 8. The Silastic slips more easily along the scala

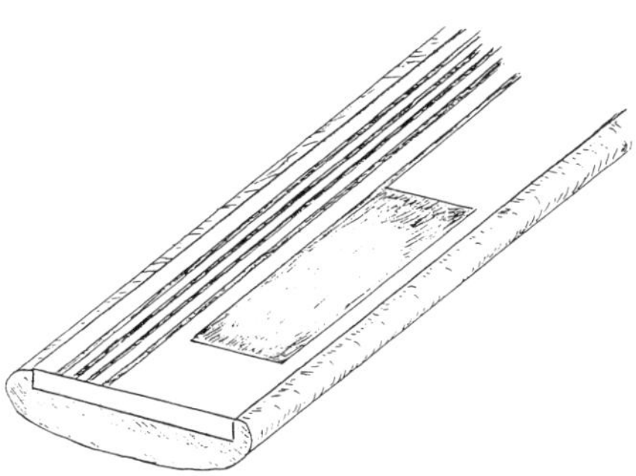

FIGURE 8. Schematic cross section of thin-film electrode on Silastic carrier.

tympani than does the polyimide, and the soft rounded edge no longer cuts the basilar membrane. Practice on cat and human cadaver ears indicates that trauma-free insertion of these electrodes can be regularly attained.

Summary and Conclusions

After a long developmental effort, we can now fabricate, using thin-film techniques, both rigid modiolar multielectrodes and flexible scala tympani multielectrodes which we believe appropriate for long-term implantation in human subjects. *In vitro* and *in vivo* life tests are in progress to confirm this expectation.

Acknowledgment

We wish to acknowledge the continuing fiscal and psychological support of Dr. F. Terry Hambrecht of the National Institute of Neurological and Communicative Diseases and Stroke.

References

1. Brummer, S. & M. J. Turner. 1975. Electrical stimulation of the nervous system: The principle of safe charge injection with noble metal electrodes. Biochem. Bioenergetics **2:** 13–25.
2. Brummer, S., J. McHardy & M. J. Turner. 1977. Electrical stimulation with Pt electrodes: Trace analysis for dissolved Pt and other dissolved electrochemical products. Brain Behav. Evol. **14:** 10.
3. Walsh, S. M. 1979. Effects of Chronic Electrical Stimulation of Auditory Nerve in Cat. Ph.D. thesis, Stanford University.
4. Mercer, H. 1976. Design Fabrication and Testing of Silicon, Molybdenum and Tungsten Microelectrode Arrays for Biostimulation. Stanford Elect. Lab. Tech. Rep. #5306–2.
5. Mercer, H. D. & R. L. White. 1978. Photolithographic fabrication and physiological performance of microelectrode arrays for neural stimulation. IEEE Trans. Biomed. Eng. (BME–25) **6:** 494–500.
6. May, G. A., S. A. Shamma & R. L. White. 1979. A tantalum-on-sapphire microelectrode array. IEEE Trans. Elect. Devices (ED–26) **12:** 1932–1939.
7. Sonn, M. & W. Feist. 1974. A prototype flexible microelectrode array for implant-prosthesis applications. Med. Biol. Eng.: 778.
8. Clark, G. M. & R. J. Hallworth. 1976. J. Laryngol. Otol. **90:** 623.
9. Shamma-Donoghue, Shihab A., G. A. May, N. E. Cotter, R. L. White & F. B. Simmons. 1982. Thin-film multielectrode arrays for a cochlear prosthesis. IEEE Trans. Elect. Devices (ED–29) **1:** 136–144.

DESIGN AND FABRICATION OF THE BANDED ELECTRODE ARRAY[a]

G. M. Clark, R. K. Shepherd, J. F. Patrick, R. C. Black, and Y. C. Tong

Department of Otolaryngology
University of Melbourne
Victoria 3052, Australia

INTRODUCTION

A multiple-channel electrode array must meet certain design requirements; these are listed in TABLE 1. First, there should be no trauma associated with the surgical insertion, and if there is a need to replace the array, this procedure should also be atraumatic. Second, it should be biologically inert. This means that it should be biocompatible with the tissues. When placed in the cochlea, the array should also not predispose the patient to local infection, and this is particularly important in children, in whom recurrent middle ear infections could spread to the inner ear. There should also be no risk of carcinogenicity with long-term implantation. Third, the electrode array should be designed so that the stimulus current can be localized to discrete groups

TABLE 1

DESIGN REQUIREMENTS FOR MULTIPLE-ELECTRODE ARRAY

1. It must be atraumatic in insertion
2. It must be biologically inert
3. Current must be localized
4. Only minimal damage should occur with chronic stimulation
5. It must have mechanical stability
6. Fabrication must be practicable

of nerve fibers, and it should also be possible to stimulate as many groups as possible from the total remaining nerve population. Fourth, with long-term stimulation, there should be no significant corrosion of the electrodes used, and the electrical stimulation should not lead to damage of the tissues in the cochlea, especially the residual nerve fibers. Fifth, the electrode array should be mechanically robust and stable. It should not be prone to break as a result of repeated stress by the acceleration of the head during everyday movements. The array should also be capable of being fixed in place so that it will not shift its position. Sixth, it is desirable that the means of fabrication of the multiple-channel array should be simple and inexpensive.

[a] Financial assistance for this work was provided by the Department of Science and Technology of the Australian Government, the National Health and Medical Research Council of Australia, and the Deafness Foundation of Victoria.

0077–8923/83/0405–0191 $01.75/0 © 1983, NYAS

The Banded Electrode Array

An Atraumatic Array

To determine the effects of certain designs and fabrication techniques in causing trauma on insertion and reinsertion, we have carried out studies on cats using our banded electrode array. Figure 1 shows an earlier banded array for cat cochleas.[1] The electrode was made from a Silastic® tube with a diameter of 0.64 mm. Wires made of 90% platinum and 10% iridium, with a diameter of 0.025 mm and coated with hexafluoropropylene (FEP), were passed through slits in the tube and along its length. These wires were welded

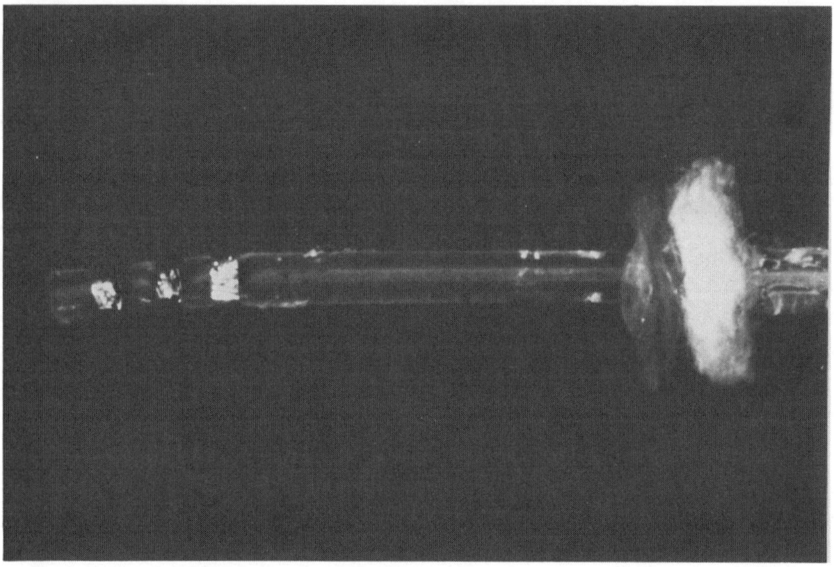

Figure 1. Banded electrode array with a Silastic disc and Teflon felt collar for experimental insertion into the scala tympani of the cat cochlea. (Original magnification × 15; reduced by 25%.)

to strips of platinum foil 0.0075 mm thick and 0.3 mm wide, which were tightly wrapped around the tube. The bands were completed by welding the ends of the strips together. The electrode was also constructed with a Silastic disc for insertion through the round window to anchor the electrode in place, and a Teflon® felt collar was glued to the electrode to seal the round window and minimize the entry of infection.[2] Figure 2 shows a photomicrograph of a cat's cochlea, where an intracochlear Silastic disc had been used to anchor the electrode. A fracture of the spiral lamina with loss of ganglion cells is apparent. This finding suggests that in anchoring the electrode more reliance should be made on extracochlear fixation, and this will be discussed later. Figure 3 provides evidence of a microfracture of a spiral lamina well away

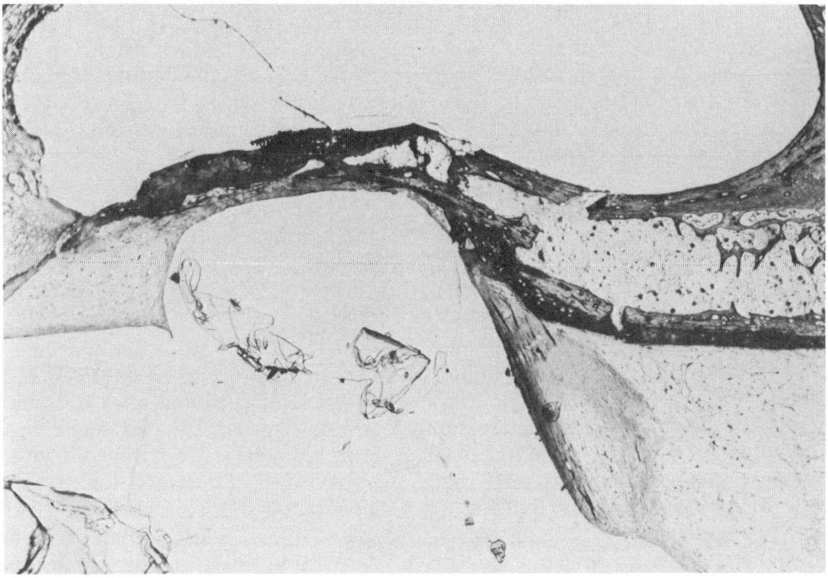

FIGURE 2. Photomicrograph of the proximal part of the basal turn of cat cochlea showing a fracture of the spiral lamina due to intracochlear fixation with a Silastic disc. (Original magnification × 80; reduced by 25%.)

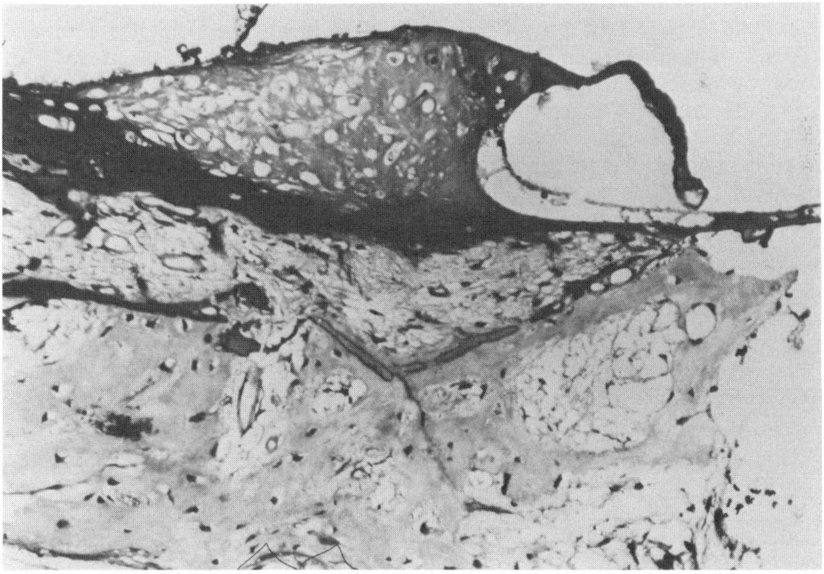

FIGURE 3. Photomicrograph of the distal part of the basal turn of a cat cochlea showing a microfracture of the spiral lamina due to electrode surface and tip irregularities. (Original magnification × 320; reduced by 25%.)

from the round window in the more distal part of the basal turn; this had led to an area of calcification. The finding suggests that the electrode tip and surface should be as smooth as possible. Furthermore, in another animal it was found that fibrous tissue had grown into a gap between the electrode band and the Silastic tube. This finding indicates the importance of carefully manufactured electrode bands, and an electrode fabrication technique that would ensure no irregularities between the electrode band and the carrier material. Injection molding is suitable and would ensure a smooth array that could be withdrawn at a later date and another one inserted.

Biological Inertness

In assessing the biocompatibility of materials for electrode fabrication a number of materials were implanted in the muscle of rats, and after a 2-week period the polymorphonuclear, mononuclear, and fibrous tissue responses were graded from 0 to 6 by an independent histopathologist who was not given information about the materials used. The averaged results are summarized in TABLE 2, which shows that Silastic MDX 4-4210 was as biologically inert as Silastic sheeting. Silastic adhesive type A, and Silastic medical-grade elastomer 382, when prepared outside the body, are also satisfactory materials.

In a separate study, specially cleaned medical-grade Silastic and FEP tubes were placed through the round-window membrane into the scala tympani of cats for periods of 16 weeks. Strict asepsis was carried out during surgery and the animals were also given a 5-day course of ampicillin to prevent infection. The cats were then sacrificed and the temporal bones sectioned, showing minimal reaction to the materials. This is illustrated in FIGURE 4, which shows the Silastic tube sectioned *in situ* after having been implanted for 16 weeks. As can be seen, there is very little fibrous tissue reaction to the electrode material.

In the design of the electrode array, importance has also been placed on preventing middle ear infections passing along the electrode track into the inner ear. This is particularly important in the case of children, in whom middle ear infections are frequent. To investigate the possibility of sealing the round-window entry point, Dacron® mesh and Teflon felt were first implanted into the subcutaneous tissue of rats to assess fibrous tissue penetration

TABLE 2

BIOCOMPATIBILITY OF MATERIALS FOR ELECTRODE FABRICATION

Electrode Materials	Polymorphonuclear Tissue Response	Mononuclear Tissue Response	Fibrous Tissue
Silastic medical-grade sheet	1	2	1
Silastic MDX–4–4210	1	2	1
Silastic medical adhesive type A	1	2	2
Silastic medical grade elastomer–382 (cured outside body)	1	2	2

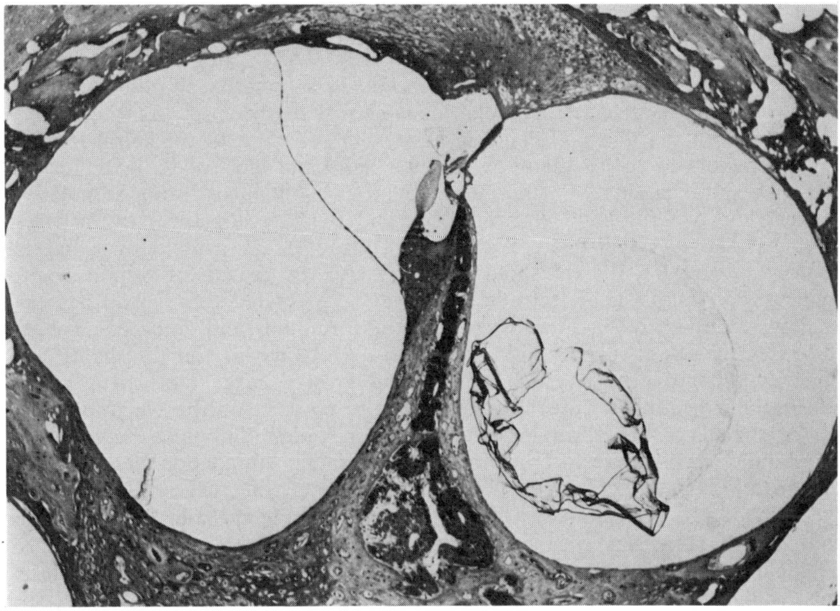

FIGURE 4. Photomicrograph of a cat cochlea after the implantation of a Silastic tube for 16 weeks. The Silastic tube sectioned *in situ* is shown in the scala tympani. (Original magnification × 62; reduced by 25%.)

and the severity of any foreign body reaction. It was found the fibrous tissue penetration of Teflon felt was adequate, and since it produced much less foreign body reaction than Dacron, it was selected as the material of choice.[3] In a subsequent study a collar of Teflon felt was then glued to the electrode array with Silastic adhesive type A, and implanted in cat cochleas for periods of up to 28 weeks. The cats were sacrificed and the temporal bones sectioned with the electrode and Teflon felt collar *in situ*. A photomicrograph of a Teflon felt collar, placed in the round window for 28 weeks, is shown in FIGURE 5. Fibrous tissue penetration of the Teflon felt and an intact epithelial lining over it can be seen.

Current Localization and Stimulus Characteristics

Studies on cats have also been undertaken to determine the stimulus characteristics on a half-band electrode compared with a full-band electrode, since a half-band electrode may lead to increased current localization if placed close to the nerve fibers. Bipolar electrodes rather than pseudobipolar electrodes were used in these studies since preliminary investigations have shown that for full-band electrodes, current distributions are similar for bipolar and pseudobipolar stimulation. In addition, because of their size, pseudobipolar electrodes are not easily implanted into cat cochleas.

The stimulus characteristics of the half-band electrode were assessed by recording the amplitude of the brainstem responses for different current intensities and different electrode configurations. An example of the results obtained can be seen in FIGURE 6. FIGURE 6a shows the amplitude growth curves for half-band electrodes placed as shown in the inset. During stimulation between the two half-band electrodes, A-A′, close to the spiral lamina, the threshold was lower than for the two half-band electrodes, B-B′, further from the spiral lamina. Furthermore, the results obtained during stimulation between the two full-band electrodes (A and B joined together) lay between those for the two half-band electrodes. During radial stimulation (that is, between A and B), the threshold was high and the growth of response with current very small. The electrode array was then rotated through 90 degrees, as shown in the inset in FIGURE 6b, and the thresholds and amplitude growth responses measured again. This resulted in a change in the thresholds and slope of the growth curves. The full-band growth curve had changed significantly, indicating an overall change in the position of the electrode relative to the nerve fibers, although there was now less difference between the half-band growth curves. The threshold for radial stimulation had dropped significantly, but its growth response function was still very small.

These results indicate that while there are inevitable variations in thresholds and growth responses with a free-fit electrode of this type, these will be significantly greater with a half-band electrode. Therefore, unless the placement and rotation of the half-band electrode can be closely controlled, the full-band electrode has advantages in providing minimum threshold and growth response variations.

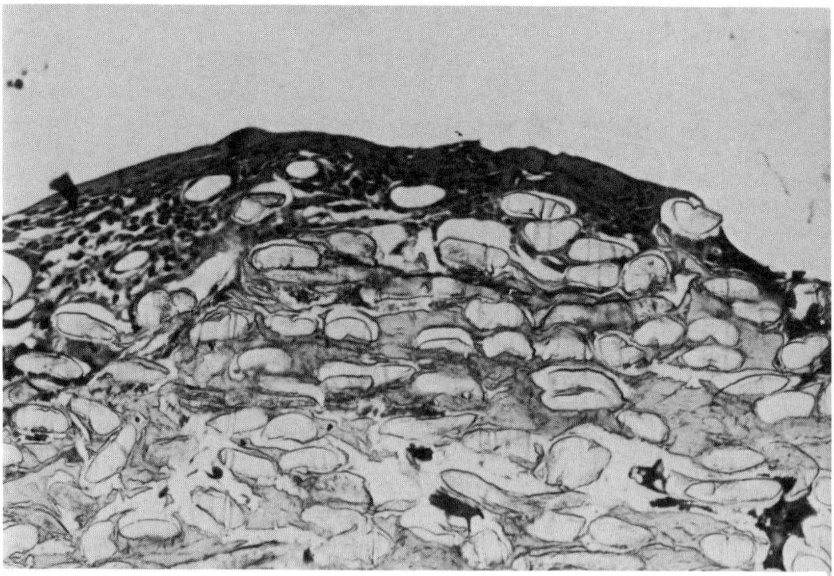

FIGURE 5. Photomicrograph of a Teflon felt collar implanted in the round window of a cat cochlea for 28 weeks. (Original magnification × 320; reduced by 25%.)

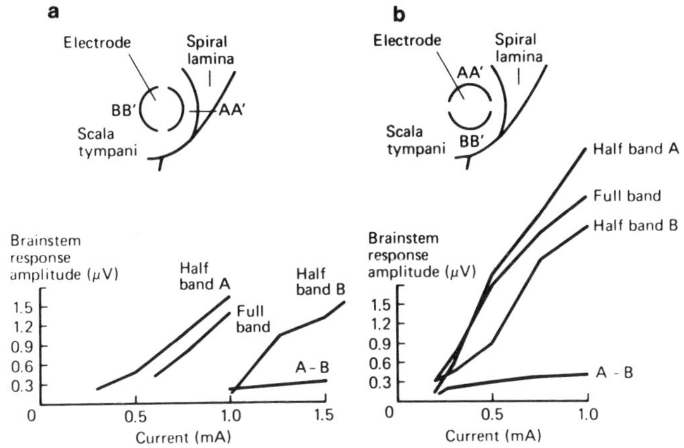

FIGURE 6. Brainstem response amplitude growth curves for full-(A and B) and half-band (A or B) electrodes in two positions (a and b) varying by 90 degrees of rotation.

With use of the technique of derived-response brainstem audiometry,[4] in which high pass filtered noise is used to mask the brainstem response resulting from electrical stimulation, the bipolar full-band electrode has been observed to produce neural excitation up to 3 mm from the stimulus site for a maximum dynamic range stimulus. Although this spread is greater than the interelectrode spacing, it may not necessarily be too great. Psychophysical data from patients implanted with the banded pseudobipolar array show that individual electrodes exhibit unique "spectral color" percepts.

Chronic Stimulation

The effect of long-term stimulation on corrosion and tissue damage has been assessed. Electrode corrosion was first measured spectrophotometrically in unbuffered saline solutions using biphasic current pulses balanced to within 1.5%. The results showed that dissolution decreased as the pulse duration was reduced, and was particularly low for durations less than 0.5 msec. Dissolution also decreased markedly with a decrease in the current density.[5] This finding means the larger surface area provided by a banded electrode should lead to less corrosion with long-term stimulation.

In vitro studies in phosphate-buffered inorganic saline solution were then carried out on the banded electrode array using biphasic, square-wave voltage source stimulation, balanced to within 0.05%. Scanning electron micrograms were taken after stimulation. The dissolution rates in this study were 4 ng/real mm^2 per C at a current density of 0.8 mA/real mm^2. The scanning electron microscopic examination showed some corrosion of the electrode for the *in vitro* study (FIG. 7). However, banded electrode arrays, implanted in cat cochleas and stimulated for long periods using the same stimulation regime and similar current densities, showed little evidence of corrosion when examined using the scanning electron microscope (FIG. 8).

In a preliminary study, the effect of long-term electrical stimulation on the cochlea, and on the ganglion cells in particular, was assessed in two cats. In this study [1] the banded electrode array was inserted into the scala tympani with strict measures to prevent infection. After 10 days electrical stimulation was commenced. The cats were stimulated continuously using a low source-impedance biphasic stimulation at 200 pulses/sec and 0.2 msec/phase. A suprathreshold stimulus current level was used that was midway between threshold and one that gave an aversive response. One cat received 250 hours of stimulation and the other 1040 hours. There was no significant loss of ganglion cells in either animal. FIGURE 9 shows ganglion cell region opposite the electrodes in the cat receiving 1040 hours of stimulation. Furthermore, in this animal, electrically evoked ABR data were recorded every 250 hours of stimulation, and the ABR thresholds and growth responses showed no significant variation during the stimulation program.

Mechanical Stability

It has been a matter of some concern to improve methods of fixing the electrode in place since the array in our first patient slipped out 10 mm because there was no adequate method of fixation. Intracochlear fixation is not favored, for our studies using an intracochlear disc of Silastic showed that it can cause trauma. Extracochlear fixation is now preferred. Further stability is later provided by the ingrowth of fibrous tissue into the Teflon felt disc in the round window.

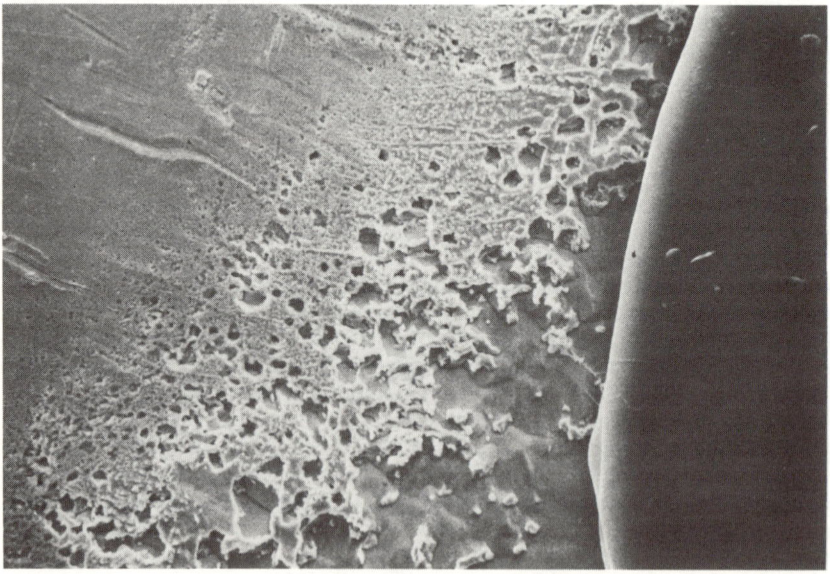

FIGURE 7. Scanning electron micrograph of the banded electrode showing corrosion after *in vitro* stimulation. (Original magnification × 1000; reduced by 25%.)

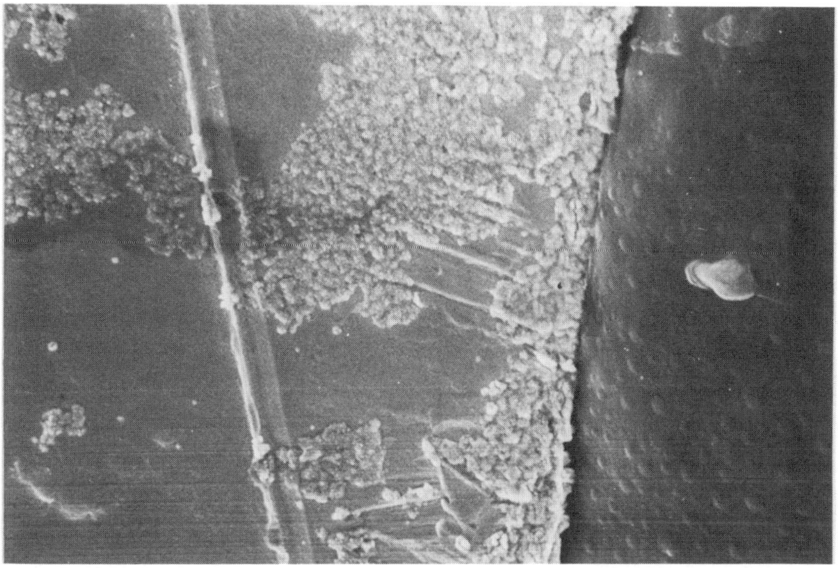

FIGURE 8. Scanning electron micrograph of the banded electrode showing a deposit, but no corrosion, after *in vivo* stimulation. (Original magnification × 1000; reduced by 25%.)

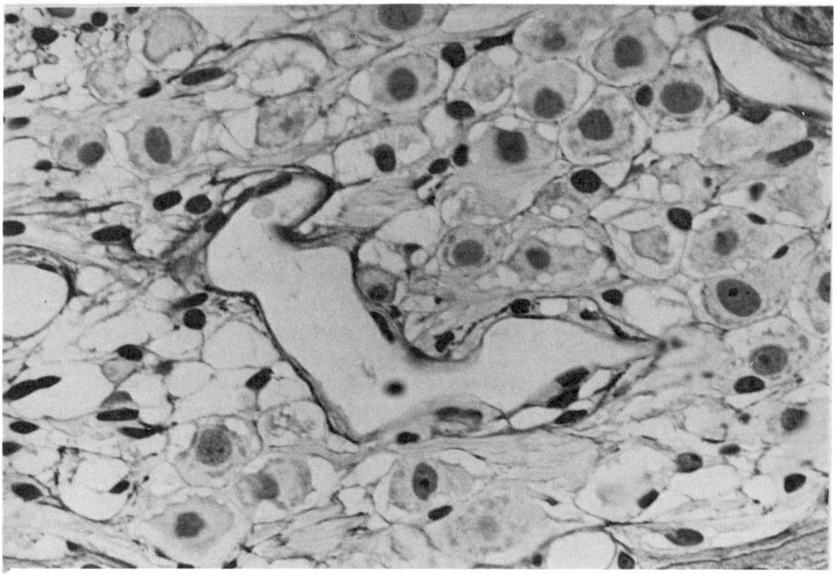

FIGURE 9. Photomicrograph of ganglion cells in the basal turn of a cat's cochlea after 1040 hours of continuous electrical stimulation. (Original magnification × 800; reduced by 25%.)

Practicability of Fabrication

The fabrication of a banded electrode array is practicable using injection molding techniques. This is achieved by placing the prefabricated electrode bands with attached electrode wires in an array mold, and by then injecting Silastic MDX 4-4210. FIGURE 10 shows a prototype molded array which is superior to the previous arrays fabricated by hand.

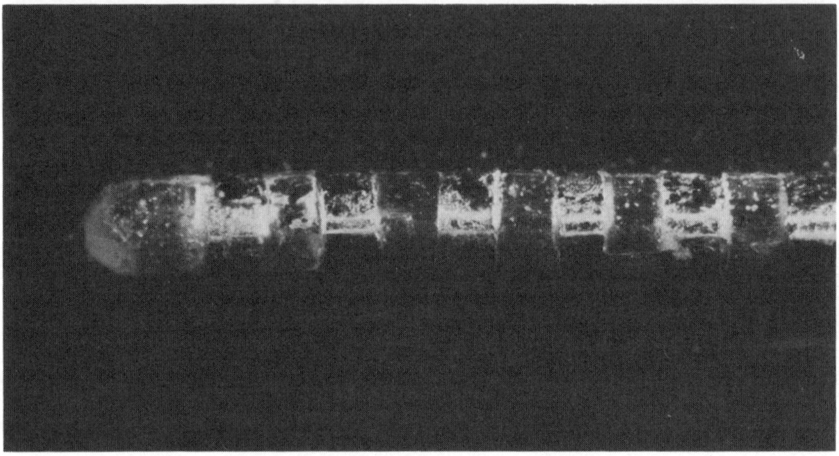

FIGURE 10. Banded array for multiple-electrode stimulation in patients. (Original magnification × 27; reduced by 15%.)

SUMMARY

The banded electrode array is a simple and effective array for multiple-channel cochlear stimulation and meets the necessary design requirements.

ACKNOWLEDGMENTS

We would like to thank Prof. G. Ryan, Dr. B. Pyman, Dr. R. Webb, Mrs. J. Ng, Mr. G. Lavery, Mr. D. Bloom, Mr. F. Rickards, Mr. G. Ewing, Mr. H. Jager, and Mr. M. Murray for their help. The Departments of Materials Science and Manufacturing Technology of the C.S.I.R.O. and the Department of Geology of the University of Melbourne provided help with the scanning electron microscopy.

REFERENCES

1. SHEPHERD, R. K., G. M. CLARK, R. C. BLACK & J. F. PATRICK. J. Laryngol. Otol. In press.
2. CLARK, G. M., J. F. PATRICK & Q. BAILEY. 1979. J. Laryngol. Otol. **93:** 107–109.

3. Clark, G. M., B. C. Pyman & R. E. Pavillard. 1980. J. Laryngol. Otol. **94:** 1377–1386.
4. Parker, D. J. & A. R. D. Thornton. 1978. Scand. Audiol. **7:** 45–52.
5. Black, R. C. & P. Hannaker. 1979. Appl. Neurophysiol. **42:** 366–374.

PART V. COCHLEAR IMPLANTS AND HISTOLOGIC DAMAGE

INTRODUCTION

Raúl Hinojosa

Section of Otolaryngology
Pritzker School of Medicine
University of Chicago
Chicago, Illinois 60637

INTRODUCTION

The development of devices that can stimulate the cochlear nerve directly brings new hope for patients who suffer from total hearing loss. The introduction of such devices into the inner ear, however, may produce lesions in the cochlea that can further destroy the remaining vital neural and sensory elements that are necessary for effective stimulation of the cochlear nerve by the cochlear implant.

Before routine implant programs are put to clinical use, extensive histologic studies of the results of various surgical approaches and electrode designs, in human subjects as well as experimental animals, are needed. Examination of both the peripheral organs and the central nervous system should give the information necessary for an understanding of the design and function of cochlear prostheses and for improvements in surgical techniques for implantation of such stimulating devices.

A histologic study of the temporal bones in man after chronic cochlear implant has been published for only one patient. This study describes the histologic damage produced by single and multichannel electrodes of an early design. Reports on the effect of newly designed implants and of new surgical techniques of implantation in human subjects are not yet available.

Even studies of histologic damage produced by cochlear implants in experimental animals are still limited in number. Such histologic studies have, nevertheless, provided some useful information on possible improvements in the design of cochlear prostheses and on the biocompatibility of various materials that have been used for the construction of electrodes. They have also been helpful in providing information on the effect of electrode manipulation, such as the distance of insertion into the scala tympani, placement in relation to specific structures of the cochlea, mechanical trauma during introduction, and short- and long-term effects of implantation and intracochlear stimulation.

The number of morphologic studies of changes produced by the implant and by electrical stimulation in the central auditory nuclei has been even more limited. In a published report, transneuronal degeneration up to the level of the inferior colliculus has been described following cochlear implants in experimental animals. This finding suggests a possible process of continuing degeneration that may severely limit the use of implants.

The papers presented in this session describe further efforts to determine the histologic changes that take place in chronically implanted ears.

COCHLEAR PATHOLOGY WITH CHRONICALLY IMPLANTED SCALA TYMPANI ELECTRODES[a]

Patricia A. Leake-Jones[b] and Stephen J. Rebscher

Coleman and Epstein Laboratories
University of California at San Francisco
San Francisco, California 94143

An experimental multichannel cochlear prosthesis developed and fabricated in the Coleman Laboratory at the University of California, San Francisco, has now been implanted in two profoundly deaf volunteers.[1-3] The 16-wire scala tympani electrode array applied in these patients is considerably different from those previously studied and applied by this group. Major alterations in design and materials include the following: use of a different silicone elastomer for the carrier, changes in the dimensions and shape of the carrier, change in size and form of electrode contact surfaces, and use of different wire and insulation materials.

In consideration of these alterations and of the fact that fabrication was to be done on-site in the Coleman Laboratory, it was deemed necessary to conduct *in vivo* tests of the biocompatibility of these new electrode materials and fabrication methods prior to their implantation in patients. The present report describes the cochlear pathology observed with chronic implantation in cats of this latest generation of scala tympani arrays. In addition, initial results with a newly developed feline electrode (which models the current human arrays) and limited materials from previous experimental series are presented for comparison.

Materials and Methods

Electrode Arrays

Cat cochleas chronically implanted with three different designs of scala tympani electrodes are included in this report (Fig. 1). The electrode currently in use for the experimental clinical series is shown in Figure 1a. The design and fabrication of these devices is discussed in detail elsewhere,[4] and will be only briefly summarized here. Figure 1b illustrates a newly designed cat electrode which models the present human device. All materials and fabrication procedures for these arrays are identical or parallel to those used for the human devices. The older-design cat electrode with a carrier formed to the contours of the scala tympani is shown in Figure 1c.

There are several major differences between the electrodes currently in use and the older designs: (1) The silicone rubber of the new arrays (MDX

[a] This work was supported by Grants NS–11804 and NS–16361 and Contract N01–NS–0–2337 from the National Institutes of Health, and by a grant from Hearing Research, Inc.

[b] Address for correspondence: Dr. P. A. Leake-Jones, Coleman Laboratory HSE 863, University of California, San Francisco, California 94143.

0077–8923/83/0405–0203 $01.75/0

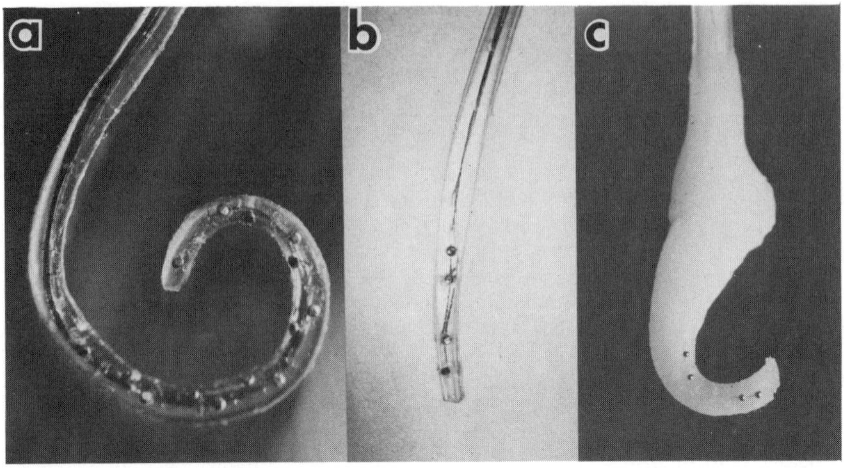

FIGURE 1. Three different designs of scala tympani electrodes used in studies of the effects of chronic implantation. (**a**) Experimental human multichannel array developed and fabricated in the Coleman Laboratory. (**b**) Feline electrode which models the human array, but is scaled to the dimensions of the cat scala tympani. (**c**) Older-design cat electrode array with carrier formed to the contours of the cat scala tympani. (Magnification × 4.)

4-4210; Dow Corning Corp.) uses a platinum catalyst (as opposed to a stannous octoate catalyst) and has no diatomaceous filler, in contrast to the elastomer used in the electrode in FIGURE 1c. (2) The intracochlear portion of the current device is cylindrical in shape, formed in a machined die to fill the middle portion of the scala tympani, leaving some fluid space around the electrode, primarily between it and the modiolar wall of the bony canal. Previous designs were molded to fit snugly in the contours of the scala, and were fabricated from casts of actual human or feline scala tympani. (3) The electrode contacts from individual wires are "mushroom"-shaped and only the center of the domed surface is flush with the carrier. In older generations electrode contacts were balls (or, even earlier, flush-cut wires) which protruded above the carrier surface. (4) Electrode wires in previous designs were Pt-Rh (90:10), while in the present arrays Pt:Ir (90:10) is used. In both cases, electrode wires are triple-coated with Pyre-ML; however, in the present generation of devices, wires are also overcoated with a 2-μm coating of Parylene-C. It should also be noted that the clean-room fabrication facilities and techniques currently in use for production of all electrodes (human and feline) were not available when the previous series of cat electrodes were fabricated.

The objective of implanting human arrays in cats was to evaluate the biocompatibility of the actual devices and all procedures leading to the final product. Since the cat scala tympani is considerably smaller than the human scala, the strategy was to insert the arrays a *shorter* distance (approximately 7 mm) into the lower basal turn. Insertion tests in cat cadaver temporal bones suggested that the most apical 6–7 mm of the human device could be accommodated by this basal portion of the cat scala tympani.

Implantation Procedure

Cats selected for this study were adult animals judged to have normal hearing as evaluated by recording auditory brainstem responses to click stimulation.[5] Thresholds lower than 50 dB peak SPL, characteristic waveform shape, and normal external ears (as evaluated in otoscopic examination) were criteria for selection of animals.

Animals were anesthetized with sodium pentobarbital for the sterile surgical implantation procedure. The bulla was exposed via a postauricular incision and opened anteriorly to allow access to the round window. The round-window membrane was carefully incised and reflected; in three cases (009R, 9157R, and 365L) the niche was enlarged by curettage of the inferior margin. Electrodes were usually anchored with dental acrylic into a groove made in the root of the zygoma immediately dorsal to the round window, and then routed to percutaneous connectors mounted on top of the skull. Alternatively, the array was simply amputated approximately 1 cm distal to the round window and the free end tucked into the bulla.

Preparation of Temporal Bones

Temporal bones included in this report were examined 1 month to 13 months postimplantation. Animals were heavily anesthetized with sodium pentobarbital. The bulla was exposed and the implanted electrode cut off at the round window. In most cases the cochlea was preserved with the implant left *in situ* in the scala tympani.

The stapes footplate was removed and a small hole made in the apex of the cochlea. Temporal bones were then preserved by gentle *in vivo* perfusion of fixative (2.5% paraformaldehyde and 1.5% glutaraldehyde in 0.1 M phosphate buffer at pH 7.4) through the cochlear fluid channels. The intracochlear perfusion was followed by cardiac perfusion of the same fixative to assure optimum preservation of the cochlear nerve and spiral ganglion. Temporal bones were removed and immersed in fresh fixative overnight. Cochlear dissection [6] was carried out in buffer. The positions of the electrode carrier and individual contacts were studied in the dissected specimen and recorded for later reference.

The implant was usually removed under visual control at this time; (alternatively, the electrode was removed after the specimen was embedded, during its preparation for the block surface technique [7]). Dissection of the cochlea was followed by postfixation in phosphate-buffered 1% OsO_4 with 1.5% potassium ferricyanide, dehydration, and embedding in Epon.

Light microscopic examination of each cochlea included analysis of the surface preparation and semi-thin (1 to 3 μm) sections stained with toluidine blue. Radial sections of the organ of Corti and spiral ganglion and tangential sections of the osseous spiral lamina were prepared from each 1-mm sector of the basal cochlear turn in the region of the implanted electrode and at predetermined intervals along the rest of the spiral apical to the electrode. To assess neural damage, counts of the myelinated radial nerve fibers were made in longitudinal photographic reconstructions of 400–600-μm segments of sections through the osseous spiral lamina.

For transmission electron microscopy in selected areas, ultrathin sections were collected on Formvar films with slotted grids and examined in a JEOL JEM-100S.

Results

As mentioned previously, the strategy for inserting human devices into the smaller cat scala tympani was to insert them a shorter distance. However, in actual practice, implantation of these arrays in four cats resulted in trauma, which ranged from severe in case #009R to mild in case #365L. For comparison, two cases of atraumatic implantation of the molded-type electrode and one case with the newly designed feline electrode are included in the present report (TABLE 1).

CASE SUMMARIES

Case #009R. Severely traumatic insertion in this case resulted in rupture of the basilar membrane and osseous spiral lamina over a 3.5-mm region located 8 to 11.5 mm from the base. FIGURE 2a shows a section from the 9-mm region in which the electrode was actually lodged above the osseous spiral lamina and limbus within the scala media and scala vestibuli.

A continuous layer of multinucleated giant cells encapsulated the misplaced electrode. The chronic inflammation and foreign body reaction induced by the trauma was characterized by invasion of the area by numerous macrophages, polymorphonuclear leukocytes, lymphocytes, and giant cells. Although implantation was for only 4 weeks, the spiral ganglion cells in the lesion area were clearly reduced in number to approximately 50% normal. Myelinated radial nerve fibers were almost totally destroyed in this area.

TABLE 1

CAT COCHLEAS CHRONICALLY IMPLANTED WITH SCALA TYMPANI ELECTRODES

Case	Duration of Implantation	Electrode Design	Trauma Site (location in mm from base)
009 R	4 wk	Coleman Lab; human array	8–11.5
9157 R	4 wk	Coleman Lab; human array	11–12
9201 R	6 wk	Coleman Lab; human array	10–11
365 L	6 wk	Coleman Lab; human array	4–5
031 R	5 wk	Coleman Lab; feline array	—
9154 R	13 mo	Contoured	—
9420 R	9 mo	Contoured	—

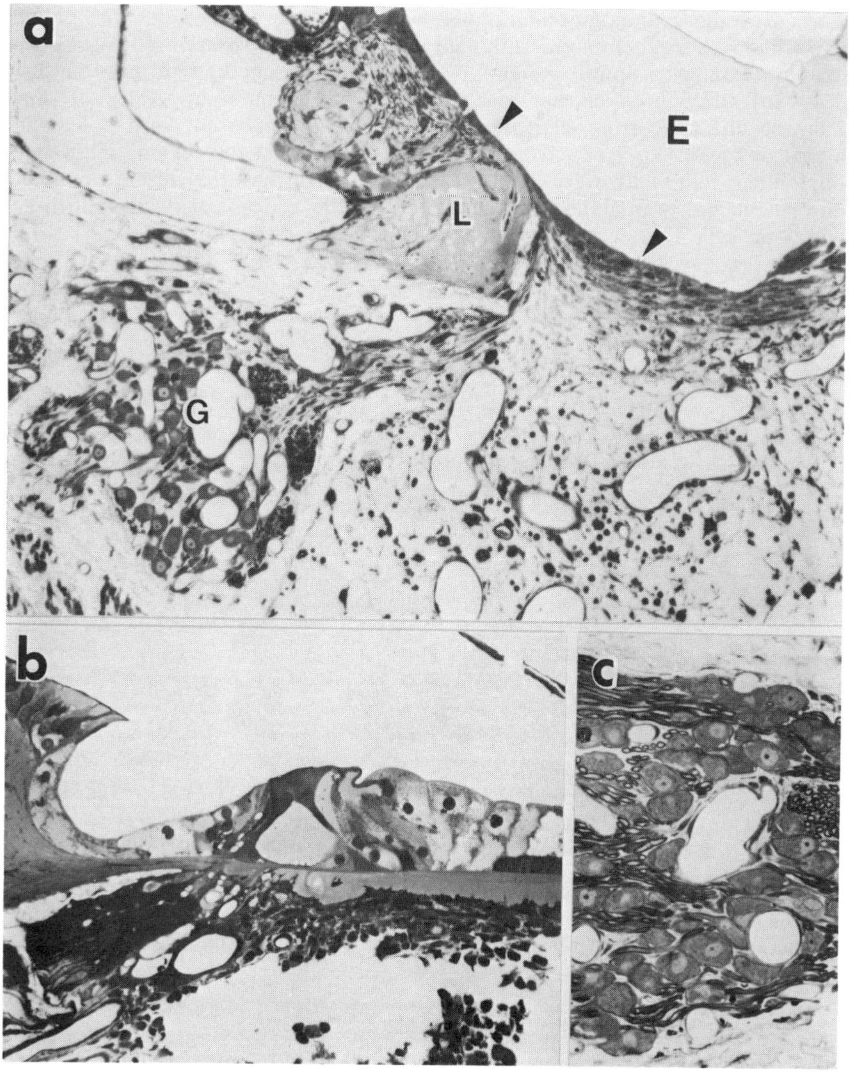

FIGURE 2. Case #009R. Pathologic alterations in the case with the most severe insertion trauma. (**a**) The electrode ruptured through the basilar partition and is lodged in the scala media and vestibuli, where it has been encapsulated by multinucleated giant cells (*arrowheads*). Section is taken approximately 10 mm from the cochlear base. E, space occupied by electrode carrier; G, spiral ganglion cells; L, spiral limbus damaged by insertion trauma. (Magnification $\times$ 125.) (**b**) Basal to the rupture (6 mm from the base) the supporting cells are better preserved, but the area under the basilar membrane contains numerous inflammatory cells. (Magnification $\times$ 250.) (**c**) The spiral ganglion basal to the lesion is normal. (Magnification $\times$220.)

Basal to the immediate trauma site there was better preservation of the cochlear duct structures (FIG. 2b). Pillars and supporting cells were present, although some pathologic alterations were observed. Likewise, the radial nerve fibers were preserved, although they appeared somewhat swollen in light microscopy. Spiral ganglion cells were present in normal density (FIG. 2c) throughout, except in the immediate lesion area. Apical to the electrode, the supporting elements and nerve array appeared normal in light microscopy less than 1 mm from the end of the traumatized region. Although some inner hair cells were also present in sections at this level, irregular sensory cell loss was noted throughout the middle and apical turns. Further, most hair cells that were present exhibited degenerative changes.

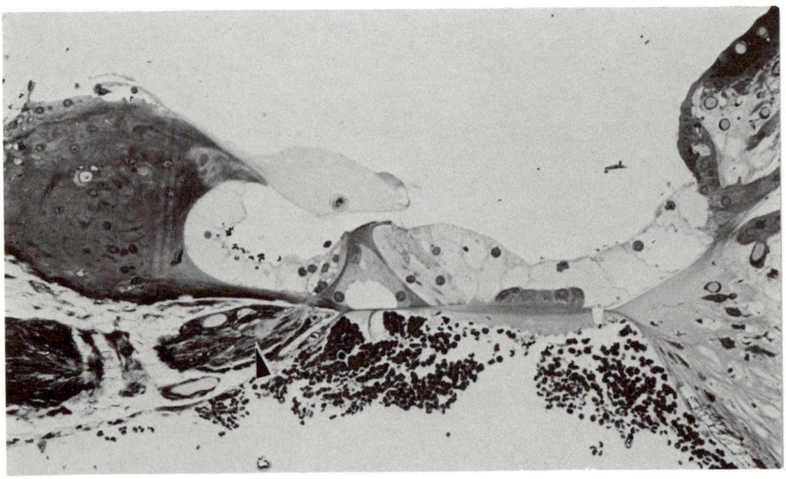

FIGURE 3. Case #9157R. With the exception of a lesion at the 11-mm position, the region occupied by the electrode showed good preservation of pillars and other supporting cells, although some consolidation of fluid spaces within the organ of Corti is seen. The radial nerve fibers were markedly thinned just at the edge of the osseous spiral lamina (*arrowhead*). (Section taken 6 mm from the base.) (Magnification × 175.)

Case #9157R. Insertion of the electrode array in this case caused moderate trauma to the osseous spiral lamina over a sector approximately 1 mm in length, from 10.5 to 11.5 mm from the base. Degeneration of the radial nerve fibers was observed adjacent to the trauma site and partial loss extended basally throughout the region occupied by the insert. FIGURE 3a shows a section from the 6-mm position of this specimen. In some sections the myelinated nerve fibers were markedly thinned at the edge of the osseous spiral lamina near the habenula perforata. However, closer to the modiolus a more normal density was seen, and spiral ganglion cells appeared to be present in normal numbers. This condition was observed in sections throughout the most basal 6 mm of the specimen. Within 1.5 mm apical to the trauma (and the upper end of the implant), the pillars and other supporting elements reappeared, although some consolidation was noted. Inner hair cells were observed in middle and apical turns, but most outer hair cells had degenerated.

Case #9201R. The only direct trauma due to insertion of the implant in this cochlea consisted of a small, partial fracture of the distal edge of the osseous spiral lamina at a point approximately 10.5 mm from the base (FIG. 4a). A focal foreign body reaction here was observed to be largely fibrotic, but with some multinucleated giant cells at the electrode tissue interface within the lesion; otherwise, inflammation and foreign body reaction were minimal. Loss of neurons was limited to a sector less than 1 mm in length at the fracture site. Otherwise, this case was characterized by excellent, uniform survival of radial nerve fibers, as evaluated in tangential sections through the limbus and underlying osseous spiral lamina (FIG. 4b). It should be noted that, as in the previous case, the distal processes of myelinated neurons were thinned at the edge of the osseous spiral lamina near the habenula, but were of normal density centrally (closer to Rosenthal's canal), where tangential sections are collected for nerve counts. Some consolidation of the fluid spaces surrounding supporting cells in the organ of Corti was noted in the implant region. However, less than 500 μm apical to the electrode tip, the organ of Corti, including the hair cells, appeared normal (FIG. 4c). Spiral ganglion cells in Rosenthal's canal were present in normal density throughout this cochlea.

Case #365L. Insertion trauma in this cochlea was restricted to apparent scraping of the lower surface of the osseous spiral lamina without actual fracture. The damage, located 4 mm from the base, resulted in thickening of the bony spiral lamina by deposition of new bone and was accompanied by nearly total degeneration of nerve fibers adjacent to the lesion.

FIGURE 5 illustrates the condition of the organ of Corti and nerve array adjacent to the electrode, but apical to the damage site. The basic architecture of the organ of Corti, the various supporting cells, and the fluid spaces (for example, tunnel of Corti and space of Nuel) were maintained throughout. A dense connective tissue formed by proliferation of fibroblasts and collagen encapsulated the implanted electrode in the scala tympani. A loose connective tissue formed between the basilar membrane and the dense connective tissue capsule. Cellular elements in this area were primarily fibroblasts, and no evidence of serious chronic inflammation was observed. Radial nerve fibers (FIG. 5b) and spiral ganglion cells were present in normal numbers (with the exception of the lesioned area).

Case #031R. This cochlea was examined after 5 weeks of chronic implantation of the electrode that was specially designed for the dimensions of the feline cochlea and fabricated with dye and electrode materials and techniques that exactly parallel the production of human electrode arrays (FIG. 1b). In the dissected cochlea the electrode was observed to be in good position in the scala tympani of the basal turn, with the lateral margins of electrode contacts visible through the basilar membrane. The electrode appeared to have been inserted atraumatically, with its tip situated at a point approximately 10 mm from the basal end of the cochlear duct.

This specimen was characterized by excellent preservation of the organ of Corti throughout most of the region overlying the implanted electrode. Pillars and other supporting cells were uniformly intact. Even most hair cells were maintained in the region of the implant, although some ultrastructural changes were noted (FIG. 6a).

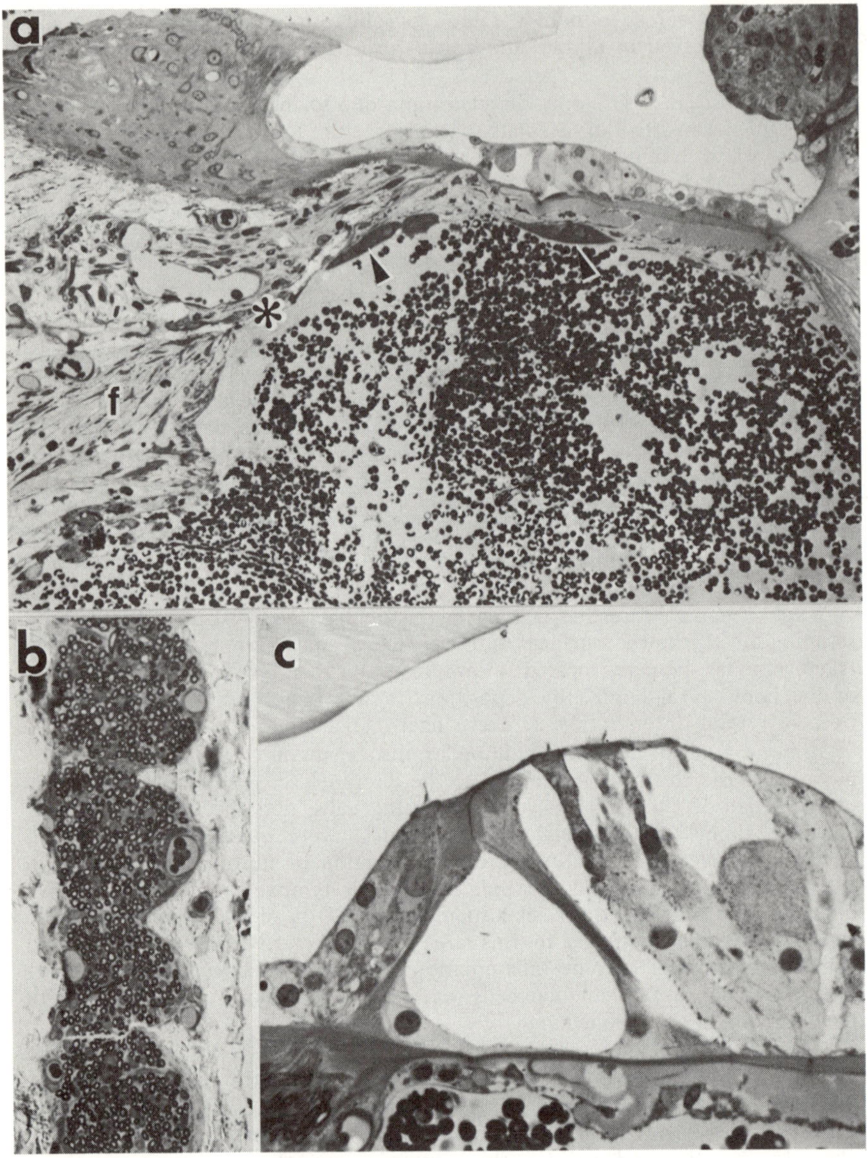

FIGURE 4. Case #9201R. (**a**) Moderate insertion trauma consisted of a small partial fracture of the osseous spiral lamina (*asterisk*) 10.5 mm from the base. Reactive fibrotic connective tissue under the osseous spiral lamina (f) and multinucleated giant cells at the electrode–tissue interface characterized the lesion site. (Cells in the scala tympani are red blood cells which entered when the electrode was accidentally removed prior to perfusion). (Magnification × 350.) (**b**) Basal to the site of trauma, radial nerve fibers adjacent to the implant are normal. (Section taken 5–6 mm from the base). (Magnification × 325.) (**c**) At 11 mm, less than 500 μm apical to the lesion shown in (**a**), preservation of the organ of Corti and hair cells are excellent. (Magnification × 500.)

Excellent, uniform preservation of the reticular lamina and hair cells was observed throughout the upper cochlear turns, from the point just apical to the electrode tip (that is, approximately 11 mm). The only exception to the relatively good condition of this cochlea occurred in the region 9.5 to 10.2 mm from the base, where a focal lesion consisted of consolidation of the fluid spaces within Corti's organ and collapse of the tunnel of Corti (FIG. 6b). In broken serial sections through this sector, the only indications of trauma were: (1) a slight distortion and displacement of the basilar

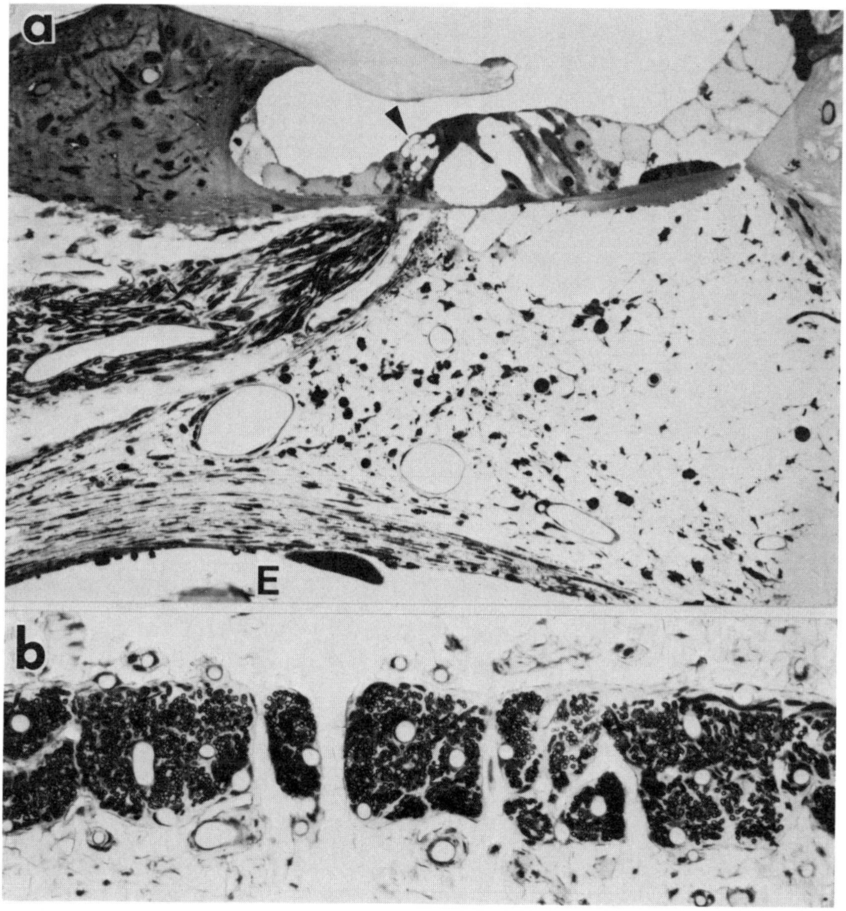

FIGURE 5. Case #365L. Micrographs taken from the region 7 mm from the cochlear base, 2 mm apical to the site of trauma. The characteristic findings with chronic (6-week) implantation of this human array are illustrated: (**a**) loss of hair cells, but intact pillars and other supporting cells in the region of the electrode and formation of a fibrotic capsule around the implant; and (**b**) normal numbers of myelinated radial nerve fibers (with variable thinning close to the habenula). *Arrowhead* indicates vacuoles in the region where the inner hair cells have degenerated; E, position of electrode carrier in the scala tympani. (Magnification × 200.)

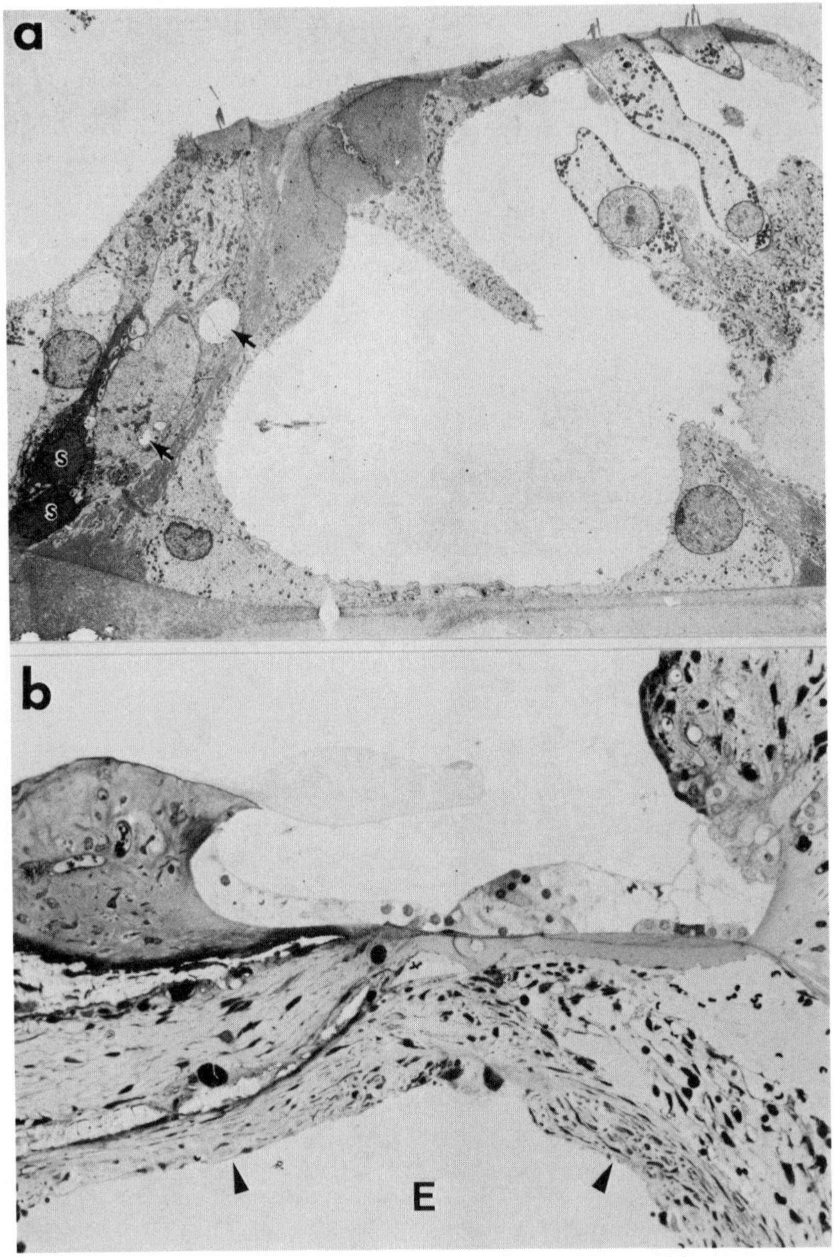

FIGURE 6. Case #031R. (**a**) Electron micrograph showing the organ of Corti in the implant region. Most hair cells appear to be normal, but the region under the inner hair cell has been invaded by Schwann cells (s). In addition, large vacuoles (*arrows*) are observed adjacent to the inner hair cells; at least some of these appear to be degenerating neural terminals. (Magnification × 1200.) (**b**) A small area of greater pathology was noted approximately 9.5 mm from the base (see text). The organ of Corti has collapsed, radial nerve fibers have degenerated, and a dense reactive fibrotic connective tissue (*arrowheads*) has formed at the electrode (E)–tissue interface. (Magnification × 200.)

membrane (not an evident tear), which might also have happened during fixation or dissection; and (2) possible slight damage to the lower bony plate of the osseous spiral lamina, evidenced by an irregular profile in some sections and disappearance of the capillaries normally found within or just under this plate.

The inflammation and foreign body reaction elicited by the electrode in this case were minimal. Proliferation of fibroblasts and formation of a dense reactive fibrotic connective tissue encapsulating the electrode was restricted to the area of the round window, where the electrode entered the scala, and to the vicinity of the lesion site (that is, 8 to 10 mm). Between these areas the scala tympani was clear. Adjacent to the sector of the organ of Corti exhibiting the greatest degree of pathologic alteration, the tissue encapsulating the electrode was infiltrated by more cells (FIG. 6b). Electron microscopy showed these cells to be almost exclusively fibroblasts, with a few macrophages and some cellular debris found immediately adjacent to the electrode surface (FIG. 7).

The condition of the radial nerve fibers in this case closely paralleled that of the organ of Corti. Density of myelinated neurons was normal throughout the entire length of the cochlea, with the exception of a focal, near total loss in the region 9 to 10.2 mm from the base (FIG. 8). The electron microscopic appearance of the intact neurons overlying the implant (examined in sections from the 7-mm region) was unremarkable.

Case #9154R. This cochlea was implanted for a period of 13 months with an older-design electrode, having a carrier molded to the contours of the scala tympani (FIG. 1c). This case represents in our experience the minimum reaction of cochlear structures to atraumatic insertion and long-term chronic implantation of this type of scala tympani electrode. In the extreme basal 3 mm of this cochlea (that is, the "hook" region), the organ of Corti was collapsed and spiral ganglion cells and their distal processes were largely degenerated. However, in the remainder of the region overlying the implanted electrode array, pillars and other supporting cells were present, although some consolidation of the organ of Corti and collapse of the space of Nuel were noted (FIG. 9a). Hair cells had degenerated from the reticular lamina above the implant. No evidence of chronic inflammation was observed and the electrode–tissue interface was characterized by minimal proliferation of fibroblasts.

Many hair cells had also degenerated in cochlear regions apical to the electrode; and of those that remained, most appeared to have undergone some pathologic alteration. The pillar cells were intact and the tunnel of Corti was maintained throughout the upper turns of the spiral. However, here again some consolidation of the fluid spaces (such as the space of Nuel and the spaces between phalangeal processes of Deiter's cells) was noted. With the exception of the extreme basal sector (the "hook" region mentioned previously), the spiral ganglion neurons and their myelinated processes in the osseous spiral lamina were present in normal numbers throughout this cochlea. Further, electron microscopic examination of these axons within the spiral lamina in the implant region revealed no degenerative changes (FIG. 9b).

Case #9420R. This case, which involved implantation for 9 months with a contoured electrode, represents the opposite end of the spectrum of pathology which has been observed with atraumatic chronic implantation. The electrode array was identical to one used in the previous case, #9154R.

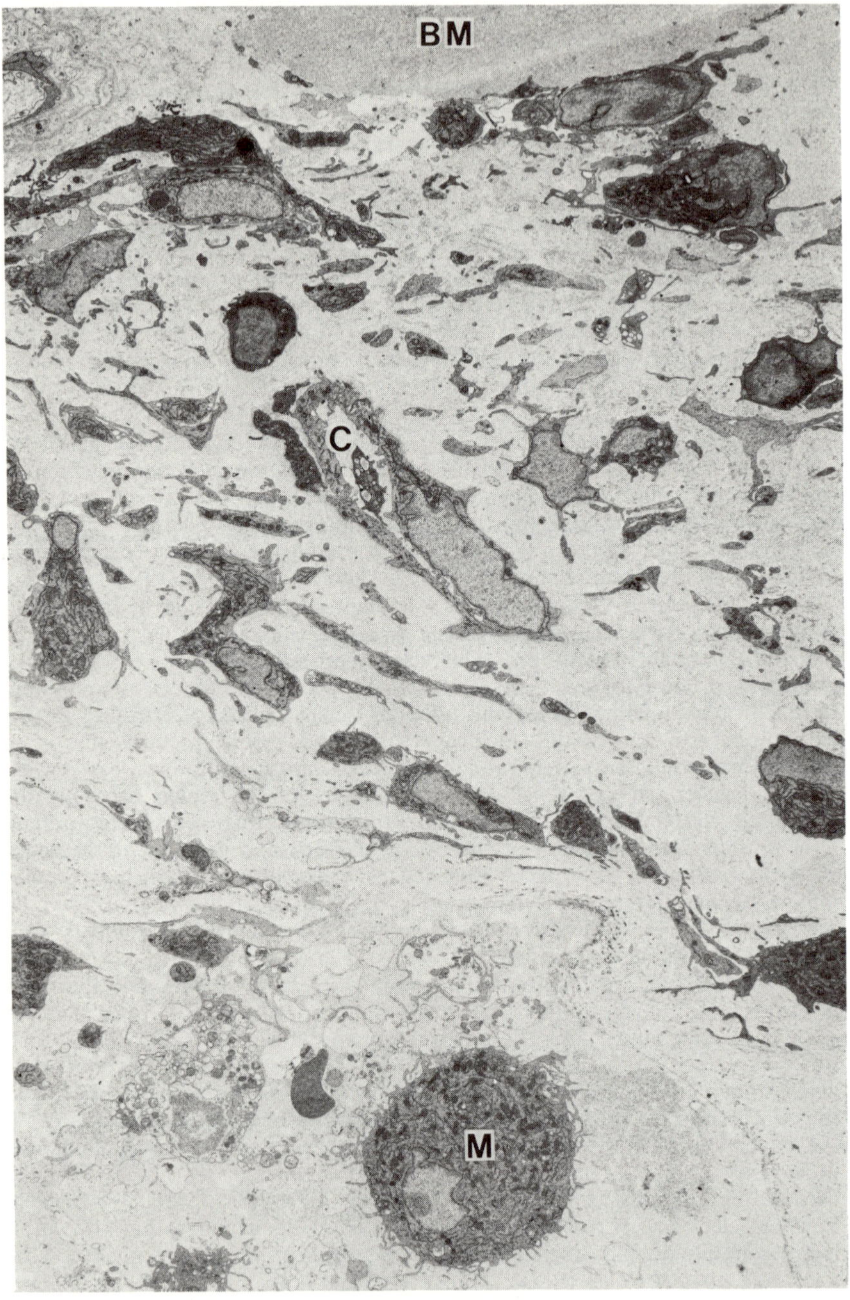

FIGURE 7. Case #031R. Dense reactive connective tissue encapsulating the electrode in the region of the damage (9.5 mm from the base) was observed in electron microscopy to consist largely of fibroblasts with a few macrophages (M) and cellular debris immediately adjacent to the electrode surface (bottom of field). BM, basilar membrane; C, capillary. (Magnification $\times$ 2500.)

Although more subtle trauma cannot be ruled out, no evident tear of the basilar membrane or fracture of the osseous spiral lamina occurred in this case. Yet severe degenerative changes were found in the region of the implant and extended into middle and upper turns as well. In the region overlying the electrode array, the condition of the organ of Corti ranged from partial consolidation with some recognizable supporting elements (FIG. 10a) to complete resorption in other sectors. It should be noted that evidence of severe chronic inflammation and foreign body response were observed to have been elicited by the implant in this case. The reactive fibrotic connective tissue was infiltrated by numerous lymphocytes, monocytes, and macrophages. At one point, a small lymphoid follicle had formed in the scala tympani adjacent to the electrode (FIG. 10a). The presence of new bone under the basilar membrane was noted throughout the most basal 6 mm of this cochlea (that is, throughout most of the region occupied by the electrode, which extended slightly more than 7 mm into the basal turn.) Near the upper end of the insert, and in middle and apical turns, the organ of Corti was better preserved (FIG. 10b). Although all hair cells had degenerated, most pillars and other supporting cells were present and the tunnel of Corti was maintained.

Neuronal degeneration in this cochlea was severe (fewer than 10% of myelinated fibers remained) throughout most of the region adjacent to the implant. Further, even with maintenance of pillars more apically, neuronal degeneration extended throughout the upper turns. Surviving radial nerve fibers never exceeded 50% of the normal number in any sector of this cochlea. Spiral ganglion cell survival paralleled that of the nerve array (FIG. 10c). Of particular interest in this case was the observation of a small fascicle of ectopic myelinated neurons in the scala tympani (FIG. 10b). Located near the inner margin of the basilar membrane, these fibers were first observed in sections from the 6-mm region, just apical to the region of osteoneogenesis under the basilar membrane and osseous lamina. The ectopic neurons apparently entered the lower scala at a point where the integrity of the lower plate of the osseous spiral lamina was compromised by new bone formation. These fibers had sprouted over a distance of at least 7 mm in the scala tympani and extended to a point more than 13 mm from the base (that is, several millimeters apical to the implanted electrode, which extended only slightly further than 7 mm into the scala tympani).

DISCUSSION

In general, the pathology observed in the four cases of implantation of human arrays in cats reflected the severity of damage to the organ of Corti. It is encouraging that even with the most extensive lesion (case #009), the chronic inflammation and serious foreign body reaction were largely restricted to the areas actually within or very close to the implant. The lack of significant acute and chronic inflammation or foreign body reaction (except in regions of direct, evident trauma) indicates good biocompatibility of materials and fabrication procedures used for these electrodes. In the cases where the trauma site was coincident with the upper end of the array (cases #009R, 9157R, and 9201R), it seems apparent that the electrodes were simply inserted too far into the scala. The nature of the damage in case #9201 (FIG. 4a) suggests that the cylindically shaped electrode was inserted until the tip fit snugly in the middle portion of the scala and that additional pres-

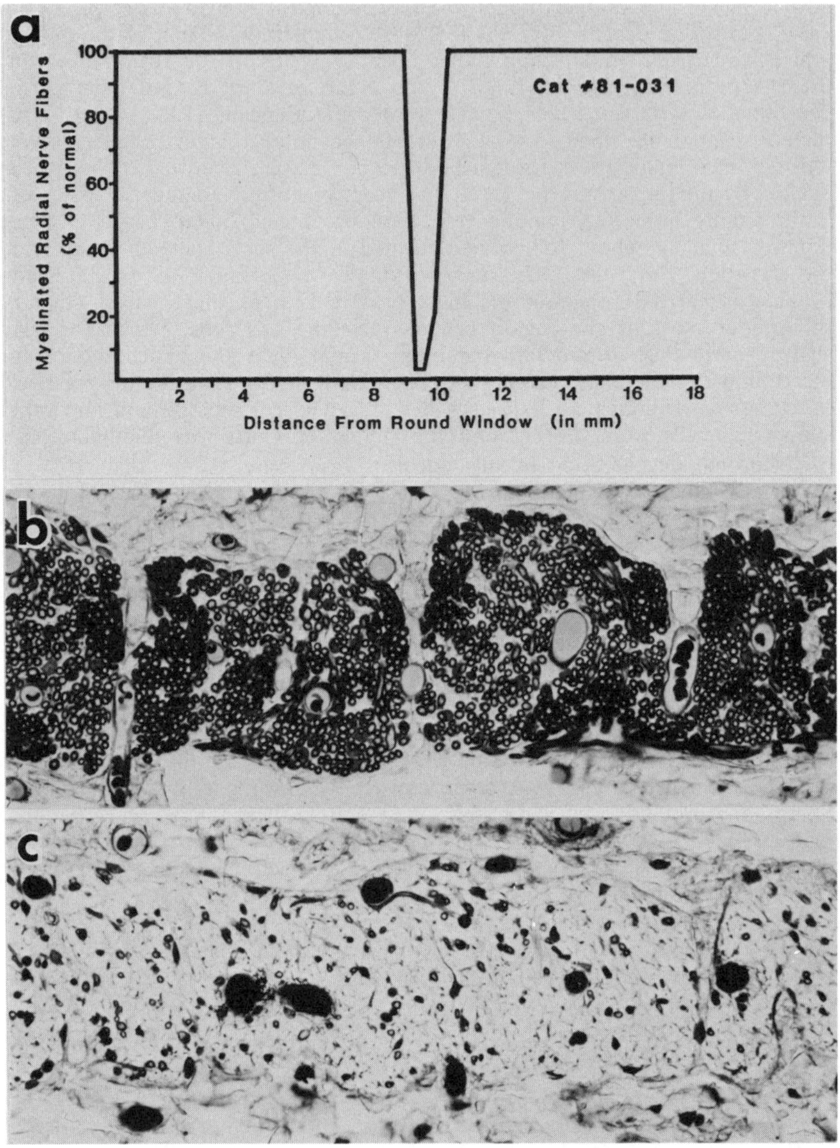

FIGURE 8. Case #031R. (**a**) The normal complement of myelinated radial nerve fibers was observed throughout this cochlea with the exception of the region 9 to 10.2 mm from the base. (**b**) Section of the osseous spiral lamina taken 6–7 mm from the base illustrates the normal appearance of the nerve array overlying the implant. (**c**) In the lesioned area 9–10 mm from the base, the majority of myelinated neurons have degenerated. (Magnification × 350).

sure on the electrode fractured the osseous spiral lamina and displaced the basilar membrane upwards. Since the scala tympani tapers much more rapidly along the spiral in the cat than in the human, there would be little frictional resistance during insertion until the tip is actually wedged between the upper and lower surfaces of the scala tympani.

It is of interest that although the spiral ganglion cells in cats have been reported to undergo retrograde degeneration 3 to 5 months after various other types of peripheral damage have occurred,[8] direct trauma to the osseous spiral lamina by a misplaced electrode may result in destruction of the ganglion over a much shorter time course. Further, the swelling of neurons noted in better-preserved regions adjacent to a lesion may indicate that they will undergo subsequent retrograde degeneration as well. The severe pathologic alterations and ganglion cell loss observed with perforation of the basilar partition in the present short-term implantation cases are consistent with previously reported results in cats in which electrodes have been implanted for longer periods.[9] It seems quite likely that traumatic electrode insertion would present an additional serious hazard to surviving neuronal elements, even in the pathologic cochleas of profoundly deaf potential implant candidates. This conclusion is supported by the findings of Johnsson *et al.*,[10] who recently described the otopathology in a patient who had received bilateral cochlear implants. Thorough assessment of the temporal bone pathology led to their conclusion that rupture of the cochlear duct by the implants (on both sides) during surgery further aggravated the ongoing sensorineural degeneration (which was probably already severe prior to implantation).

The pathologic alteration ("thinning") of neuronal processes at the edge of the osseous spiral lamina may represent an initial step in a process eventually leading to total retrograde degeneration of these cochlear neurons. Similar damage to the distal ends of myelinated processes of first-order neurons in human temporal bones has been reported with aminoglycoside-induced cochlear pathology.[11] In that report, the phenomenon was attributed to recent severe insult to the organ of Corti and it was suggested that this alteration was secondary to destruction of sensory and supporting cells. In the present study in cats, although hair cells were destroyed, supporting cells were frequently preserved in regions where the distal dendrites showed this degenerative pattern. It has been suggested that these early changes in cochlear neurons may be accompanied by simultaneous or earlier degenerative changes in the ganglion cells.[11] Therefore, it is of interest to note that the light microscopic appearance of the spiral ganglion was normal in the present plastic-embedded material in regions showing these changes in the distal dendrites. Further, Hinojosa [12] has observed that in temporal bones from profoundly deaf patients (from various causes) total degeneration of the myelinated peripheral processes may be associated with a wide range in percentages of surviving spiral ganglion cells. The precise time course and sequence of degenerative alterations in spiral ganglion cells and their peripheral processes after damage to the organ of Corti must vary with the type of peripheral injury.

The loss of hair cells from the organ of Corti in the region overlying the implanted electrode is an interesting finding that is fairly consistent throughout the series. The better preservation of sensory cells in case #031R with the new feline electrode (and an implantation period similar to the cases with the human array) suggests that when insertion trauma is minimal,

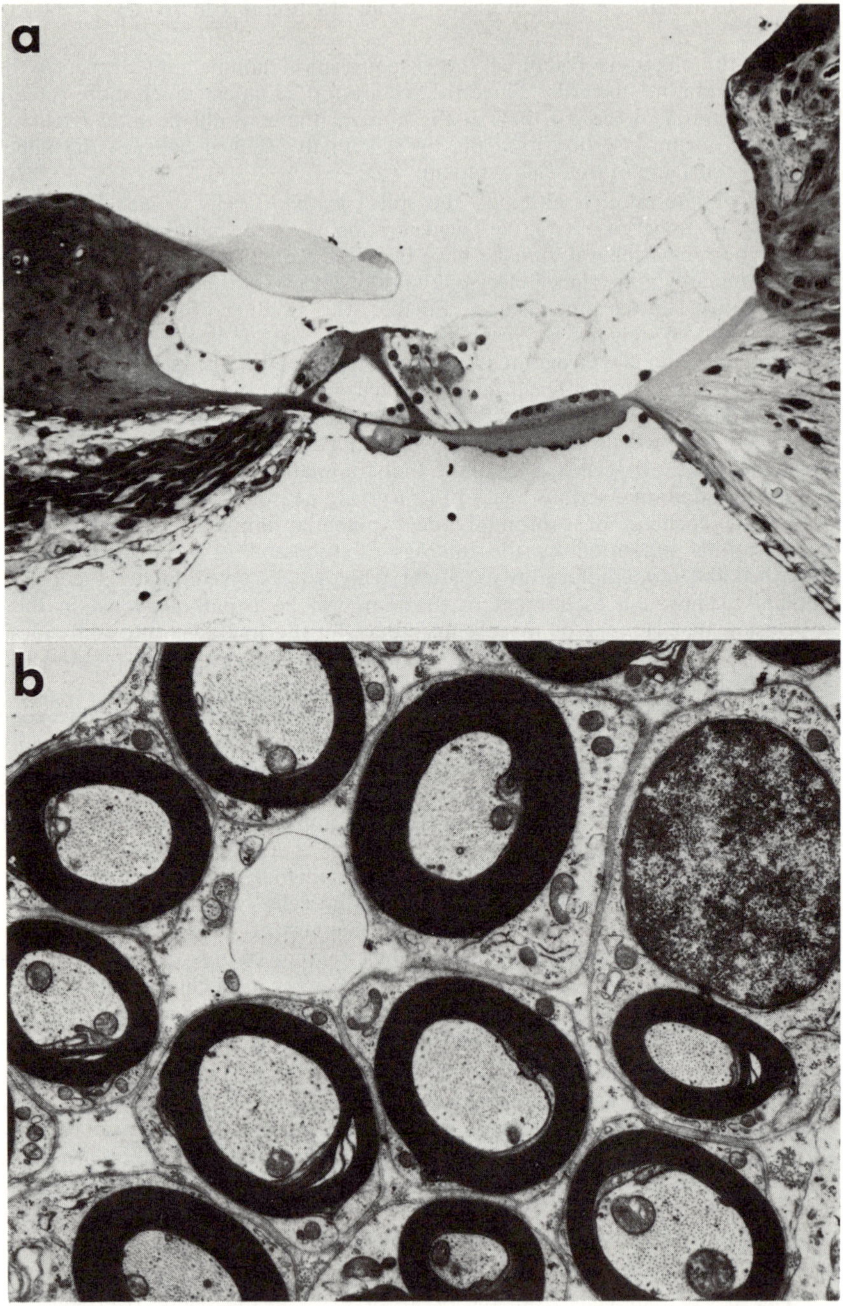

FIGURE 9. Case #9154R. (**a**) Section of the organ of Corti in the region of the electrode array (5–6 mm from the base), which was implanted for 13 months. Pillars are intact, although hair cells have degenerated and obliteration of the fluid spaces is noted. (Magnification × 225.) (**b**) No significant loss of myelinated radial nerve fibers in the osseous spiral lamina occurred (with the exception of the most basal 3 mm, or "hook" region) and the electron microscopic appearance of these myelinated axons is within normal limits. (Section taken 5–6 mm from the base.) (Magnification × 13,000.)

hair cells in the implant region may survive for at least several weeks. However, it should be pointed out that some ultrastructural changes were observed in case #031R within the organ of Corti and in regions around the hair cells, although the condition of the sensory cells themselves appeared to be within normal limits. It is not known what factor(s) are responsible for the hair-cell loss in these cochleas. No correlation between the condition of the stria vascularis and the survival of sensory cells could be demonstrated. The loss appears to occur first at the base in the region of the implant; and it may be important to note that in cases with little or no trauma, degeneration of hair cells in regions apical to the electrode may be considerably delayed (for example, for more than a year in case #9154). The focal lesion in case #031 associated with the close proximity of the electrode carrier to the upper surface of the scala suggests that impairment of adequate perilymph circulation may be a causative factor in loss of hair cells, and (for example, if blockage is complete enough) perhaps it may even precipitate collapse of the organ of Corti and neural degeneration. However, other etiologic factors, such as compromise of the local blood supply, cannot be ruled out, and more data will be necessary before any conclusion can be drawn.

The final two case studies reported in this series, #9154 R and 9420R, represent the extremes of a spectrum of pathology observed in individual cochleas with atraumatic chronic implantation of the contoured type of scala tympani electrode. The minimal reaction of cochlear structures in case #9154R illustrates that supporting elements in the organ of Corti and myelinated peripheral dendrites of cochlear neurons can withstand atraumatic insertion and chronic implantation of this type of electrode for periods of more than a year. On the other hand, the extensive neural degeneration in case #9420R (9-month implantation), accompanied by evidence of severe chronic inflammation, demonstrates the worst extreme of a range of cochlear pathology observed in individual cats in a long series designed to evaluate the consequences of chronic implantation of these arrays. The electrodes used in these cases were assumed to be identical. However, the severe inflammatory response and neural damage in the latter case appears to be most consistent with a biotoxicity problem with this particular electrode. Possible sources of contamination in these older-generation contoured electrodes include: (1) leaching of unbound stannous octoate catalyst from the Silastic® carrier; (2) leaching of ethylene oxide from the carrier as a result of an inadequate out-gassing procedure after gas sterilization; (3) contamination of electrode materials or final product due to, for example, inadequate clean fabrication techniques and facilities. The sequence of pathologic changes in this cochlea may be different from that observed in other types of peripheral cochlear damage. The preservation of the pillar cells has been reported to effectively delay secondary neural degeneration, yet in case #9420R, apical to the implant region, the tunnel of Corti and space of Nuel were preserved, while profound neural loss was evident. According to Spoendlin,[13] damage to the unmyelinated distal neural processes in the organ of Corti is the factor that precipitates degeneration. It may be that hair cells and their neurons are particularly sensitive to the suspected contamination or biotoxicity problem, while the supporting cells are more resistant.

The finding in this last case of ectopic myelinated neurons, which had sprouted into the scala tympani at a point where the integrity of the osseous spiral lamina was compromised by osteoneogenesis, is of interest. Similar

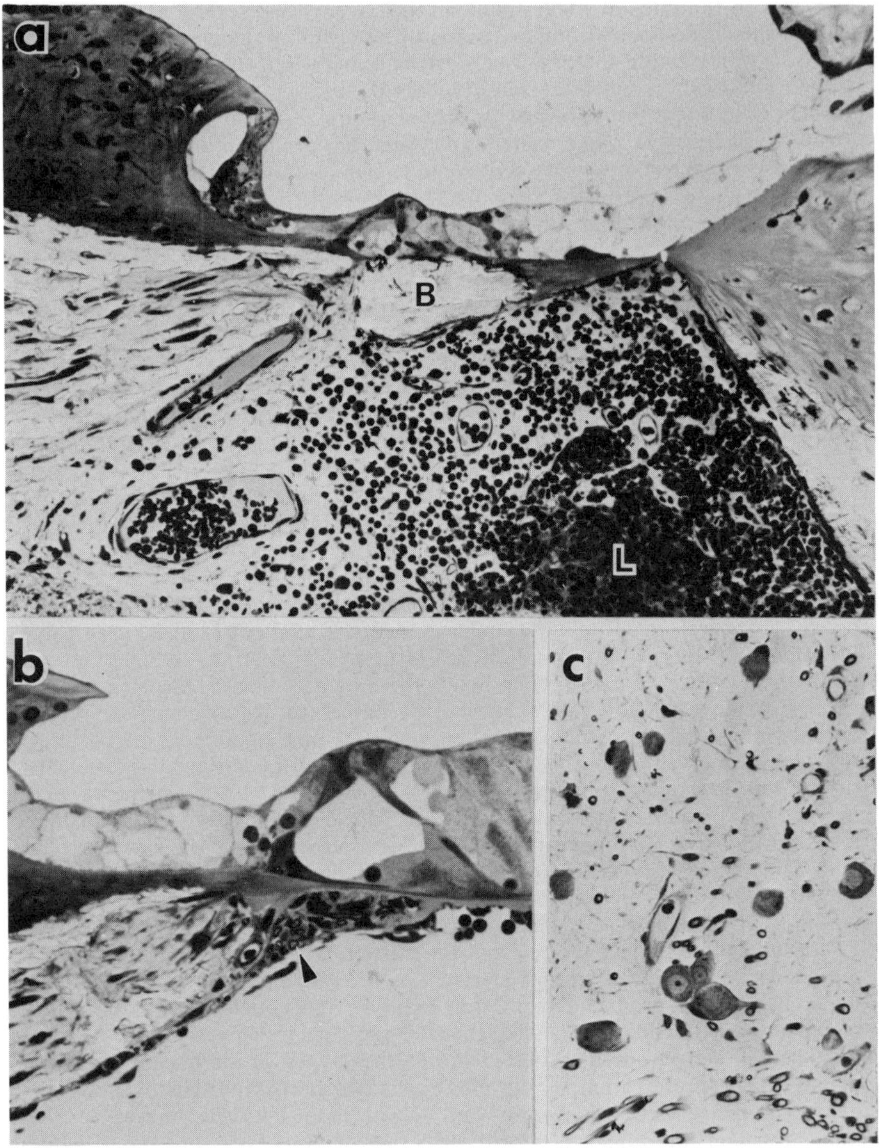

FIGURE 10. Case #9420R. (**a**) Five mm from the base, the organ of Corti over the implant has collapsed and the tectorial membrane is resorbed. Evidence of chronic inflammation is seen in osteoneogenesis (B) under the basilar membrane and in the infiltration of the scala tympani by numerous lymphocytes, monocytes, and macrophages. L, lymphoid follicle. (Magnification × 200). (**b**) Apical to the electrode (8 mm from the base) some pillars are preserved, but the neuronal degeneration is still severe here (and throughout the length of spiral). (Magnification × 225.) *Arrowhead* shows ectopic myelinated neurons which had sprouted for over several millimeters in the scala tympani. (**c**) Spiral ganglion cell degeneration paralleled that of the nerve array, and was extensive throughout the specimen, as illustrated in this section from the 8-mm position. (Magnification × 275.)

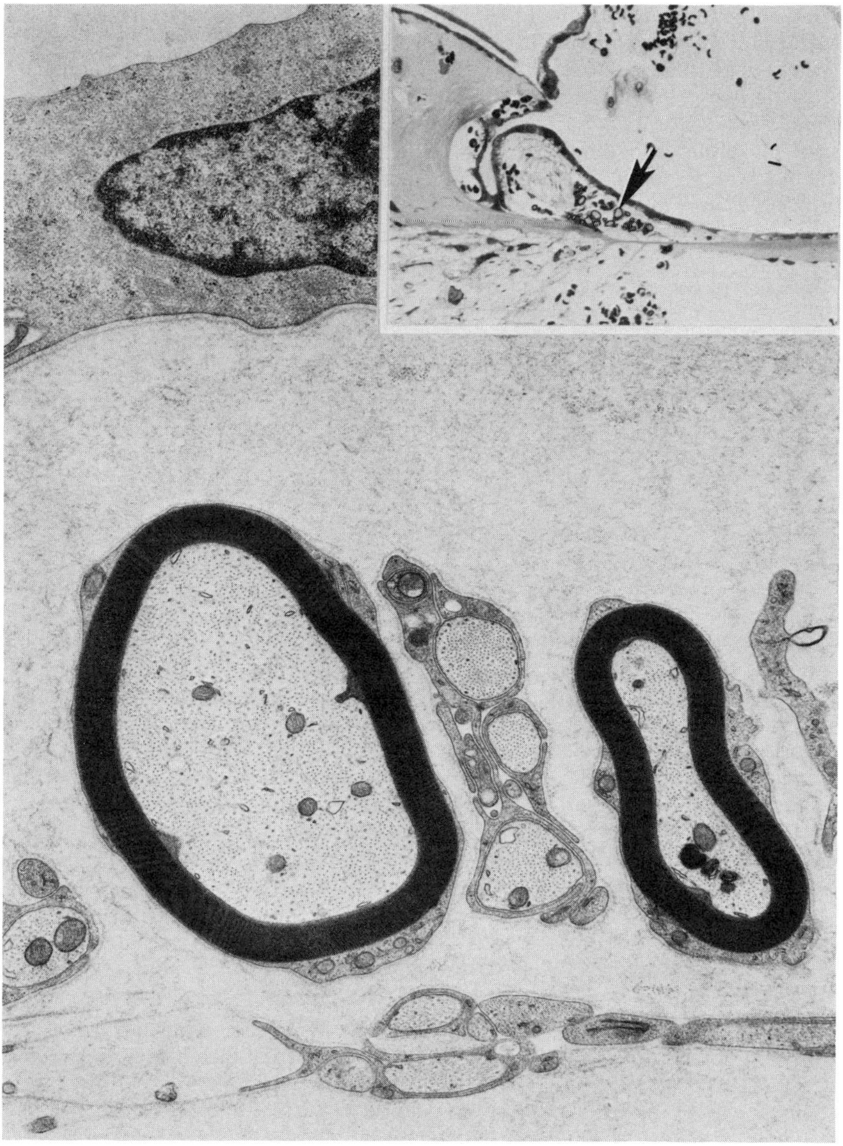

FIGURE 11. Ectopic myelinated neurons are seen in the region of the collapsed organ of Corti 8 months after pretreatment of the cochlea by perilymph perfusion of neomycin, implantation of a contoured type of scala tympani electrode, and subsequent continuous electrical stimulation for a period of 500 hours. Electron micrograph illustrates the sprouting myelinated neuronal processes as well as several unmyelinated fibers. *Inset* shows the position of these fibers (*arrow*) near the habenula perforata. The tectorial membrane is detached from the limbus and appears as a round mass on the tympanic lip invested with the simple epethelium that formed in the region of the resorbed organ of Corti. (Magnification × 12,325; magnification of inset × 250.)

ectopic neurons have been observed in the scala media (FIG. 11) and scala tympani in cases of continuous bipolar stimulation at high current levels when cochleas were pretreated with perilymphatic infusion of an ototoxic antibiotic (neomycin sulfate).[14] Terayama *et al.*[15] have described a similar phenomenon after perilymphatic perfusion of streptomycin. With intracochlear electrical stimulation, such fibers appear to persist beyond expected survival periods and even to sprout into other cochlear regions. The cochlea illustrated in FIGURE 11 was pretreated with perilymph perfusion of 50 μl of 10% neomycin sulfate,[5,6] implanted for 8 months with a contoured type electrode, and subsequently exposed to 500 hours of continuous electrical stimulation (charge-balanced biphasic pulses at 40 μC/phase per cm^2 real surface area; 100 μsec/phase at 20–25 pulses/s).[16,17] Although this initial observation suggested that the sprouting might be induced by intracochlear electrical stimulation, it is now evident that other conditions, such as chronic inflammation or irritation, may also induce sprouting. The phenomenon is probably worthy of further investigation. The possibility of a trophic effect of electrical stimulation in delaying ongoing sensorineural degeneration should not be overlooked.

SUMMARY

In summary, these results with chronic implantation of three types of scala tympani electrode indicate the critical importance of two factors in reducing the risk of additional damage to cochlear structure by implantation surgery: (1) The shape and mechanical characteristics of the array must be precisely controlled such that insertion can be performed with an acceptably low incidence of trauma; and (2) the specific electrode materials and fabrication procedures must be demonstrated to be highly biocompatible in *in vivo* animal control studies. It appears that the neuronal elements of a prior normal cochlea (in the cat) can withstand chronic implantation of scala tympani electrodes (for at least 1 year) if these two prerequisites are met. The effects of chronic electrical stimulation with these arrays at current levels appropriate for the operation of such devices in patients is not known at present.

ACKNOWLEDGMENTS

We wish to thank Drs. R. F. Gray and S. M. Walsh, who performed the surgical implantation procedure in some of the animals included in this study.

REFERENCES

1. MERZENICH, M. M. 1983. Coding of sound in a cochlear prosthesis. Some theoretical and practical considerations. This volume.
2. WHITE, M. W. 1983. Formant frequency discrimination and recognition in subjects implanted with intracochlear stimulating electrodes. This volume.
3. OWENS, E. O., D. KESSLER & M. RAGGIO. Results for some patients with cochlear implants on the Minimal Auditory Capabilities (MAC) battery. This volume.

4. LOEB, G. E., C. L. BYERS, S. J. REBSCHER, D. E. CASEY, M. M. FONG, R. A. SCHINDLER, R. F. GRAY & M. M. MERZENICH. The design and fabrication of an experimental cochlear prosthesis. Med. Biol. Eng. Comp. In press.
5. LEAKE-JONES, P. A., M. C. VIVION, B. F. O'REILLY & M. M. MERZENICH. Deaf animal models for studies of a multichannel cochlear prosthesis. Hearing Res. In press.
6. LEAKE-JONES, P. A., B. F. O'REILLY & M. C. VIVION. 1980. Neomycin ototoxicity: Ultrastructural surface pathology of the organ of Corti. SEM/1980/ **III:** 427–434. SEM Inc., AMF O'Hare, IL 60660.
7. SPOENDLIN, H. & J. P. BRUN. 1974. The block-surface technique for evaluation of cochlear pathology. Arch. Otorhinolaryngol. **208:** 137–145.
8. SPOENDLIN, H. 1975. Retrograde degeneration of the cochlear nerve. Acta Otolaryngol. **79:** 266–275.
9. SCHINDLER, R. A. & M. M. MERZENICH. 1974. Chronic intracochlear electrode implantation: Cochlear pathology and acoustic nerve survival. Ann. Otol. Rhinol. Laryngol. **83**(2): 202–215.
10. JOHNSSON, L.-G., W. F. HOUSE & F. H. LITHICUM, JR. 1982. Otopathological findings in a patient with bilateral cochlear implants. Ann. Otol. Rhinol. Laryngol. **91** (Suppl 91): 74–89.
11. JOHNSSON, L.-G., J. E. HAWKINS, JR., T. C. KINGSLEY, F. O. BLACK & G. J. MATZ. Aminoglycoside-induced cochlear pathology in man. Acta Otolaryngol. Suppl. 383.
12. HINOJOSA, R. & M. MARION. 1983. Histopathology of profound sensorineural deafness. This volume.
13. SPOENDLIN, H. 1978. The afferent innervation of the cochlea. *In* Evoked Electrical Activity in the Auditory Nervous System. R. A. Naunton and C. Fernandez, Eds.: 21–41. Academic Press. New York, NY.
14. LEAKE-JONES, P. A., S. M. WALSH, B. F. O'REILLY, M. C. VIVION & M. M. MERZENICH. 1980. Development of a multichannel auditory prosthesis: Cochlear pathology in animal models. Abstracts of the Third Midwinter Research Meeting, Association for Research Otolaryngology, St. Petersburg Beach, FL.
15. TERAYAMA, Y., Y. KANEKO, K. KAWAMOTO & N. SAKAI. 1977. Ultrastructural change of the nerve elements following destruction of the organ of Corti. Acta Otolaryngol. **83:** 291–302.
16. WALSH, S. M., P. A. LEAKE-JONES, L. S. VUREK & M. M. MERZENICH. 1981. Chronic electrical stimulation with intracochlear electrodes: Electrophysiological results. Ann. Otol. Rhinol. Laryngol. **90** (Suppl 82): 27–29.
17. WALSH, S. M. & P. A. LEAKE-JONES. 1982. Chronic electrical stimulation of auditory nerve in cat: Physiological and histological results. Hearing Res. **7:** 281–304.

RELATION OF COCHLEAR IMPLANT FUNCTION TO HISTOPATHOLOGY IN MONKEYS [a]

Bryan E. Pfingst [b] and Dwight Sutton

Department of Otolaryngology and
Regional Primate Research Center
University of Washington
Seattle, Washington 98195
and
Virginia Mason Research Center
Seattle, Washington 98101

Although a number of patients are currently benefiting from cochlear implants, it is widely believed that considerable improvement can be made in this method of providing hearing to the deaf. Many investigators are currently gathering data with this goal in mind. We believe that one of the most fruitful approaches is to examine the relations between implant function, measured psychophysically, and the condition of the implanted cochlea, measured histologically.

This approach yields data that are applicable at several levels: (1) Observing the relation of implant function to various levels and types of pathology will aid in establishing criteria for selection and treatment of implant candidates. (2) These observations yield data relevant to physiological models of implant function. If we can model what neural elements are being excited by electrical stimulation, and how various percepts are encoded, we will be in a much better position to specify optimal electrode placements and parameters for electrical stimulation. (3) Studies of hearing in the absence of hair cells and basilar membrane mechanics, and in many cases in the absence of a large percentage of the normal complement of eighth nerve fibers, provide unique opportunities to analyze central neural mechanisms. A better understanding of central auditory processing would be of great benefit to those who are trying to devise paradigms for translating acoustic stimuli into electrical signals that can be delivered by single- or multichannel cochlear implants.

Realistically, achievement of these goals will require data from both implanted human patients and laboratory animals. The human data ultimately demonstrate the relevance of the animal data, and in addition, some percepts are more readily tested in humans than in animals. On the other hand, the procurement of human histological data is naturally very slow, and the human psychophysical data are often inadequate owing to a variety of complicating factors. For example, human data are usually collected from patients who have been deaf for a number of years and whose ability to perform the required psychophysical experiments is not known, whereas animal data can often be obtained from a deafened, implanted ear and a normal hearing

[a] This work was supported by Grants NS 13056 and RR 00166 from the National Institutes of Health and by the William G. Reed Fund.

[b] Address for correspondence: Dr. Bryan E. Pfingst, Regional Primate Research Center SJ–50, University of Washington, Seattle, Washington 98195.

0077–8923/83/0405–0224 $01.75/0 © 1983, NYAS

ear in the same subject. Animal experiments can be conducted on a relatively large number of subjects under well controlled laboratory conditions, and histologic material can be obtained quickly and under optimal conditions.

Our initial exploration of the relation of psychophysical measures to histopathology indicated that the degree of pathology was related to the level of detection-threshold current and was inversely related to dynamic range.[1] More recent results have been consistent with these findings. We have also measured other aspects of implant function, and found that they, too, were related to the degree of pathology.

METHODS

Overview

Cases were selected from a series of monkeys undergoing a variety of tests of cochlear implant function. Selection was based on the following criteria: (1) The implants were located in the scala tympani; we have found that placement of electrodes in other parts of the cochlea can significantly affect some psychophysical measures, such as threshold. (2) Stable threshold data were available at a variety of frequencies of sinusoidal stimulation for several electrode spacings, and other psychophysical data were available as well. (3) Implants remained in place for 9 months or more so that at least the initial trauma of neomycin poisoning and implantation as well as any initial effects of electrical stimulation could be manifest in the histopathology. (4) The animal was sacrificed within 1 month of the last behavioral testing, with no disturbance of the implant up to the point of sacrifice. (5) Histologic evaluations of at least the cochlea and spiral ganglion were available. In order to model the presumed condition of the cochlea in implant candidates, we used only cases in which no healthy-appearing hair cells were present at the time of sacrifice.

The subjects were adolescent or adult male rhesus macaques (*Macaca mulatta*). The monkeys were trained first to perform a simple reaction-time task, which was used for measuring detection thresholds and dynamic ranges, and then to perform intensity and frequency discrimination tasks (see below). Training with acoustic stimuli continued until (1) the monkey's performance was stable, and (2) measures of thresholds and difference limens for acoustic stimuli were comparable to those obtained previously in this species.[2,3] After initial training and testing with acoustic stimuli, the monkeys underwent surgery. One ear was poisoned with neomycin sulfate (with one exception, see TABLE 1) followed by insertion of a multichannel implant in the scala tympani. Thresholds, dynamic ranges, and various discrimination functions were then measured for various parameters of electrical stimulation using a constant-current source[4] connected directly to the electrodes.

After behavioral testing was completed, the animals were sacrificed and the cochleas were prepared for histologic examination as described below.

Psychophysical Procedures

Detection thresholds were measured while the monkeys performed a simple reaction-time task. Monkeys were trained to press a telegraph key at the onset of a visual cue and to release the key after onset of an acoustic cue occurring after a variable foreperiod. Responses were divided into two categories: releases within 1 sec of stimulus onset were "hits," and failures to release within 1 sec were "misses." Various threshold intensities were presented by the method of constant stimuli, and the intensity to which the monkey responded correctly on 50% of the trials was defined as "threshold" (see Pfingst *et al.*[5] for details).

Dynamic ranges were measured using the subjects' reaction times. During training, subjects were taught, using differential reinforcement techniques, to release the key quickly after the onset of the acoustic cue.[6] Suprathreshold stimuli were presented by the method of constant stimuli. Previous studies in humans and monkeys have shown that reaction times in well-trained subjects reflect stimulus loudness.[7-11] Thus, equally loud stimuli tend to produce equal median reaction times. For electrical stimuli, the upper limit of the dynamic range was defined as the intensity of electrical stimulation producing a median reaction time equivalent to that obtained for a white-noise acoustic stimulus of 100 dB SPL delivered to a normally hearing ear in the same subject.[12,13]

Frequency and intensity discrimination were measured using a slight modification of the simple reaction-time task. When the monkey depressed the telegraph key, a train of stimulus bursts at the initial stimulus frequency and intensity was presented during the variable foreperiod. At the end of the foreperiod, stimulus intensity or frequency was changed to the test stimulus value with the change in frequency-synthesizer or attenuator settings being made during an interburst interval. The difference limen was defined as the intensity or frequency change to which the monkey responded correctly (that is, within 1 sec after the change) on 50% of the trials (see Pfingst *et al.*[14] for details).

Electrode-place discrimination was tested in a manner similar to frequency and intensity discrimination except that the electrode pair to which stimuli were delivered was changed during an interburst interval at the end of the variable foreperiod, and the monkey was required to detect this change. In some cases, the intensity of the stimulus was also changed simultaneously with the electrode-place change in an attempt to test for the use of intensity cues in making this discrimination.

Guess rate (that is, the percentage of "hits" on catch trials when there was no change in the stimulus) and percentage of premature releases were monitored during each session. These variables were brought under experimental control by varying the duration of a "penalty time-out" that was contingent on premature releases. We attempted to hold the guess rate within criterion limits of 1–15%, and collected data only when the monkey was performing within these limits. Once initial estimates of thresholds or difference limens were made, we attempted to select stimuli in such a way that the monkey would be reinforced on roughly 75% of the trials. We have found that keeping this reinforcement density constant also helps to maintain a consistent guess rate.

Implant Procedures

Each implant consisted of four platinum–iridium spherical electrodes, approximately 200 μm each in diameter, in silicon (Silastic®) rubber carriers (see Figure 1 in Pfingst *et al.*[12]). The silicon carriers were smooth, tapered tubes with diameters roughly one-half to three-quarters the diameter of the scala tympani (TABLE 1). The tubes were flattened slightly on the side where the electrodes rested. The electrodes were arranged longitudinally along the carriers, separated by 0.4 to 5.0 mm. The implants were inserted into the scala tympani via the round window, and advanced so that the most distal electrode was approximately 10 mm from the round window. Details of the surgical procedure are given elsewhere.[12]

Histology

After behavioral testing was completed, the animals were deeply anesthetized with pentobarbital. The middle ears were infused with cold phosphate-buffered 10% formalin, and the monkeys were perfused systemically with 10% saline solution followed by phosphate-buffered 10% formalin. The brainstems and temporal bones were separately removed and immediately stored in cold formalin.

The cochleas were decalcified in 10% EDTA (Versene®, Dow Chemical), embedded in celloidin, and serially sectioned (18 μm) in a paramodiolar orientation. Every tenth section, or in some cases every fifth section, was stained with Harris' hematoxylin and eosin-Y. Selected intermediate sections were stained with Luxol fast-blue or Holmes' silver stain.

The sections were examined by light microscopy to determine the presense or absence of hair cells, and to estimate the number of remaining myelinated nerve fibers. Spiral ganglion cells in each segment of Rosenthal's canal were counted in each section. All cells identified by a nucleus and a perikaryon were counted. The resulting numbers were compared with numbers at comparable sites from control ears. These values were plotted in terms of percent of cells remaining along the length of the spiral ganglion. Since normal cochleas contain varying numbers of elements, estimates of the percentages of surviving elements are only approximate.

In cochleas that showed extensive fibrosis or ossification, bony or fibrous capsules loosely enveloping the implant often were clearly seen in the serial sections. Dome-shaped intrusions in the capsules spaced at intervals corresponding to the electrode spacing in the Silastic carrier indicated the locations of the spherical platinum–iridium electrodes, which rested on the surface of the carrier (see Figure 6 in Pfingst *et al.*[1]).

RESULTS AND DISCUSSION

Overview

Four cases met the criteria described in METHODS. For ease of presentation we have labeled these A–D with A representing the least severe pathology and D representing the most severe. Identification of these four implants together with details regarding their size, duration of implantation, and so forth, are given in TABLE 1. In the following sections we will describe first the histopathology (illustrated in part in FIGURE 1) and then the psychophysical data for these four implants. Observations made in other implants that did not meet the five criteria are consistent with the observations for these four cases if certain assumptions are made.

TABLE 1

DESCRIPTION OF THE FOUR IMPLANTS FOR WHICH PSYCHOPHYSICAL AND HISTOLOGIC RESULTS ARE PRESENTED

Case	Implant Diameter (mm)		Ease of Insertion [a]	Neomycin Concentration [b] (w/v)	Implant Duration (mo.)	Codes	
	Proximal End	Distal End				Implant	Cochlea
A	0.83	0.73	No comment	None	11.1	PU-R-1	264R
B	0.80	0.76	Very easy	10%	23.2	BE-R-1	075R
C	0.64	0.55	Easy	10%	32.6	MA-R-1	229R
D	0.73	0.50	Difficult	100%	27.7	RI-L-1	251L

[a] Judged by comments in surgeon's report.
[b] 10% w/v equals approximately a 0.1 molar concentration. 100% w/v equals approximately 1 molar.

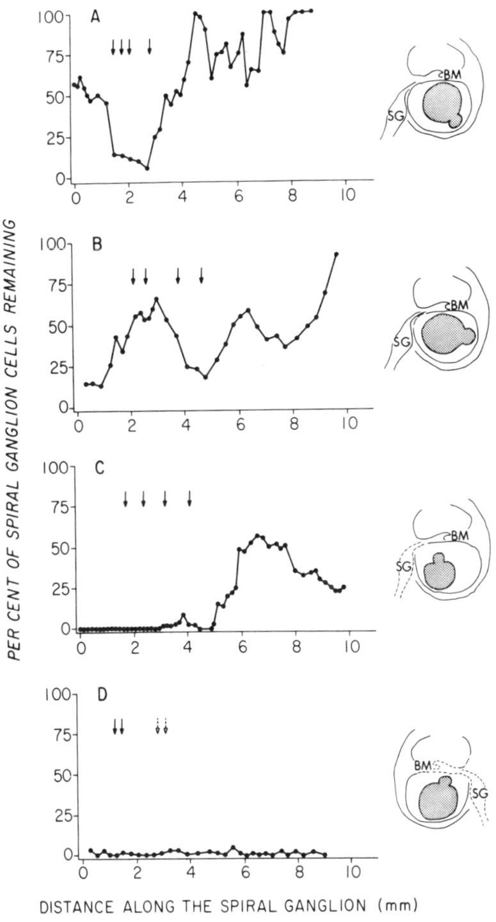

FIGURE 1. The left side of this figure shows the percent of spiral ganglion cells found in paramodiolar sections taken at 200-μm intervals throughout the cochleas in cases A–D. On the abscissa, the base is to the left and the apex to the right. The *solid arrows* indicate the locations of the stimulating electrodes as determined by indentations in the bony or fibrous capsules that surrounded the implants, and the *dashed arrows* indicate probable locations, based on implant design, of two electrodes for which no capsule was found. Schematic drawings to the right of each graph indicate the orientations of the implants in the scala tympani. SG = spiral ganglion; BM = basilar membrane. A, B, and C are right cochleas and D is a left cochlea.

Histopathology

Case A had the least severe histopathology in the series. Some hair cells remained (about 5% in the base of the cochlea, increasing to about 15% in the upper turns) but none seemed to be entirely intact. About 30% of the normal complement of myelinated nerve fibers remained in the base adjacent to the implant, increasing to 85% in the upper turns. About 50% of the normal complement of spiral ganglion cells remained in the basal turn except near the region where the electrodes were located. In this area, the spiral ganglion cell counts dropped to about 15% of normal. Apical to the implant, spiral ganglion cells increased in density to about 80% of normal in the upper turns. The implant was oriented with the most proximal (that is, most basal) electrode facing the floor of the scala tympani opposite the basilar membrane, and was twisted slightly so that the most distal (that is, most apical) electrode was directly opposite the spiral ganglion.

In case B, the organ of Corti was absent from the base; pillar cells were collapsed in the second and third turns leaving limited patches of support cells. Hair cells were absent throughout the cochlea. Five to ten percent of the normal complement of myelinated nerve fibers remained in the first half of the basal turn, increasing to 30% in the second half, 40–60% in the second turn, and 70% in the apex. Spiral ganglion cell loss was less prominent, and most of the remaining cells appeared healthy. The implant rested on the floor of the scala tympani, with the electrodes oriented toward the lateral wall. New bone enveloped most of the implant.

Case C showed extensive degeneration, particularly in the basal turn. No hair cells were found. Virtually no myelinated nerve fibers remained in the basal turn, but patchy regions of surviving fibers were seen in the upper turns, giving an overall density of 20–30% of normal in this region. Spiral ganglion cells were absent from the first half of the basal turn, and the few remaining cells in the second half seemed to be degenerating. In the upper turns, spiral ganglion cell counts increased to a maximum of about 55% and the majority of the cells seemed healthy. The basal turn of this cochlea was filled with collagen and new bone, which surrounded the implant. There was a lesser degree of ossification in the basal turn of the scala vestibuli, and both scalae were free of infiltration in the upper turns. The implant in this cochlea lay close to the floor of the scala tympani, with electrodes facing the habenula perforata but separated by 60–70 μm from the osseous spiral lamina.

Case D was the most severely impaired cochlea in the series. No organ of Corti structures were found in any part of the cochlea. Only a few patches of myelinated nerve fibers remained. Our samples yielded an estimate of 180 spiral ganglion cells remaining (out of a normal complement of 32,000 cells), of which one-third gave evidence of degenerative changes. Those cells that remained were evenly distributed throughout the cochlear turns. Extensive osteogenesis was found throughout scala tympani and scala vestibuli. This obliterated the basilar membrane and organ of Corti in the basal turn. The implant in this cochlea was oriented with the electrodes facing the osseous spiral lamina and surrounded by new bone.

Detection Thresholds

Thresholds for the four implants are shown in FIGURE 2. Results for cases A, B, and C were consistent with our previous findings that higher thresholds were correlated with more severe cochlear damage.[1] Thresholds for case D were unexpectedly low, given that this subject had very few remaining spiral ganglion cells. However, the low thresholds relative to the other curves were probably due in part to the fact that these data were for a very widely spaced pair of electrodes (4.8 mm compared with a maximum of 3.0 mm for the other cases); thresholds decrease as a function of electrode separation.[12] When electrode separation is taken into account (FIGURE 3), the thresholds for case D are generally higher than those for the other three cases.

It is clear from FIGURES 2 and 3 that the correlation between pathology and threshold level is more marked at low frequencies (<100 Hz) than at higher frequencies of sinusoidal stimulation. At the low frequencies, the thresholds for these four cases varied over a range of about 20 to 30 dB, whereas at the higher frequencies, the range averaged only about 10 dB.

Thresholds for cases C and D were very similar, despite the considerably better morphologic picture apical to the implant in case C. This suggests that proximity of the electrodes to the remaining neurons may be of some importance.

In cases A, B and C, we tested thresholds for monopolar stimulation (that is, stimulation between a single electrode in the scala tympani and a reference electrode in the skull). In cases A and C, where more nerve fibers survived apical to the electrodes than basal to the electrodes, the thresholds for the more apical electrodes (open symbols in FIGURE 3) were lower than thresholds for the more basal electrodes (solid symbols). In case B, which had a somewhat more symmetric distribution of neurons in the vicinity of the electrodes, no difference in thresholds was found for the apical compared with the basal electrode. In case C, comparisons were made between more apically and more

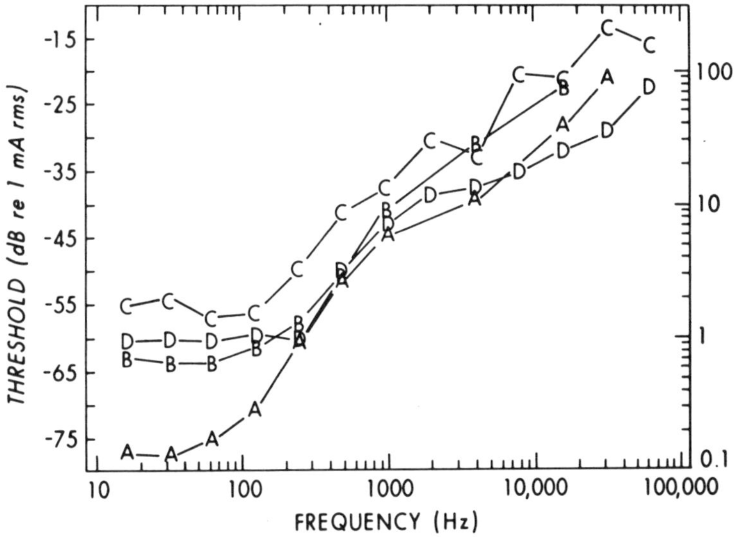

FIGURE 2. Detection threshold versus frequency of sinusoidal stimulation for one intracochlear electrode pair from each of the four cases. Electrodes were separated by 2.9 mm in monkey A, 2.0 mm in monkey B, 3.0 mm in monkey C, and 4.8 mm in monkey D. Data points are averages of thresholds measured throughout the stable period using 20 trials per stimulus per measurement.[12] Ranges of values obtained over repeated measurements for a given frequency and electrode pair averaged 3.1 dB.

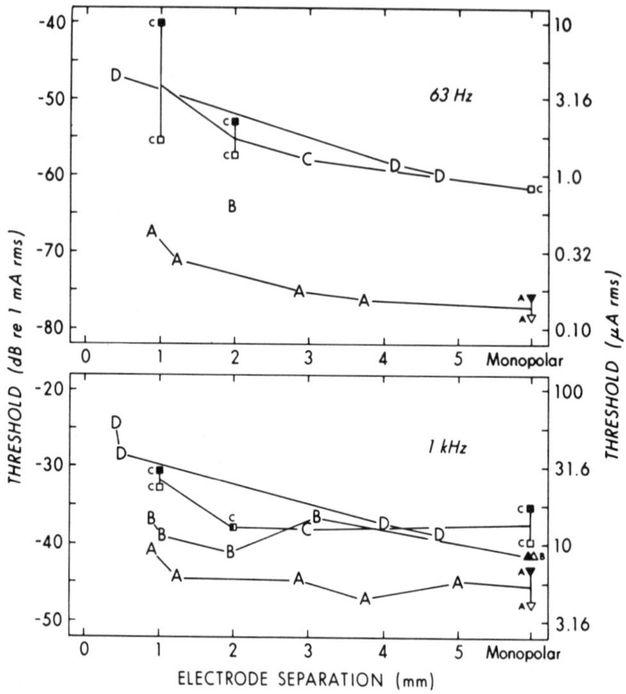

FIGURE 3. Detection threshold versus electrode separation for the four cases discussed in the text. Data are for 63-Hz (upper graph) and 1-kHz (lower graph) sinusoids. *Open symbols* represent more apically located electrodes and *solid symbols* represent more basally located electrodes. Apical-based distinctions are made only in cases where data were available for two equally spaced pairs of electrodes in the implant, and for monopolar stimulation. For monopolar stimulation of a single electrode within the scala tympani, the reference was a stainless-steel wire wrapped around a screw in the parietal bone. Means are shown. Ranges averaged 3.0 dB.

basally located pairs of scala tympani electrodes with equal spacing. Again, the more apically located electrode pairs had lower thresholds than the more basally located pairs (FIG. 3). This effect was more marked at 63 Hz than at 1 kHz, and was larger for the more closely spaced electrode pair.

Threshold Stability

Previous studies in both humans and monkeys have indicated that thresholds for electrical stimuli remain stable over a long period of time, except for some initial changes in the first few months after surgery.[12, 15, 16] This applies to the majority of cases we have studied. We have seen only a few instances of fluctuations in thresholds after the first few months and even fewer cases in which thresholds increased systematically as a function of time. Increases, when they occurred, were usually limited to a few decibels. These observations, coupled with the large differences in threshold correlated with histologic damage, suggest that much of the functional damage to the neural population occurred at the time of implantation rather than during the long-term stimulation period.[1] With regard to this hypothesis, two observations in the present cases are of interest. First, there is a correlation between our pretreatment of the cochleas and the amount of neural degeneration seen. Case A, which had the least degeneration, received no neomycin treatment, while case D, which had the most degeneration, received a highly concentrated dose of neomycin (TABLE 1). Second, the surgeon's comments at the time the implants were inserted are of interest. While no comments about the ease of insertion of implant A were made, the surgeon noted that implant B entered the scala tympani more easily than any others that he had implanted up to that time. Case D, which subsequently showed severe neural degeneration, presented difficulties requiring multiple attempts before all four electrodes were inside the cochlea.

Implant Orientation

Orientation of electrodes away from the nerve fibers projecting to the organ of Corti (cases A and B) did not seem to cause a major elevation in thresholds relative to the effects of neural degeneration. Since the diameter of the scala tympani is small compared with its length, and since, in many cases, the number of nerve fibers in the immediate vicinity of the implant is greatly reduced, it is reasonable to expect that in most cases, implant orientation would not be of major importance. On the other hand, the possibility of more subtle effects of implant orientation should not be ignored. For example, it may be that the relative proximity of the electrodes to the spiral ganglion in cases C and D caused the thresholds in these cases to be somewhat closer to the thresholds for cases A and B than would otherwise have been true. Also, it is likely that some orientations yield more shunting of currents than others. Clearly, more data are needed to address these issues.

Dynamic Range

Dynamic ranges for one electrode pair from each of the four cases are given in FIGURE 4. Consistent with previous findings,[1] dynamic ranges are larger in cases with greater numbers of surviving neural elements than in cases with more severe degeneration, although in these cases the effect is seen only at the low frequencies. The upper limits of the dynamic range for the four cases in this study using electrode pairs described in FIGURE 2 were fairly uniform, varying over a range from implant to implant of only about 12 dB compared with variations of 20 dB or more in threshold at low frequencies. If the electrode spacings had been uniform, we would expect the range of these upper limits to have been even smaller and the range of low-frequency thresholds to have been slightly larger. This, coupled with other observations,[17] suggests that the major differences in dynamic range that are correlated with histopathology occur in the low-intensity region of the dynamic range (near threshold), particularly at the low frequencies.

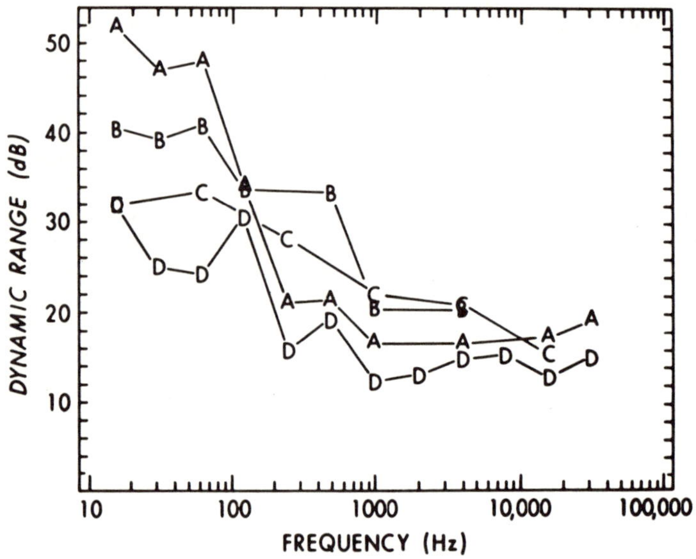

FIGURE 4. Dynamic range versus frequency of sinusoidal stimulation for a single intracochlear electrode pair for each of the four cases discussed in the text. Electrode pairs are the same as in FIGURE 2. Means are shown. Ranges averaged 7.7 dB.

Intensity Discrimination

Intensity difference limens were measured in cases B and C, and the results for three initial stimulus intensities at two frequencies are shown in FIGURE 5. Interestingly, intensity difference limens for the more severely damaged of these two ears are lower than those for the less severly damaged ear.[14]

Electrode-Place Discrimination

Electrode-place discrimination was studied in case C. The results (FIG. 6) indicate that the ability of the monkey to detect a change of stimulation from one electrode to another is a function of electrode location. To test whether changes in perceived loudness might account for the ability to discriminate one electrode from another, we varied the intensity presented to the second electrode in 0.5-dB steps for 5 dB above and below the intensity of the stimulus presented to the first electrode. This procedure caused no reduction in the percent of correct detections, suggesting that intensity was not a primary cue.

In case C, and in several previous cases, changing stimulation among more apically located electrodes was more readily discriminated than similar changes among more basally located electrodes. One hypothesis that might account for the reduced discriminability between the more basally located electrodes is that there are fewer fibers available for stimulation by the basal electrodes than by the more apical electrodes. This hypothesis is consistent with the morphologic picture seen in FIG. 1. Previous studies have shown that electrode-place discrimination is better at higher intensities than at lower intensities of stimulation.[18] Taken together, these two observations suggest that a minimum number of fibers must be stimulated in order to produce a percept that is distinguishable from percepts produced by stimulation of a partially overlapping population of fibers. Thus, in patients with few remaining nerve fibers we would expect that fewer channels of a multichannel implant could be utilized than in patients with larger populations of surviving fibers.

Relation to Human Cases

These four cases cover a reasonably wide range of pathologic conditions. The percentage of surviving spiral ganglion cells covers a range that is roughly comparable to that seen in humans who would be acceptable candidates for cochlear implants (see the paper by Hinojosa [19] in this volume). The pathologic conditions observed in our cases C and D are roughly comparable, in pattern of surviving neural elements, to the right and left ears respectively of House and Brackman's patient, C.R.[20] To date, the data on C.R. comprise the only published results on histopathology in a human cochlear implant patient. The multielectrode implant in C.R.'s left ear was tested psychophysically 2 years before the patient died, at which time both place pitch and

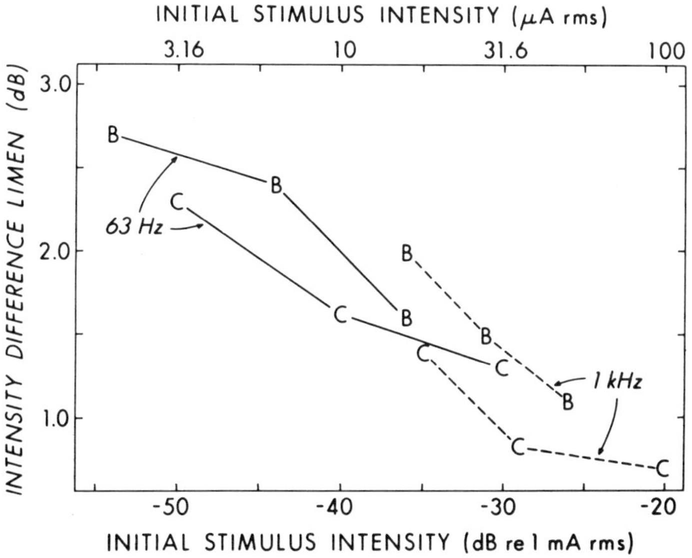

FIGURE 5. Intensity difference limens plotted as a function of initial stimulus intensity at two sinusoidal frequencies for cases B and C. Intensities were selected at 25%, 50%, and 75% of the dynamic range ± 2 dB. Means for three repeated measurements (20 trials per stimulus per measurement) are shown. Ranges averaged 16% of the means.

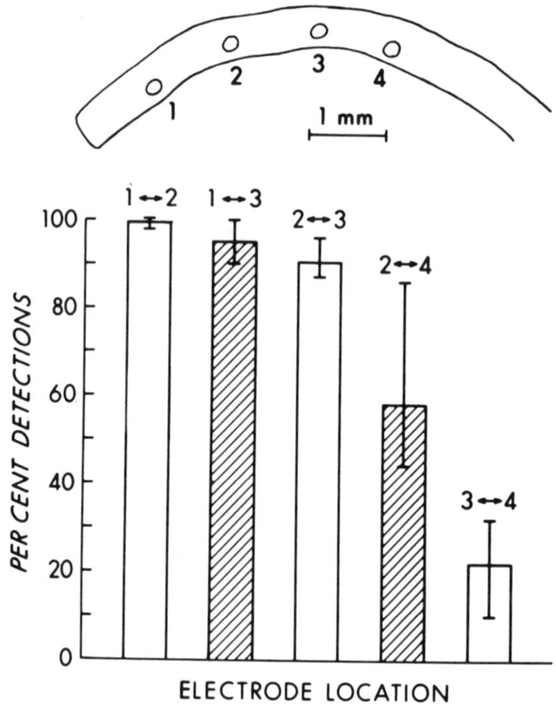

FIGURE 6. Percent discrimination of changes in stimulation from one electrode to another for case C. Monopolar stimulation was used. Stimuli were pulsed 1-kHz sinusoids (pulse duration = 200 msec) with the intensity set at the middle of the monkey's dynamic range. Stimulation was changed from one electrode to another during the interpulse interval. A scale drawing of the implant is shown at the top of the figure, with the electrodes numbered 1 through 4, 1 being the most apical. The change involved in each case is represented by the numbers above each bar in the graph. The *open bars* represent changes in electrode position over a distance of 1 mm and the *shaded bars* are for changes over 2 mm. Direction of change made no difference in the results. The mean percent correct detections for 4 separate days of testing (50 trials per stimulus per day) and the range of values obtained over the 4 days are shown.

periodicity pitch perception were found.[21] It is not clear, however, whether the extensive degeneration seen at C.R.'s autopsy was present at the time these psychophysical measurements were made. In the two years from the time these measurements were made until he died, C.R. primarily used a wearable single-channel stimulator.

Thresholds for monopolar stimulation of C.R.'s left ear are compared in FIGURE 7 with thresholds for a widely spaced pair of electrodes for our case D. Although there are some interesting differences between these two threshold contours, the similarity in threshold level in the two cases is striking. No psychophysical data are available for C.R.'s right ear.

C.R.'s left ear was tested about 1 year before his death by Starr and Brackmann,[22] who measured evoked potentials, and by Bilger *et al.*,[23] who conducted a variety of tests with the subject's wearable single-channel stimulator. The patient was last seen in the clinic 5 months before he died, and the implant was presumably working up until the time of his death.[24] These results are remarkable in light of the almost total absence of neural elements in the patient's left cochlea at the time of death.[20] This, together with the data reported in the present paper, suggests that either (1) very few nerve fibers are necessary for at least some elementary aspects of implant function or (2) the site of neural activation in severely damaged cochleas is remote from the site of the electrodes. This is not to say that implants function optimally in severely damaged ears. The increased thresholds and reduced dynamic ranges are undesirable for obvious reasons. Furthermore, it seems that more complex functions such as electrode-place discrimination are poorer in cases with more severe neural degeneration.

Clinical Implications

A variety of factors influence measures of implant function, including stimulus waveform, electrode placement and the subject's ability to perform the task. Therefore, considerable care must be taken when comparing one implant with another. In this presentation we compared implants in cochleas exhibiting a range of pathologic features, taking these variables into account,

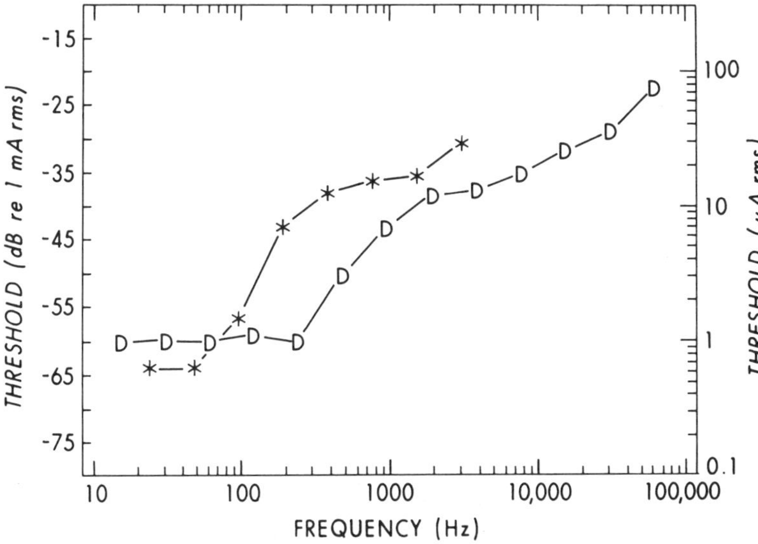

FIGURE 7. Detection threshold versus frequency of sinusoidal stimulation for a widely spaced pair of electrodes (4.8 mm) for case D compared with thresholds for monopolar stimulation in human patient C.R. (The human data were supplied by D. K. Eddington.)

and we continue to find relations between degree of pathology and functional measures.

This correlation, of course, does not prove causality, but one may hypothesize causality in either direction. The correlation could result from animals with higher thresholds receiving more stimulation. However, since the upper limits of the dynamic ranges for these four cases were similar, this argument holds only for near-threshold intensities, where damage from stimulation is less likely. From a physiological point of view, it is certainly reasonable to hypothesize that higher thresholds would result from decreasing the number of nerve fibers available for stimulation. The clinical implications of such a causal relation are worth considering.

These clinical implications are two-fold. First, the results suggest that implants may be expected to function differently in different patients, depending on the nature and degree of temporal bone pathology. Current levels and the factors for adjusting current as a function of frequency may vary over ranges of 20 dB or more from patient to patient, especially at low stimulation levels. Spacing of electrodes in a multichannel implant, and even the patient's ability to use a multichannel device, may depend on the patient's pathology.

Second, our results suggest that it may be possible to establish tests for diagnosing the degree of neural loss on the basis of some simple functional measures. Probably the easiest test to implement, and one of the most fruitful in light of the present results, would be a detection threshold test using round-window or other extracochlear placements. Our results suggest that low-frequency stimuli (or similarly, long-duration pulsatile stimuli [13]) would yield the greatest differentiation near threshold. Placement that minimizes current spread would be desirable. Care must be taken at low frequencies of stimulation to avoid charge-related damage, but at near-threshold intensities and with extracochlear stimulation these problems should be minimal. Good differentiation should be possible at about 80 Hz, so lower frequencies could be avoided.

Acknowledgments

We thank James A. Donaldson for performing the implant surgery, and Donald K. Eddington for supplying the human data in Figure 7. We are also particularly grateful to the many members of the Department of Otolaryngology and the Regional Primate Research Center at the University of Washington who have collaborated in this project.

References

1. Pfingst, B. E., D. Sutton, J. M. Miller & B. A. Bohne. 1981. Cochlear implants: relation of psychophysical measures to histological findings. Acta Oto-laryng. (Stockholm) **92:** 1–13.
2. Stebbins, W. C. 1973. Hearing of old world monkeys (Cercopithecinae). Am. J. Phys. Anthropol. **38:** 357–364.
3. Pfingst, B. E., J. Laycock, F. Flammino, B. Lonsbury-Martin & G. Martin. 1978. Pure tone thresholds for the rhesus monkey. Hearing Res. **1:** 43–47.
4. Spelman, F. A., B. E. Pfingst & J. M. Miller. 1978. A constant-current stimulator for use with chronic cochlear implants. Proc. San Diego Biomed. Symp. **17:** 1–3.

5. Pfingst, B. E., R. Hienz & J. M. Miller. 1975. Reaction-time procedure for measurement of hearing: II. Threshold functions. J. Acoust. Soc. Am. **57:** 431–436.
6. Miller, J. M., M. Glickstein & W. C. Stebbins. 1966. Reduction of response latency in monkeys by a procedure of differential reinforcement. Psychon. Sci. **5:** 177–178.
7. Chocholle, R. 1940. Variation des temps de réaction auditifs en fonction de l'intensité a diverses fréquences. Ann. Psychol. **41:** 65–124.
8. Stebbins, W. C. 1966. Auditory reaction time and the derivation of equal loudness contours for the monkey. J. Exp. Anal. Behav. **9:** 135–142.
9. Moody, D. B. 1970. Reaction time as an index of sensory function. *In* Animal Psychophysics: The Design and Conduct of Sensory Experiments. W. C. Stebbins, Ed.: 65–124. Appleton-Century-Crofts. New York, NY.
10. Pfingst, B. E., R. Hienz, J. Kimm & J. M. Miller. 1975. Reaction-time procedure for measurement of hearing: I. Suprathreshold functions. J. Acoust. Soc. Am. **57:** 421–430.
11. Marshall, L. & J. F. Brandt. 1980. The relationship between loudness and reaction time in normal hearing listeners. Acta Oto-Laryng. (Stockholm) **90:** 244–249.
12. Pfingst, B. E., J. A. Donaldson, J. M. Miller & F. A. Spelman. 1979. Psychophysical evaluation of cochlear prostheses in a monkey model. Ann. Otol. (St. Louis) **88:** 613–625.
13. Pfingst, B. E., F. A. Spelman & D. Sutton. 1980. Operating ranges for cochlear implants. Ann. Otol. (St. Louis) **89** (Suppl. 66): 1–4.
14. Pfingst, B. E., P. A. Burnett & D. Sutton. Intensity discrimination with cochlear implants. J. Acoust. Soc. Am. In press.
15. Michelson, R. P. 1971. Electrical stimulation of the human cochlea: A preliminary report. Arch. Otolaryng. **93:** 317–323.
16. Eddington, D. K., W. H. Dobelle, D. E. Brackmann, M. G. Mladejovsky & J. L. Parkin. 1978. Auditory prosthesis research with multiple channel intracochlear stimulation in man. Ann. Otol. (St. Louis) **87** (Suppl. 53): 5–39.
17. Miller, J. M., B. E. Pfingst, B. M. Clopton, F. A. Spelman & D. Sutton. 1982. Loudness growth functions for electrical stimulation of scala tympani implants. Abstracts of the Fifth Midwinter Research Meeting, Association for Research in Otolaryngology: 51–52.
18. Pfingst, B. E., D. Sutton & J. M. Miller. 1981. Electrode-place discrimination by monkeys with cochlear and modiolar implants. Abstracts of the Fourth Midwinter Research Meeting, Association for Research in Otolaryngology: 64.
19. Hinojosa, R. Pathology of profound sensorineural deafness. This volume.
20. Johnsson, L. G., W. F. House & F. H. Linthicum. 1979. Bilateral cochlear implants—histological findings in a pair of temporal bones. Laryngoscope **89:** 759–762.
21. Mladejovsky, M. G., D. K. Eddington, W. H. Dobelle & D. E. Brackmann. 1975. Artificial hearing for the deaf by cochlear stimulation: pitch modulation and some parametric thresholds. Trans. Am. Soc. Artif. Int. Organs **21:** 1–6.
22. Starr, A. & D. E. Brackmann. 1979. Brain stem potentials evoked by electrical stimulation of the cochlea in human subjects. Ann. Otol. (St. Louis) **88:** 550–556.
23. Bilger, R. C. 1977. Evaluation of subjects presently fitted with implanted auditory prostheses. Ann. Otol. (St. Louis) **86** (Suppl. 38): 3–176.
24. Berliner, K. I. Personal communication.

INTRODUCTION

Robert C. Bilger

Department of Speech and Hearing Science
University of Illinois
Champaign, Illinois 61820

There are two reasons why it is important to study speech perception as mediated by cochlear implants. The most obvious reason is that the ultimate goal of such implants is to restore to the individual the ability to understand speech. The second reason for studying speech perception directly is less obvious and is somewhat convoluted. Since the relation of psychoacoustic abilities (such as frequency discrimination, intensity discrimination, and rhythmic perception) to the perception of speech is not really understood for the normal and impaired auditory system and since the basis upon which psychoacoustic tasks are performed by subjects wearing implants is not known, it does not seem reasonable to continue psychoacoustic investigations as correlative studies of speech perception. Because it is obvious that an implant that will not allow for the discrimination of frequency or intensity, for example, can hardly provide signals for intelligible speech, there is a place for some psychoacoustic study of implants. That place, however, involves establishing that independent channels for encoding speech do exist for the implant-wearer, not in predicting that speech will be intelligible.

Given the importance of studies of speech perception in the future of auditory prostheses, two comments seem warranted: First, as one scans the schemes for encoding speech into *n*-channel implants, there is a surprise dependence on vocoder-like strategies. It would be refreshing to encounter encoding strategies that were less dependent on wide-spectrum assumptions.

My second comment on speech perception deals with how the nervous system processes information. We should all be aware of the observer's ability to label meaningless stimuli.[1] That is, the typical human subject can categorize a unidimensional stimulus continuum into five to nine categories and can use those categories consistently. For a two-dimensional signal array, the same subject can handle as many as 40 or 50 categories. This kind of categorization of stimuli is not a replacement for speech perception, because speech is neither a uni- nor bidimensional stimulus array. The unique aspect of speech perception is not the number of categories that are processed; rather, it is the speed with which they are processed. Future researchers in the area of speech perception by implanted subjects should take care to differentiate between slow and rapid processing of categorical signals.

REFERENCE

1. MILLER, G. A. 1956. The magical number seven, plus or minus two: Some limits on our capacity for processing information. Psychol. Rev. **63:** 81–97.

SPEECH RECOGNITION IN DEAF SUBJECTS WITH MULTICHANNEL INTRACOCHLEAR ELECTRODES[a]

Donald K. Eddington

Artificial Hearing Project
Institute for Biomedical Engineering
University of Utah
Salt Lake City, Utah 84112

Introduction

Although an effective treatment for the sensorineural deaf does not exist, results of experiments using cochlear implants indicate that these devices may eventually make speech communication possible for some profoundly deaf individuals. The goal of this area of research is to use electrical stimulation of the auditory nerve to elicit the patterns of neural activity the brain requires to understand speech. Several research groups are working to attain this goal and as a result several different stimulation systems have been developed. This paper briefly describes the basic elements of these stimulation systems and reports the results of recent speech recognition experiments conducted with two deaf volunteers using multichannel systems. Finally, results and analyses that give some insight about the possible cues these volunteers use to recognize speech will be described.

The Basic Stimulation System

Even though the experimental devices used to stimulate the auditory nerve take many forms, most are composed of three basic elements: a microphone that produces an electrical representation of the acoustic stimulus (such as speech), a processor that transforms the output of the microphone to the desired electrical stimuli, and one or more pairs of "stimulating" electrodes that deliver the stimuli to the neural tissue.

Several criteria may be used to group these devices into classes. One useful criterion is the number of different processing channels included in the device. A multichannel system employs a customized processing channel for each stimulating electrode. A single-channel device has only one processing channel and therefore delivers the same stimulus to all active electrodes.

Implanted electrode configurations take many forms and may be classified by characteristics such as number of electrodes, anatomic placement, and the use of a common ground electrode.[1] A single-channel device may include a configuration of one or more electrodes. Multiple electrodes (at least one for each processing channel) are required for multichannel systems. When the electrodes are implanted in the cochlea, the devices are known as cochlear implants.

[a] This work was supported by grants from the American Telephone & Telegraph Corporation, Mountain Bell, and the Deafness Research Foundation.

0077-8923/83/0405-0241 $01.75/0 © 1983, NYAS

Two-Syllable Word-Recognition Experiments

Because the goal of cochlear implant research is to restore speech communication to the deaf, most groups working in this area have used word-recognition tests as one method to evaluate implants. The results of such tests indicate a wide range of effectiveness for different devices and suggest that the effectiveness of some devices may depend greatly on the patient using them. In this section a brief summary of these word-recognition scores is presented and the most recent results of word-recognition experiments conducted in our laboratory are described.

On the basis of results of experiments with 13 subjects fitted with single-channel implants,[2] it is probably safe to assume that most of the 200 to 300 patients who have received single-channel implants are able to score higher on tests of lipreading and recognition of environmental sounds with their prostheses than without them. Speech-recognition results remain, in general, poor. Data reported by Bilger [2] for 13 subjects show an overall average of about 16% recognition of closed-set (16 words), spondaic word lists. Open-set word recognition would likely be worse.

Recently published results of experiments conducted with two subjects (each subject working with a different research group and using a different system of single-channel stimulation) have shown significantly higher speech recognition than has been reported for the usual single-channel implant subject. Hochmair-Desoyer *et al.*[3] report that their subject, C. K., scored 43% recognition on an open-set, unpracticed word list (German). Owens and Telleen [4] report a recognition score of 35% for their subject, L. Y., using an unpracticed, open-set, spondee word list. It should be noted that both C. K. and L. Y. (as well as the 13 subjects cited earlier) had extensive experience with their portable stimulation devices before these tests were conducted: L. Y. had been using his device for more than 1 year and C. K. had been using hers for at least 9 months.

The scores on word-recognition tests using multichannel systems also exhibit a wide range. Using open-set, unpracticed word lists, Chouard [5] reported 9% recognition by subjects using his multichannel system. Clark [6] reported 37% recognition using open-set, consonant–vowel–consonant syllables. I reported recognition scores between 40 and 80% for open-set, unpractised two-syllable word lists for two subjects using a multichannel system.[7] These same two volunteers served as subjects for the following speech recognition experiments.

Subject D. C. suffered two, sudden-onset hearing losses (one in each ear) coincident with sudden episodes of prolonged vertigo and was subsequently diagnosed as having Ménière's disease. J. S. suffered a gradual-onset loss of undiagnosed origin. Both subjects suffer from profound, bilateral hearing losses. Four years before these speech recognition experiments were conducted, six platinum electrodes (spaced approximately 4 mm apart) were implanted in one cochlea of each subject by Dr. Derald E. Brackmann. The implant and basic psychophysical experiments conducted with these and other patients have been described in a previous report.[8] Because these volunteers are not equipped with a portable stimulation system, the only time they are stimulated is during testing in the laboratory. Each subject had logged approximately 30 hours of laboratory experience with speech stimuli over a 2-year period before the following experiments were conducted. This represents significantly less experience than the subjects using the portable single-channel and multichannel systems described earlier.

The 4-channel processing system used during the speech-recognition experiments is much like the one used for previous discrimination and recognition experiments [1, 7] and is shown in FIGURE 1A. The microphone was positioned approximately 4 feet from the male speaker and its output was connected to the processing electronics. The output of the automatic gain control (AGC) stage (including the pre- and post-gain elements) served as input to each of the 4 bandpass filters (BPF). FIGURE 1B shows the magnitude of the amplitude response for each of the four bandpass filters. Electrode 1 in FIGURE 1 is the most apical, scala tympani electrode and is located approximately 22 mm from the round window in each subject. The spacing between electrodes is about 4 mm; the higher the electrode number, the closer its position to the round window.

Three speech-recognition tests were administered to each subject. During each test an open-set, unpractised list of 36 two-syllable words (see APPENDIX I) was read in random order by a male speaker. Each word was repeated three times, after which the subject gave his response. The subjects did not receive feedback concerning the accuracy of their responses. During the first test, the stimulation system (as shown in FIGURE 1) was connected to the subject's electrodes and the subject was positioned so he was unable to see the lips of the speaker. This condition is identified as "4 channels with

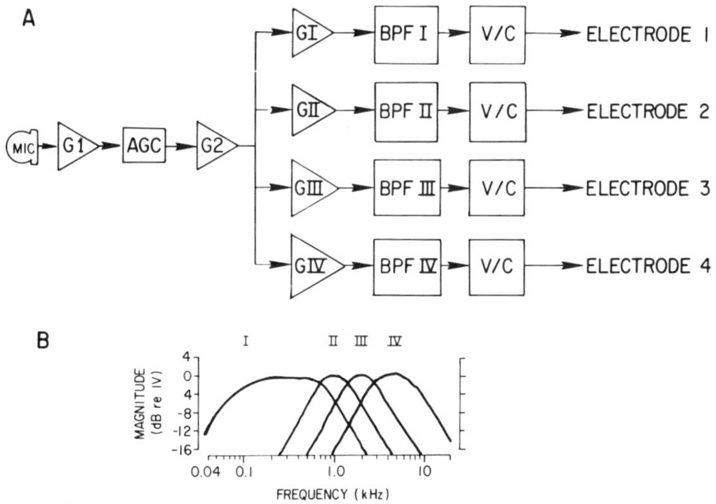

FIGURE 1. (A) The four-channel processing scheme used to transform speech stimuli to electrical stimuli. The acoustic waveform is transformed to an electrical analogue by the microphone (MIC). This waveform passes through two gain stages (G1 and G2) and an automatic gain control stage (AGC) before it is presented as input to each of the four processing channels. Each processing channel consists of a gain stage (GI), bandpass filter stage (BPS I), and a voltage-to-current source converter (V/C I). (B) The magnitude of the frequency response for each of the four bandpass filters of the processing system.

filters." The second test was conducted like the first except that only one of the channels (with the bandpass filter removed) was used. This scheme is identified as "single-channel without filter." The third test was conducted like the first, except that the subject faced the speaker (from a distance of approximately 8 feet). This condition is identified as "4 channels with filters, with lipreading."

TABLE 1 shows a summary of the results of the two-syllable recognition tests for each subject for each of the three conditions (see APPENDIX I for the data). The results for the "4 channels with filters" case fall within the 40 to 80% range previously reported.[7] Since this initial report,[7] scores as low as 30% and as high as 85% have been obtained with these two subjects using the "4 channels with filters" processing scheme. This variability has not been observed for the "single-channel without filter" and the "4 channels with filters, with lipreading" conditions.

Although changes in the "4 channels with filters" processing scheme may account for the large range of scores we have experienced, lack of specific data makes it impossible to identify this, rather than other possible candidates (for example, patient alertness or some inherent subject variability) as the primary cause. The data presented here are the most recent results of speech-recognition experiments and are (to date) typical for the current processor configuration.

Because normal patterns of spike activity on the auditory nerve are very complex, some argue that single-channel systems that tend to excite all fibers alike will not be as effective as multichannel systems that are able to elicit more complex activity.[9] Although the results shown in TABLE 1 (when compared with the single-channel results described at the beginning of this section) are consistent with this postulate, they are by no means conclusive. Because the details of the two single-channel processing schemes use by L. Y. and C. K. were not available, a direct comparison of these schemes was not possible. It is possible that if these single-channel processing systems were substituted for the "single-channel without filter" configuration used in the current experiments, the scores for single-channel stimulation would be much higher.

CVC/CDC Syllable Recognition Experiments

The results of tests like those just described give some information about a subject's ability to recognize speech and are useful when comparing the

TABLE 1

TWO-SYLLABLE WORD RECOGNITION

Subject	Four Channels with Filters	One Channel with No Filter	Four Channels with Filters and with Lipreading
D.C.	67%	3%	94%
J.S.	64%	6%	94%

effectiveness of different implant systems. They are, however, of little value when trying to identify the cues implant patients use to perform the task of speech recognition. It is likely that if these cues were identified, they would suggest modifications of current implant systems that would enhance appropriate cues and eliminate inappropriate ones, resulting in an overall improvement in speech-recognition scores.

One technique that has been used successfully to identify the perceptual attributes of speech sounds subjects use to recognize speech is the analysis of data that represent the degree of similarity between a set of such sounds.[10-13] The similarity measures between sounds are usually obtained by direct scaling or by their confusability. In the next set of experiments confusabilitly measures were made with two subjects using a set of 10 single-syllable words. These data were subjected to a preliminary analysis to determine whether the cues used to recognize these words could be identified. Although these initial experiments and analyses are far from complete, they do provide some information about the cues the implant subjects use to recognize speech.

Seven consonant–vowel–consonant (CVC) syllables and three consonant–dipthong–consonant (CDC) syllables were used as the speech stimuli for the following tests. A test consisted of 100 presentations (each of the 10 stimuli presented 10 times in random order). During a presentation, the stimulus was spoken three times by a male speaker, after which the subject wrote down his response. The duration of each utterance was varied randomly between approximately 0.8 to 1.5 sec. The subjects did not know which syllables were on the list and did not receive feedback concerning the accuracy of their responses. Both J. S. and D. C. were tested with the "4 channels with filters" processing scheme. D. C. was also tested with the "single-channel without filter" scheme. The results of these three tests are given in Tables 2, 3, and 4.

The data represented in these tables may be thought of as similarity matrices. The value of each matrix element (the number of times the subject gave a particular response to a particular stimulus) represents the relative similarity between two elements of the stimulus set. The diagonals of the matrices represent stimulus–response pairs that are the same, so for high recognition scores these elements should be large. The other matrix elements represent confusions. Note that the response "book" used by D. C. (TABLES 2 and 3) is not an element of the stimulus set.

Averages of the first and second formant (F1 and F2) frequencies of the stimuli (and of "book," a response not part of the stimulus set) are plotted in FIGURE 2 (see APPENDIX II for computational details). Notice that the dashed lines marking the channel boundaries (based on "effective stimulus;" see caption of FIGURE 5) divide the F1 versus F2 frequency space into six regions. If the place cue (that is, which electrode or combination of electrodes is activated) were the principal cue used by the subjects to recognize the stimulus syllables, one would expect to see at least two relationships between the syllables located within the six regions. First, the number of confusions between syllables within a region should be significantly greater than the number of confusions between syllables in different regions. Second, the CDC syllables that move across regions should be confused more often with other CDC syllables than with the "stationary" CVC syllables. Since neither of these relationships is significant (90% confidence limit), the data are con-

TABLE 2

CVC CONFUSIONS IN SUBJECT D.C.: ONE CHANNEL WITHOUT FILTERS (18%)

		Response										
		Boot	Boat	Bet	Beet	Bit	Bought	Bait	Bite	Bat	But	Book
Stimulus	Boot		1	1			1				4	3
	Boat						2		8			
	Bet						5		1		2	2
	Beet		1				1	1	4			3
	Bit					1	2		4		2	1
	Bought		2				5		3			
	Bait		1				2		6	1		
	Bite		1	1			1		6			1
	Bat		1				6		1	1	1	
	But					1	1		2	1	5	

TABLE 3

CVC CONFUSIONS IN SUBJECT D.C.: FOUR CHANNELS WITH FILTERS (53%)

		Response										
		Boot	Boat	Bet	Beet	Bit	Bought	Bait	Bite	Bat	But	Book
Stimulus	Boot	7	1		1	1						
	Boat		7				1					2
	Bet			1		2	2				1	4
	Beet							7	3			
	Bit			1		8			1			
	Bought		3				5			2		
	Bait				1			9				
	Bite								10			
	Bat		3				3		1	3		
	But					1	2				3	4

TABLE 4

CVC CONFUSIONS IN SUBJECT J.S.: FOUR CHANNELS WITH FILTERS (58%)

		Response									
		Boot	Boat	Bet	Beet	Bit	Bought	Bait	Bite	Bat	But
Stimulus	Boot	9									1
	Boat		1					5	4		
	Bet			5		4				1	
	Beet				4			6			
	Bit					10					
	Bought						5		2	3	
	Bait							9	1		
	Bite					1			7	1	1
	Bat						7			3	
	But			4					1		5

sistent with the hypothesis that place of stimulation alone is not a dominant cue for this multichannel stimulation scheme.

One class of analysis techniques that is useful for identifying the perceptual attributes used by subjects to scale, order, or categorize (for example, recognize) a set of objects (spoken syllables in this case) is that of multidimensional scaling (MDS).[14] MDS uses similarity measures between a particular set of stimuli as input to compute a spatial configuration of points in a particular stimulus space. Each point of the configuration in the stimulus space represents one element of the stimulus set. The greater the similarity between a pair of elements of the stimulus set, the smaller their separation in the stimulus

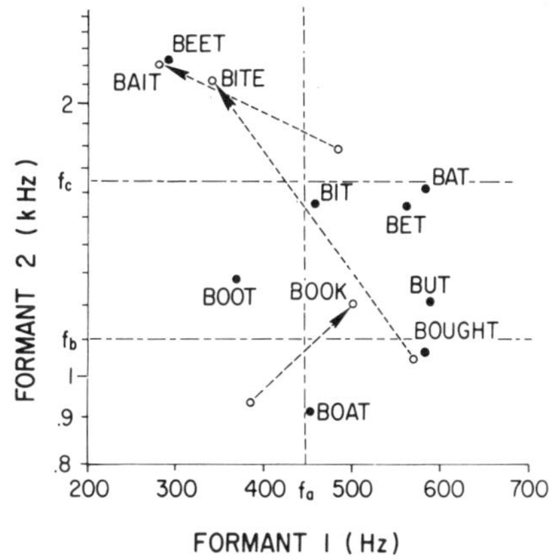

FIGURE 2. Plot of the averaged first and second format (F1 and F2) frequencies for each of the CVC and CDC syllables. The CVC syllables are represented by *solid circles.* The *open circles* connected by *dashed lines* represent the beginning and endpoints of the F1 and F2 frequency excursions for diphthongs (see APPENDIX II for computational details). The vertical and horizontal *dashed lines* represent the boundaries between channels computed by combining the frequency reponse of each bandpass filter (FIG. 1B) and the threshold-versus-frequency relationship of its respective electrode (see FIGURE 5 for a plot of "effective stimulus" versus frequency for channels I and II). The "effective stimulus" boundary (see caption of FIGURE 5 for definition) between channels I and II is identified by f_a, between II and III by f_b, and between III and IV by f_c.

space. The goal of the analysis algorithm is to compute the spatial configuration that best reflects the similarity data (see Kruskal and Wish [14] for details). When the MDS analysis is properly applied, each of the perceptual attributes used by a subject to produce the measures of stimulus similarity will typically be represented by a dimension in the stimulus space.

The specific technique used to perform the initial MDS analysis of the data of TABLES 2, 3 and 4 is the individual differences model,[15] as implemented in the ALSCAL-4 computer program.[16] The two-dimensional stimulus configuration computed by ALSCAL is shown in FIGURE 3, and the scattergram of the linear fit is plotted in FIGURE 4. Computation was halted after 14 iterations because the stress improvement was less than 0.001. TABLE 5 shows

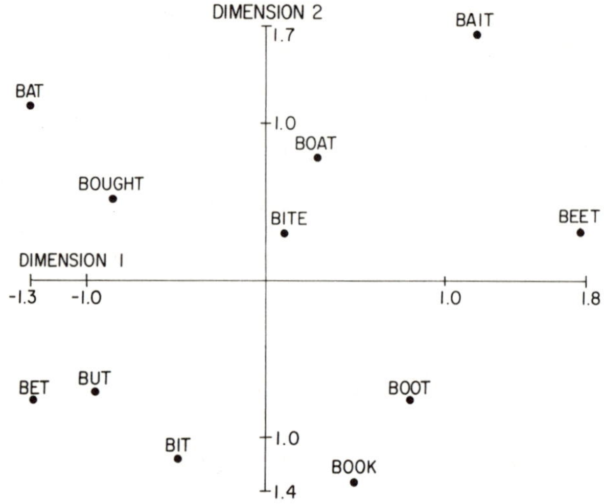

FIGURE 3. Plot of the two-dimensional stimulus configuration computed by the MDS computer analysis for the data shown in TABLES 2, 3, and 4.

that the overall squared correlation (in distance) was 0.856 (the stress was 0.147).

Inspection of the stimulus configuration (FIG. 3) reveals at least two possible interpretations of dimension 1. The first associates dimension 1 with the first formant frequency of the stimulus syllables. This relationship is clear when the CVC and CDC syllables are listed with their respective first, second and third formant frequencies as ordered by the MDS dimension 1 (see TABLE 6). The correlation between the frequency of F1 and the coordinate of dimension 1 is 0.962.

A second interpretation [b] associates dimension 1 with the F1 intensity of the stimulus syllables. Notice that for each stimulus, the frequency of F1 lies on the low-frequency skirt of BPF II. If the F1 intensities for all stimuli are within 5 dB (a definite possibility [17, 18]), the relative intensities of F1 in channel II will be highly correlated with both the frequencies of F1 and with the stimulus coordinate for MDS dimension 1. Although the F1 amplitudes will be greatly reduced, this correlation will also be present in channels III and IV.

One interesting aspect of the second interpretation is that the F1 intensity cue in channel II is not consistent with the F1 intensity cue in channel I. In channel I, the intensity of F1 tends to fall with increasing frequency, while in channel II this relationship is reversed. The relative saliency of the intensity cues produced by these two channels for each stimulus can be assessed by combining the amplitude responses of bandpass filters I and II (see FIGURE 1B) with the threshold-versus-frequency relationships of their respective electrodes. Such a combination describes the relationship between "effective

[b] Murray Sachs suggested the possibility of this interpretation.

TABLE 5

MDS DATA: OVERALL SQUARED CORRELATION (0.856)

Subject Weights

Subject	Dimension 1	Dimension 2
D.C., 4-channel	0.812	0.509
J.S., 4-channel	0.794	0.475
D.C., 1-channel	0.423	0.784

stimulus" and stimulation frequency for each channel. A plot of "effective stimulus" as a function of frequency for channel I and channel II is shown in FIGURE 5.

Notice that F1 is most strongly represented in channel I for the stimuli "beet," "bait," and "boot." The F1 intensity cue for these stimuli should be decreasing intensity for increasing F1 frequency. Channel II provides the strongest F1 representation for "bat," "bet," "but," and "bought." The F1 intensity cue for these stimuli should decrease with decreasing F1 frequency. The F1 intensity cue for "bit," "bite," and "boat" is difficult to predict since F1 intensity is essentially equally represented in channels I and II. Although F1 intensity cannot be rejected as an interpretation of MDS dimension 1, the

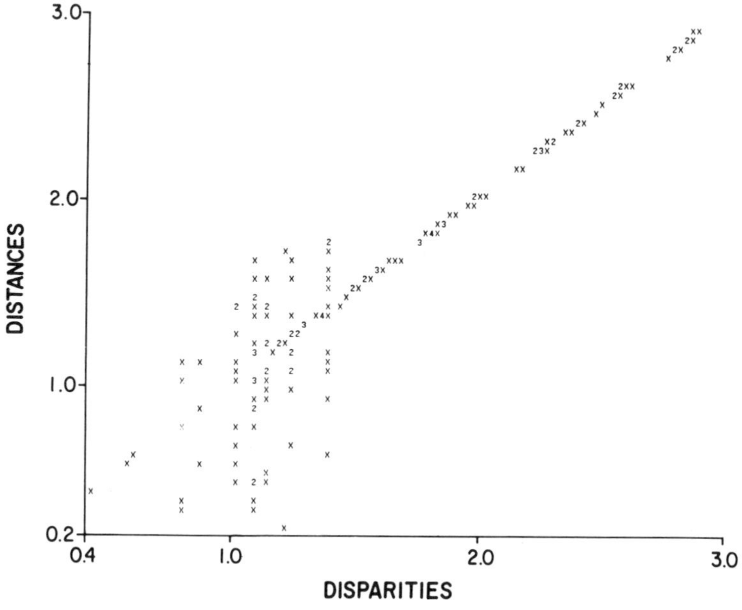

FIGURE 4. Plot of the scattergram computed by the MDS analysis for the stimulus configuration shown in FIGURE 3.

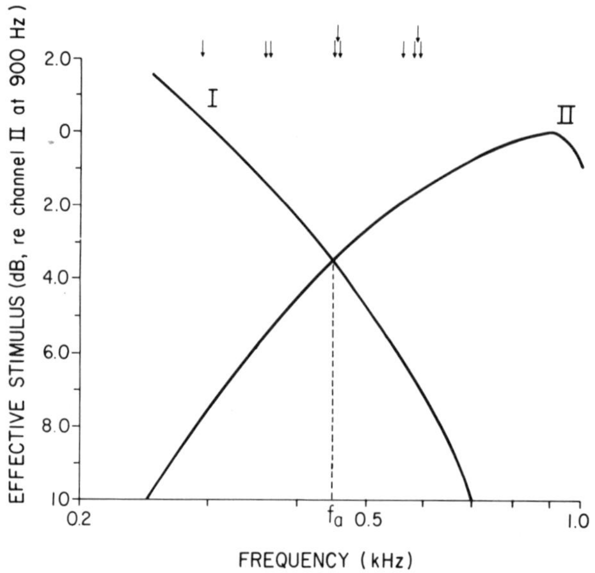

FIGURE 5. Plot of "effective stimulus" as a function of stimulus frequency for processing channels I and II. The "effective stimulus" was computed by combining the magnitude of the frequency response for BPF I and BPF II (see FIGURE 1B) with the threshold-versus-frequency relationships of their respective electrodes. The dynamic ranges of these electrodes (threshold to maximum comfortable loudness) is between 9.5 and 12 dB. The boundary between channels I and II is identified as f_a. The *arrows* at the top of this plot indicate the F1 frequency position of the stimulus syllables.

fact that its representation is not consistent across all stimuli makes it an unlikely candidate.

Dimension 2 of this analysis (also dimensions higher than 1 for analyses using 3- and 4-dimensional object spaces) has remained uninterpretable using conventional relationships such as second or third formants or articulatory features. Because a wide variety of other attributes still remains to be investigated as possible correlates of both dimension 1 and the higher order dimensions, the interpretations presented here should not be thought of as exhaustive.

Notice that the subject weights of TABLE 5 indicate that the two "4 channel with filters" cases emphasize dimension 1 (an appropriate cue?), while the "single-channel without filters" case emphasizes dimension 2. If dimension 2 remains uninterpretable (is noise, for example) or correlates with some other inappropriate cue, this would be consistent with the higher scores for the multichannel stimulation system.

Examination of the F1 frequency values in TABLE 6 reveals at least two clusters of syllables (a cluster is defined as a group of syllables whose mean of F1 frequency is separated from the means of adjacent sets by more than 10 standard deviations and by more than 5 times its range). One cluster includes syllables with F1 frequency between 588 and 573 Hz and a second includes syllables with F1 frequency between 458 and 442 Hz. When schematic spectrograms of the syllables are arranged in order of their position along MDS dimension 1 (FIG. 6), it is apparent that the first cluster is arranged in descending order of second formant frequency ($r = 0.993$). Although this ordering hints that F2 frequency may also be used as a cue for recognition of some syllables, more work is needed to determine whether it is truly significant. If F2 frequency is a significant cue, it could account for the gross misordering (in terms of F1 frequency) of "bet" as shown in TABLE 6.

CONCLUSION

The frequency boundaries between channels of the multichannel stimulation system used in the present experiments result in the partitioning of F1 versus F2 frequency space into six regions. Analysis of the confusions between syllables in the same regions and between syllables in different regions produces results consistent with the hypothesis that place of stimulation alone is not a dominant cue used by the subjects to recognize the CVC and CDC syllables.

The MDS analysis of the confusion data reveals that F1 intensity and F1 frequency are two possible cues that would account for the confusions experienced by the two subjects during the CVC and CDC recognition experiments. Because the F1 frequency cue is consistent across channels (and the F1 intensity cue is not), it is the most likely cue used by the subjects to recognize the speech stimuli tested. Even though the F1 intensity cue seems unlikely, it cannot, on the basis of the present data, be rejected as a possible cue.

The speech-recognition results for the open-set, unpracticed list of two-syllable words (67 and 64%) are better than the best single-channel results reported (43 and 35%). Because of the small number of subjects and because the processing schemes used by the single-channel patients of other groups were not available for testing with the current multichannel subjects, it is

TABLE 6

FORMANT COMPARISON FOR CVC SYLLABLES [a]

CVC	Formant 1	Formant 2	Formant 3
Bat	583	1607	2420
Bet	563	1541	2391
But	588	1227	2353
Bought	580	1063	2402
Bit	458	1543	2427
Bite	570–342 (456)	1048–2128	2351
Boat	452	915	2399
Book	385–499 (442)	934–1196	2390
Boot	371	1284	2261
Bait	486–272 (379)	1771–2221	2500
Beet	293	2236	2706

[a] Ordered as in MDS dimension 1.

difficult to draw any firm conclusions regarding the relative merits of the single-channel and multichannel stimulation schemes. It should be noted that scores for the multichannel subjects were obtained when the subjects had virtually no experience with the device. Their scores are likely to improve significantly when they have logged the 9 to 12 months of daily experience that the single-channel subjects had accumulated before they were tested.

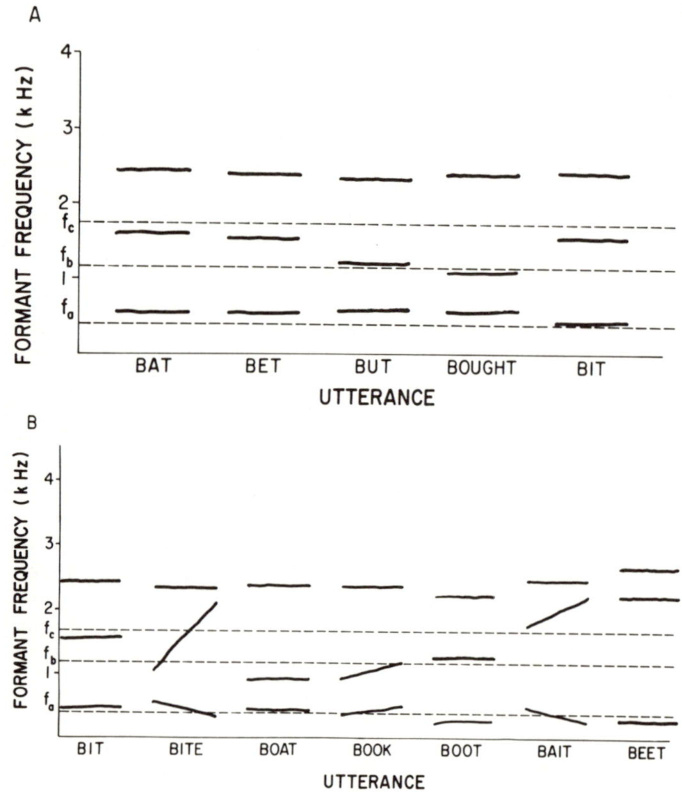

FIGURE 6. Schematic spectrograms of the vowel and diphthong portions of the CVC and CDC syllables used in the recognition experiments. The utterances are ordered as in dimension 1 of the MDS stimulus configuration. (See APPENDIX II for computational details.)

Although the speech recognition results cited for the two single-channel subjects (C. K. and L. Y.) and the results reported for D. C. and J. S. are remarkable, caution should be exercised when advising patients to undergo surgery for a cochlear implant. Prospective patients should realize that the majority of subjects fitted with single-channel devices are not able to approach the scores of C. K. and L. Y. Also, because the multichannel results reported here are based on only two subjects, prospective patients should not expect (with any degree of certainty) to match the performance of D. C. and J. S. The remarkable ability of some implant patients to recognize speech should, however, give the hearing-impaired hope that as our understanding of cochlear implants increases, a device will be developed that will be of real benefit to a significant population of the deaf.

Appendix I

Word-Recognition Data

Tables 7 and 8 give the data from the two-syllable word-recognition experiments conducted with D. C. and J. S. The stimulus words are given in alphabetical order in the tables, but were presented in random order for the experiments.

Table 7

Two-Syllable Word Recognition in Subject D.C.

Word	Four Channels with Filters	One Channel with No Filters	Four Channels with Filters and with Lipreading
Airplane	Airplane	Airplane	Airplane
Armchair	Armchair	NR [a]	Armchair
Baseball [b]	Baseball	NR	Baseball
Birthday	NR	NR	Birthday
Cowboy	Cowboy	Doorbell	Cowboy
Daybreak	Daybreak	NR	Daybreak
Doormat	Doormat	NR	Doormat
Drawbridge	Drawbridge	NR	Drawbridge
Duckpond	Duckpond	NR	Duckpond
Eardrum	Eardrum	NR	Eardrum
Farewell	NR	NR	Farewell
Grandson	NR	NR	Grandson
Greyhound	NR	NR	Greyhound
Hardware	Hardware	NR	Hardware
Headlight	NR	NR	Ink light
Horseshoe	Horseshoe	NR	Horseshoe
Hotdog [b]	NR	NR	Hotdog
Hothouse	Hothouse	NR	Outhouse
Iceberg [b]	Iceberg	NR	Iceberg
Inkwell	Inkwell	NR	Inkwell
Mousetrap	Mousetrap	NR	Mousetrap
Mushroom	NR	NR	Mushroom
Northwest	NR	Ballpark	Northwest
Oatmeal	Oatmeal	Airplane	Oatmeal
Padlock	NR	NR	Padlock
Pancake	NR	NR	Pancake
Playground	NR	NR	Playground
Railroad	Railroad	NR	Railroad
Schoolboy	Schoolboy	NR	Schoolboy
Sidewalk	Sidewalk	Airplane	Sidewalk
Stairway	Stairway	NR	Stairway
Sunset	Sunset	Ballpark	Sunset
Toothbrush	Toothbrush	NR	Toothbrush
Whitewash [b]	Whitewash	NR	Whitewash
Woodwork	NR	NR	Woodwork
Workshop	Workshop	NR	Workshop

[a] No response.
[b] Word had been used on a previous word list.

TABLE 8

TWO-SYLLABLE WORD RECOGNITION IN SUBJECT J.S.

Word	Four Channel with Filters	One Channel with No Filters	Four Channels with Filters and with Lipreading
Airplane	Airplane	NR [a]	Airplane
Armchair	Armchair	NR	Armchair
Baseball [b]	Baseball	NR	Baseball
Birthday	Birthday	NR	Birthday
Cowboy	Cowboy	NR	Cowboy
Daybreak	Boardwalk	NR	Daybreak
Doormat	Doorbell	NR	Doorbell
Drawbridge	Drawbridge	NR	Drawbridge
Duckpond	NR	NR	NR
Eardrum	Eardrum	NR	Eardrum
Farewell	NR	NR	Farewell
Grandson	Grandson	NR	Grandson
Greyhound	NR	NR	Greyhound
Hardware	Hardware	NR	Hardware
Headlight	NR	NR	Headlight
Horseshoe	Horseshoe	NR	Horseshoe
Hotdog [b]	NR	NR	Hotdog
Hothouse	NR	NR	Hothouse
Iceberg [b]	NR	Iceberg	Iceberg
Inkwell	Inkwell	NR	Equal
Mousetrap	Mousetrap	NR	Mousetrap
Mushroom	Mushroom	NR	Mushroom
Northwest	NR	NR	Northwest
Oatmeal	Oatmeal	NR	Oatmeal
Padlock	NR	NR	Padlock
Pancake	NR	NR	Pancake
Playground	NR	NR	Playground
Railroad	Railroad	NR	Railroad
Schoolboy	Schoolboy	NR	Schoolboy
Sidewalk	Sidewalk	NR	Sidewalk
Stairway	Stairway	NR	Stairway
Sunset	Sunset	NR	Sunset
Toothbrush	Toothbrush	NR	Toothbrush
Whitewash [b]	Whitewash	Whitewash	Whitewash
Woodwork	Woodwork	NR	Woodwork
Workshop	Workshop	NR	Workshop

[a] No response.

[b] Word had been used on a previous word list.

APPENDIX II

Formant Computation for the CVC and CDC Syllables

The formant values for the CVC and CDC syllables in TABLE 6 were computed in the following manner. First, several utterances of each syllable were digitized (10-kHz sample rate). The vowel and diphthong segments were identified by finding the voiced segment of each utterance using an algorithm much like SIFT.[19] A linear predictive coding (LPC) spectrum was then computed every 8 msec over the length of each voiced segment and the peaks (formants) of each LPC spectrum were computed by an algorithm much like FINDPK.[19] The frequency of each formant for the CVC syllables listed in TABLE 6 was computed by averaging the formant frequencies computed for the middle 80 msec of the voiced segment of each syllable. When the frequency of F1 made a consistent upward or downward excursion over the voiced segment (not including the first 40 msec), the syllable was classified as a diphthong. The beginning, ending, and average frequencies for F1 are listed in TABLE 6 for diphthongs.

REFERENCES

1. EDDINGTON, D. K. 1980. Speech discrimination in deaf subjects with cochlear implants. J. Acoust. Soc. Am. **68:** 885–891.
2. BILGER, R. C. 1977. Evaluation of subjects presently fitted with implanted auditory prostheses. Ann. Otol. Rhinol. Laryngol. **86** (Suppl. 36): 1–176.
3. HOCHMAIR-DESOYER, I. C., E. S. HOCHMAIR, K. BURIAN & R. E. FISHER. 1981. Four years experience with cochlear prostheses. Med. Progr. Technol. **8:** 107–119.
4. OWENS, E. & C. C. TELLEEN. 1981. Speech perception with hearing aids and cochlear implants. Arch. Otolaryngol. **107:** 160–163.
5. CHOUARD, C. H. 1980. The surgical rehabilitation of total deafness with the multichannel cochlear implant. Audiology **19:** 137–145.
6. CLARK, G. M., Y. C. TONG, L. F. A. MARTIN & P. A. BUSBY. 1981. A multiple-channel cochlear implant. An evaluation using an open-set word test. Acta Otolaryngol. **91:** 173–175.
7. EDDINGTON, D. K. 1982. Multiple channel intracochlear stimulation. *In* Neurological Surgery of the Ear and Skull Base. D. E. Brackmann, Ed. Raven Press. New York, NY.
8. EDDINGTON, D. K., W. H. DOBELLE, D. E. BRACKMANN, M. G. MLADEJOVSKY & J. L. PARKIN. 1978. Auditory prosthesis research with multiple channel intracochlear stimulation in man. Ann. Otol. Rhinol. Laryngol. **87**(Suppl. 53). 1–39.
9. KIANG, N. Y. S., D. K. EDDINGTON & B. DELGUTTE. 1979. Fundamental considerations in designing auditory implants. Acta Otolaryngol. **87:** 204–281.
10. DRESCHLER, W. A. & R. PLOMP. 1980. Relation between psychophysical data and speech perception for hearing-impaired subjects. J. Acoust. Soc. Am. **68:** 1608–1615.
11. BILGER, R. C. & M. D. WANG. 1976. Consonant confusions in patients with sensorineural hearing loss. J. Speech Hear. Res. **19:** 718–748.
12. FRANKS, J. R. & R. G. DANILOFF. 1973. A review of audiological implications of testing vowel perception. J. Aud. Res. **13:** 355–368.

13. WALDEN, B. E. & A. A. MONTGOMERY. 1975. Dimensions of consonant perception in normal and hearing-impaired listeners. J. Speech Hear. Res. **18:** 444–454.
14. KRUSKAL, J. B. & M. WISH. 1978. Multidimensional Scaling. Sage Publications. Beverly Hills, CA.
15. CARROL, J. D. & M. WISH. 1974. Multidimensional perceptural models and measurement methods. *In* Handbook of Perception, vol. 2. E. C. Carterette and M. P. Friedman, Eds. Academic Press. New York, NY.
16. TAKANE, Y., F. YOUNG & J. DE LEEUW. 1976. Nonmetric individual differences multidimensional scaling: An alternating least squares method with optimal scaling features. Psychometrika **42:** 7–67.
17. PETERSON, G. E. & H. L. BARNEY. 1952. Control methods in a study of the vowels. J. Acoust. Soc. Am. **24:** 175–184.
18. LEHISTE, I. & G. E. PETERSON. 1959. Vowel amplitude and phonemic stress in American English. J. Acoust. Soc. Am. **31:** 428–435.
19. MARKEL, J. D. & A. H. GRAY. 1976. Linear Prediction of Speech. Springer Verlag. New York, NY.

PERCEPTS FROM MODIOLAR (EIGHTH NERVE) STIMULATION [a]

F. Blair Simmons

Division of Otolaryngology/Head and Neck Surgery
Stanford University School of Medicine
Stanford, California 94305

When we began to use electrical stimulation several years ago, we selected the modiolus as the most promising site to place electrodes. We did so for two reasons, the probability that being closer to nerve fibers would require less current for excitation, and the possibility of more discrete fiber stimulation. There are now sufficient data on both scala tympani and modiolus stimulations to ask whether one site is "better" than the other, either in safety or in the range of percepts produced. The basic answer to this question seems to be *no,* even though one can say in general terms that thresholds are typically lower for modiolar stimulation.

Stimulation at both sites seems to produce comparable upper limits of rate–pitch discrimination with a maximum upper limit (optimistically) of 450 Hz. There is a considerable difference in this upper limit among individual subjects and even among electrodes in the same subject, but no clear difference with location. It is almost impossible to guess whether there are differences in "place" or "characteristic pitch" sensations. Both sites produce electrode-specific pitches in subjects who seem to use similar anectodal descriptors in describing them. Neither sounds are pure tones, but seem rich in harmonic content. We have not produced any "voice-like" vowel sounds of the sorts described by Eddington, but we presume that this is a subject difference, rather than a stimulus location phenomenon.[1]

Loudness phenomena, when produced by stimulation of a single electrode, also seem to be about the same. Thresholds for comparable waveforms are between 4 and 45 nC/pulse for modiolar and 6 and 60 nC/pulse for scala tympani stimulations. "Maximum loudnesses" are 7 to 30 dB (modiolar) and 6 to 17 dB (scala tympani) above these thresholds. (These comparisons are for stimulation rates above 200 Hz.) Loudness difference limens, as reported in the literature, tend to favor scala tympani electrodes, wherein a 2% change in stimulus intensity produced a loudness change.[2] Modiolar stimulation requires about a 5% change for a noticeable difference in loudness.[3] While this may be a real difference between stimulus locations, the data available need a lot more statistical rigor before the difference becomes accepted fact.

A troublesome feature of modiolar loudness growth is that it is not uniform across all electrodes. This also seems true for at least some multielectrode scala tympani implants.[4] This semi-unpredictability is not surprising since some electrodes are bound to have different positions relative to viable nerve fibers than others. However, it has presented real problems during multi-

[a] This work was supported by Grant NS 10532 from National Institutes of Health, Bethesda, Maryland.

0077–8923/83/0405–0259 $01.75/0 © 1983, NYAS

channel stimulation in knowing when a percept change is due strictly to loudness or to another perceptual quality. There are some suggestions that loudness summations may be different in the modiolus than in the scala tympani. Subthreshold modiolar stimulations do not usually add. In the scala tympani they do.

Specifically, in the modiolus, if thresholds are established individually for each of two (or more) electrodes, simultaneous in-phase stimulation of both will produce no change in thresholds. Further, subthreshold stimuli on two (or more) electrodes do not "add" to produce threshold when stimulated together. Finally, even if both electrodes are initially above threshold by perhaps as much as 30% of their dynamic ranges, simultaneous stimulation with identical pulses will cause no change in loudness.[3] Loudness does begin to summate at intensities in the vicinity of 50% of dynamic range. That is, simultaneous stimulations are louder than either singly. Then, if one electrode is substantially louder than the other, the loudness increment added by the weaker of the two is quite small, just as it is with normal hearing.

FIGURE 1 shows one set of typical loudness summations for two modiolar electrodes during monopolar stimulation. The subject estimated loudness between two fixed points using a money scale, where 1¢ was the softest and 100¢ was the loudest sound. The subject had considerable practice with this scale. The loudness he assigned for stimuli to each electrode singly is shown along the ordinates. Note that combined stimulation loudness increases only occurred when intensities on both electrodes were well above threshold. These magnitude estimations were later verified by direct balancing of various two-electrode trial sounds against a single-electrode standard, using A/B comparisons.

One insightful exception to the above was for two electrodes in one of the subjects. There was strong evidence for an overlap in the suprathreshold pool of neurons excitable from each. When these two were stimulated with the same paradigms just described, the combined stimulation loudness functions were quite different from the typical ones. Suprathreshold loudness did add, according to the total charge on the two electrodes ($E_3 + E_4$). Data from these electrode stimulations are shown in FIGURE 2 as iso-loudness contours (loudness for combined stimulations was compared to a reference loudness

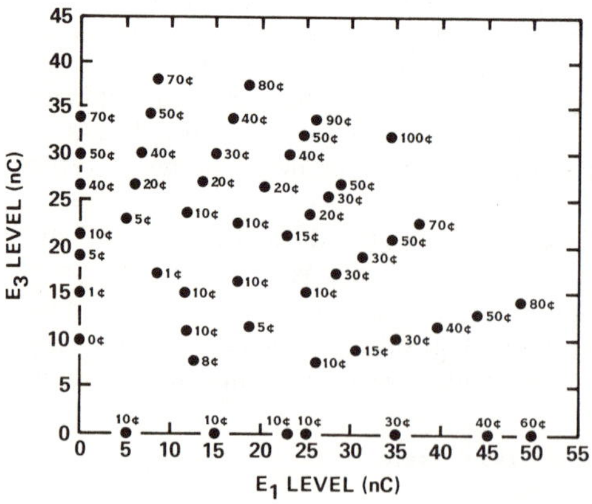

FIGURE 1. Loudness judgments for simultaneous stimulation of two electrodes. The subject (R.F.) was instructed to assign a 1¢ value to the softest and a 100¢ value to the loudest possible 200-Hz pulse train. These judgments appear along the ordinate and abscissa for electrodes E_1 and E_3 when stimulated separately at the indicated charge levels. Both electrodes were then stimulated simultaneously and the subject was asked for a 1¢–100¢ loudness judgment.

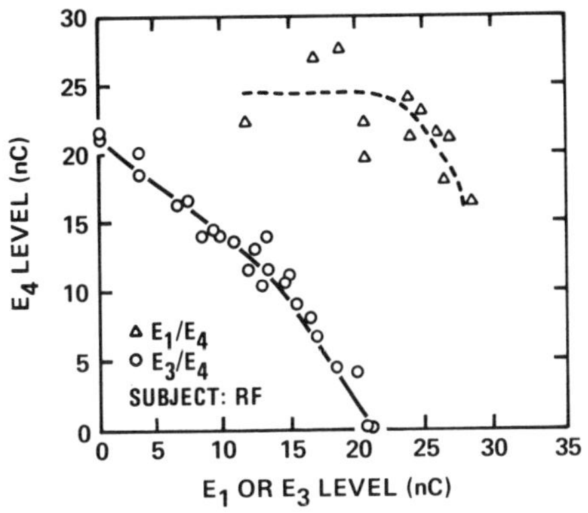

FIGURE 2. Iso-loudness contours for the anomalous ($E_3 + E_4$) and for a typical ($E_1 + E_4$) electrode pair during simultaneous stimulation. The subject compared the combined stimulation loudness to a standard 20¢ sound of a reference electrode. Pulse rate was 200 Hz.

on a single electrode). The typical two-electrode loudness behavior is illustrated by stimulations of $E_1 + E_4$ in the upper right part of FIGURE 2.

Electrode stimulations from within the scala tympani seem to behave differently. Two individually subthreshold stimulations produce a lower threshold when stimulated simultaneously.[2, 5] Intensities (for rectangles) can be reduced as much as 30%, and even more for sinusoids. One presumes that suprathreshold loudness is affected in a similar manner, but this is not specifically stated in the literature available.

Nonsimultaneous Multielectrode Stimulation

All of the foregoing results were produced when pulses or sines exactly overlapped in time on both electrodes. The threshold, subthreshold summations described by Eddington did not occur when pulses did not overlap, at least by some degree.[2] What happens to loudness of nonoverlapping pulses considerably above threshold has not been reported in print. Unpublished observations suggest that for one recently implanted subject with a multielectrode scala tympani array, there is some degree of loudness summation until pulses to individual electrodes are separated by about 3 msec.[4]

In the modiolus, using rectangles and either mono- or bipolar stimulation, there was no substantial effect upon loudness when trains of pulses were symmetrically alternated between electrodes at total rates up to 400 Hz—an interpulse interval of 2 msec for the pulses used. Shorter interpulse intervals caused loudness to increase.[6]

Herndon has examined the interpulse interval question in considerable detail in another subject and with slightly different results.[7] He used 0.25 msec/phase at rates of 100 or 200 Hz, and a loudness standard whereby stimulus intensity was increased in one electrode until it equaled the loudness of the two-electrode condition. Least loud were 100/sec pulses on a single electrode. Simultaneous in-phase two-electrode stimuli were usually slightly louder. Much louder were two-electrode pulses separated by more than the biphasic periods of the pulses (intervals exceeded 0.5 msec). Loudest were two-electrode pulses which partially overlapped in their phase relationships.

FIGURE 3 shows a typical set of loudness relationships for 0.25 msec/phase, 100/sec pulse trains delivered to two electrodes. Loudness on each electrode separately was balanced at about 20¢ (1–100¢ scale). Loudness changes are shown on the y axis as the current required to produce a loudness equal to the two-electrode condition on a single electrode. The loudness of nonoverlapping pulses remained at about the same levels for interpulse intervals of 1 to 5 msec. Note especially that the lead-lag loudness relation is not symmetrical. In fact, at 0.3 msec in one phase relationship, we were unable to balance loudness with the single electrode without exceeding what we consider to be the safe limit of charge. Longer intervals were not examined. Similar experiments done using three electrodes showed additional loudness increases for three separate pulses.

While the data in FIGURE 3 may be taken as a typical example, other combinations of electrodes produce a different magnitude of the same types of interactions. I will leave it to your imagination what might happen with

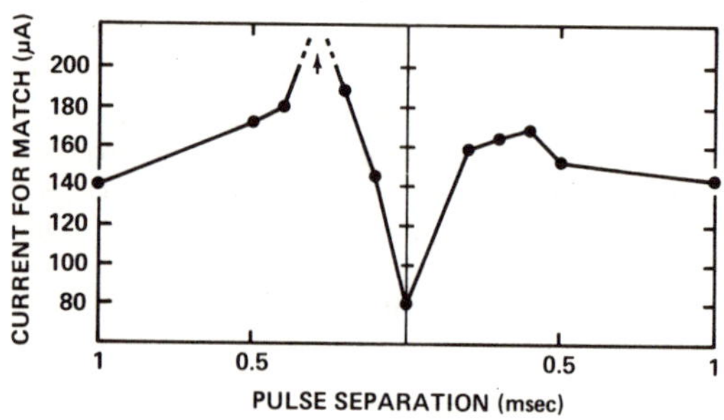

FIGURE 3. Relative loudness for time-separated trains of pulses on two electrodes. Trains were of 0.25 msec/phase rectangular pulses at 100/sec to two monopolar electrodes, E_1 and E_4. Loudness on each stimulated separately was balanced beforehand ($E_1 = 72$ μA, $E_4 = 149$ μA). The y axis shows the current required on a single electrode (E_1 here) to equal the loudness of the two-electrode stimulation. The x axis is the time separation of the leading edges of the two-electrode pulses. Thus, when the pulses overlapped exactly their loudness was the same as E_1 stimulated alone at 78 μA. E_1 led E_3 by 0.2 msec; E_1 alone required 165 μA for an equal loudness balance.

eight or more simultaneous stimulations whose interpulse intervals or phase relations are continually changing. It is indeed complex. It may well be that if predictability is demanded by a given coding scheme, stimuli will have to be serially multiplexed, as they have been in the Melbourne projects.[8] Clearly, we need more information.

There is one final perceptual result with modiolar stimulation which may be subject-specific and might also occur with scala tympani multielectrode stimulation. I do not know; perhaps someone has contrary information. In both our subjects we have been unable to obtain a description of hearing more than one sound, even when simultaneous stimulations on two electrodes have been quite different. We have tried every type of stimulus available and these subjects consistently refuse to report hearing two separate sounds, except from temporal cues. Is this consistent with percepts in other subjects, and if so, how might it affect speech-coding strategies?

References

1. Eddington, D. K. 1980. Speech discrimination in deaf subjects with cochlear implants. J. Acoust. Soc. Am. **68:** 885–891.
2. Eddington, D. K., W. H. Dobelle, D. E. Brackman, M. G. Mladejovsky & J. L. Parkin. 1978. Auditory prosthesis research with multiple channel intracochlear stimulation in man. Ann. Otol. Rhinol. Laryngol. **87** (Suppl 53): 1–39.
3. Mathews, R. G. 1978. Sound processing for an auditory prosthesis (Ph.D. dissertation). Technical report 5306–4, Stanford University, Department of Electrical Engineering.
4. Shannon, R. J. 1981. Personal communication.
5. White, M. W. 1982. Personal communication.
6. Simmons, F. B. 1966. Electrical stimulation of the auditory nerve in man. Arch. Otolaryngol **84:** 2–54.
7. Herndon, M. H. 1982. Personal communication.
8. Tong, Y. C., R. C. Black, G. M. Clark, I. C. Forster, J. B. Millar, B. J. O'Loughlin & J. F. Patrick. 1979. A preliminary report on a multiple channel cochlear implant operation. J. Laryngol. Otol. **93:** 679–695.

PERCEPTS FROM SCALA TYMPANI STIMULATION

Y. C. Tong and G. M. Clark

Department of Otolaryngology
University of Melbourne
Victoria 3052, Australia

This report summarizes the characteristics of the hearing sensations produced by electrical stimulation using scala tympani electrodes in a postlingually deaf patient (MC1) at the University of Melbourne. An array of 10 electrodes, spaced 1.5 mm apart, was inserted through the round window for a distance of 15 mm around the scala tympani. Biphasic current pulses with each phase fixed at 180 μsec were used. Fifteen current levels from 67 μA to 1 mA could be assigned in 67-μA steps, and a maximum repetition rate of 1000 rep/sec was possible. More detailed descriptions of the stimulation hardware and the patient's history can be found in previous reports.[1-3]

Stimulation Using One Electrode at a Time

A. Sensations Produced by Time-Invariant Signals

Time-invariant signals are those whose signal parameter values do not vary over the duration of the signal. The results are summarized as follows:

1. Loudness by magnitude estimation was a power function of current level with exponent greater than 10 in comparison with the acoustic exponent of 0.6.[2,4]
2. The loudness growth as a function of electric repetition rate was much more gradual and was similar to the loudness growth with acoustic sound pressure.[4]
3. Pitch increased with repetition rate up to 300 rep/sec and then saturated very rapidly.[2,4] This behavior is different from the pitch variation with acoustic pure tones, but is similar to the "nonspectral pitch" perception described by Burns and Viemeister,[5] who reported pitch-like variations achieved with amplitude-modulated noise bands.
4. Relative difference limens of repetition rate in the range from 2.6 to 3.4% at 100 rep/sec and 4.7 to 6.2% at 200 rep/sec were obtained.[4] These limens are larger than those for acoustic fundamental frequency (0.5 to 1%)[6] and pure tones (0.2 to 1.5%).[7]
5. At a fixed repetition rate, pitch varied from low to high and sharpness from dull to sharp for individual electrodes ordered in the apical to basal direction.[2,3,8]
6. Vowel labels could be assigned to the sensations produced by individual electrodes, and the second formant frequency of the vowel is consistent with the characteristic frequency of the location of the activated electrode.[2]
7. A perceptual study by the method of triadic comparisons provided evidence that the sensations produced by repetition rate and electrode position are perceptually separable. The stimuli were the nine possible combinations

0077–8923/83/0405–0264 $01.75/0 © 1983, NYAS

of three electrodes, spaced 3 mm apart, and three repetition rates. A two-dimensional solution by nonmetric multidimensional scaling showed that the stimulus points were ordered approximately on a rectangular grid with axes corresponding to the two physical dimensions, electrode position and repetition rate.[9] This configuration for the nine electric stimuli is similar to that reported by Plomp and Steeneken[10] for nine acoustic stimuli generated by the excitation of three bandpass filters with three repetition rates.

B. Sensations Produced by Trajectories of Electrode and Repetition Rate

1. The discriminability of repetition rate trajectories on a single electrode deteriorated with decreases in the duration of the trajectory, while excellent discrimination of electrode trajectories at a fixed repetition rate was maintained when the duration of the trajectory was reduced to as short a period as 25 msec.[8]
2. The hearing sensations produced by electrode trajectories were associated with those produced by acoustic speech signals characterized by second formant frequency transitions, while repetition rate trajectories were associated with variation in acoustic fundamental frequency.[8]
3. The patient was able to categorize increasing and decreasing repetition rate trajectories superimposed on electrode trajectories as "Questions" and "Statements," respectively.

C. Speech-Processing Considerations

For electrodes implanted in the basal coil of the human cochlea and for repetition rates below 300 rep/sec, the results described in the two foregoing sections indicated that it may be possible to convey low-frequency acoustic information by electric repetition rate, and higher-frequency information by electrode position. This dichotomy of pitch coding has been used in a speech-processing strategy in which the fundamental frequency of the acoustic speech signal was converted to electric repetition rate, the second formant frequency to electrode position, and the acoustic intensity to current level. With this strategy, the auditory system will discriminate the rapidly changing electrode trajectories required to convey segmental speech information. The slowly time-varying suprasegmental information contained in the fundamental frequency of a speech signal, on the other hand, is encoded in the electric repetition rate. In addition, the results in *A*7 and *B*3 provided evidence that the hearing sensations produced by repetition rate and electrode position are perceptually separable, and closely paralleled those produced by acoustic fundamental frequency and spectral envelope.

This speech-processing strategy has been implemented in a wearable speech processor, and speech evaluation results showed that it improves significantly the patient's ability in speech communication.[12, 13]

Two-Electrode Stimulation[14]

For the two-electrode studies, 300-msec pulse trains with 50-msec rise–decay times were used. The pulse trains on the two electrodes were at the same repetition rate with the pulse train on the more apical electrode leading by 0.5 msec. The current levels were chosen so that the loudness produced by either electrode was approximately the same.

A. A perceptual study by the method of triadic comparisons showed that a two-component sensation was produced by two-electrode stimulation. The stimuli were the following 10 electrode pairs: 1–2, 1–4, 1–6, 1–8, 2–4, 2–6, 2–8, 4–6, 4–8 and 6–8. A repetition rate of 166 rep/sec was used, and loudness was balanced across the electrode pairs. The dissimilarity matrix was analyzed by nonmetric multidimensional scaling, and a two-dimensional configuration was found to be suitable in representing the dissimilarity data. The two axes of the spatial configuration can be interpreted as corresponding to the position of: (1) the more apical electrode, and (2) the more basal electrode, and they closely parallel those corresponding to the first and second formant frequencies in the analysis of acoustic vowel confusion data by multidimensional scaling.[15]

B. Discrimination of repetition rate on two individual electrodes [2, 8] and five electrode pairs (2–4, 2–6, 2–8, 4–8, 6–8) was investigated. A same–different paradigm was used with repetition rates of 100 rep/sec and 108 rep/sec presented randomly as A–A, A–B, B–A and B–B in four blocks of 32 randomized trials. As suggested by Macmillan *et al.,*[16] the hit and false-alarm rates were analyzed and a modified sensitivity measure, d′, was obtained for each of the individual electrodes and electrode pairs. The d′ values were 3.3 and 2.2 for individual electrodes 2 and 8, respectively, while d's ranging from 2.5 and 4.8 were obtained for electrode pairs. These results suggested that the discriminability of repetition rate for two-electrode stimulation is as good as or better than that for single-electrode simulation.

C. These two-electrode results indicate that, in addition to the fundamental frequency and second formant that were presented by activating one electrode at a time, as described in this section, further speech information, such as the first formant, can be presented to implant patients by two-electrode stimulation.

Summary

The characteristics of the sensations produced by activating one electrode at a time are summarized as follows: (a) Loudness was found to increase with current level and pitch with repetition rate. (b) Pitch and sharpness increased in the apical-to-basal direction, and vowel labels could be assigned to sensations produced by individual electrodes in accordance with the tonotopical organization of the cochlea. (c) Results from triadic comparisons provided evidence that the sensations produced by repetition rate and electrode position are perceptually separable. (d) For short-duration stimuli, the discrimination performance for electrode trajectories was much better than that for repetition rate trajectories. For noncoincidental two-electrode stimulation, triadic comparisons showed that two perceptual components, one related to the more basal electrode and the other to the more apical one, could be discerned. Speech-coding considerations based on these psychophysical results are discussed.

References

1. Clark, G. M., R. C. Black, I. C. Forster, J. F. Patrick & Y. C. Tong. 1978. Design criteria of a multiple-electrode cochlear implant hearing prosthesis. Technical notes and research brief. J. Acoust. Soc. Am. **63**: 631–635.
2. Tong, Y. C., R. C. Black, G. M. Clark, I. C. Forster, J. B. Millar, B. J. O'Loughlin & J. F. Patrick. 1979. A preliminary report on a multiple-channel cochlear implant operation. J. Laryngol. Otol. **93:** 679–695.
3. Tong, Y. C., J. B. Millar, G. M. Clark, L. F. A. Martin, P. A. Busby & J. F. Patrick. 1980. Psychophysical and speech perception studies in two multiple-channel cochlear implant patients. J. Laryngol. Otol. **94:** 1241–1256.
4. Blamey, P. J., Y. C. Tong, R. C. Dowell & G. M. Clark. 1981. Pitch and loudness studies on a multiple-channel cochlear implant patient. J. Acoust. Soc. Am. (Suppl. 1) **70:** S53.
5. Burns, E. E. & N. F. Viemeister. 1976. Nonspectral pitch. J. Acoust. Soc. Am. **60:** 863–869.
6. Flanagan, J. L. 1955. A difference limen for vowel formant frequency. J. Acoust. Soc. Am. **27:** 288–291.
7. Wier, C., W. Jestaedt & D. M. Green. 1977. Frequency discrimination as a function of frequency and sensation level. J. Acoust. Soc. Am. **61:** 178–184.
8. Tong, Y. C., G. M. Clark, P. J. Blamey, P. A. Busby & R. C. Dowell. 1982. Psychophysical studies for two multiple-channel cochlear implant patients. J. Acoust. Soc. Am. **71:** 153–160.
9. Tong, Y. C., P. J. Blamey, R. C. Dowell & G. M. Clark. 1981. The effects of electrode position and stimulus period on the hearing sensations in a multiple-channel cochlear implant patient. J. Acoust. Soc. Am. (Suppl. 1) **70:** S52.
10. Plomp, R. 1976. Aspects of Tone Sensation. Academic Press. London.
11. Tong, Y. C., G. M. Clark, P. M. Seligman & J. F. Patrick. 1980. Speech-processing for a multiple-electrode cochlear implant hearing prosthesis. J. Acoust. Soc. Am. **68:** 1897–1899.
12. Tong, Y. C., G. M. Clark, R. C. Dowell, L. F. A. Martin, P. M. Seligman & J. F. Patrick. 1981. A multiple channel cochlear implant and wearable speech-processor: An audiological evaluation. Acta Otolaryngol. **92:** 193–198.
13. Clark, G. M., Y. C. Tong, L. F. A. Martin, P. A. Busby, R. C. Dowell, P. M. Seligman & J. F. Patrick. 1981. A multiple-channel cochlear implant: An evaluation using nonsense syllables. Ann. Otol. Rhinol. Laryngol. **90:** 227–230.
14. Dowell, R. C., Y. C. Tong, P. J. Blamey & G. M. Clark. 1981. Perceptual dissimilarity and discrimination studies using two-electrode stimulation with a multiple-channel cochlear implant patient. J. Acoust. Soc. Am. (Suppl. 1) **70:** S53.
15. Shepard, R. N. 1972. Psychological representation of speech sounds. *In* Human Communication: A Unified View. E. E. David and P. M. Denes, Eds. McGraw-Hill. New York, NY.
16. Macmillan, N. A., H. L. Kaplan & C. D. Greelman. 1977. The psychophysics of categorical perception. Psych. Rev. **84:** 452–471.

PERCEPTS ELICITED BY DIFFERENT SPEECH-CODING STRATEGIES[a]

Erwin S. Hochmair and Ingeborg J. Hochmair-Desoyer

Department of Electrical Engineering
Technical University of Vienna
A-1040 Vienna, Austria

INTRODUCTION

A number of remarkably different speech-coding strategies exist that were developed or suggested for the electrical stimulation of the auditory nerve. The considerable differences among those strategies may reflect both (1) the relative importance attached by the various groups to the place and periodicity principle, and, to a certain degree, (2) the varying abilities and limitations of the different implants used.

The second point may need some explanation: Without doubt, a percutaneous plug is the most advantageous from the point of view of coding, but many groups do not use it for good reason. The implanted receiver circuits necessary for the transcutaneous transmission are severely restricted in size, power consumption, and complexity. This limits the number and bandwidth of independent stimulation channels. Often some low-power digital circuits are used.[1, 2] Their incompatibility with analog stimulation waveforms may explain the preponderance of pulsatile stimulation schemes. Fortunately, speech seems to be so redundant that even a considerable degree of processing leaves some cues sufficiently intact to enable the listener to partly reconstruct the information. This may explain why widely differing coding schemes *may* achieve similar results.

There is no agreement on the number of independent stimulation channels necessary or feasible. Existing devices feature from one to fifteen channels.[3] The stimulation sites used include the scala tympani, the modiolus, the cochlear nucleus, the round window and the promontory, and sites along, but external to, the cochlea. The stimulation signals themselves span the range from fixed-frequency, variable-duration pulses[4] to modulated carriers[5] and to completely analog waveforms.[6] There are schemes using varying amounts of feature extraction from voiced/unvoiced-coding only, to heavily coded signals on several channels.[7] In this paper the speech processing used with the Vienna auditory prosthesis is described and results are presented. In addition, some results of our ongoing investigations of further single- and multichannel strategies are given.

THE VIENNA AUDITORY PROSTHESIS

The four-channel implant presently used is shown in FIGURE 1, together with the external sound processor. It consists of a four-channel bipolar stimulation electrode (described elsewhere[8]) inserted into the scala tympani and an

[a] This work is supported by the Austrian Science Research Fund.

0077-8923/83/0405-0268 $01.75/0 © 1983, NYAS

implantable passive receiver set featuring four independent transmission channels. The transcutaneous transmission is achieved by four independent rf-transmission paths arranged in two pairs. By spatial separation (by using two different transmission frequencies [12 MHz and 31 MHz]) and by special shaping of the receiver coils, cross coupling is kept to less than −45 dB in 10 of the 12 possible channel combinations and to −20 dB in two combinations. Conventional amplitude modulation is used for the transmission. In order to achieve the stable transfer function necessary for psychoelectric measurements, critical coupling is maintained between the tuned circuits of the receiver and the transmitter for each channel. With a transmitter coil diameter of 18 mm,

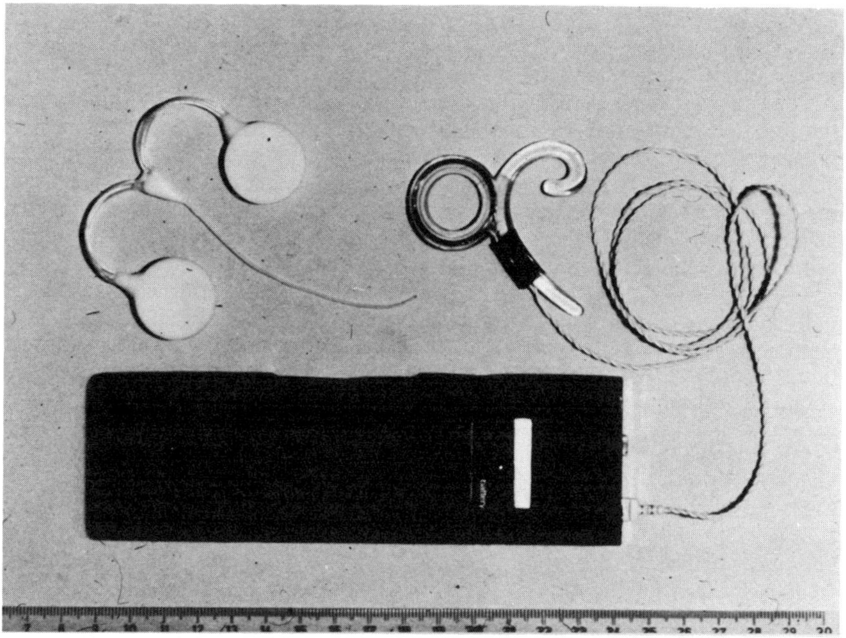

FIGURE 1. Auditory prosthesis consisting of a scala tympani implant featuring four independent channels and a single-channel external sound processor.

lateral displacements of ± 8 mm and distance changes of ± 2 mm can be tolerated when assuming an 0.4-dB allowable tolerance in stimulation current. The received signals are demodulated and fed to the electrode via capacitive coupling.

In the laboratory four transmitters are used, each feeding its own transmission coil. When the device is used as an auditory prosthesis, only one of the four channels is used as described in Hochmair-Desoyer *et al.*[9] The wearable single-channel speech processor measures 12.5 by 4.5 by 2 cm and weighs 110 g and includes a 9-V rechargeable battery. The battery lasts for one day and is recharged overnight. A small amplitude-modulated rf-transmitter is directly mounted to an ear-hook fixed over the implanted receiver selected.

The system developed gradually from more complex, but less effective predecessors as described by Hochmair.[3] The main goal was to achieve a simple system, easy to manufacture and capable of supporting many different coding schemes. In other words, the "intelligent" parts of the system are transferred from the receiver to the external processor, thus leading to a passive, highly signal-transparent receiver, which allows research on many single- and multichannel strategies. However, four channels are about the maximum that can be achieved this way. If it should turn out that more than four channels would be necessary for optimum speech coding, which we consider somewhat unlikely, one would have to return to implant active circuitry.

Speech Processing of the Vienna Auditory Prosthesis

The earlier work performed with several different versions of implants[10] showed that stimulation using a somewhat modified analog speech signal results in superior speech understanding as compared with that achieved with pulsatile stimulation schemes. From these experiments it may be concluded that the waveform of the electrical stimulus does, to some extent, determine the percept. This finding was supported at a later date by phase experiments using multicomponent stimulation signals.[11]

The necessary processing of the signal is quite straightforward. It essentially consists of amplitude compression and frequency equalization. This is in contrast to various types of feature extractions performed for pulsatile stimulation. Hence, we have obtained a simple system that easily fits the power and volume constraints of a wearable stimulator and that results in more or less natural-sounding percepts, which makes rehabilitation easier.

We believe that, besides the dependence of percepts on wave shape, there is another reason why pulsatile stimulation signals (of frequencies less than a few kHz) are not well suited for speech coding. The coding process involves a considerable amount of feature extraction, the consequences of which are not very well defined. Furthermore, coding that involves speech feature extraction frequently destroys the natural appearance of environmental sounds. Finally, because of this lack of naturalness, rehabilitation takes a longer period of time.

The simple sound processing performed in our wearable speech processor is detailed in FIGURE 2. The amplified audio signal is compressed by a syllabic compressor, that is, a gain-controlled amplifier (GCA) with a very short attack time (0.5 msec) and a release time of approximately 20 msec. The compression ratio is around 6. Adjustments according to the patient's dynamic range can be made. This compression ratio derives from a comparison of the Stevens function's exponents for electrically and acoustically induced hearing (approximately 3.5 and 0.6, respectively).

The exact shape of the amplitude compression function over the whole dynamic range is important in everyday life, with its varying amplitude levels and its constantly changing amount of background noise. This circumstance is in contrast to that of similar devices suggested for hearing aids, where compression sets in only at a fairly high output level.

Much of the frequency response of the stimulation current is already corrected as a byproduct of driving the frequency-dependent, somewhat capacitive impedance of the stimulating electrodes by a source impedance of

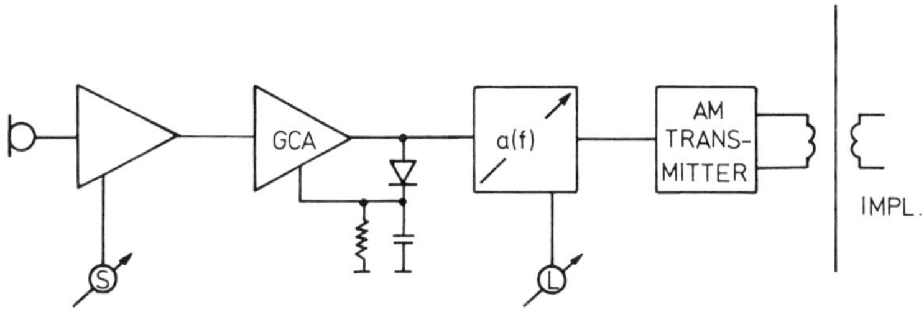

FIGURE 2. Single-channel sound processor including an AM transmitter for transcutaneous transmission. The gain-controlled amplifier (GCA) performs the dynamic range compression. Preamplifier and modulation amplifier gains are variable to control sensitivity (S) and loudness (L), respectively. The frequency response of the equalization network, a(f), is detailed in FIGURE 4.

roughly 3 kΩ of the receiver. This results in a frequency-dependence of threshold, 40% equal-loudness contour, and uncomfortable listening level, measured at the rf-transmitter input, as shown in FIGURE 3. The residual frequency response is corrected by an adjustable equalization circuit following the amplitude compressor. It is adjusted to the subject's characteristics by a fitting procedure that locates three poles and one zero in such a way that the 40% equal-loudness contour (most comfortable loudness) corresponds to constant microphone output voltage for frequencies from 100 Hz to 4 kHz (FIG. 4). This fitting of the frequency response is very important for speech understanding.

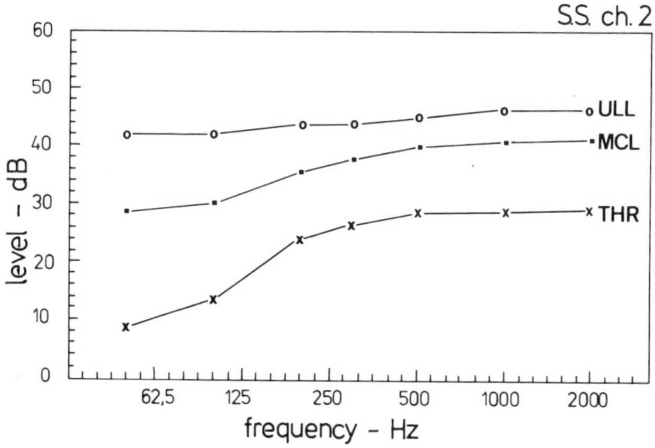

FIGURE 3. Threshold (THR), most-comfortable loudness level (MCL), and uncomfortable listening level (ULL) for a sinewave stimulus in dependence of frequency. The ordinate is the voltage at the transmitter modulation input. The actual stimulation current increases approximately by an additional + 3 dB/octave with frequency.

SPEECH PERCEPTION RESULTS

Of the subjects implanted with a multichannel scala tympani electrode, we have mainly worked with four: L.P., C.K., F.W. and S.S., who could afford to spend considerable time in test sessions. Most of the results from those subjects have been already described in another article,[10] but part are repeated here for completeness.

For the patient, the improvement of lipreading by additional electrical stimulation is important. Our postlingually deafened patients reach aided lipreading scores between 60 and almost 100% in open-list tests using 200 one-syllable words (Freiburger Test). This reflects a mean improvement of 25% over lipreading alone. Nevertheless, it is better to compare different prostheses by open-list speech-understanding tests without lipreading, that is, through stimulation only. For such a test 100 sentences not used in any of the preceding sessions were selected. Because only very little standardized speech test material is available in German, a list of everyday sentences was set up that does not contain first names or brand names or any uncommon expressions. These sentences were completely unknown to the subject. There are four to eight words per sentence. The test material was presented from good-quality tapes using a Revox B 77 tape recorder, the output of which was directly connected to the patient's wearable unit. Thus, no sound was present in the room. The sentences were presented by an unfamiliar male speaker. With the four subjects tested, the percentages of correctly understood words ranged from 18%, through 31 and 34%, to 80% (for our best subject, C.K.). With C.K. an additional open-speech comprehension test consisting of 100 one-syllable adjectives unknown to her has been performed. She reached a score of 40% on that test. The difference in this score from that of the score in the sentence test can be attributed to the lack of context in the one-syllable word list.

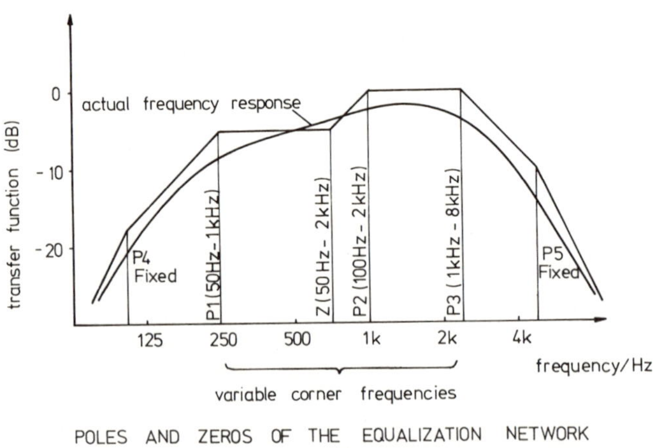

FIGURE 4. Example of the transfer function of the equalization network. Poles P1 . . . P3 and zero (Z) are varied for best equalization when the sound processor is fitted to the patient.

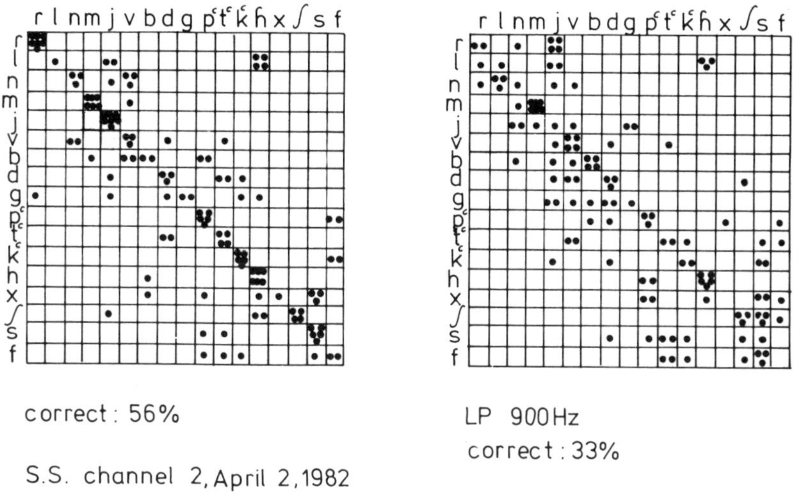

FIGURE 5. Consonant confusion matrices for two different signal bandwidths. On the *left* the stimulation signal had the full bandwidth of 4 kHz; on the *right* it is low-pass-filtered at 900 Hz. The items were presented in citation form as [a:Xa:]. (Electrical stimulation only [without lipreading].)

It should be stressed that there is an enormous difference between good closed-list results and even the restricted open-speech understanding of 18 or 30%.

We are convinced that it is very important to produce as naturally sounding hearing impressions as possible and not to rely on a learning process by the patient. According to our experience, patients do not readily accept a totally different-sounding speech, which contradicts their memory. Furthermore, such a rehabilitation program would take too much time and it would be too costly, even if it eventually achieved its goal.

In order to find out whether frequencies above the saturation frequency in the pitch scaling [12] do contribute at all to speech understanding, confusion matrices have been obtained with lowpass filters inserted into the signal path. FIGURE 5 shows a comparison of two consonant confusion matrices (for subject S.S.) with upper frequency limits of 4 kHz and 900 Hz, respectively. The 900-Hz lowpass filter had a fourth-order Butterworth response.

Frequencies above 900 Hz increased the score from 33% to 56%. This demonstrates that the frequency range above 900 Hz, where frequency discrimination becomes very poor,[12] does indeed contribute to the understanding of speech. This was also confirmed in tests with S.S. using two-digit numbers.

The results obtained with the single-channel analog stimulation described herein compare favorably with the scores obtained with single-channel pulsatile stimulation (FIG. 6) used earlier. No open-speech understanding was obtained with the latter strategy. In a reduced five-item consonant confusion matrix ([d], [n], [z], [s], [t]) scores increased from 48% to 88% when processors were changed.[10] (FIG. 7).

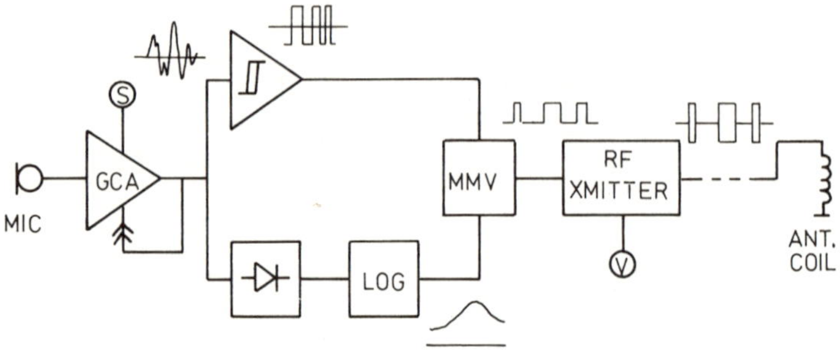

FIGURE 6. Block circuit diagram of an earlier version of the sound processor using pulsatile stimulation. The pulse rate is determined by the zerocrossings and the pulse width depends logarithmically on the audio signal amplitude.

OTHER SINGLE-CHANNEL SPEECH-PROCESSING SCHEMES

FIGURE 8 lists four amplitude compression schemes together with a schematic representation of the distortions of a two-frequency signal as seen in time and frequency domain. The dashed curves in the right column represent threshold and uncomfortable-loudness level of the subject.

Each method improves the consonant-to-vowel ratio. The syllabic compression (as just discussed, this method is used in our portable sound processor) introduces comparatively little distortion. For sufficiently small attack times it practically leaves the waveshape within one phoneme unchanged. However, since the dominant component of the signal scales the spectrum (that is, determines the gain of the gain-controlled amplifier), the lower amplitude components may fall below threshold.

The second method avoids any effects due to the time constants involved with automatic gain control, albeit at the cost of considerable distortion.

Our comparison of these two methods showed the syllabic compression to give superior results. FIGURE 9 compares the confusion matrices for the two

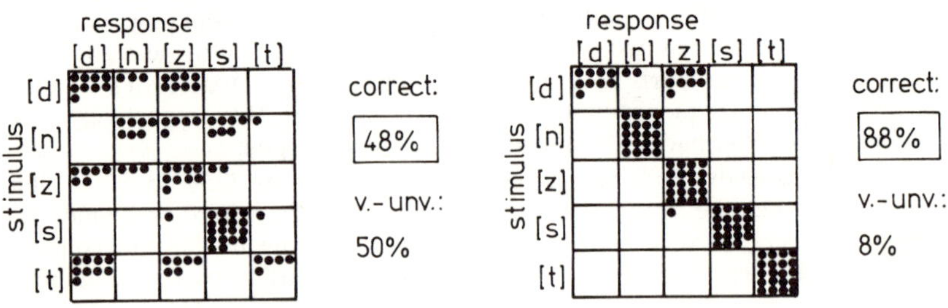

FIGURE 7. Comparison of pulsatile (*left*) and analog stimulation (*right*), both without lipreading. Beneath the percentage of correct answers, the percentage of voiced–unvoiced errors with respect to the total numbers of errors is given. (Data are for C.K., channel 3, bipolar, female speaker I.H.) The same confusion matrices were also used by Fourcin *et al.*[14]

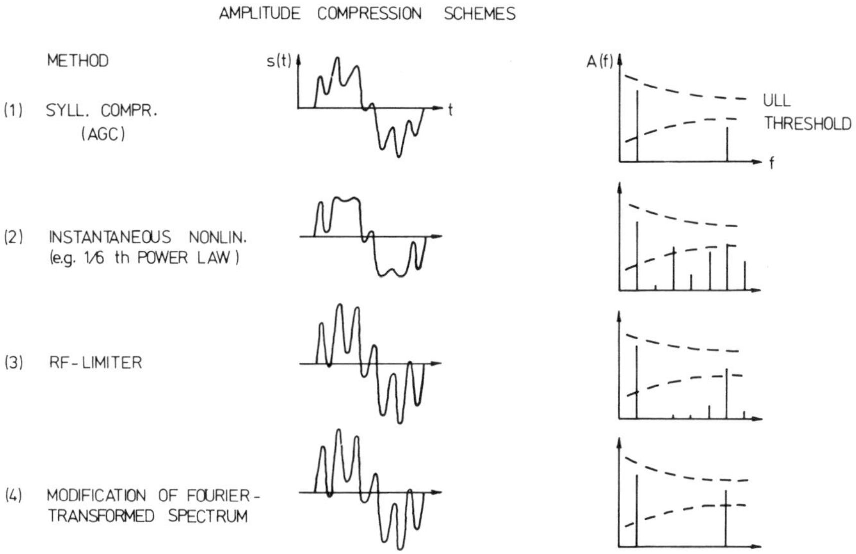

FIGURE 8. Examples of amplitude compression schemes. The time function and the amplitude spectrum at the output of the compression circuit for a two-component input signal are indicated in the second and third column.

methods using plosives as stimuli. The syllabic compression also sounded more pleasant to the patient.

The nonlinear distortion is considerably reduced by method 3: up-conversion of the signal before the nonlinear compression, and down-mixing of the bandfiltered compressed signal.

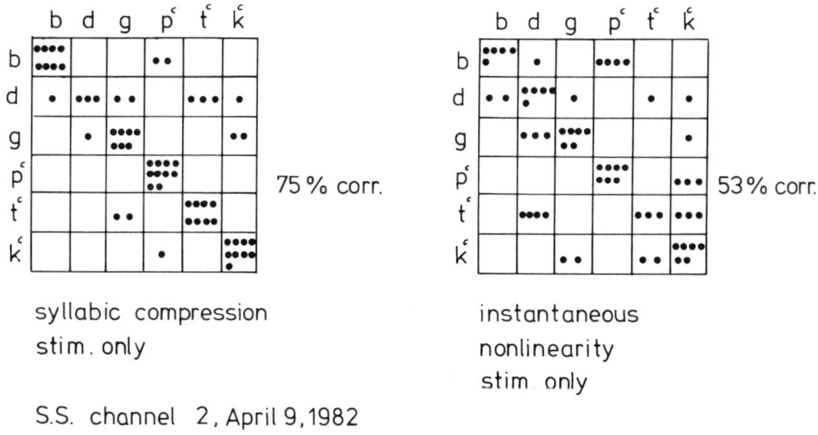

FIGURE 9. Stimulation-only plosives-confusion matrices for syllabic compression and for instantaneous nonlinearity.

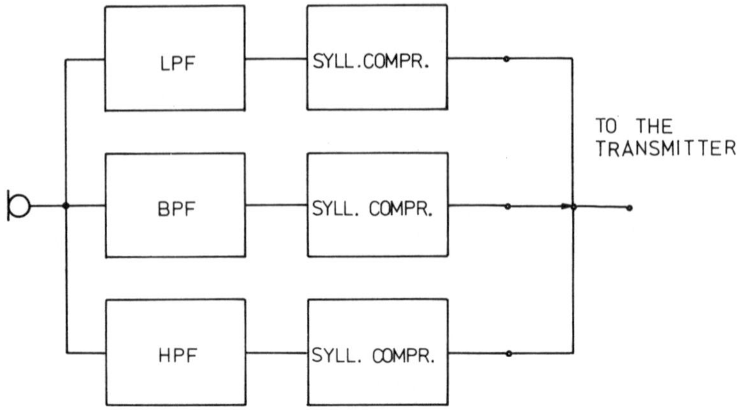

FIGURE 10. Three-band compression scheme.

A theoretically superior method should be the direct modification of the signal's Fourier transform, which allows amplitude ratios of simultaneously occurring components to change. We have not yet investigated the last two methods, but we looked into three-band-compression (FIGURE 10), which approximates method 4. No significant improvements over single-channel syllabic compression have been found independent of whether the filters are linear phase or not.

The latter result shows a difficulty encountered in comparing different speech processors, and this difficulty is even more pronounced when multichannel strategies are compared: Since the subjects are so used to their single-channel syllabic compressor, it is difficult for a competing strategy being tried in the laboratory during one or two test sessions to score significantly better. Also, some patients are more responsive than others to different processing strategies. In particular, subjects who have been deaf for many years before implantation do not discriminate well among different strategies. Fortunately, the contrary is also true: a good subject can make use of the potential of a good speech processor. At any rate, the development of sensitive speech tests is very important. These tests should uncover different error modes in different strategies which might otherwise result in similar overall scores. The confusion matrix test mentioned earlier is a step in this direction.

An unexpected low score was obtained by the preemphasis of 3 and 6 dB/octave inserted before an instantaneous compressor (logarithmic nonlinearity). The test with 243 minimal pairs led to only 69% correct answers (63% chance at 1% significance). The subject's response time was markedly increased, and when asked, she gave her answers a very low confidence rating.

The considerable compression of dynamic range involved in signal conditioning of auditory prostheses raises a number of yet unanswered questions: Which of the various characteristics of complex waveforms (such as spectral distribution [like location of peaks or center of gravity], zerocrossings, or amplitude density distribution) determine to some extent the sensations elicited? Which parameters can be modified without destroying the information content? Which ones have to be modified in a specific way? To what extent can nonlinear distortions be tolerated? We are confident that more-sensitive tests can be developed in the future to answer some of those questions.

Multichannel Experiments

Although single-channel stimulation does provide usable information to the subject and has been shown to result in comparatively good speech understanding, we cannot exclude the possibility that results with multichannel coding strategies could eventually surpass these results.

The term "multichannel" is used here for strategies using multiple stimulation sites as opposed to single-channel stimulation devices, which may also use multichannel coding schemes and/or multiple transmission channels.

The adherents of place theory propose to achieve this goal by dividing the speech band into several critical-band-wide channels. This strategy necessitates roughly 15 independent stimulation channels.

In simulations with normal-hearing subjects it has been shown [13] that at least 12 channels would be necessary for good speech understanding. Besides the presently unresolved problem of achieving the necessary channel separation, there is also the question of whether the percepts elicited by different channels do differ sufficiently from each other and in some usable way. Although pitch differences between channels are rather small compared with what could be expected from place theory, channels can be distinguished from each other to some extent by their timbre or dullness. But even so, it may well be possible that multichannel stimulation is better than single-channel stimulation merely because of the increased channel capacity, which thus avoids interaction between simultaneously present components of complex signals. If this is the case, then just a few—or even two—channels should show some improvement over single-channel stimulation.

In our investigation of multichannel coding strategies we confined ourselves for the time being to band-filtered analog signals without feature extraction. The number of channels used was between 2 and 4. Figure 11 shows the pertinent schematic diagram. The amplitude compression was achieved separately in each channel, either by logarithmic compression or by syllabic compression. In some experiments linear phase filters were used and in one experiment, the delay of the traveling wave withing the cochlea was modeled. Table 1 summarizes preliminary results obtained with minimal-pair tests. No particular improvement over that of a single-channel stimulation is seen. Note that the delay introduced between channels did not have any significant effect on scores.

Conclusion

Among the various single-channel coding strategies investigated, stimulation schemes using a somewhat modified analog speech signal rank highest in speech understanding. Within this group, the method used for dynamic range compression is also important. Syllabic compression seems to work best with most of our patients. At the present state of the art, these single-channel sound processing strategies can be implemented by small low-power circuits, and hence are well suited to be used in wearable prosthetic devices.

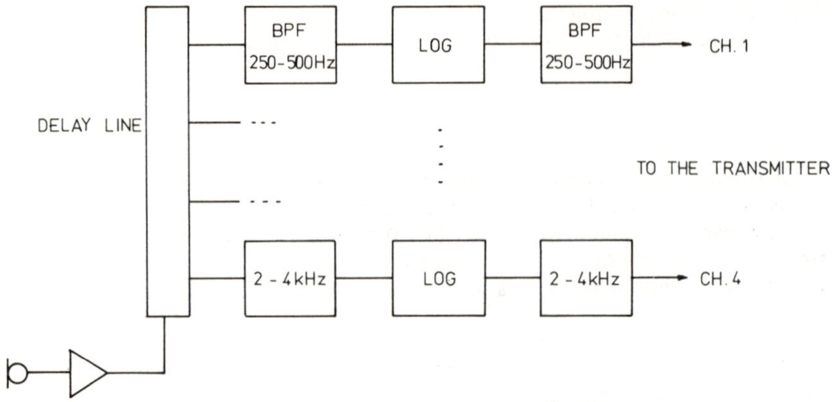

FIGURE 11. Vocoder-type coding for four independent stimulation channels. The logarithmic amplitude compressors may be replaced by any of the other three schemes of FIGURE 8. An optional delay line simulating the delay of the traveling wave within the cochlea is also shown.

Theoretically, vocoder-type multichannel strategies should give an improvement in speech understanding over single-channel devices, but so far none of the pertinent strategies investigated gave superior results.

TABLE 1

MINIMAL-PAIR SPEECH DISCRIMINATION SCORES USING MULTICHANNEL STRATEGIES

Subject	Type Vocoder-Filter Bank 3–4 Channels	Filter Bank with Delay (60 μsec–1.36 msec 2–4 Channels	Phase Linear Filters 3 Channels	LP/HP-Filters (700-Hz Crossover) 2 Channels	Single-Channel Processor (Comparison)
S.S.					
Consonants	73	72	75	81	78
Vowels	75	78	73	79	83
Total	73	74	75	80	80
S.O.					
Consonants	—	71	78	73	77
Vowels	—	—	70	69	77
Total	—	—	76	72	77

NOTE: 243 pairs were compared for each system. The numbers indicate percent correct. Error bounds are 37% at 1% significance.

ACKNOWLEDGMENTS

This research is conducted in cooperation with the Second ENT Department of the University of Vienna (K. Burian). The minimal-pair test was developed by B. Eisenwort and E. Benkö. J. Steurer conducted the multichannel speech tests.

REFERENCES

1. HOCHMAIR, E. S. 1980. An implantable current source for electrical nerve stimulation. IEEE Trans. Biomed. Eng. BME-**27:** 278–280.
2. GHEEWALA, T. R., R. D. MELEN & R. L. WHITE. 1975. A CMOS implantable multielectrode auditory stimulator for the deaf. IEEE SC–**10:** 472–479.
3. HOCHMAIR, E. S. 1981. Engineering aspects of auditory implant research. Proceedings of the Twelfth ORL World Congress, Budapest, Hungary: 477–481. The Hungarian Academy of Sciences.
4. CHOUARD, C. H. 1983. Multichannel cochlear implant: Surgical technique, signal processing and clinical results. This volume.
5. HOUSE, W. F. 1976. Cochlear Implants. Ann. Otol. Rhinol. Laryngol. (Suppl. 27) **27:** 85.
6. HOCHMAIR, E. S., I. J. HOCHMAIR-DESOYER & K. BURIAN. 1981. Results of the Vienna cochlear prosthesis for the deaf program. Proceedings of the Third Meeting of ISAO, Paris, France. Supplement to Vol. 5 of Artificial Organs.
7. CLARK, G. M., R. BLACK, D. J. DEWHURST, I. C. FOSTER, J. F. PATRICK & Y. C. TONG. 1977. A multiple-electrode hearing prosthesis for cochlear implantation in deaf patients. Med. Progr. Technol. **5:** 127–140.
8. HOCHMAIR-DESOYER, I. J. & E. S. HOCHMAIR. 1980. An eight-channel scala tympani electrode for auditory prostheses. IEEE Trans. Biomed. Eng. BME-**27:** 44–50.
9. HOCHMAIR-DESOYER, I. J., E. S. HOCHMAIR & K. BURIAN. 1981. Four years of experience with cochlear prostheses: A review. Med. Progr. Technol. **8:** 107–119.
10. HOCHMAIR-DESOYER, I. J., E. S. HOCHMAIR, FISCHER, R. E. & K. BURIAN. 1980. Cochlear prostheses in use: Recent psychophysical data and speech comprehensions results. Arch. Otorhinolaryngol. **229:** 81–98.
11. MÜLLER, C. G. Personal communication.
12. HOCHMAIR-DESOYER, I. J., E. S. HOCHMAIR, K. BURIAN & H. K. STIGLBRUNNER. 1983. Percepts from the Vienna cochlear prosthesis. This volume.
13. HARTMANN, R. 1979–1981. Grundlagenstudien zur Hörprothese. *In* Arbeitsbericht des Sonderforschungsbereiches 45: 167–200. Vergleichende Neurobiologie des Verhaltens. Frankfurt-Darmstadt.
14. FOURCIN, A. J., S. M. ROSEN, B. C. J. MOORE, E. E. DOUEK, G. P. CLARKE, H. DODSON & L. H. BANNISTER. 1979. External electrical stimulation of the cochlea: Clinical, psychological, speech-perceptual, and histological findings. Br. J. Audiol. **13:** 85–107.

SPEECH PERCEPTION WITH PROMONTORY STIMULATION [a]

A. J. Fourcin,[b] E. E. Douek,[c] B. C. J. Moore,[d] S. Rosen,[b] J. R. Walliker,[b] D. M. Howard,[b] E. Abberton,[b] and S. Frampton [c]

[b] *University College, London*
London NW1 2HE, England

[c] *Guy's Hospital*
London SE1, England

[d] *Cambridge University*
Cambridge, England

Introduction

The present work of the EPI [e] group is characterized by a combination of four features. First, our patients are essentially all adults who have had largely normal speech communication ability prior to total bilateral loss of hearing. Second, the electrical stimulation that we use to give them a new sensation of hearing is always applied externally at the round window or on the cochlear promontory by means of a single active electrode. Third, the information that is transmitted along this single channel is designed to give maximum assistance to the deaf lipreader and is organized in terms of speech pattern components rather than the whole speech signal. These speech pattern components can be used separately or in combination, and are transformed to match the patient's electrical hearing. Finally, our program of rehabilitation involves work with the patient's speaking ability as well as the new sensation of hearing, and quantitative measures of both speech and hearing are made routinely.

Physical Basis of Stimulation

The simplest means that we use to apply an input to the cochlea is shown in Figure 1. A conventionally formed ear mold provides a mechanical base for a ball-ended electrode assembly. The ear mold is gold-coated on its external meatal surface to provide an electrical return path and to reduce any possibility of allergic reaction.[1] The electrode assembly itself comprises an axially sprung stem which is adjusted for each individual patient so that the contact made by the 1–2-mm-diameter spherical end is on an appropriate part of the promontory. A stimulation level of not more than 10 μC/cm^2/pulse is involved.

The speech pattern information is typically derived from any of a variety of different signal sources. At home, the patient would rely primarily on a microphone input, but would also use speech signals from a television receiver.

[a] This work is primarily supported by the British Medical Research Council.

[e] The External Pattern Input group is composed of the above workers in collaboration with Drs. L. H. Bannister and H. Dodson of Guy's Hospital.

0077–8923/83/0405–0280 $01.75/0 © 1983, NYAS

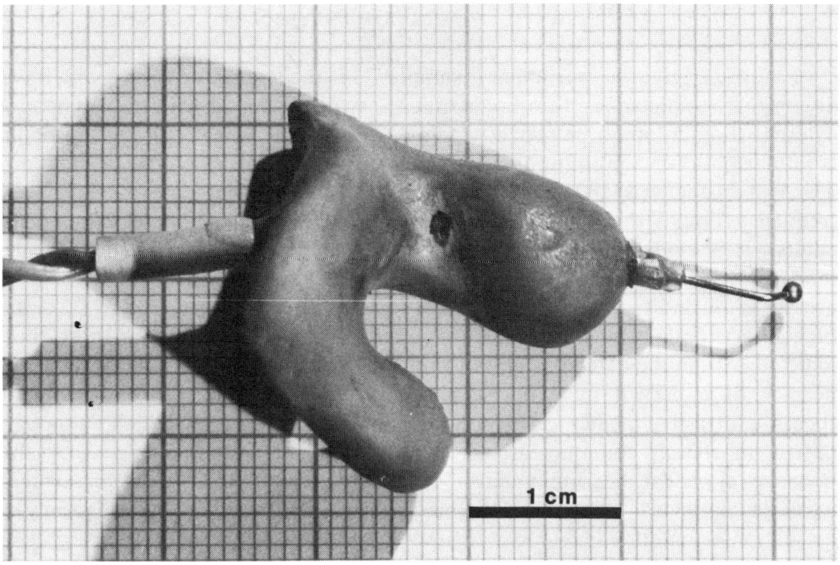

FIGURE 1. Ear mold electrode assembly.

In each case, at present, the frequency of laryngeal vibration is the main pattern component. Considerable use is made of infrared transmission since this gives excellent patient isolation and is relatively immune to (and itself causes little) external interference. Constant-current, zero net charge transfer stimulating pulses are provided at present by a body-worn device no matter what the signal source. The pulse amplitude is automatically varied, as a function of the particular laryngeal period that it terminates, so that it corresponds to the individual patient's comfortable loudness level. Although a microphone-based laryngeal frequency extractor is also body-worn, both of these devices could, in due course, be combined in a single meatal or behind-the-ear placement.

In surgical terms, two classes of totally deaf patient are provided for.[2] The first group of patients has an open middle ear as the result of, for example, the treatment of mastoiditis. In this group, the electrode contact is made directly with the surface of the cochlear promontory. Once adjusted and fitted, the mold electrode assembly is removed and reinserted by the patient without supervision.

Patients in the second group have a closed auditory meatus in which the tympanic membrane has been displaced by tympanopexy[2] so that it is in intimate contact with the promontory. These patients present with a wide range of etiologic factors, but all have essentially normal middle ears. The same ear-mold electrode assembly (FIG. 1) used for the "open-ear" patients is used for these patients, but now electrical contact is made between the spherical end of the electrode and the epithelial surface of the membrane. The contact point is chosen to be at the region where the membrane is grafted on to the promontory so that the direction of current flow is primarily into the cochlea.

SINEWAVE STIMULATION THRESHOLDS

FIGURE 2 gives a particular example [3] of the constant-current sinewave discomfort and detection thresholds that are typically found with single-channel external stimulation at the round window. The overall shape of these thresholds is similar both for a promontory electrode site and for intracochlear stimulation. The two histograms above the thresholds in FIGURE 2 indicate the laryngeal frequency ranges that are typically found in the speech of male and female adults. It is evident that the made voice is likely to be more readily accommodated within these threshold ranges than is the female voice. (The analyses are based on individual vocal-fold closure counts [4] and give a bias in favor of higher laryngeal frequencies). The thresholds do not, however, do more than indicate magnitude-detection ability and any potential speech-processing competence of a patient must be assessed by techniques that relate directly to speech-contrastive ability. This requires the use of stimuli which, although of use in speech communication, are yet capable of being detected by the patient's electrical hearing ability. The first part of our patient assessment work has, in consequence, been directed towards the use of larynx frequency—intonation—contours.

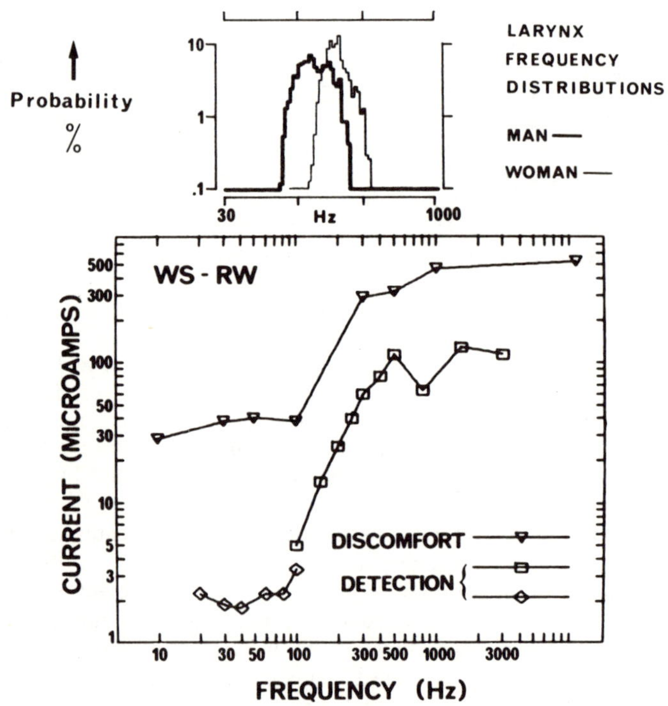

FIGURE 2. Sinewave extracochlear stimulation thresholds (rms current).

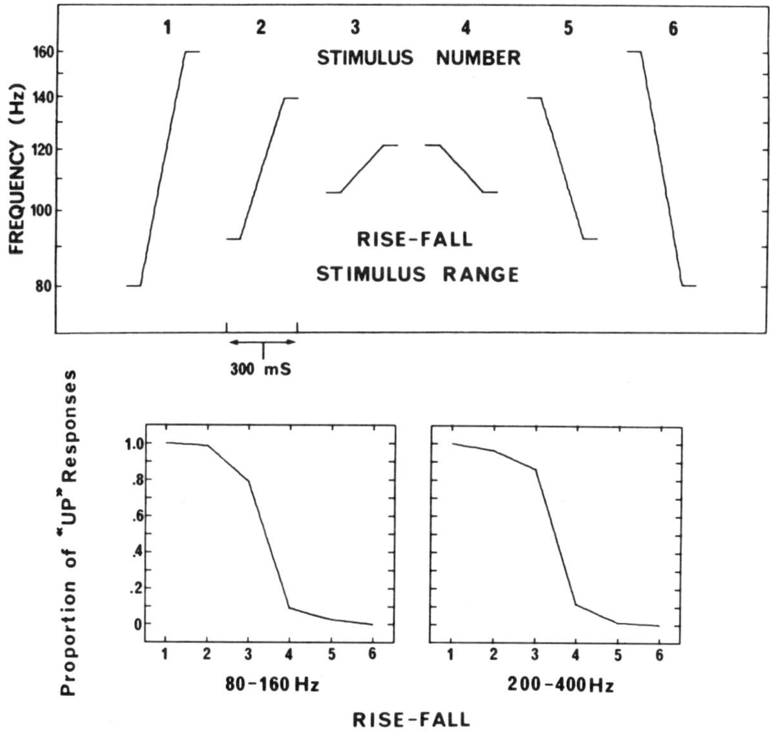

FIGURE 3. Average rise-fall labeling responses from 31 normal listeners.

SPEECH RECEPTIVE ABILITY

Larynx Frequency Contours

The upper half of FIGURE 3 shows a set of intonation stimuli progressing from an extreme rise in fundamental frequency, Fx,[f] to an extreme fall.[5] The maximum range of Fx, 80–160 Hz, corresponds to what might be obtained in a citation form taken from a man (see, for example, the left-most Fx distribution in FIGURE 2). These fundamental frequency contours were used in the synthesis of [ɑ] sounds with appropriate formant frequencies, and normally hearing listeners (18–22 years old) were asked to give either an "UP" or "DOWN" label to five tokens of each of the resulting randomly presented stimuli. The average labeling responses are shown in the lower half of FIGURE 3. The Fx range for the labeling response on the right goes beyond what is ordinarily found for a woman and corresponds to that for a child. In each case, however, an orderly, symmetrical changeover in labeling is found with the boundary sharply defined in the middle of the stimulus range; this is the expected form of response from a group of normal listeners.

[f] Fx is used to designate an unsmoothed, period-by-period, measurement of vocal fold frequency.

FIGURE 4 shows the individual labeling responses obtained from two open-ear patients with promontory stimulation in the 80–160 Hz range (positive-going constant-current pulses with zero net charge transfer). Two weeks before the responses recorded for subject DS in FIGURE 4(1), he was quite unable to hear the difference between an extreme rise and an extreme fall. For subject IH, FIGURE 4(1) shows her first labeling responses to the stimuli. In each case the responses on the right (FIG. 4[2]) were obtained after practice in only one clinical session. We have found it to be of great value to associate the patient's speech-productive and -receptive abilities. Productive training, using a visual intonation pattern display [6] can, in fact, be crucial in eliciting appropriate labels. Once familiarity has been established—or, in a sense, restored, since our patients are postlingually deaf—these tests can be applied without difficulty either, as here, with prerecorded stimuli or interactively under computer control. The effects of practice can easily explain the otherwise anomalous responses to question–statement lists that have been reported elsewhere.[7] We find that sentence lists of this type do not present real difficulty to our practiced patients.

Our patients seem less able to hear the intonation contrasts in the speech of children, for example, than in men. Stimuli of the type shown in FIGURE 3 provide a speech-based evaluation of this ability. Adaptive computer-controlled testing is used to find the symmetrical pair of stimuli that have 75% correct labeling. The use of this technique for different octave ranges of the stimulus extremes provides the basis for a quantitative estimate of the sharpness of the

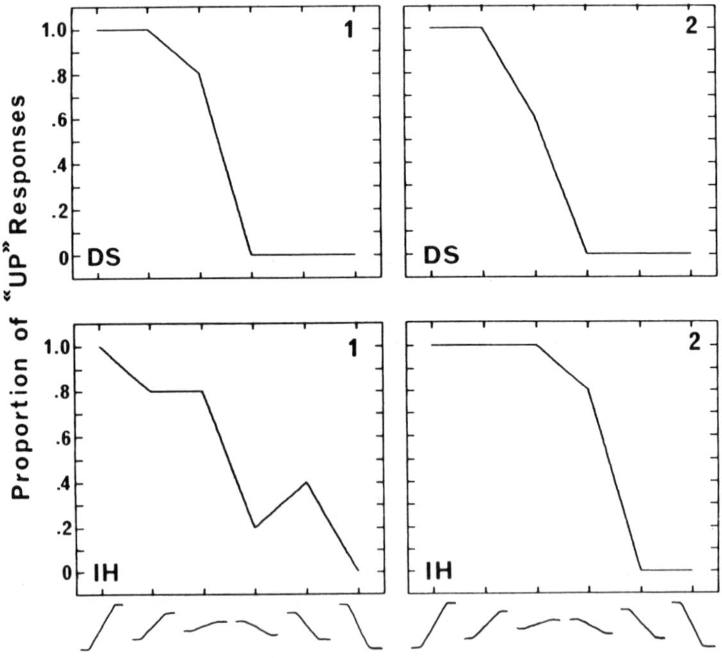

FIGURE 4. Rise-fall labeling with electrical promontory stimulation in two "open-ear" patients.

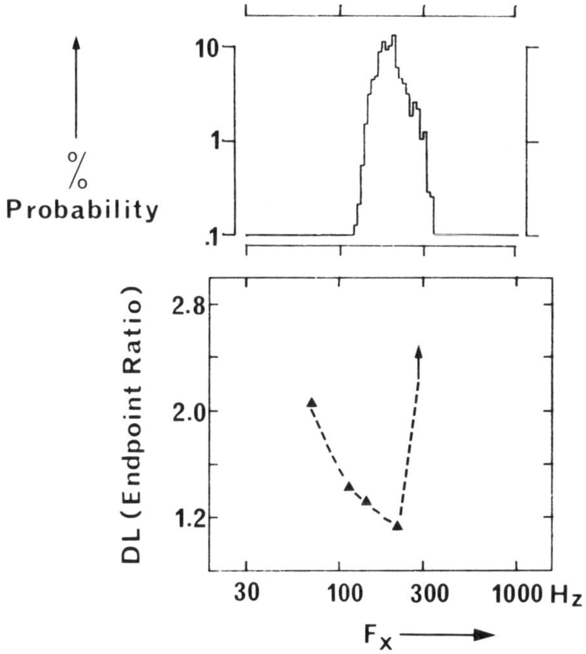

FIGURE 5. Labeling sharpness and laryngeal frequency range in patient IH with promontory stimulation.

corresponding labeling boundary, and this is plotted in the lower half of FIGURE 5 for four center frequencies of the Fx stimulus ranges used. The fifth stimulus set (200–400 Hz) went beyond the range at which the patient, IH, could respond usefully. The upper half of FIGURE 5 makes it possible to relate the laryngeal frequency range of the normal woman's voice shown in FIGURE 2 to these responses, and it is evident that much of this range and nearly all of the range of the man's voice shown in FIGURE 2 is available for perceptual processing. Indeed, IH's younger child cannot always easily communicate with his mother using her home prosthesis. Although it is quite possible that IH will extend her useful Fx range with further practice, it seems likely with present stimulation techniques that both she and many other patients will have a low upper limit to their perception of laryngeal frequency. (We have now developed a simple laryngeal frequency transposing option for our patients' "take-home" prostheses which can both bring higher-pitched voices within the range of electrical hearing and can increase their proportional Fx variation. This is done on a laryngeal period-by-period basis in the initial signal analysis, and in the final output it involves, for example, a simple constant shift in frequency by subtraction. Linguistic information is still provided by this transformation and speaker-identification is still possible.[8] We call this processing Mapitch.)

These particular tests, although speech-based, are intermediate between speech and psychophysical assessments, and they form part of a more complete array of speech test material that we have developed to cover, at least in part, the use of prosodic contrasts involving question–statement contrasts, stressed word placement, and syntactic structure.

Voiced–Voiceless Oppositions

Part of the ability to perceive prosodic contrasts stems, of course, from the patient's capacity to detect changes in time as well as frequency. Although our present concentration on laryngeal frequency patterning does not make it possible to transmit the many detailed consonant and vowel features in speech that depend broadly on place of articulation, contrasts that depend in part on temporal differences can be perceived—at least in principle. Figure 6 shows some results from a temporal perceptual test which, although it is psychophysi-

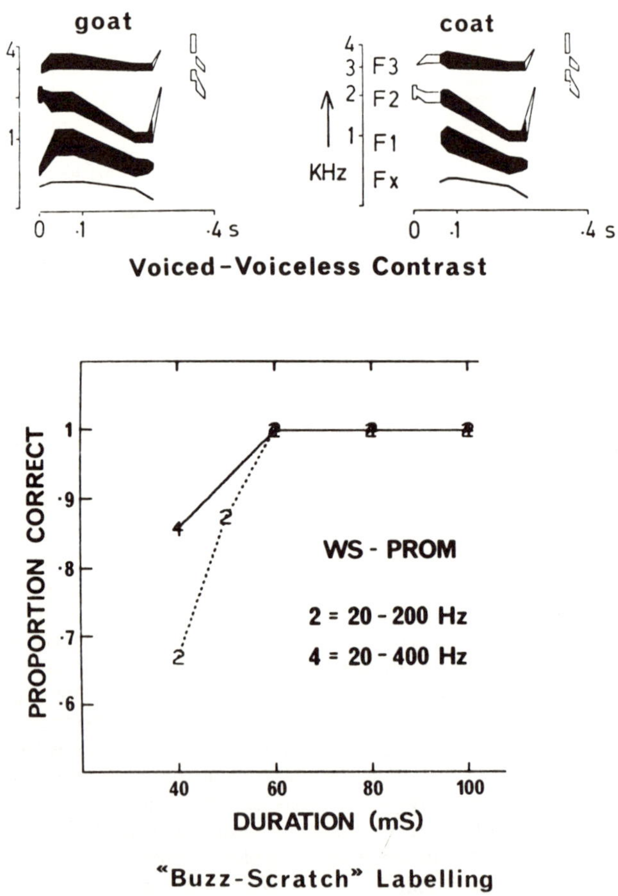

Figure 6. Aspects of temporal processing in relation to a speech contrast.

cal, bears directly on important speech oppositions. English, in common with many other speech systems, makes use of a large proportion of consonantal oppositions which are primarily characterized by the presence or absence of vocal-fold vibration during otherwise largely identical articulations. The upper part of FIGURE 6 illustrates a particular example of this contrast.[5] The filled-in portions of the formant patterns relate to those parts of the utterances that have vocal-fold vibration. The open sections are, in physical terms, noise-excited. Labeling tests with a stimulus range having these extremes typically give a sharply defined boundary in the region of 30 msec. When only voicing information is transmitted, the presence of, for example, a voiceless segment like [k] in *coat* or of a voiceless fricative results in a brief interval of silence. We have found that listeners with electrical stimulation devices can detect correspondingly brief silent intervals in psychophysical tests.[3] FIGURE 6 shows results from a related test which now contrasts random with periodic stimulation as a function of stimulus duration.[3] In each of the presentation conditions, a 200-Hz sinewave is paired, at equal loudness level, with a random noise of the indicated bandwidth. When the noise band covers the frequency range available to the patient, very good (2I–2 AFC) discrimination is obtained with stimulus durations down to 60 msec. This makes it highly likely that fricative intervals and plosive consonant stop durations will be well perceived. It is possible also for the recognition of voiced–voiceless plosive consonant oppositions to be assisted by lipreading in this way, especially when noise is also used for pattern stimulation.

CONSONANT IDENTIFICATION

A simple but usefully representative format for assessing a patient's consonantal lipreading ability is provided by the use of meaningless vowel–consonant–vowel (VCV) combinations.[9] In our work video recordings of two phonetically trained speakers, a man and a woman, have been used in order to assess the relative utility of a variety of associated acoustic and electrical speech pattern presentations. Two sorts of test situation have been used. The first involves the use of normal subjects in order to obtain a normative reference. Results from a group of normally hearing subjects are shown in FIGURE 7. In each situation there were 144 presentations of each stimulus. Presentations were of the form [ˈɑCɑ]. With lipreading alone, 41% of the responses were correct, while the addition of voice pitch derived from 4-kHz high pass filtering of 20-μsec larynx-synchronous pulses gave an overall score of 72%. The same pattern of results is also obtained for a totally deaf lipreader when presented with a useful laryngeal frequency stimulation. FIGURE 8 shows that patient DS has an average score of 35% with lipreading alone (24 presentations/stimulus), while the provision of laryngeal frequency information reduces confusion and increases his score to 62% (12 presentations/stimulus from only one speaker). In each case the availability of laryngeal frequency information tends to reduce all sources of error, not only those that come from the lack of voicing discrimination. This effect comes from the additional temporal information carried by the pulse train and it operates essentially just as well—in this VCV condition—for artificially constant pitch as for the naturally varying condition. These results are given as an indication of what can be obtained, rather than as an example of the best that could be achieved in this condition with

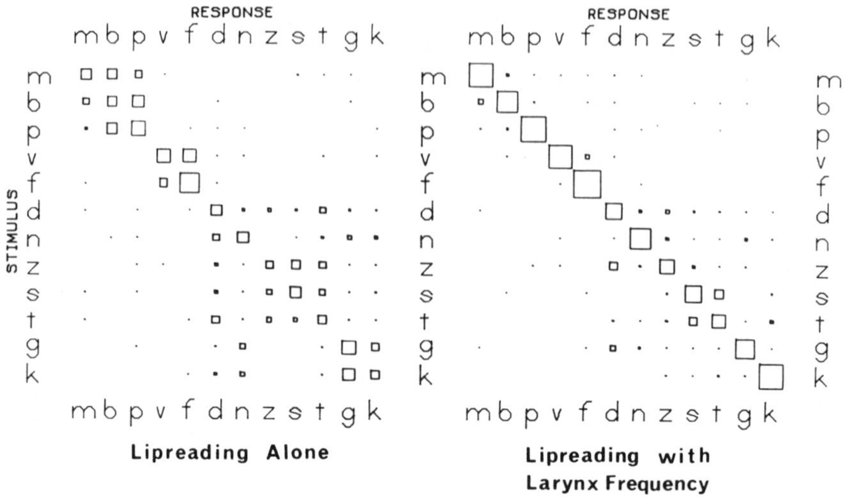

FIGURE 7. Consonant confusions in VCV responses from normal subjects.

single-channel stimulation. Quite simple coding changes could substantially improve the overall score for many deaf patients. Even so, these results are as good as those reported for invasive multichannel stimulation by Clark and Tong [10] (and their patient 2 [but not their patient 1] in this volume).

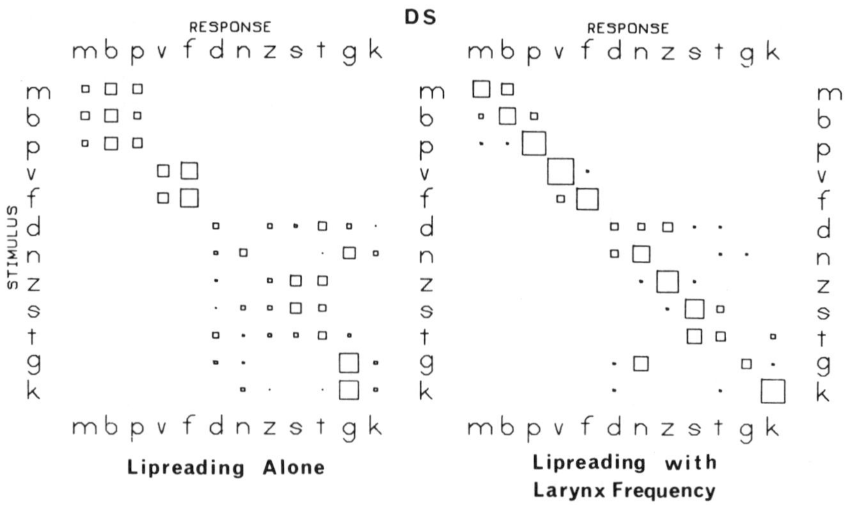

FIGURE 8. Consonant confusions in VCV responses from a patient with promontory stimulation.

CONVERSATION

Although the use of synthetic speech tests and lipreading with a defined set of consonants provides a well-controlled, quantitative basis for assessment, we also need, and are now beginning to make use of, an approximation to a natural conversational situation.[11, 12] In this connected discourse tracking (CDT) test, the lipreader must correctly repeat back every word spoken by the talker. When normally hearing subjects are used, they are separated by a soundproof transparent screen and the lipreader hears only an associated sound provided via headphones. Each test session lasts 5 minutes, and in FIGURE 9 each subject has had 6 hours' experience with laryngeal frequency information (LF) as both talker and receiver when first exposed to the lipreading alone (LA) condition. In spite of this relatively intensive prior experience, the lack of laryngeal frequency information more than halves the lipreaders' communication ability, expressed in words/minute. In FIGURE 9 the particular LF condition shown is associated with a laryngograph[g] output from the speaker. Essentially the same difference between the LA and LF conditions is obtained from a real-time

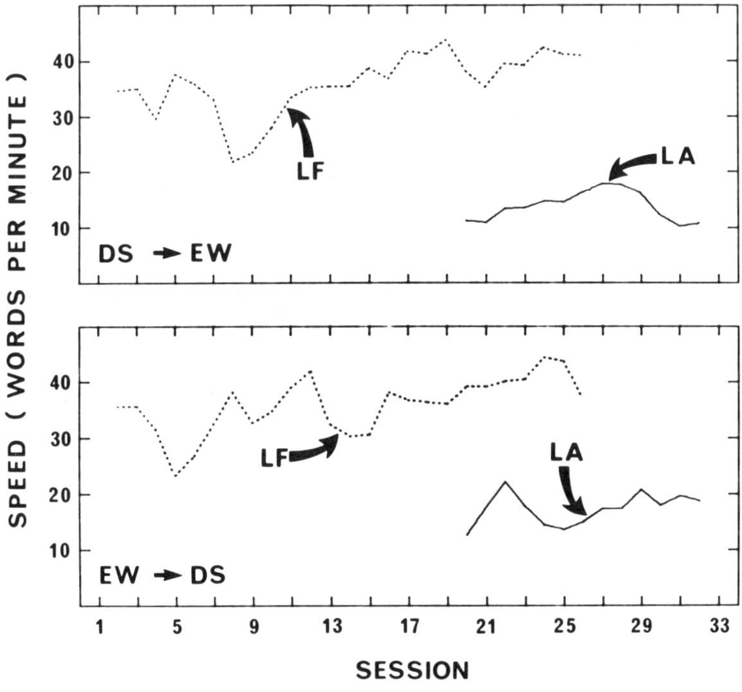

FIGURE 9. Lipreading rates for normal subjects with (LF) and without (LA) laryngeal frequency.

[g] Laryngograph equipment and Voiscope® Fx training equipment are manufactured by Laryngograph, Ltd.

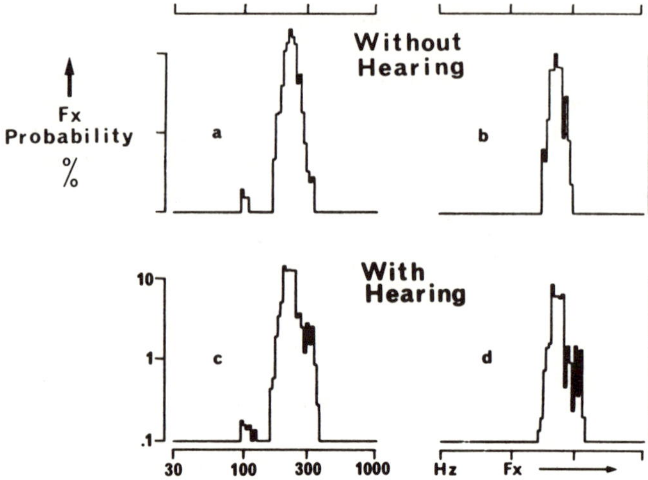

FIGURE 10. An effect of electrical hearing on laryngeal frequency range in patient IH.

acoustic (peak-picking) measurement. Reduction of the temporal accuracy of laryngeal frequency sensing reduces the words/minute score of the LF condition, and this occurs, for example, if cepstral processing with a basic time window of 50 msec is used. Similarly if the LF information is represented only by a constant frequency, the word rate in this test is now severely reduced and may, depending upon the lipreader, be little better than in the LA condition. Our present experience indicates that these results also apply to the patients with electric stimulation devices, and we have been careful to design clinical and home equipment that provides laryngeal frequency information on a period-by-period basis.

Speech Control with Electrical Hearing

Prolonged total deafness always has some influence on speaking, although there is a large variation in degree of disturbance from one patient to another. Both voice excitation and articulatory abilities are influenced. Just as laryngeal frequency information can contribute to the improvement of receptive ability, it can also assist prosodic control in speech production. The speech and simultaneous laryngograph recordings that we make routinely make it possible to follow the changes that occur as the result of the daily use of an extracochlear stimulator. Although patient IH lost her hearing completely only 1½ years ago, she has a long history of hearing disability and her voice control is a little abnormal. FIGURE 10a shows her laryngeal frequency histogram [4] based on a read text without electrical stimulation, but following a speech therapy session using an interactive fundamental frequency display.[6, g] The distribution is rather narrow (178–282 Hz at the 1% level). FIGURE 10c is based on a reading of the same text immediately before the same therapy session, but with self-monitoring using a microphone and laryngeal frequency analyzer as input to the electrical stimulator. This distribution is one-third of an octave broader at the 1% level (178–338 Hz) and has a flat peak; kurtosis for these distributions is also very different, having a value of 23 without hearing in FIGURE 10a and 15 with hearing in FIGURE 10c. The triple-period histograms [4] in FIGURES 10b and 10d provide a simple indication of laryngeal frequency regularity. It is especially worth comparing FIGURE 10d with the lower half of FIGURE 5 for the same patient. Vocal-fold vibration regularity is markedly poorer above about 270 Hz, and this corresponds to the sharp reduction in pitch-discriminative ability in this frequency region.

An attempt to give a combined picture of laryngeal frequency range and regularity is shown in FIGURE 11, where the instantaneous frequency of each laryngeal period is plotted against that of the period immediately following.[4] It is now easier to see that both range and regularity have improved in the with-hearing condition. We can expect that these changes will be consolidated with continued use of auditory feedback. (It was a privilege, at this meeting, to discuss these results in the presence of Dr. C. A. Black, the inventor of the feedback amplifier.)

The improvements in laryngeal frequency control shown in these figures are very similar to those that can occur when profoundly deaf children are taught to use their residual hearing,[5] and it is possible that the same temporal mechanisms are involved, electrically for our patients and from an acoustic input with the children.

CENTRAL PITCH AND ELECTRICAL HEARING

FIGURE 12 gives the results from two early pitch-matching experiments made in New York in 1958 at Haskins Laboratories.[13] Low-pass filtered random noise

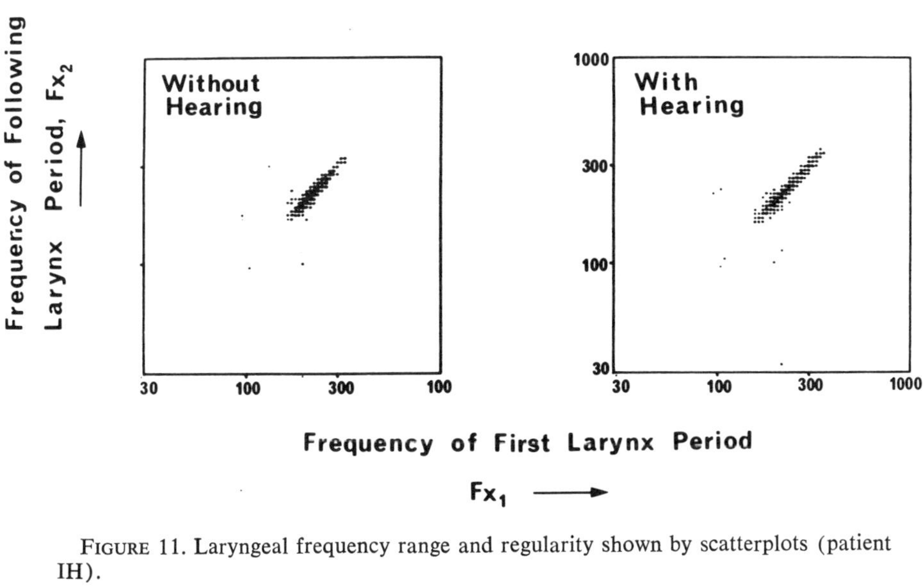

FIGURE 11. Laryngeal frequency range and regularity shown by scatterplots (patient IH).

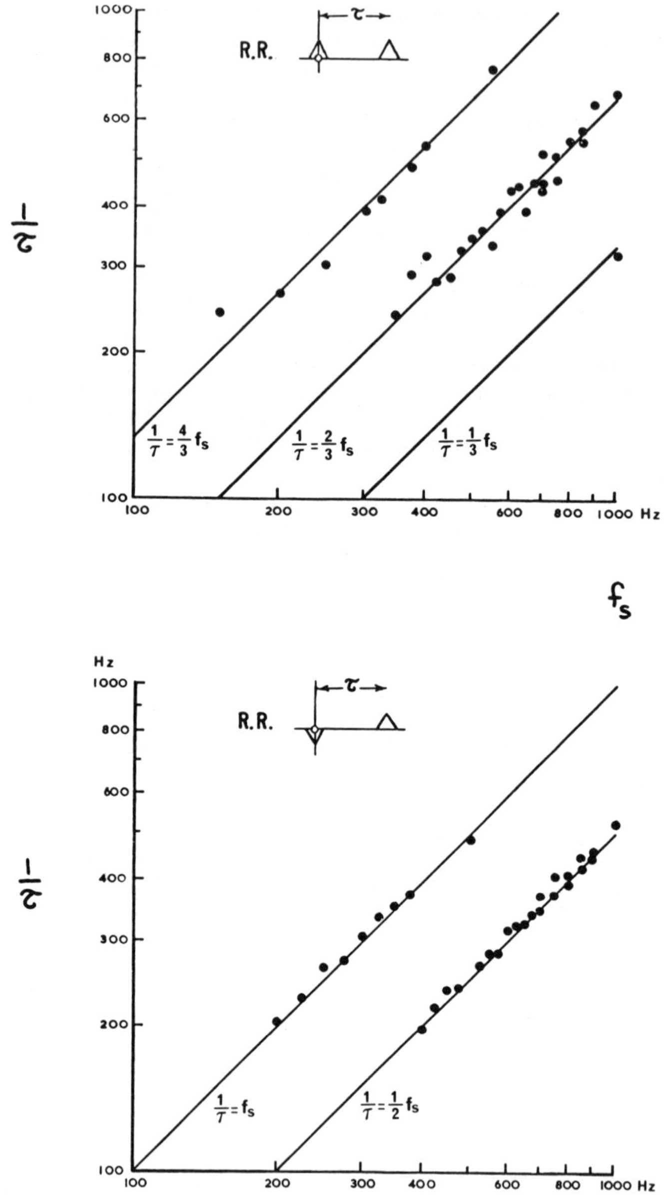

FIGURE 12. Central pitch-matching for pure tone references.

stimuli from two independent sources were binaurally presented using a single variable delay line so that one noise source gave a fixed central auditory image, while the other produced a lateralized image, the displacement of which was controlled by the variable delay, τ. Although listening with either ear alone gave an auditory sensation of an unvarying noise, attention to the central percept that accompanied binaural stimulation provided a relatively distinct pitch sensation, with the pitch increasing as the delay, τ, decreased. Each point in FIGURE 12 comes from one pitch match against a pure tone source of frequency, f_s, and the difference in the overall pattern of matching between the upper and lower graphs results from a reversal of the interaural phase of the common, undelayed, noise. This is only one example of a family of central pitch phenomena [14-16] that can only be explained in terms of temporal auditory analysis rather than peripheral place processing. The electrical stimulation results described earlier similarly depend on the direct neural transmission of temporal information and, in this respect, are related to the central pitch phenomena. There is, however, an important difference, since central pitch matches of this type typically extend to a little beyond 1 kHz, while electrical stimulation does not ordinarily yield a sensation of pitch much beyond 300 Hz. In addition, central pitch can be associated with a neurally mediated qualitative sensation of timbre, and this has also not so far been found with our patients.

These binaural, and related, central pitch results may indicate a deficiency in our methods of stimulation for single-channel work with the electrically stimulated ear, with respect to both fundamental frequency and spectral contrast, since although the results depend on auditory nerve processing of temporal features of an acoustic input, we cannot yet attain a comparable range of auditory ability for our patients.

DISCUSSION

Although the methods of stimulation described in this paper are simple and noninvasive, they are capable of bringing a measurable improvement in both receptive and productive abilities.

Quite straightforward extensions of our present methods of encoding seem likely to bring further improvement since both the mapping of input voice frequencies into the patient's useful auditory range and the provision of noise-excitation to signal voiceless sounds will enhance contrastive ability. It seems quite possible that further developments in speech-signal processing will bring additional benefits since the present limits of patient performance may well be considerably inferior to those capable of being achieved on the basis of a purely temporal transmission of information.

Even though our present patients have considerable speech ability, the speech-training component of our rehabilitation program is useful both in regard to speech improvement and, even more importantly, with respect to the training of the new sense of hearing given by electrical stimulation. Part of our present speech-encoding work can also be used to enable the residual hearing of the profoundly deaf to be more usefully employed. It may be even more important in future work to see electrical stimulation as part of a whole range of interrelated approaches to deafness. Similar speech-pattern-based training and prosthetic techniques can then be applied, but using different modalities—electric, acoustic, and visual (at least for training), and possibly tactile.

We have not worked systematically with totally deaf children, but the availability of an effective noninvasive method of stimulation would be of even greater potential value to them than to the already-developed adult, and the developing child could perhaps make greater use of binaural presentations and special speech signal-processing.

Acknowledgments

Our research could not proceed without the contributions made by our own institutions and colleagues. In particular, we would like to thank Dr. C. A. Greatorex and his staff in the Department of Clinical Physics and Bioengineering at Guy's Hospital.

References

1. Walliker, J. R., E. E. Douek, A. J. Fourcin, B. C. J. Moore & S. M. Rosen. 1983. Speech signal presentation to the totally deaf. *In* High Technology Aids for the Disabled. W. J. Perkins, Ed. Butterworths. London.
2. Douek, E. E. *et al.* 1983. Clinical aspects of extracochlear electrical stimulation. This volume.
3. Fourcin, A. J., S. M. Rosen, B. C. J. Moore, E. E. Douek, G. P. Clarke, H. Dodson & L. H. Bannister. 1979. External electrical stimulation of the cochlea: Clinical, psychophysical, speech perceptual and histological findings. Br. J. Audiol. **13**(3): 85–107.
4. Fourcin, A. J. 1981. Laryngographic assessment of phonatory function. ASHA Rep. **11:** 116–127.
5. Fourcin, A. J. 1980. Speech pattern audiometry. *In* Auditory Investigation. H. A. Beagley, Ed.: 170–208. Clarendon Press. Oxford.
6. Abberton, E. & A. J. Fourcin. 1975. Visual feedback and the acquisition of intonation. *In* Foundations of Language Development, Vol. 2. E. H. Lenneberg and E. Lenneberg, Eds.: 157–165. Academic Press. New York, NY.
7. Hendon, M. K. 1981. Psychoacoustics and speech processing for a modiolar auditory prosthesis. Stanford Electronics Laboratories Technical Report No.G906–5.
8. Abberton, E. & A. J. Fourcin. 1978. Intonation and speaker identification. Lang. Speech **21**(4)**:** 305–318.
9. Rosen, S. M., B. C. J. Moore & A. J. Fourcin. 1979. Lipreading with fundamental frequency information. Proc. Inst. Acoust. (U.K.) Autumn, paper A12.
10. Tong, Y. C. & G. M. Clark. 1980. Speech comprehension with multiple-channel electrical stimulation of human auditory nerve fibres. Proc. Austral. Phys. Pharm. Soc. **11:** 201P.
11. De Filippo, C. L. & B. L. Scott. 1978. A method for training and evaluating the reception of ongoing speech. J. Acoust. Soc. Am. **63:** 1186–1192.
12. Rosen, S. M., A. J. Fourcin & B. C. J. Moore. 1981. Voice pitch as an aid to lipreading. Nature **291:** 150–152.
13. Fourcin, A. J. 1958. Speech perception and bandwidth compression. *In* Haskins Laboratories Progress Report. (See also Signals Research and Development Establishment, Report 112 (1958), U.K.)
14. Fourcin, A. J. 1970. Central pitch and auditory lateralization. *In* Frequency Analysis and Periodicity Detection in Hearing. R. Plomp and G. F. Smoorenburg, Eds.: 319–328. A. W. Sijthoff. Leiden.
15. Raatgever, J. & F. A. Bilsen. 1977. Lateralization and dichotic pitch as a result of spectral pattern recognition. *In* Psychophysics and Physiology of Hearing. E. F. Evans and J. P. Wilson, Eds.: 443–454. Academic Press. London.
16. Schroeder, M. R. 1977. New viewpoints in binaural interaction. *In* Psychophysics and Physiology of Hearing. E. F. Evans and J. P. Wilson, Eds. 455–468. Academic Press. London.

PERCEPTS FROM THE VIENNA COCHLEAR PROSTHESIS [a]

Ingeborg J. Hochmair-Desoyer,[b] Erwin S. Hochmair,[b]
Kurt Burian,[c] and Helmut K. Stiglbrunner [b]

[b] *Department of Electrical Engineering*
Technical University of Vienna
A-1040 Vienna, Austria

[c] *Second ENT Department*
University of Vienna
A-1090 Vienna, Austria

INTRODUCTION

The auditory prosthesis project in Vienna started with the development of an eight-channel implant realized in hybrid technology and encapsulated in a hermetic glass package. This concept was in agreement with the then-dominant opinion that to possibly reach speech understanding by means of electrical stimulation of the auditory nerve, 8 to 20 or more stimulation channels would be necessary. This approach turned out to be premature because it required sound-coding strategies as well as electrode connection schemes to be decided upon before they had been sufficiently compared.

It was therefore decided not to put a lot of effort into reproduction and redesign of complex hybrid implants, but to first use simple, quickly designed, and easy-to-modify implants and to use those for basic stimulation experiments with deaf volunteers. These would enable a decision to be made between different electrode connection schemes. Basic data on the prosthetic hearing would first be gathered and different sound-coding strategies compared. In the course of this program, it turned out that stimulation of one single channel of a multichannel intracochlear electrode using a simple correlate of the analog speech signal did result in some very useful speech understanding [1, 2] in our patients C.K. and L.P. This sound-coding strategy was then implemented in a small portable sound-processor/stimulator and is now used to activate the one of four implant channels that gives the best possible speech understanding. This system (a scala tympani electrode [3] with four bipolar pairs of electrode contacts driven by a four-channel implant, and the external portable single-channel sound-processor/stimulator) is the currently used version of our auditory prosthesis (FIG. 1). In addition to this system, a single-channel implant driving an extracochlear pair of electrodes has been developed. This extra-cochlear implant has been used since early 1980. The main rationale for this system was to avoid damage to the inner ear in patients with some residual hearing. It has thus been mainly used in patients with limited residual hearing that was to be preserved. The external portable sound-processor is the same as that used with the intracochlear electrode.

So far, a total of 19 patients have been equipped with one of the implant versions described. A clinical study including 100 patients has been started to evaluate intracochlear and extracochlear auditory prostheses. The protocol includes a battery of presurgical tests, with some of them serving patient-

[a] This research is funded by Grant 4151 from the Austrian Science Research Fund.

0077-8923/83/0405-0295 $1.75/0 © 1983, NYAS

selection purposes and others giving data for comparison with postoperative results.

Patients

Since 1977, 19 patients have been equipped with an auditory prosthesis; these patients are listed in Table 1. The type of implant used in each case is included (a more detailed description of implants will be given later).

Of the 13 patients who received intracochlear electrodes, two are prelingually, possibly congenitally, deaf, and of the remaining 11 patients four had been deaf for less than 5 years before implant surgery.

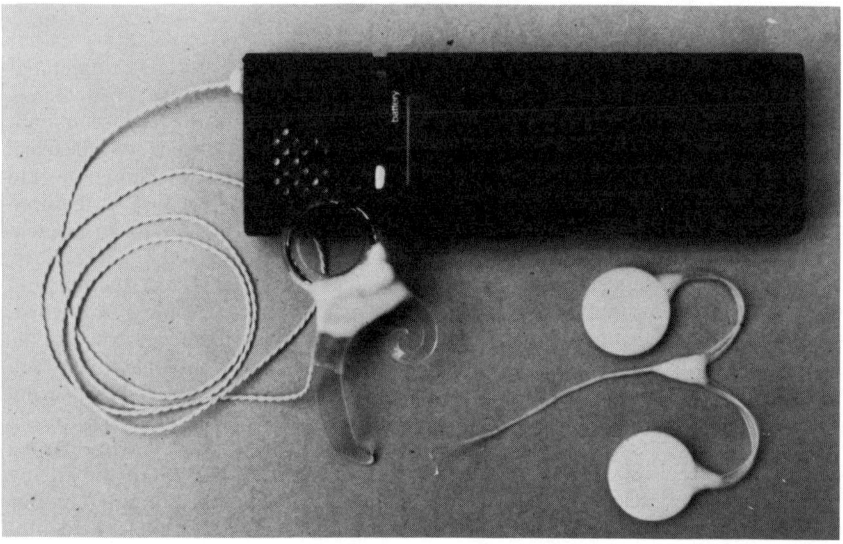

Figure 1. Auditory prosthesis consisting of four-channel bipolar scala tympani electrode, four-channel implantable receiver/stimulator electronic device, and external single-channel sound-processor.

Of the six patients who received extracochlear electrodes, four are prelingually or congenitally deaf, and the remaining two have been deaf for more than 5 years. All of these patients have some residual hearing, which is useful to the extent that it should not be destroyed.

Implants

Table 2 lists the different implant versions in the order they were designed and also implanted. "SC" stands for an implant comprising a scala tympani electrode. "E" stands for an implant with an extracochlear pair of electrodes. The implants always couple to an external portable support system via a wireless inductive link. A percutaneous plug has never been used.

TABLE 1

DATA IN PATIENTS RECEIVING COCHLEAR IMPLANTS

Patient	Year of Birth	Sex	Deaf since:	Cause of Deafness	Year of Implantation	System Implanted
1 (H.R.)	1953	M	1959	Hereditary	1977	8-channel hybrid c.g.
2 (V.K.)	1955	M	(postlingually deaf)	Hereditary	1978	8-channel hybrid c.g.
3 (R.B.)	1957	M	(prelingually deaf)	Infection at 2 wk(?)	1978	6-channel c.g.
4 (L.P.)	1939	F	1977	Bacterial infection	1978	6-channel bipolar
5 (C.K.)	1956	F	1978	Hereditary	1979	4-channel c.g./bipolar
6 (R.M.)	1931	F	1978	? (slow degradation)	1980	Extracochlear, round-window niche
7 (E.K.)	1939	F	(prelingually deaf)	Otitis(?)	1980	Extracochlear, round-window niche
8 (F.W.)	1951	M	1968	Head trauma	1980	4-channel c.g./bipolar
9 (S.S.)	1962	F	1969	Mumps	1980	4-channel c.g./bipolar
10 (S.H.)	1967	F	1973	Meningitis	1980	4-channel c.g./bipolar
11 (G.W.)	1961	M	(prelingually deaf)	Smallpox vaccination (1 yr)	1981	Extracochlear, promontory
12 (E.L.)	1939	M	1979	Round-window rupture	1981	4-channel monopolar
13 (S.O.)	1952	F	1964	Head trauma	1981	4-channel, 2 bipolar 2 monopolor
14 (M.B.)	1961	F	(prelingually deaf)	? (prior to 1 year)	1982	4-channel bipolar
15 (Ch.K.)	1963	F	(prelingually deaf)	? (prior to 1 year)	1982	Extracochlear, promontory
16 (W.T.)	1938	M	1944	Meningitis	1982	4-channel bipolar
17 (W.R.)	1924	M	1980	Hydrops	1982	4-channel bipolar
18 (S.P.)	1964	F	(prelingually deaf)	?	1982	Extracochlear, round-window niche
19 (H.F.)	1968	M	(prelingually deaf)	?	1982	Extracochlear, round-window niche

ABBREVIATION: c.g. = Common distributed intracochlear ground.

NOTE: In three cases the implant was removed: in 1979 in patient H.R. because of failure; and in V.K. in 1978 because of tinnitus and lack of motivation; and in R.B. in 1980 because sensations were too soft, and thus of not much use. F.W. underwent successful revision surgery in 1982, 616 days after initial implant surgery.

Implant Version SC 1

This implant is a complex hybrid thin-film circuit. The circuit comprises eight stimulation channels. The system uses a "common distributed intracochlear ground" (c.g.) (for electrode connection schemes, see FIGURE 2). The maximum stimulation frequency is 5 kHz, the dynamic range of the output signal is 30 dB, and the modulation scheme used is PAM/FM (combined pulse amplitude/frequency modulation).[4]

Implant Version SC 2

This implant [5] contains a tuned AM receiver circuit and an array of latching reed switches. These switches can be switched on or off by small external magnets, thus selectively connecting the electrode channels to the receiver circuit. Several or all channels can also be connected simultaneously, but then the signal in all channels is the same. This reed switch array also uses an intracochlear distributed ground.

Implant Version SC 3

In order to also try bipolar stimulation as suggested in Merzenich and White,[6] the reed switch array was slightly modified so that, with one magnet, two reed switches selecting a bipolar pair of electrode-contacts could be switched.

TABLE 2

VERSIONS OF IMPLANTS USED AS PART OF AUDITORY PROSTHESIS

Implant Version	Description	Number of Channels	Electrode Configuration	Timing between Channels
SC 1	Hybrid circuit	8	Common ground	Time multiplex with 10-kHz update rate
SC 2	Reed switch array with AM receiver	6	Common ground	One channel at a time (switchable) or several channels in parallel
SC 3	Reed switch array with AM receiver	6	Bipolar	
SC 4a	AM receivers	4	Common ground/bipolar switchable	Simultaneous independent stimulation with no restriction; 20-kHz bandwidth
SC 4b	AM receivers	4	Two monopolar, 2 bipolar	
SC 4c	AM receivers	4	Bipolar	
E	AM receiver	1	Bipolar	20-kHz bandwidth

ABBREVIATIONS: SC = scala tympani; E = extracochlear.

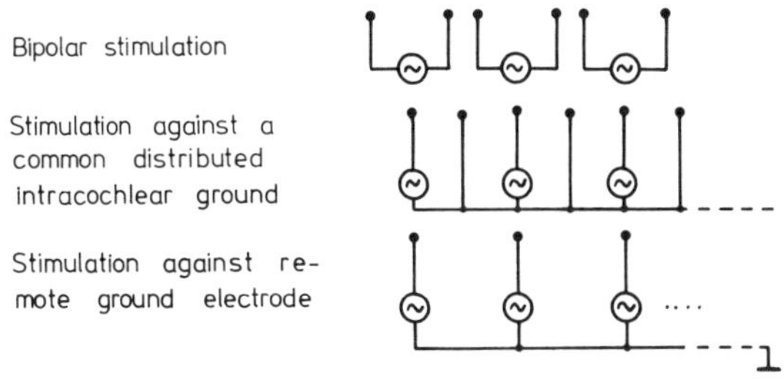

FIGURE 2. Connection schemes used with intracochlear electrodes.

Implant Version SC 4

The current version, first implanted in 1979,[1] uses a four-channel implant comprising only passive components. It consists of four AM-receivers with two different carrier frequencies arranged in two disks.

A theoretical optimization of the rf transmission via inductively coupled coils [7] allowed lateral and axial position tolerances for the ear hook antenna coil of ±8 mm and ±2 mm, respectively, at a distance of 8 mm between implanted and transmitting coil.

Despite—or because of—its simplicity, this implant imposes nearly no restrictions on the stimulation signals that can be used. The signal bandwidth is 20 kHz and the four channels can be simultaneously addressed with four different signals.

It is easy to vary the connection scheme of the electrode between bipolar, common intracochlear ground, unipolar against a remote ground, or any combination of these configurations. In four cases, three additional latching reed switches allowed switching from bipolar to common intracochlear ground stimulation in the same patient.

We have now settled on the bipolar configuration and intend to stick to the SC 4 version four-channel implant for scala tympani stimulation. We find it very useful to have a four-channel implant and to be able to select the channel that gives the best speech results to be chronically stimulated.

Only one channel is chronically activated through the patient's sound processor. In addition to that, psychophysical experiments and multichannel speech-coding experiments over four channels are performed with volunteer patients. As soon as some multichannel-coding strategy can be found that works significantly better than our single-channel strategy, the already-implanted patients will only need to get a different sound-processor; the implant can stay the same.

Implant Version E

This single-channel implant (FIG. 3) comprises an AM receiver and a pair of Pt–Ir electrodes that are intended for extracochlear placement. The ball-shaped active electrodes has been placed either on the bony promontory or in the round-window niche.

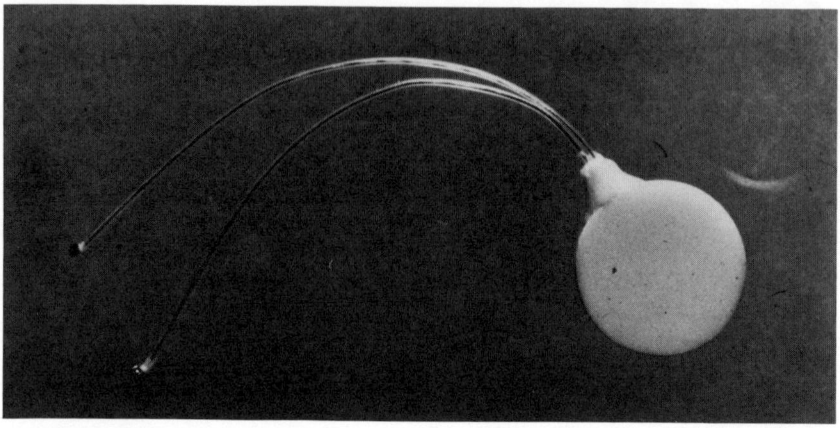

FIGURE 3. The extracochlear single-channel implant. As a prosthesis, the extracochlear implant is used in connection with the same external sound-processor as the intracochlear-electrode implant.

CHARACTERISTICS OF THE PROSTHETIC HEARING

In all patients (with scala tympani electrodes and with extracochlear electrodes) percepts described as auditory can be evoked with stimulation frequencies between 50 Hz and 2.5 kHz (the frequency range normally used in the psychophysical stimulation tests). This holds true up to 20 kHz in those few patients in whom it was tried.

Patients who received a scala tympani electrode do not experience any other than auditory sensations. There are two patients, however, who are an exception to this: F.W. and S.O. Patient S.O. experiences nystagmus (which is not accompanied by vertigo) when her channel 3 is activated. The neighboring channels do not cause any noticeable nystagmus. Patient F.W. experienced hearing sensations and vertigo when his channel 2 was activated. F.W. is the first patient we had who underwent revision surgery (a report is in preparation). He received a system similar to the one he had before. With the new scala tympani electrode that was inserted 2 mm further (approximately 20 mm total) than the first one, he experiences a twitching of his mouth at the side of the implant when channel 1 at the tip of the electrode is activated at levels that evoke hearing sensations of comfortable loudness. His other three channels evoke hearing sensations only and work well. Both patients (S.O. and F.W.) are deaf because of trauma to the head.

Psychophysical stimulation tests are performed using a computer-controlled stimulation system. From the psychophysical data collected with our patients, only those data are included here that have some impact on the adjustment of the speech-processor and represent part of the basic set of data that are now collected for every patient.

Usually the data collected are expressed in dB re 20 mV_{pp} at the input of the transmitter. Inductive coupling and transcutaneous transmission characteristics are stable enough for accurate measurements. The electrode channels are numbered such that channel 1 is at the tip of the electrode.

Range of Hearing

For most of the patients wearing an intracochlear electrode, the thresholds, as well as uncomfortable listening levels (FIG. 4), are similar with respect to their dependence upon stimulation frequency. The frequency-dependence of the stimulation current is partly compensated for by the implant. The frequency-dependence of the actual stimulation current is slightly steeper. A correction of +3 dB/octave has to be taken into account for the intracochlear-electrode implant. For the extracochlear-electrode implant, the correction is approximately +5 dB/octave for frequencies below 800 Hz. In all cases, the upper limit of the dynamic range is a true uncomfortable listening level, where the sensation gets too loud to be tolerated for more than a few seconds. There was no pain felt at this level in any case. Beyond this level (for example, when a patient turns up too high the volume control of his stimulator), some of the patients with extracochlear devices feel a stinging sensation in the throat, especially for high-frequency sounds.

The dynamic range decreases towards higher frequencies. The slope of this decrease is steeper for the patients with extracochlear electrodes (FIGS. 5 and 6). In two patients, the extracochlear active electrode was placed in a cavity drilled into the bony promontory. This site gave the smallest dynamic ranges (traces 2 and 5 in FIGURE 6).

Placement of the extracochlear active electrode in the round-window niche is preferable because it results in larger dynamic ranges, some of which (traces

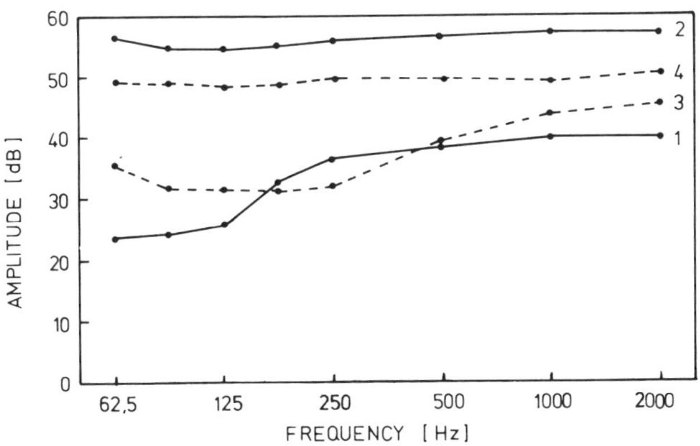

FIGURE 4. Threshold (traces 1 and 3) and uncomfortable listening level (traces 2 and 4) for a patient with an intracochlear electrode (F.W., channel 3, 176 days post revision surgery) and a patient with an extracochlear electrode (S.P., round-window niche, 22 days post operation). *Signal:* sine, 300-msec burst, 300-msec pause, 25-msec rise and fall time. *Procedure:* Threshold is determined using the Bekesy alogrithm at fixed frequency; amplitude change: 0.1 dB/sec. The first two responses are not taken into account. A mean value is computed from six upper and six lower response values. Then the patient, using a slide potentiometer, adjusts the stimulus amplitude to the uncomfortable listening level. This is done four times, and again the first value is not taken into account. The same procedure is repeated for 8 frequencies: 62.5, 88, 125, 176, 250, 500, 1000, and 2000 Hz.

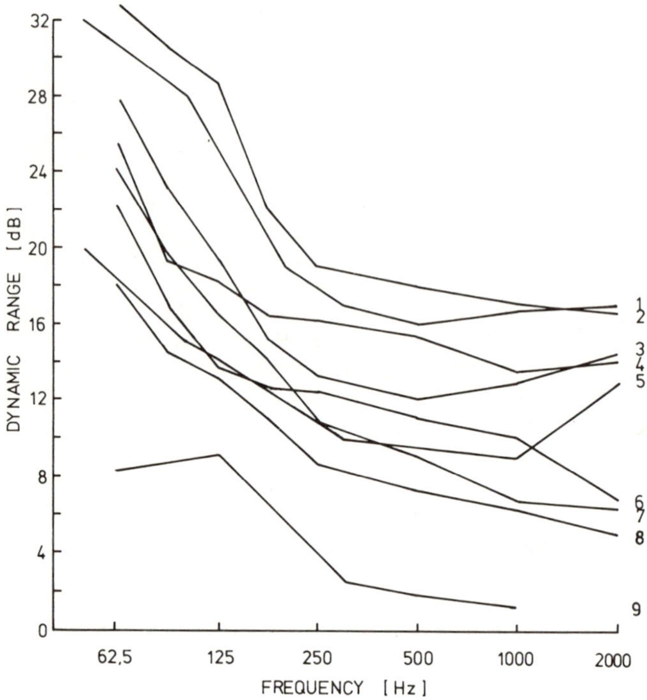

FIGURE 5. Dynamic ranges versus stimulation frequency for patients with intracochlear electrodes. 1 = patient S.S., channel 2, 648 days post operation; 2 = patient F.W., channel 3, 180 days post revision; 3 = F.W., channel 2, 179 days post revision; 4 = S.S., channel 2, 731 days post operation; 5 = F.W., channel 4, 93 days post revision; 6 = W.R., channel 3, 22 days post operation; 7 = S.O., channel 3, 464 days post operation; 8 = S.O., channel 4, 463 days post operation; 9 = W.T., channel 3, 36 days post operation. For stimulus and procedure, see FIGURE 4.

1 and 3 in FIGURE 5) are comparable to the majority of dynamic ranges of the scala tympani electrode in the midfrequency range.

Amplitude Discrimination

With a number of patients, the smallest detectable amplitude difference (amplitude difference limen) has been measured. TABLE 3 summarizes values taken at most comfortable loudness. Amplitude DLs expressed in dB are, in many cases, considerably smaller than they are for normal subjects. When expressed as a percentage of measured dynamic range, the amplitude discrimination in most of our cochlear prosthesis wearers turns out to be comparable to that of normal subjects.

Gap Detection

The ability to detect short gaps within noise-bursts has been measured with a number of patients (FIG. 7). Some results for patients with intracochlear electrodes almost fall into the 3- to 6-msec range obtained for normal subjects,[9] and some are considerably worse.

Pitch Perception and Frequency Discrimination

These factors represent difficulties for patients with a cochlear prosthesis, as has been reported before by all investigators who have looked into these problems. Several characteristics of pitch perception by the patient with a cochlear prosthesis have been described by Hochmair-Desoyer *et al.*[2]

FIGURE 8 contains pitch scalings of two patients. Some of our patients show an increase in subjective pitch when stimulation frequency decreases in the

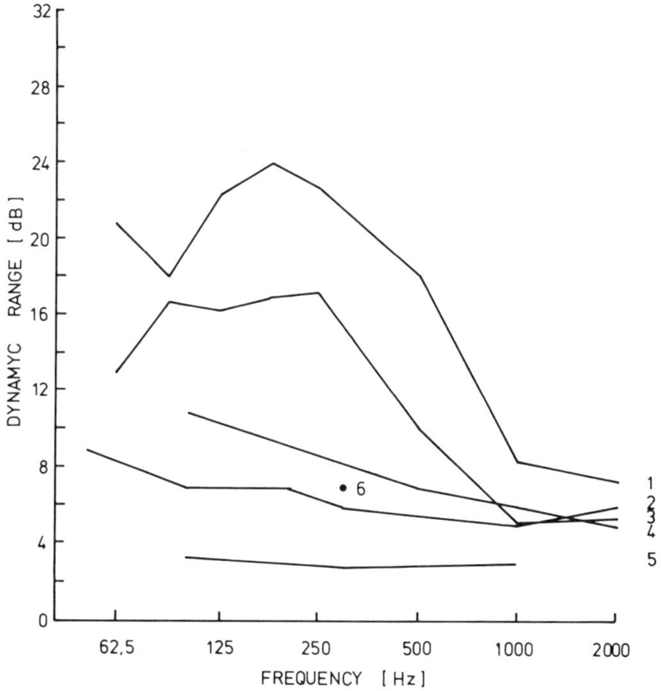

FIGURE 6. Dynamic ranges versus stimulation frequency for patients with extracochlear electrodes. 1 = H.F., round window, 10 days post operation; 2 = G.W., promontory, 35 days post operation; 3 = S.P., round window, 22 days post operation; 4 = R.M., round window, 9 days post operation; 5 = Ch.K., promontory, 17 days post operation; 6 = E.K., round window, 287 days post operation. For stimulus and procedure, see FIGURE 4.

TABLE 3

AMPLITUDE DIFFERENCE LIMENS DETERMINED AT MOST-COMFORTABLE LOUDNESS

Patient/Channel	Days post Operation	Difference Limens %	dB	% of Dynamic Range
C.K., channel 3	692	2.0	0.18	1.6
S.S., channel 2	563	2.6	0.22	1.7
S.S., channel 3	233	2.4	0.2	1.7
F.W., channel 2	179(795)	1.4	0.12	0.9
F.W., channel 3	180(796)	1.6	0.14	0.7
F.W., channel 4	178(794)	2.1	0.18	2.5
S.O., channel 3	466	1.7	0.15	1.4
S.O., channel 4	463	0.7	0.06	0.7
W.T., channel 3	15	1.9	0.17	8.3
S.P., round window	49	9.9	0.82	5.0
H.F., round window	24	7.6	0.64	2.8

NOTE: *Stimulus:* sine, 500-msec burst, 500-msec pause, 500-msec burst, 250 Hz; rise and fall time: 25 msec. *Procedure:* PEST algorithm [8]: target probability: 75%, deviation limit 0.90, louder/softer decision with feedback. An amplitude difference limen is only included in this table when the dynamic range was determined for 250 Hz on the same day. The burst duration for the dynamic range determination was 300-msec (see FIG. 4).

frequency range below 100 Hz. Within this range, percepts are described as noises and the variance of pitch estimates is large there. The saturation onset in subjective pitch very often lies around 350 Hz, or even lower, during the first 4 to 10 weeks postoperatively. After this period, the majority of patients show pitch saturation onset around 1000 Hz. This is true not only for the one channel chronically activated via the sound processor, but most often for all the channels.

Frequency difference limens are determined for most comfortable loudness at 250 Hz and at 1000 Hz. In the pitch scalings in FIGURE 8 the frequency difference limens are included.

FIGURE 9 summarizes frequency difference limens for several patients with intracochlear or extracochlear electrodes.

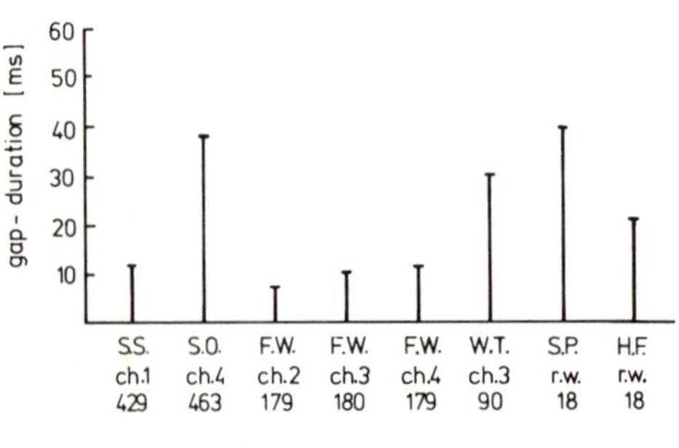

FIGURE 7. Detection of temporal gaps in noise. *Stimulus:* white noise: 16 Hz–22 kHz; burst duration: 320 msec; rise and fall time: 20 msec. 50% of the stimuli contain pauses starting 160 msec after the onset of the burst with 10-μsec fall and rise time. *Procedure:* A same/different decision for pairs of stimuli using the PEST algorithm with feedback is used.

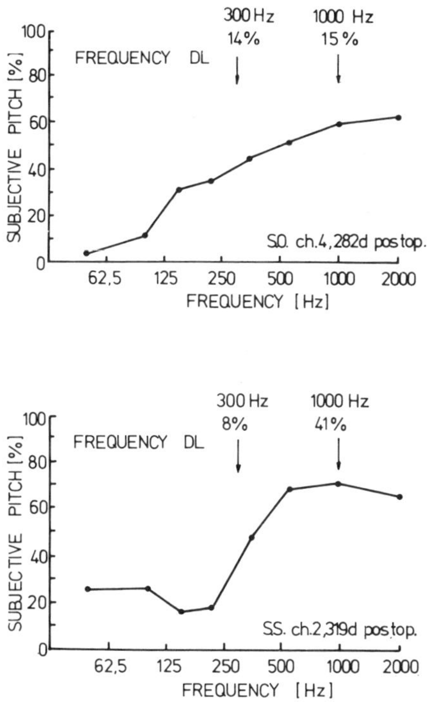

FIGURE 8. Pitch scalings for two patients. *Stimulus:* sine, burst duration: 500 msec, rise and fall time: 25 msec, all stimuli balanced in loudness. Twenty-four data points per frequency. The frequency difference limens (DL) determined at 300 Hz and at 1000 Hz are indicated. These were determined using a PEST algorithm.

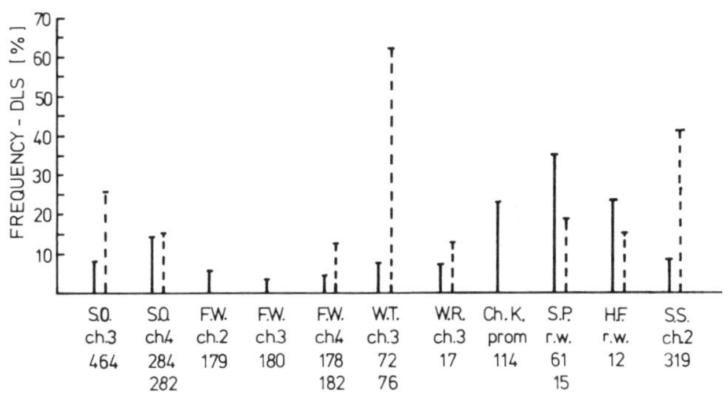

FIGURE 9. Frequency difference limens determined at 250 Hz (*solid bars*) (except for S.O. [channel 4], Ch.K., and S.S. [channel 2], where solid bars indicate values at 300 Hz) and at 1000 Hz (*dashed bars*). Data are mean values from three runs (preceded by a practice run) using PEST (target probability 75%, higher/lower decision with feedback). Loudness balance was achieved by linear interpolation of amplitudes. *Signal:* sine, 500-msec burst, 500-msec pause, 500-msec burst; rise and fall time: 25 msec. The numbers beneath the patients' initials and channel number indicate days after implant surgery (for F.W., the number gives days after revision surgery) for the value at 250 Hz, and beneath that, if determined on a different day, for the value at 1000 Hz. 250 Hz and 1000 Hz are not the center frequency, but the higher frequency for the frequency difference limen determination.

Summary

This report includes psychophysical data on some of the 13 patients who have been equipped with intracochlear electrodes and the 6 patients who have received an extracochlear electrode. Thresholds and uncomfortable listening levels versus frequency, amplitude difference limens, and gap detection in noise and frequency difference limens have been determined and represent some essential characteristics of prosthetic hearing.

References

1. Hochmair-Desoyer, I. J., E. S. Hochmair, R. E. Fischer & K. Burian. 1980. Cochlear prostheses in use: Recent psycho-physical data and speech comprehension results. Arch. Otorhinolaryngol. **229:** 81–98.
2. Hochmair-Desoyer, I. J., E. S. Hochmair & K. Burian. 1981. Four years of experience with cochlear prostheses: A review. Med. Progr. Technol. **8:** 107–119.
3. Hochmair-Desoyer, I. J. & E. S. Hochmair. 1980. An eight-channel scala tympani electrode for auditory prostheses. IEEE Trans. Biomed. Eng. BME-**27:** 44–50.
4. Hochmair, E. S. & I. J. Hochmair-Desoyer. 1981. An implanted auditory eight-channel stimulator for the deaf. Med. Biol. Eng. Comput. **19:** 141–148.
5. Hochmair, E. S., I. J. Hochmair-Desoyer & K. Burian. 1979. Un implant cochleaire a 8 canaux. Cah. ORL XIV (7):691–695.
6. Merzenich, M. M. & M. W. White. 1977. Cochlear implant: The interface problem. *In* Functional Electrical Stimulation. T. Hambrecht and B. Reswick, Eds. Marcel Dekker, Inc. New York, NY.
7. Hochmair, E. S. 1983. System of optimization for improved accuracy in transcutaneous signal and power transmission. IEEE Trans. Biomed. Eng. BME **29:** in press.
8. Taylor, M. M. & C. D. Greelman. 1967. PEST: Efficient Estimates on Probability Functions. J. Acoust. Soc. Am. **41:** 782–787.
9. Penner, M. J. 1977. Detection of temporal gaps in noise as a measure of decay of the auditory sensation. J. Acoust. Soc. Am. **61** (2): 552–557.

PART VII. CLINICAL RESULTS WITH COCHLEAR PROSTHESES

INTRODUCTORY REMARKS

T. Spillmann

Audiology Division
ENT Department
University Hospital
CH-8091 Zurich, Switzerland

When we compare the results of electrical prosthetic auditory implants achieved at different centers, we are still left with many questions. Some answers may emerge from this conference, and to that end I will just note a few ideas conceived while compiling the latest results at our center and while attending a recent cochlear implant conference in Germany.

Since the time of Volta,[1] artificial stimulation of sensory organs has been known to produce sensations of specific modality. Therefore the fact that hearing percepts can be elicited by electricity is neither a new nor an exceptional finding, let alone a therapeutic success in this last decade of otology. Rather, these hearing sensations are to be expected and only confirm an old law established in the very early days of physiological science. There is no question, then, that environmental sounds and speech can be transformed to such percepts. The field of electronics is now at the point where electrical stimuli can be safely delivered to the inner ear by surgically implanted electrodes and by careful adjustment of the electrical signal to the restricted range between hearing and the limits of discomfort.

Time has passed, and assessment of the results of more than 200 human cochlear implants should help us to answer this question: How much progress has been attained since the time of Volta?

The answer will come from study of those deaf humans with auditory electric implants who have learned to use their prostheses in many different communication situations. The total number of man-hours of use of implants may have exceeded 1 Mio., and yet the question has still not been settled as to whether these devices only provide basic cues for speech understanding and support for some prosodic speech features and recognition of environmental sounds, or whether they stimulate hearing in a manner that physiologists have failed to detect and denominate as yet. The well-known psychophysical theories (for example, critical bands or two-tone interaction) and the physiological models (such as tuning curves and PST-histograms) could not account for the efficiency with which some totally deaf persons are using the prosthesis, as shown by recent experiments in Vienna[2] or Melbourne.[3] The lack of tuning revealed by auditory nerve fiber studies in totally deaf ears[4] lets us conclude that the role of stimulation relative to the tonotopy of the normal hearing nerve might not be critical. Rather, it is the temporal structure of the stimulation that might drive a third, yet unknown, physiological mechanism that is apart from the well-known principles of periodicity and place-coding. Alternatively, the construct of periodicity has to be revised, and it must be admitted that the simultaneous stimulation of a larger group of nerve fibers by the same pulse code could be more informative than the stimulation of smaller groups of fibers each with different codes.

0077–8923/83/0405–0307 $1.75/0 © 1983, NYAS

Thus, to test all these new and unorthodox ideas, more information about persons with such implants is indispensable. Conferences such as this one can help to provide us with the results of many different tests performed at the major centers, eliminating the necessity for time-consuming experiments on every implanted person. Nevertheless, we must treat our patients as deaf persons whose hearing problem must be dealt with first, and thus we must regard them as individuals to be fitted with sensory aids, not as subjects in whom to implant cochleas for experimentation. Ethical rules exist for both selection of individuals and for postimplantation training.

Because of the great differences between individuals in our own small sample of three persons,[5] we believe that the effect of such variables such as etiology and duration of hearing loss, and linguistic proficiency, outweigh the possible effects of different electrode placements, of increasing the channel number over one, and maybe also of different coding options. The only common feature of all three persons is that they are becoming accustomed to the prosthesis and training, which makes benefits increasingly measurable with time. However, training is not a goal per se, but the appreciated consequence of the successful use of the aid. Therefore, in order not to falsify the results, training should be directed towards the person's attaining better proficiency with the implant in many communication situations, rather than towards familiarizing the patient with lists of words (possibly the same words that will be used later to establish the success of the implant in terms of discrimination scores).

To obtain comparable results between centers, a general scheme of testing might be useful (FIG. 1). We propose to give special consideration to the following contrasting test paradigms (in increasing order of redundancy):

- Parametric/nonparametric signals
- Threshold/suprathreshold stimuli
- Speech/nonspeech stimuli
- Segmental/suprasegmental speech material
- Closed/open speech presentation

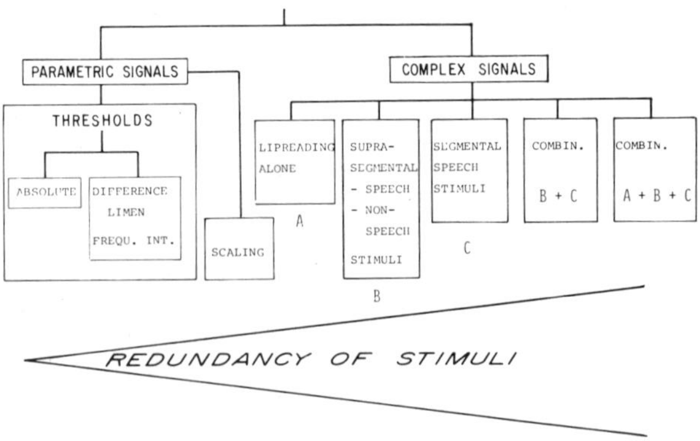

FIGURE 1. Implanted cochlear electrode testing: Overview of testing paradigms with different levels of redundancy.

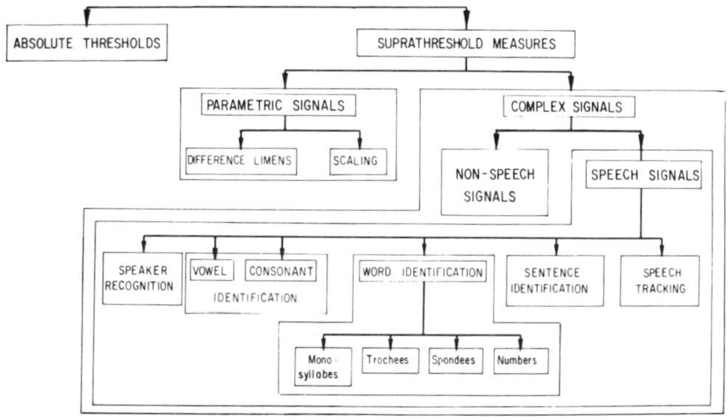

FIGURE 2. Implanted cochlear electrode testing: Tests used to evaluate perceptions with implanted electrodes.

Parametric signals (for thresholds, difference limens, scaling) should be used primarily to estimate the theoretical information capacity as expressed in terms of "just noticeable differences" (jnd's) or bits per second. These signals do not resort to a speech code and give only a coarse picture of the real-life benefit of an electronic aid. Nevertheless, such measures are badly needed since they are nearly independent of linguistic and sociocultural conditions.

The more complex the signals, the more likely they are to be supported by lipreading, and the more carefully their testing has to be watched with regard to open or closed application. Suprasegmental features, such as prosody, rhythm, and intonation, are represented by variations of the fundamental frequency which are easily dealt with by the periodicity mechanism of hearing. Our preliminary results allow us to conclude that coding of speech by the fundamental frequency is preferable, both in subjective scoring and in terms of spondee discrimination, to the coding of speech by second-formant-derived pulse sequences. This might be explained by the fact that prosody is better represented by the fundamental frequency than by formants; or it may be assumed that fundamental frequency gives more cues to the identification of consonantal segmental features than formant frequencies.

Lipreading assists in the recognition of both segmental and suprasegmental distinctions. Segmental distinctions of speech are subdivided into place and manner of articulation, and nasality and voicing contrasts. The former two features are easily obtained by visual cues, the latter two are not. Therefore, nasality and voicing contrasts are more needed from a cochlear prosthesis than place and manner contrasts.

In our opinion, the term "open discrimination" should only be used strictly. Neither the use of familiarized word lists nor the repetition of words not understood should be permitted in discrimination testing. Also, the fact that so-called "open speech discrimination" with implants is mostly achieved with familiar speakers only points to a need for tape-recorded standard speech test material in addition to the usual live testing.

FIGURE 2 illustrates a scheme adopted to test our patients with implants. By selecting different coding features, we try to get an optimal signal processing for every individual and for different types of information. Only records of monosyllables can be considered as true open testing, since familiarization, context, and limited size of spondee and number words in the lists provide many cues for recognition to the attentive examinee that can remain unnoticed by the examiner.

My final point refers to the number of individuals in whom results are reported. Results in the literature are mainly "best case" presentations. The practical advantage of implants might preferably be considered with respect to "average cases," taking into account the moderate and poor cases as well. Mean results could then be compared with the results in patients with conventional acoustic aids or communication training without use of prostheses. Realistic success figures are more informative to the prospective user than are exceptional ones and help to prevent unrealistic anticipation.

Realistic experiences and careful investigations of the expectations of the deaf person are the first steps in acquiring the comparable prosthetic results that are urgently needed now. I hope that this session will be another step towards this objective.

Summary

Reports on results of cochlear prostheses have left open many questions. More information on implanted persons is needed to counterbalance the fact of small sample size and heterogeneous makeup of the implanted patient groups. The precise use of audiological and phonetic terms in reporting on postimplantation test results could help to clarify the influence of different electrode setups, electrode locations, and coding features, and to make results comparable between different centers.

References

1. Volta, A. 1800. On the electricity excited by the mere contact of conducting substances of different kinds. Trans. Roy. Soc. Phil. **90:** 403–431.
2. Hochmair-Desoyer, I. J., E. S. Hochmair & R. E. Fischer. 1981. Four years of experience with cochlear prostheses. Med. Progr. Technol. **8:** 107–119.
3. Tong, Y. C., J. B. Millar, G. M. Clark, L. F. Martin, P. A. Busby & J. F. Patrick. 1980. Psychophysical and speech perception studies on two multiple channel cochlear implant patients. J. Laryngol. Otol. **94:** 1241–1256.
4. Evans, E. F. 1978. Peripheral auditory processing in normal and abnormal ears. Physiological considerations for attempts to compensate for auditory deficits by acoustic and electrical prostheses. Scand. Audiol. Suppl. **6:** 9–47.
5. Dillier, N., T. Spillmann & J. Güntensperger. 1983. Computerized testing of signal-encoding strategies with round-window implants. This volume.

THE EFFECTS OF SIGNAL PROCESSING BY THE HOUSE–URBAN SINGLE-CHANNEL STIMULATOR ON AUDITORY PERCEPTION ABILITIES OF PATIENTS WITH COCHLEAR IMPLANTS

Bradly J. Edgerton, Karen Jo Doyle, Judith A. Brimacombe, Michael J. Danley, and Robert J. Fretz

House Ear Institute
Los Angeles, California 90057

The House–Urban single-channel cochlear implant (CI) was first implanted in a patient in 1972 after an extensive investigation of multiple-electrode hard-wired systems in three patients. The major goal in the design of the single-channel, single-electrode system was to provide a prosthesis that was safe, had a high degree of clinical efficacy, and was biologically stable. To begin, we should consider the rationale that forms the basis for the engineering decisions which resulted in the present House–Urban CI. There are three key components of the House–Urban CI device that will be briefly reviewed: (1) bandpass filtering of the input speech spectrum; (2) amplitude modulation of a 16-kHz carrier wave; and (3) transmission of the AM signal to the implanted electrodes via a magnetic induction coil system.

The design of the input filter section is based on data collected from patients using speech and environmental sound tests, as well as subjective evaluations under everyday listening conditions. The 3-dB downpoints for the low- and high-frequency cutoffs of the filter are $\approx$ 200 and 4000 Hz, respectively. Our experience has demonstrated that lowering the low-frequency cutoff results in interference and annoyance due to environmental sound with no improvement in speech discrimination or environmental sound recognition. Increasing the high-frequency cutoff above 4 kHz also does not improve performance with this CI system.

The amplitude-modulated high-frequency carrier system was originally selected because (1) it was believed that there would be negligible net DC; (2) it allowed efficient energy transfer across the skin via the induction coils; and (3) it allowed frequency coding over the entire speech spectrum with little effect from the induction coil transfer characteristics. The decision to use a 16-kHz carrier signal was based primarily on threshold considerations and patient preference.

A magnetic induction system was designed for transmitting signals from the processor to the implanted electrodes since it was believed that to be useful as a long-term clinical device, that is, to avoid tissue reaction and rejection, the conncction should not protrude through the skin. It was also felt that by keeping the implanted device as simple as possible, with a minimum of implanted electronic components, the chance of internal device failure would be substantially reduced. From the standpoint of safety and clinical efficacy these bioengineering decisions have stood the test of time.

0077–8923/83/0405–0311 $1.75/0

The Processor

We will now trace a signal as it moves from the microphone, through the processor, to the implanted coil (Fig. 1). An electret microphone with a standard operational amplifier circuit, followed by the bandpass filter, shapes the analog spectrum. Recall that at moderate input levels the frequency response of the input stage of the processor is relatively flat over the 200 to 4000 Hz range.

From the output of the filter section, the signal is routed to a "modulator control" and then to a 16-kHz amplitude modulator. The "modulator control" serves to vary the sensitivity of the device. That is, it allows the patients to increase or decrease the signal level entering the modulator. Increased sensitivity is usually obtained at the cost of increased background noise.

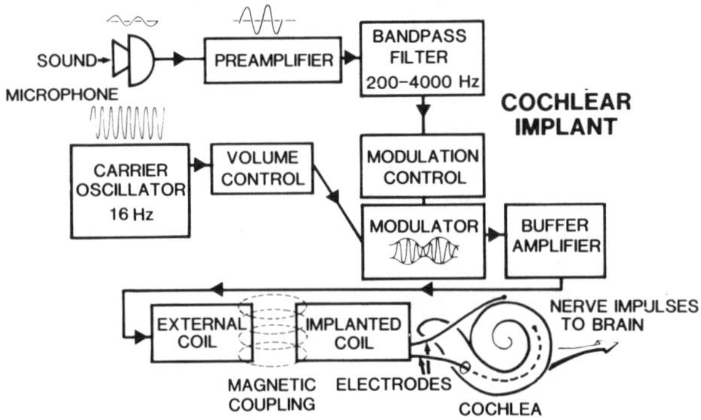

Figure 1. Block diagram of the House–Urban single-channel cochlear implant system.

After leaving the modulator control, the signal enters the modulator. At this stage the 16-kHz ($\pm$1.5 kHz) signal (generated by a free-running multivibrator) is amplitude-modulated using a voltage divider network with a field effect transistor (FET). When the auditory signal enters the modulator, it changes the resistance of the FET, which then varies the amplitude of the 16-kHz carrier. The modulator is highly nonlinear; the nonlinearity of the modulator is shown in Figure 2. In this figure the voltage amplitude at the external coil (appropriately loaded) is plotted as a function of sound pressure level at the microphone. The shape of this curve can be varied by the patient using the volume and modulation controls and by the audiologist using controls inside the stimulator. In Figure 2, three distinct regions in the function can be identified. The first region (A) occurs when input levels are less than about 45 dB SPL, usually below threshold. In the region between 45 and 65 db SPL input (B), the unit output increases dramatically with small changes in input level. The third region (C) occurs for input signals greater than 65 dB SPL. In this region the peak amplitude does not increase beyond the clipping level, but there is a slight increase in the duty cycle of the 16-kHz burst.

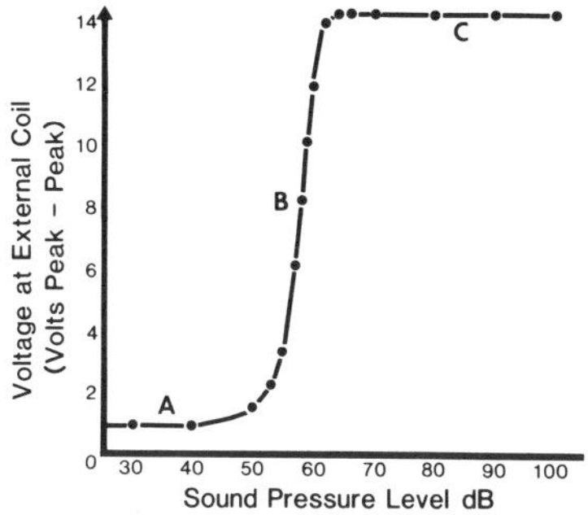

FIGURE 2. Input–output function for the House–Urban CI stimulator. Input is a 1-kHz sinewave at sound-pressure levels from 30 to 100 dB. Output is in peak-to-peak volts at the external coil.

Following the modulator is a buffer amplifier, which drives the external coil with an amplified version of the modulator output. The patients' volume control functionally varies the gain of this buffer amplifier. The buffer drives the coil differentially. In general, driving the coil differentially allows a maximum of 36 volts peak-to-peak (p–p) to be generated across the external coil, using two 9-volt batteries as a power source.[1]

FIGURE 3 presents a diagrammatic summary of the input–output response of a typical CI unit with references to voltage at the external coil, estimated current at internal electrodes, and subjective loudness perceptions. It should be noted that the patients' external volume control can be used to bring signals similar to those obtained at the 70- or 80-dB input levels into a more comfortable listening range. It should also be pointed out that in the natural listening environment, sound is most likely driving the CI stimulator at levels at or above 65-dB SPL, which yields a corresponding clipped waveform.

As discussed earlier, the coupling of signals from the external processor to the implanted electrodes is achieved using an induction coil system. The ex-

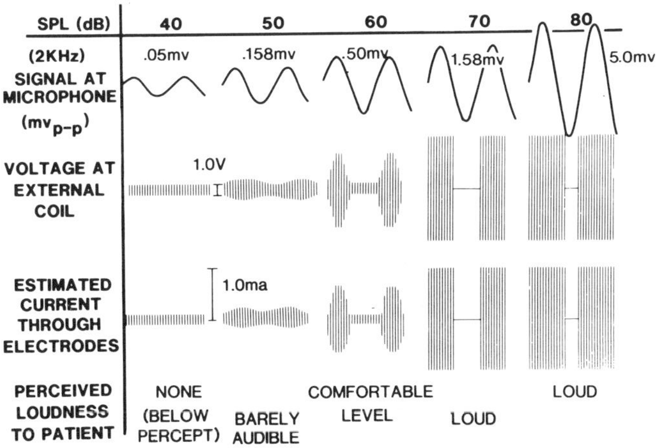

FIGURE 3. Relationships of signal intensity at the microphone to voltage at the external coil, current at the electrodes, and perceived loudness for a 2000-Hz sinusoid.

ternal and implanted coils are physically distinct and different, but electrically can be treated as parts of one transformer. The coupling coefficient is low between the coils over the normal range of skin thicknesses (3 to 6 mm). The low coupling coefficient results in the buffer amplifier seeing an external coil impedance equal only to the coil itself. Likewise, the internal impedance driving the electrode is that of the internal coil. The coupling coefficient drops off as coil separation or misalignment increases. The final step in the transmission sequence is at the electrodes. FIGURE 4 shows the electrode system and internal induction coil used with the House–Urban CI stimulator. It consists of an active electrode which is placed about 15 mm into the scala tympani and a ground electrode placed in the eustachian tube or temporalis muscle. The surface area of the intracochlear electrode is very large (0.14 cm^2 real), which greatly reduces the risk of damage due to high charge densities. At the levels of stimulus intensities typically used, the charge density will be less than 0.2 $\mu C/cm^2$ per phase.

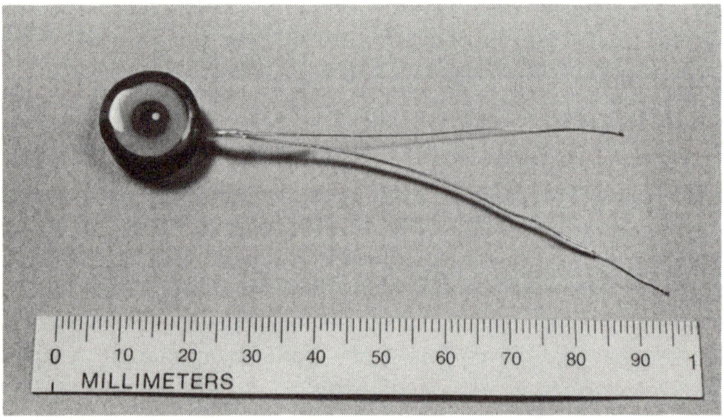

FIGURE 4. Internal electromagnetic coil with active and ground platinum electrodes.

The exact current levels at the electrodes have always been very difficult to ascertain because of the induction method of coupling the signal across the skin. Recently, however, we have developed a technique of estimating the current levels at the electrodes on the basis of: (1) a known internal–external coil separation and (2) an estimation of the electrode impedance characteristics made on the basis of hard-wired (direct access) measurements in one patient.

FIGURE 5 summarizes the process of electrode current estimation for a 16-kHz AM signal. To interpret this figure, one estimates the coil separation (for example, 4 mm), measures the voltage at the external coil and multiplies it by the corresponding ratio (150 in this case), resulting in the current estimate. This technique of current estimation was verified in a patient who was first implanted with a hard-wired system and then later with induction coils without disturbing the original scala tympani or ground electrodes. We estimate that patients report sound to be uncomfortably loud at signal (16 kHz) intensity levels less than 1000 μA rms. Conversion from current to discharge density ($\mu C/cm^2$ per phase) reveals that these levels are well under conservative damage-risk criteria.[2]

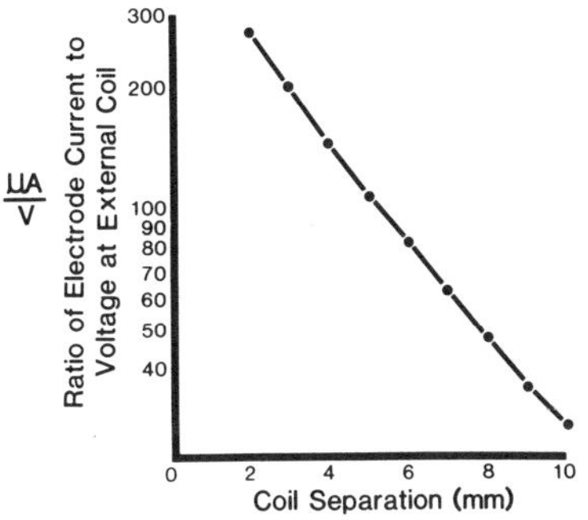

FIGURE 5. *In vitro* estimate of the ratio of electrode current to voltage at the external coil for a 16-kHz sinusoid as a function of the distance between the internal and the external coils.

AUDITORY PERCEPTUAL RESULTS

The results that are obtainable with single-channel, single-electrode cochlear implants are influenced by both the signal processing and the physiologic limitations and variations among patients. The work at the House Ear Institute [3, 4] and the results of other researchers [5–7] has revealed that patients with multiple- or single-channel implants are unable to code frequency or intensity in a normal fashion. FIGURE 6 provides a brief summary of the operating range that we have found for patients with single-channel CI devices. In FIGURE 6 the heavy dark line at the top represents the approximate loudness tolerance limit for normal listeners. The area under this line represents the discriminable space of the normal listener. From this figure it can be seen that the cochlear implant user, indicated by the box entitled "nerve operating range," is severely limited by the number and distribution of the surviving neural population as well as the physiologic response characteristics of the nerves. Note that the frequency limitation at 500 Hz is related to discrimination, not detection. That is, patients can generally detect frequencies over the entire auditory range, but have difficulty discriminating pitch beyond about 500 Hz. Because frequency resolution is very important for vowel and consonant discrimination, the results of a recent study of frequency discrimination will be presented.

In this study, six patients with cochlear implants were tested. The patients varied in terms of the etiologic factors associated with their deafness and their experience with the CI. All testing was done at a "comfortable listening level."

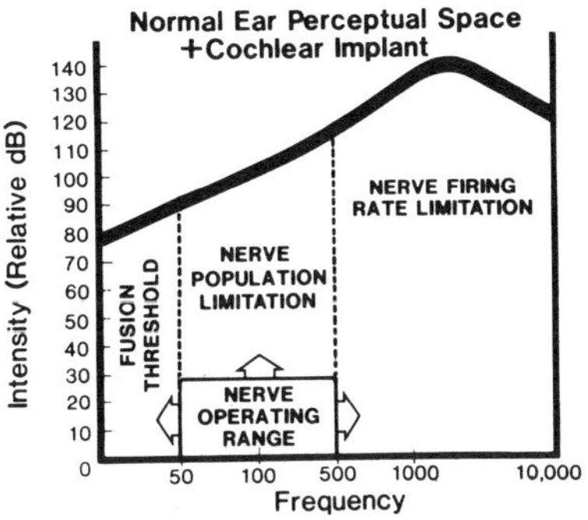

FIGURE 6. Discrimination limitations of the patient with a single-channel cochlear implant (nerve operating range) as contrasted to the perceptual space of normal-hearing listeners.

The standard and comparison tones were adjusted to equal loudness prior to the frequency limen measurement. Loudness was controlled because previous experience has demonstrated that pitch changes can occur with relatively small changes in signal intensity.[8]

Frequency difference limens were studied using analog and 16-kHz amplitude-modulated (100%) and clipped stimuli. The 16-kHz amplitude-modulated (AM) stimuli were not processed through the House-Urban CI stimulator in an effort to obtain a more standardized signal. Stimuli were presented in pairs, with the standard tone at a fixed frequency and a variable comparison tone. The standard tones were 50, 100, 200, 315, 500, and 630 Hz. The comparison tones were varied in 1-Hz steps for standards of 50, 100, 200 and 315 Hz, and 5-Hz steps for 500- and 630-Hz standards. Ascending and descending trials were used. If the distance between the comparison tone and the standard tone exceeded one octave, the test was terminated.

Patients were instructed to determine whether the pitch of the comparison tone was lower or higher than the pitch of the standard tone. The frequency limen was taken as the point at which the patients correctly responded to at least 75% of the comparison stimuli.

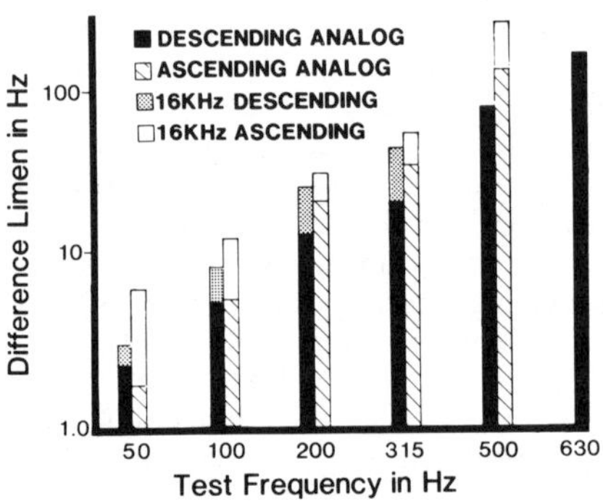

FIGURE 7. Frequency difference limens for sinusoids and amplitude-modulated and clipped stimuli at 50, 100, 200, 315, 500, and 630 Hz. Data from ascending and descending trials are presented.

FIGURE 7 presents the mean ascending and descending frequency limens for the analog and 16-kHz stimuli. In this figure, both ascending and descending frequency limens are presented, since large differences existed between them, particularly at high frequencies. Also, as the standard frequency increased, the number of patients successfully completing the task decreased. For example, at 500 Hz, only three patients could complete the analog task and only one patient could complete the 16 kHz AM task.

When both the average of the frequency limens and the number of patients successfully completing the task are considered, the analog frequency limens were better at all frequencies than the 16-kHz AM frequency limens. The analog frequency limens were within normal limits at 100 Hz and below. At 200 Hz, analog frequency limens were obtained from all patients, although they were larger than normal (> 5 Hz). Above 200 Hz, the analog frequency limens increased rapidly, and not all patients could complete the task. For the 16-kHz AM stimuli, the frequency limens were slightly poorer than normal, even at the very low frequencies. At 200 Hz and above, not all patients could complete the task. It should be noted that all of the preceding data are pooled across subjects. For one patient, frequency limens were consistently better for the 16-kHz AM stimuli than for the analog, and for another patient, there was no appreciable difference in frequency limens between the two stimuli. We are currently doing a more extensive evaluation of frequency discrimination using a variety of stimuli and the House–Urban CI system. In the future we will attempt to relate these findings directly to speech perception results.

Given the basic limitations of single-channel cochlear implants, there has been a great deal of clinical benefit obtained by patients using the House–Urban CI system. To date, however, cochlear implant patients have been unable to process conversational speech using only audition. Little is known regarding the perceptual features of speech that are retrieved by CI patients. At the House Ear Institute, we are interested in determining whether certain features of consonant phonemes are salient for single-electrode CI patients. By determining the perceptual feature systems of cochlear implant users and by correlating these features with known CI signal processing characteristics, we may be able to determine the effects of the House–Urban single-channel processor on speech perception.

At present, a series of studies are underway to investigate the consonant perceptions of cochlear implant patients using a paired-comparison interval-scaling task and the Symmetric Individual Differences Scaling Analysis (SINDSCAL) technique. SINDSCAL takes input matrices and determines by an iterative least-squares procedure the stimulus coordinates that account for the maximum variances in the patients' dissimilarity data. The analysis yields individual and group stimulus spaces which demonstrate the dimensions in which the patients perceive the stimuli. For this preliminary study, test stimuli were consonant–vowel (CV) combinations consisting of six sonorants (/w, l, r, j, m, n/), six stops (/b, p, d, t, g, k/) and six fricatives (/v, f, ð, s, ʃ, z/, followed by the vowel /a/. Analog recordings of a midwestern American male producing four repetitions of each CV were digitized and stored in computer files, and one representative production of each CV was chosen for the stimulus tape. The vowel portion of each CV was edited so as to keep vowel duration constant (240 msec). Each CV was paired with every other CV in the set, plus itself, six times, for a total of 1026 pairs.

Four patients with cochlear implants were instructed to listen to each stimulus pair and to rate the degree of dissimilarity of the stimuli on a 7-point scale. The scale was anchored such that 1 was used when the stimuli were perceived to be very similar and 7 when they were very dissimilar. The test stimuli were presented at a level of 70 dB SPL with the individual patient stimulators adjusted to "typical" comfortable listening settings.

The patients' data were analyzed individually and also pooled for group analysis. Dissimilarity judgments were converted to 18×18 lower-half dissimilarity matrices and submitted to the multidimensional scaling program SINDSCAL. The solutions were interpreted and labeled by the experimenters according to perceptual features such as voicing, manner, and place of articulation as well as the acoustic correlates of these features.

TABLE 1 shows feature interpretations of SINDSCAL dimensions for the pooled cochlear implant matrices. Four dimensions were interpretable: the features of sonorancy, frication, plosion (stop), and duration. Frequency-related features such as sibilancy and place of articulation were not salient to this group as they are to normal-hearing listeners. In TABLE 2 the dimensions that were retrieved for our best patient are presented. This is the only patient

TABLE 1

FEATURES INTERPRETED FOR SINDSCAL DIMENSIONS FOR FOUR CI PATIENTS [a]

	Features
Dimension 1	Sonorant
Dimension 2	Duration
Dimension 3	Stop/continuant
Dimension 4	Fricative +/t/, sonorant, stop—/t/

[a] Data pooled; most-interpretable solutions only. Sixty-five percent of the total variance was accounted for.

that yielded four interpretable dimensions (the other three patients provided only three).

FIGURES 8 and 9 give examples of the dimensions provided by the output of program SINDSCAL for the dissimilarity matrices of our best patient. FIGURE 9 shows dimension 1 (D1) versus D4. The D1, on the horizontal axis, separates the stop consonants /p, t, k, b, d, g/ from the nasal and continuant consonants. On the vertical axis, D4, the voiceless consonants plus one error /b/ are divided from the voiced consonants. In FIGURE 9, D2 on the horizontal axis divides the sonorants /m, n, w, r, l, j/ plus one error /t/ from the obstruent consonants. Along the vertical axis, D3 separates those consonants having the longest measured durations /ð, z, ð, v/ from the remainder of the stimuli.

To further understand the relationship of the perceptual dimensions that were retrieved in the SINDSCAL analysis to the actual processed signals, we have begun an extensive electric analysis of the CV stimuli used in this study. At the present time the Interactive Laboratory Systems (ILS) analysis package is being used to examine the waveforms. As a representative sample of the type of analysis underway we have selected the CVs/ma/,/ʃa/, and /pa/ for discussion; recall from FIGURES 8 and 9 that these stimuli were perceptually dissimilar. In the FIGURES 10 through 13, unprocessed (*top*) and processed (*bottom*) waveforms are presented. The sampling rate was 20 kHz for the analog stimuli and 40 kHz for the processed stimuli. The waveforms are displayed over the same time period; however, because of the increased sampling

TABLE 2

FEATURES INTERPRETED FOR SINDSCAL DIMENSIONS FOR ONE PATIENT'S MOST-INTERPRETABLE SOLUTION [a]

	Features
Dimension 1	Stop/continuant
Dimension 2	Sonorant +/t/
Dimension 3	Duration
Dimension 4	Voiced/voiceless +/b/

[a] Sixty-six percent of the total variance was accounted for by this solution.

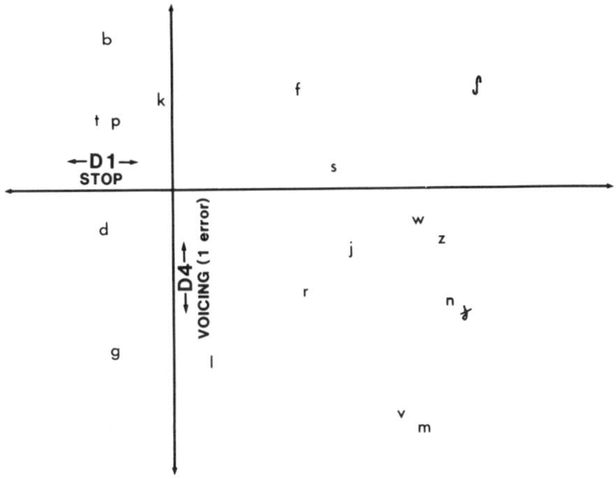

FIGURE 8. Dimension 1 versus dimension 4 for the four-dimensional solution, using our best patient's perceptual data.

rate necessary for analyzing the processed stimuli, they have more data points per unit time. The input amplitude of the analog and AM-modulated signals was equal to or less than 8 volts p–p to avoid oversaturation of the analog to digital converter.

In FIGURE 10 the waveform for the CV /ma/ is presented; the analog in the upper portion and the processed in the lower portion. Although the envelope of the analog stimulus varies from 0 V to 8 V, the processor is driven into saturation with inputs on the order of 2 V and is thus unable to duplicate the envelope, except at the initial portion of the phoneme /m/. Although the dis-

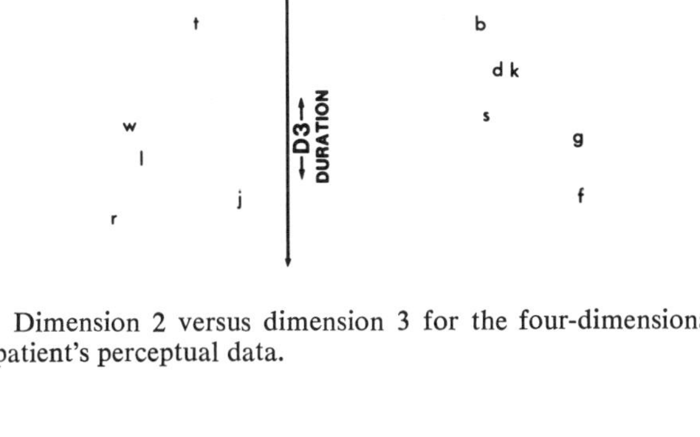

FIGURE 9. Dimension 2 versus dimension 3 for the four-dimensional solution, using our best patient's perceptual data.

play does not clearly indicate that the processor follows the periodicity of the vowel portion of the syllable, FIGURE 12 (to be discussed later) suggests that it does. It can be seen in FIGURE 10 that the low-frequency, low-intensity periodic waveform of the consonant /m/ is followed by the processor. The articulatory features of sonorancy and nasality, which have such low-frequency periodicity, as their acoustic correlates, were shown in the perceptual portion of the experiment to be salient to our patients. The ability of the processor to code low-frequency periodic waveforms with low-frequency bursts may explain the perceptual results obtained.

FIGURE 11 shows the processed and unprocessed versions of /ʃa/. As in the previous example, the processor is unable to follow the envelope of the stimulus except at the very low-amplitude portions of the consonant /ʃ/. In the analog portion of this figure, the characteristic turbulence or noisy source present in fricatives such as /ʃ/ is seen. The resolution in this slide, however,

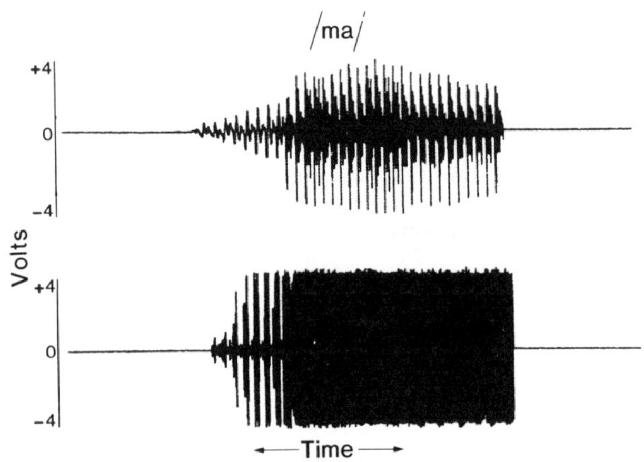

FIGURE 10. Analog (*top*) and processed (*bottom*) time–intensity envelope for /ma/.

does not provide sufficient detail for us to determine whether the processor differentiates the noise source from the periodic source in the vowel /a/. In FIGURE 12, 8 milliseconds of the original sample is provided for detail, showing the end of the consonant /ʃ/ and the first five periods of the vowel /a/. The greater resolution in the slide reveals that the AM processor decodes the random noise in the consonant /ʃ/ differently from the way in which it decodes the periodic pulses of the vowel. That is, there is distinct periodicity in the vocalic portion of the CV, which roughly corresponds to the envelope peaks of the vowel. In the perceptual portion of the study, frication was found to be a salient feature for our patients. The fact that speech stimuli that have a noise source are processed differently from periodic speech stimuli by the 16-kHz AM system supports this perceptual finding.

In FIGURE 13 the CV /pa/ is presented. We can see that during the time after the release of the burst there is a corresponding period of reduced activity in the processed signal; the amplitude of the modulated signal is reduced nearly to the base carrier level. It can also be seen, as with /ʃa/,

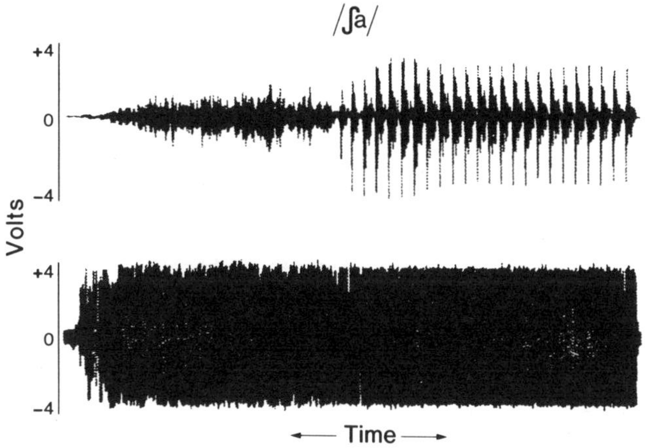

FIGURE 11. Analog (*top*) and processed (*bottom*) time–intensity envelope for envelope for /ʃa/.

that the noise-burst after the stop release is coded as noise by the processor. Consistent with the other stimuli, only the lowest-amplitude portion of the analog signal is not driven into clipping by the processor. Recall from the perceptual study that the feature stop versus continuant was salient for this group of patients.

From the preceding brief review it can be seen that through the House–Urban cochlear implant there are definite temporal-intensity patterns that correlate with the original analog waveform and may be used by CI patients in speech-perception tasks. However, additional pilot experiments using consonant and vowel identification tasks have revealed that patients using the

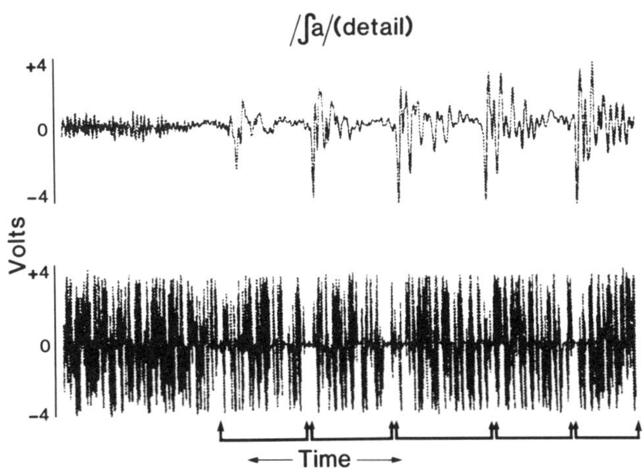

FIGURE 12. Analog (*top*) and processed (*bottom*) time–intensity envelope for 8 msec of /ʃa/. This sample includes random noise from /ʃ/ and five periods of /a/.

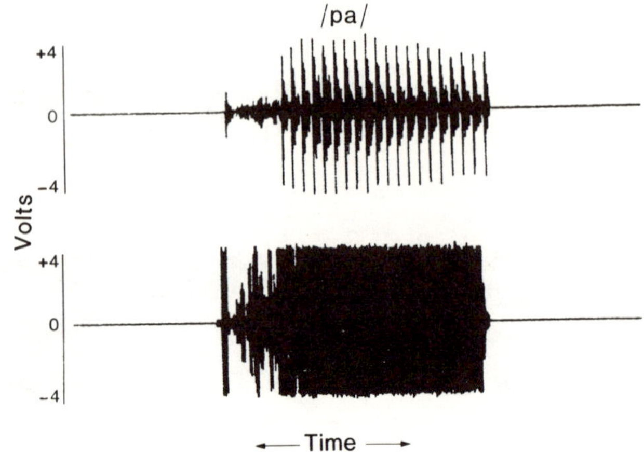

FIGURE 13. Analog (*top*) and processed (*bottom*) time–intensity envelope for /pa/.

House–Urban CI cannot identify speech stimuli presented in an open set with any high degree of accuracy. Apparently the features of voicing and the manner of articulation that were recovered from the paired-comparison interval-scaling experiment reported herein are not sufficient for consonant identification. To achieve consonant identification we will have to code the frequency-related information that correlates with the perceptual feature, place of articulation.

REFERENCES

1. GRAEME, J. 1973. Applications of Operational Amplifiers: Third Generation Techniques. : 50–52. McGraw-Hill. New York, NY.
2. WALSH, S. M., P. A. LEAKE-JONES, L. S. VUREK & M. M. MERZENICH. 1981. Chronic electrical stimulation with intracochlear electrodes: Electrophysiological results. Ann. Otol. Rhinol. Laryngol. (Suppl.) **82:** 27–29.
3. HOUSE, W. F., K. I. BERLINER, W. G. CRARY, *et al.* 1976. Cochlear implants. Ann. Otol. Rhinol. Laryngol. (Suppl. 27) **85:** 1–93.
4. HOUSE, W. F. & K. I. BERLINER, EDS. . 1982. Cochlear implants: Progress and perspectives. Ann. Otol. Rhinol. Laryngol. **91** (Suppl. 91): 1–124.
5. BILGER, R. C., F. O. BLACK, N. T. HOPKINSON, *et al.* 1977. Evaluation of subjects presently fitted with implanted auditory prostheses. Ann. Otol. Rhinol. Laryngol. (Suppl. 38) **86:** 1–76.
6. EDDINGTON, D. R., W. H. DOBELLE, D. E. BRACKMANN, *et al.* 1978. Auditory prostheses research with multiple channel intracochlear stimulation in man. Ann. Otol. Rhinol. Laryngol. (Suppl. 53) **87:** 1–39.
7. SIMMONS, F. B., M. G. WALKER, R. G. MATHEWS & R. L. WHITE. 1978. Percepts and discrimination by auditory nerve stimulation: A summary of results and some proposals for nerve viability evaluation. *In* Advances in Prosthetic Devices for the Deaf: A Technical Workshop. E. L. McPherson, Ed.: 271–274. National Institute for the Deaf. Rochester, NY
8. HOUSE, W. F. & B. J. EDGERTON. 1982. A multiple-electrode cochlear implant: Ann. Otol. Rhinol. Laryngol. (Suppl. 91) **91:** 104–116.

STATUS OF THE ADULTS' AND CHILDREN'S COCHLEAR IMPLANT PROGRAMS AT THE HOUSE EAR INSTITUTE

Laurie S. Eisenberg, Karen I. Berliner, William F. House, and Bradly J. Edgerton

House Ear Institute
Los Angeles, California 90057

The single-electrode cochlear implant used at the House Ear Institute (HEI), Los Angeles, California, is currently in the clinical trials phase of investigation.[1] The clinical trials program is directed towards gathering information on the safety and efficacy of the single-electrode cochlear implant. The principal investigator is William F. House, who directs the Los Angeles-based team and the coinvestigator teams located around the United States and in foreign centers. The coinvestigators enlarge the data pool as well as making the implant available closer to home for those patients who might be suitable candidates. An important result of this program is the finding that the implant procedure is clinically feasible and can be performed adequately in a variety of clinical settings. The implant program allows the clinician to offer something to the patient he or she has not been able to help in the past.

Patient Description and Status

As of March 15, 1982, 214 deaf patients have undergone surgery to receive a single-electrode cochlear implant. The surgical procedures were performed by William F. House, M.D., and 23 other otologists working as coinvestigators with the HEI cochlear implant program.

The patients ranged in age at time of implant from 3.5 to 75 years of age, with a mean age of approximately 43 years. The age at onset of profound hearing loss varied from birth to 64 years, with a mean age at onset of 30 years. The patients had experienced profound deafness for an average of 15 years prior to receiving the implant. One patient had had a profound loss for only 6 months prior to receiving the implant, while another had been profoundly deaf for almost 50 years.

Patients with a wide variety of etiologic factors have been found suitable for cochlear implantation. The most commonly occurring reasons for deafness in the patients who have had the implant are otosclerosis (21%), meningitis (18%), unknown causes (23%), and ototoxic causes (7%). The remaining cases included patients with Ménière's disease, congenital lues, trauma, and Usher's syndrome, among others.

The current status of patients with an HEI single-electrode cochlear implant is presented in Table 1. Patients have been grouped according to age at onset of profound hearing loss. Patients suffering a profound loss at or prior to age 5 have been listed as those with "early childhood" losses. The majority of patients selected for an implant have postlingual losses that occurred in at least late childhood and more often into adulthood.

0077-8923/83/0405-0323 $1.75/0 © 1983, NYAS

The implant cases have been classified with respect to how much the patients use their implants. Those who use their device on a regular basis are considered "users." Those who have chosen to use their implants only sporadically, or not at all, are termed "nonusers." Some patients cannot use their implant because the internal device has failed due to such occurrences as wire breakage or leakage of fluid into the coil. These failures can be corrected by replacing the failed coil with a new system, with the patient under a local anesthetic. Also classified as "device failure" would be patients in whom stimulation cannot occur for physiological reasons. For example, bone growth in the lower basal turn of the cochlea may be too dense to allow flow of the electric current.

Patients are categorized as "in process" if they are within the 2-month period after completion of the basic guidance rehabilitation program. The last classification is "deceased." Five patients with implants are now deceased. One died before receiving the external device, and therefore never used the implant.

TABLE 1

SINGLE-ELECTRODE COCHLEAR IMPLANT PATIENTS (MARCH 15, 1982)

	Number of Patients with:		
	Late Loss	Early Loss	Total
Users	136	28	164
Nonusers	13	7	20
In process	13	0	13
Device failure	10	2	12
Deceased	5	0	5
Total	177	37	214

As shown in TABLE 1, the vast majority of cochlear implant patients use their prosthesis regularly. Most use it all day, every day. In total, patients have received more than 900,000 hours of electrical stimulation. This is approximately 180 "person-years" of use of the implant for a 14-hour waking day. One patient has had electrical stimulation for 10 years, with daily use for 9 years—about 45,000 hours of electrical stimulation. Eight patients have each used the implant daily for 7 or more years. There has been no deterioration over time in audiological performance or electrical thresholds. Psychological and neuropsychological assessments show no evidence of organic brain damage or other psychological problems. Studies at HEI have shown that the electric current does not even seem to spread to or affect the vestibular [2] or the facial nerves.

Surgical and postoperative complications have been minimal with few measurable adverse effects. Likewise, there have been no significant adverse effects in patients after beginning use of electrical stimulation.

TABLE 2

MEAN PREOPERATIVE UNAIDED WARBLE TONE AND SPEECH DETECTION THRESHOLDS FOR 135 ADULT PATIENTS WITH COCHLEAR IMPLANTS (IN dB SPL RE: 20 μPA)

	Frequency (Hz)					
	250	500	1000	2000	3000	SDT
Mean [a]	123	122	125	127	129	120
Percentage with No Response	71%	57%	76%	84%	94%	56%

[a] Mean thresholds were calculated using 130 dB SPL when no response was obtained.

AUDIOLOGICAL RESULTS IN ADULT PATIENTS

The following results represent findings to date on 135 adult patients. The test procedures used have been described in detail in a previous publication.[3] A summary of the results is presented in the following discussion.

Preoperative audiometric tests are performed to confirm profoundness of hearing loss. TABLE 2 presents the mean unaided warble tone and speech detection thresholds (SDT) for the ear that was chosen for the implant. A large percentage of these patients had no measurable hearing at any of the frequencies tested.

Patient selection for implant surgery is dependent primarily on auditory thresholds and performance with powerful hearing aids. It should be noted that many patients with the level of loss that would be considered appropriate for an implant will not or cannot wear an aid. They may have little or no tolerance for the vibrotactile sensations accompanying used of the aid. They may experience increases in tinnitus or vertigo. They may have a temporary threshold shift, with the aid activated, that leads to loss of sensation after a short time period. Or they may require a greater power input than could be in their best interests. The level of amplification required is such that it may

TABLE 3

MEAN PREOPERATIVE WARBLE TONE (N = 73) AND SPEECH DETECTION (N = 91) THRESHOLDS FOR THE IMPLANTED EAR WITH A HEARING AID (IN dB SPL RE: 20 μPA)

	Frequency (Hz)					
	250	500	1000	2000	3000	SDT
Mean [a]	86	83	84	99	108	68
Percentage with No Response	25%	23%	40%	62%	78%	14%

[a] Mean thresholds were calculated using 120 dB SPL when no response was obtained.

TABLE 4

MEAN WARBLE TONE AND SPEECH DETECTION THRESHOLDS WITH THE COCHLEAR IMPLANT AT BASIC GUIDANCE TRAINING (N = 74) AND MOST RECENT AUDIOLOGICAL TESTING (N = 65) (IN dB SPL RE: 20 μPA)

	Frequency (Hz)					
	250	500	1000	2000	3000	SDT
Basic Guidance						
Mean	64	60	58	57	60	56
Percentage with No Response	0%	0%	0%	0%	0%	0%
Recent [a]						
Mean	61	56	56	57	59	53
Percentage with No Response	0%	0%	0%	0%	0%	0%

[a] Most recent test was an average of 2 years post implant.

actually produce further damage to the auditory system.[4,5] Preoperative thresholds on 73 patients with hearing aids (in the ear undergoing surgery) are presented in TABLE 3. Mean aided warble tone thresholds ranged from 83 to 108 dB SPL across the frequencies tested, with a large percentage of "no responses" (NR) at the limit of the audiometer at 2000 and 3000 Hz. Mean audiometric thresholds with the cochlear implant are displayed in TABLE 4. They ranged from 53–64 dB SPL across the frequencies tested. These results are consistent over time.

Auditory thresholds with an implant did not correlate significantly with any of the following: (1) age at onset of profound deafness; (2) years of profound deafness; or (3) age at time of cochlear implant. In addition, unaided warble tone thresholds and thresholds with a powerful hearing aid were not predictive of cochlear implant auditory thresholds. Etiology also does not appear to be a major factor. However, statistical analysis does show some relationship of etiology to implant performance. For example, the patients with otosclerosis tend to have better auditory thresholds with the implant at 1000 and 2000 Hz than do patients with other causes of deafness ($p \leq 0.0025$ and $p \leq 0.001$, respectively).

Speech and environmental sound discrimination scores on multiple-choice tasks have been obtained for 86 patients with the cochlear implant. Mean scores for the Monosyllable Trochee Spondee (MTS) test were 34.5% for word discrimination and 73.9% for stress discrimination. The mean Environmental Sounds test score was 55.1%. Paired-comparisons of scores from a select group of 37 patients who were tested preoperatively with hearing aids and postoperatively with the implant were statistically analyzed. This group included only those patients who were able to detect speech with a hearing aid at levels better than 70 dB SPL. Since the majority of the patients tested had aided SDTs poorer than 70 dB SPL, this group represents those patients with the best preoperative aided thresholds. TABLE 5 indicates that MTS word and stress scores, as well as Environmental Sounds test scores were all significantly better with the implant than with a hearing aid ($p \leq .001$), and were better than those attributed to chance with both prostheses.

A moderate correlation ($r = 0.44$, $p \leq 0.05$) was found between MTS stress discrimination scores with a hearing aid preoperatively in the ear to be implanted and those with the cochlear implant. The same was found for environmental sound discrimination. That is, those patients who scored higher on these measures with a hearing aid were also the highest-scoring cochlear implant patients. No relationship was found between MTS word discrimination with a hearing aid and with the implant. MTS word and stress scores were found to correlate negatively with years of profound deafness ($r = -.40$ to $-.54$, $p \leq 0.01$). That is, discrimination scores were found to be poorer as years of profound deafness increased, although the relationship was small. There was also a tendency for patients whose deafness was caused by meningitis or unknown causes to perform more poorly than did patients with ototoxic or otosclerotic deafness on discrimination tasks. However, there was considerable overlap in the distributions, and minimum and maximum scores were similar for all groups. Thus, etiology does not seem to be a major predictor of implant performance.

While the cochlear implant at this stage in its development does not provide even near-normal speech discrimination, it is of benefit to the profoundly deaf. It gives enough clues from timing and intensity information to aid in speechreading. Additionally, it allows the deaf individual to hear his/her own voice for purposes of monitoring volume and pitch. Thus, communication is enhanced, giving the subject more confidence and less reason to withdraw from social settings. With the implant, the majority of the profoundly deaf patients attain thresholds for warble tones from about 50–70 dB SPL. This enables the individual to come into contact with many sounds within the environment, and gives a greater sense of security and independence in the ability to perceive and recognize warning signals, and to use the telephone for emergency situations.

The Cochlear Implant in Children

On the basis of findings in adults using the cochlear implant, and given the greater ability of children to learn to use new information, it might be expected that the potential benefit to be gained by the child is even greater than that obtained by the adult.[6]

Table 5

A Paired Comparison of Mean Percent Correct Discrimination Scores with a Hearing Aid (HA) and the Cochlear Implant (CI)

	N	Chance	HA	CI	*t* Test
MTS word	37	8%	18.0%	33.8%	$p \leq .001$
MTS stress	37	33%	50.6%	72.4%	$p \leq .001$
Environmental sounds	32	20%	34.1%	53.3%	$p \leq .001$

Note: Chance performance is also shown.

It is consistently found that the child with a severe hearing loss (80–90 dB) who can make use of that residual hearing with a hearing aid is much more successful in acquiring oral skills than is the profoundly deaf child. The hearing-impaired child (60–80 dB) does better yet, and can often be successfully "mainstreamed" rather than educated in schools for the deaf. Even minimal auditory input can make a significant difference in language acquisition and educational success. This is why educators of the deaf feel so strongly about the necessity of fitting hearing aids on children with hearing losses at as young an age as possible, in spite of the potential risk that powerful aids may further damage residual hearing. The cochlear implant can provide auditory thresholds that would put the profoundly deaf child into the range of the hearing-impaired. This does not mean that the child was an implant would be able to discrimination sound as well as the child with better hearing who is using a hearing aid, but it certainly means that auditory input from speech and environmental sounds can be detected.

It is to be expected that children will receive the same information from the implant as the adults receive. Therefore, we can assume that they will get timing and intensity information. The importance of this information cannot be underestimated with respect to speech reception and production. Simmons [7] reports three patients with no hearing above 750 Hz, but normal hearing below that frequency. All three of the patients developed the losses prior to age 2, yet are able to communicate effectively. He attributes this to an ability to make use of rate–pitch coding during the early years. This situation is not unsimilar to that provided by the implant.

Early auditory experience may be important in developing basic concepts about sound and its meaningfulness. Some early opportunity to learn that objects produce sounds, that sounds signal an action in the environment, and therefore that sound contains meaningful information about events in the environment may be an important determinant in whether a child can later in life make effective use of auditory input. Thus, a potential benefit for children receiving implant while they are young may be a greater ability to benefit maximally from improved auditory prostheses developed later in their lives.

Finally, there is some reason to believe that stimulation of the system as early as possible may help to prevent further degeneration or in some way have a positive physiological effect.[8] Furthermore, studies on auditory deprivation indicate that absence of acoustic stimulation in early developmental years can result in the inability of the auditory neural system to reach full maturity.

To date, thirteen profoundly deaf patients under the age of 18 have been selected to undergo cochlear implant surgery as part of a pilot study at HEI.[9] The children chosen for the study were tested under headphones, with hearing aids and impedance audiometry, and auditory brainstem tests (in those under age 5), to confirm bilateral profound deafness. The children were additionally given otologic, psychological, and speech/language evaluations preoperatively.

The ages of these patients at the time of beginning stimulation ranged from 3.5 to 17 years, with a mean age of 10.1 years. Six patients were born deaf, while the other seven were deafened because of either meningitis or trauma. Eight of the 13 children utilize manual communication (sign language) as their primary means of communication, while the other five use oral means (speech and lipreading). All of the children have had some experience with high-powered amplification. Eight of the children were still wearing aids at the time of receiving the implant.

Results

Twelve of the 13 children have successfully undergone cochlear implant surgery and are receiving electrical stimulation. The one child in whom results were unsuccessful underwent surgery with no complication, but then did not respond to electrical stimulation. This child had been deaf for five years (since age 2) as a result of meningitis. Preoperative x-rays revealed extreme bone growth in the cochlea. Nevertheless, the parents decided to give the implant a try as a "last chance" for their child to hear. It should be noted that the other children whose deafness was caused by meningitis also showed some formation of bone growth, but not to the extent of this one child.

From the experience we have had with congenitally deaf adults, we know that initial reaction to the implant can be disturbing.[10] The sensation is often first perceived as "dizziness" and feelings in the chest or throat. As the signal is made a little stronger, the sensation is perceived as a feeling or vibration in the center of the forehead. With time, patients report that the vibration decreases and the sensation is perceived in the ear. This trend has also been observed in children. The congenitally deaf children have indicated that the sensation was perceived as a feeling in the forehead. Two of these young patients have noted that the sensation localized to the ear some months later. The children with acquired loss described the sensation as being in the ear.

Test results on the children as a group are consistent with those found in the adults. The mean warble tone thresholds across the frequency range fall between 59 and 64 dB SPL for the children. This is comparable to those of the adults, whose thresholds range from 57 to 64 dB SPL.

With the implant, the children have demonstrated the ability to perform specific timing and intensity differentiations, none of which could be done with hearing aids. Specifically, they can discriminate between sounds that are loud and soft, continuous and interrupted, long and short, fast and slow. They are able to count and tell differences in numbers of sounds, and then to carry this over to numbers of syllables in words and sentences. As with the adults, the children can differentiate between two and three sounds within the environment, such as a door knock versus a siren versus their name being called.

In general, all of the children's voices become much quieter and more modulated when the implant is activated. In fact, it has been this voice change that has helped us in setting the units on the very young children. Teachers and speech therapists of the children have remarked that the voices have become more relaxed and natural sounding with the implant. Practicing with speech is easier and more progressive now that the children are able to auditorily monitor their voices. Parents have observed that objects in the environment are treated with more gentleness. Some of the parents have also noted that their children seem to focus more on the faces when conversation is going on, and seem very curious about speech.

Current Status

Eleven of the twelve children are considered to be successful implant users in that they use the implant on a daily basis, approximately 8 to 10 hours a day. The one child, a 12-year old boy, currently not using the implant is the first child to have received an implant. This child had a difficult time adjusting to sound from the very beginning. He also had a history of rejecting hearing aids. Prognosis with the implant was believed to be good, because after 2 weeks he was using the implant up to 11 hours a day, and performing simple discrimination tasks. After leaving the Institute, he had great difficulty in adjusting to sound, particularly in the school setting. From his reactions to both the implant and to hearing aids in school, there is evidence that the addition of an auditory stimulus somehow interferes with his processing of other information. On the other hand, another of the children (of the same age as this first child) demonstrated a hyperactive-type behavior prior to receiving the implant. With the implant, he is more relaxed and can better focus on school activities.

Our youngest subject is a 3½-year-old child who had been deaf for 6 months (from meningitis) before receiving the implant. After being deaf for only 6 months, this child's speech had completely deteriorated. After 6 months of daily electrical stimulation with the implant, the child's speech is now much more understandable (although by no means normal), and she is talking in sentences. Like adult postlingually deaf patients, she is speechreading better with the implant, and is responding to moderate-intensity sounds from a distance of about 15 feet. She is becoming much more responsive to sound in a noisy environment. Also, similarly to the responses of the adults, this child has become more social, whereas prior to the implant she was much more socially withdrawn as a result of the sudden profound deafness.

To date, no measurable adverse effects have been observed in the children. Surgery and the postoperative period have been unremarkable. Two of the children have experienced otitis media in the ears with the implant. Both were treated with antibiotics, and the problem was resolved without any further complication.

Conclusion

Clinical experience is now considerable with the single-electrode cochlear implant. A coinvestigator program has broadened the pool of data, as well as making the implaint available closer to home for suitable patients. More than 150 patients are wearing the device on a daily basis. Auditory thresholds with the implant are such that patients can hear conversational level speech and a wide variety of sounds in the environment. Although they cannot understand speech, they can discriminate at an above-chance level on closed-set discrimination tasks.

Experience with cochlear implantation in profoundly deaf adults suggests that in deaf children the benefit to be expected far outweighs the potential risks involved. Pilot results on a small group of children receiving implants have shown that the cochlear implant is feasible for this population. Adults' and children's performances are comparable. How the implant can influence the speech and language of the child must now become the main inquiry of this long-term investigation.

References

1. Berliner, K. I. & W. F. House. 1982. The cochlear implant program: An overview. *In* Cochlear Implants: Progress and Perspectives. W. F. House and K. I. Berliner, Eds. Ann. Otol. Rhinol. Laryngol. (Suppl. 91) **91:** 11–14.

2. Eisenberg, L. S., J. R. Nelson & W. F. House. 1982. Effects of the single-electrode cochlear implant on the vestibular system of the profoundly deaf adult. *In*: House and Berliner (see Ref. 1). Ann. Otol. Rhinol. Laryngol. (Suppl. 91) **91:** 47–54.
3. Thielemeir, M. A., J. A. Brimacombe & L. S. Eisenberg. 1982. Audiological results with the cochlear implant. In: House and Berliner (see Ref. 1). Ann. Otol. Rhinol. Laryngol. (Suppl. 91) **91:** 27–34.
4. Humes, L. E. & F. H. Bess. 1981. Tutorial on the potential deterioration in hearing due to hearing aid usage. J. Speech Hear. Res. **24**(1): 3–15.
5. Rintelmann, W. F. 1976. Effects of over-amplification on hearing of children. Presented at International Symposium on Childhood Deafness, Michigan.
6. Berliner, K. I. 1982. Risk versus benefit in cochlear implantation. In: House and Berliner (see Ref. 1). Ann. Otol. Rhinol. Laryngol. (Suppl. 91) **91:** 90–98.
7. Simmons, F. B. 1974. The electrical stimulation of the acoustic nerve. *In* Proceedings of the First International Conference on Electrical Stimulation of the Acoustic Nerve as a Treatment for Profound Sensorineural Deafness in Man. M. Merzenich, R. Schindler and F. Sooy, Eds.: 123–125. University of California. San Francisco, CA.
8. Wong-Riley, M. T. T., S. M. Walsh & P. A. Leake-Jones *et al.* 1981. Maintenance of neuronal activity by electrical stimulation of unilaterally deafened cats demonstrable with the cytochrome oxidase technique. Ann. Otol. Rhinol. Laryngol. (Suppl. 82) **90:** 30–32.
9. Eisenberg, L. S. & W. F. House. 1982. Initial experience with the cochlear implant in children. In: House and Berliner (see Ref. 1). Ann. Otol. Rhinol. Laryngol. (Suppl. 91) **91:** 67–73.
10. Eisenberg, L. S. 1982. Use of the cochlear implant by the prelingually deaf. Ann. Otol. Rhinol. Laryngol. (Suppl. 91) **91:** 62–66.

CLINICAL ASPECTS OF EXTRACOCHLEAR ELECTRICAL STIMULATION

Ellis Douek,[a] A. J. Fourcin,[b] B. C. J. Moore,[c] S. Rosen,[b] J. R. Walliker,[a] S. L. Frampton,[a] D. M. Howard,[b] and E. Abberton [b]

[a] *Guy's Hearing Research Group*
Guy's Hospital
London SE1, England

[b] *University College, London*
London WC1E 6BT, England

[c] *Cambridge University*
Cambridge, England

The history of attempts to help the totally deaf by electrical stimulation of the cochlea is well known.[1-4, 8] Our own interest in this question stems from a new approach reported in 1977.[5] The principle therein is that by using single-channel electrical stimulation applied externally to the cochlea, useful speech communication may be obtained. The reasons for using an external stimulus rather than one applied by an intracochlear electrode were the following:

1. The insertion of an intracochlear electrode would inevitably damage what remained of functioning tissue in the cochlea. This must happen through tearing by the electrode, through local inflammatory reaction, and through new bone formation in the presence of a metallic foreign body. The only question was whether this damage would be severe or slight, and although at that time evidence, at least in the short term, suggested that it would be slight, it seemed reasonable to seek a noninvasive alternative.
2. All the work concerned, by ourselves as well as others, involved an associated obsolescence. Both electronic systems and biocompatible materials were obviously in the process of development. Not one prosthesis could be made without improvements suggesting themselves in the process.
3. Our own experiments [6] showed that the use of external cochlear stimulation applied either at the round window or the promontory does not appear to involve a limitation of information transfer compared with that of intracochlear procedures.
4. The fact remained that this comparability applies only to single-channel transmission. In the theory, at least, an intracochlear multiple-channel system should give a wider range of pitch information. This, however, would only be the case provided that enough neuronal elements were still viable. Histologic material from the organ of Corti of totally deaf ears was obtained during operation on the internal auditory meatus in patients in whom records of the response to electrical stimulation had been previously obtained.[7] Even though limited in number, the variation in residual structure of myelinated and unmyelinated nervous elements was such as to imply that the value of introducing many channels into a cochlea remains a hit-or-miss procedure at the present time. The procedure for the development of an extracochlear prosthesis has

followed these steps: (*a*) a temporary experimental and testing system; (*b*) a system for patients with radical mastoid cavities; (*c*) tympanopexy for patients with intact tympanic membranes.

Material and Methods

Temporary System

The incision was made somewhat distal and inferior, as compared with a stapedectomy incision, and a stainless steel ball electrode inserted into the round window niche, but not through the membrane (Fig. 1). A reference electrode was placed elsewhere. In other cases, the electrode was inserted through a needle-prick at the back of the ear and passed through a tympanotomy incision in the same manner. This procedure proved more stable and allowed

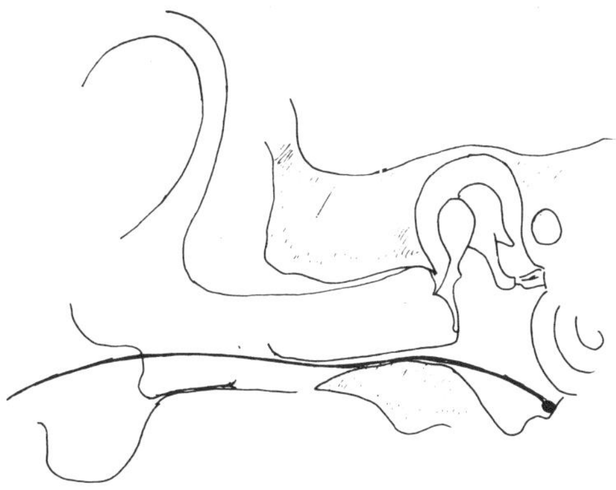

Figure 1. Diagram showing electrode placed into round-window niche through tympanotomy.

testing over a period of weeks. In some cases, a cavity was also made on the surface of the promontory that was small enough to hold the ball of the electrode without penetrating the bone (Fig. 2). (In one patient, this was done in both ears so as to present bilateral stimulation.)

Patients with Exposed Promontory ("Open") Ears

These patients were totally deaf as a result of inner-ear infection and had all had radical mastoidectomies in the past. Consequently, a tympanic membrane was not present and the promontory, covered by thick fibrous tissue, was exposed to the outside. An electrode could then be held in place on to this area without surgical intervention. This was possible in seven patients.

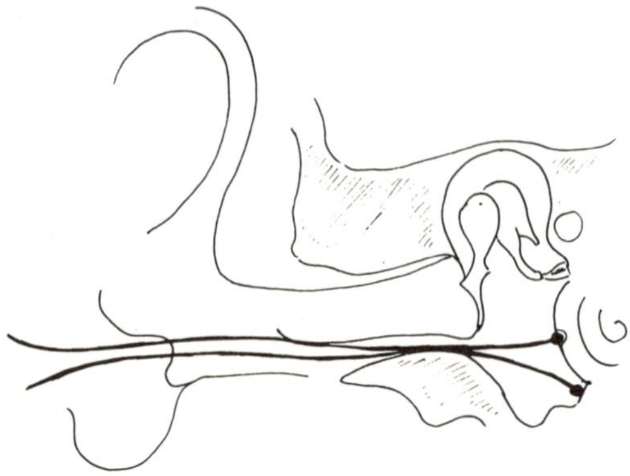

FIGURE 2. Two electrodes—one in round-window niche and one on promontory—introduced by endomeatal incision.

Tympanopexy

Stimulation in the "open" ears was successful despite the thick fibrous covering of the promontory. The fact that the patients were able to put in and take out the prosthesis as they would a hearing aid and that they could use it and complain about it at will introduced a quality so satisfying and so unexpected that we decided to extend the procedure to patients with intact tympanic membranes.

A simple operation was devised and carried out endomeatally by a distally placed tympanotomy-type incision. The handle of the malleus was detached from the tympanic membrane and excised, and the incus was also excised. The mucosa over the promontory was removed together with the tympanic plexus of nerves and the tympanic nerve of Jacobson. The tympanic membrane with its inferior cuff of meatal skin was displaced medially to adhere to the promontory (FIG. 3) and held there by proflavine cotton-wool pledgets for two weeks.

This operation was carried out in two patients, the first of whom had had an original perforation of the tympanic membrane.

The Prosthesis

The prosthesis consists of two boxes and an ear mold assembly. The first box is an acoustically driven fundamental frequency extractor wtih a microphone receiver. It triggers an infrared transmitter. These infrared light pulses, corresponding to each vocal-fold closure, reflect off the walls and ceiling of a room so that this box can be discreetly placed.

The second box is carried in the breast pocket as a body-worn hearing aid. This box contains an infrared receiver that triggers off an electrical stimulus for each infrared pulse. The on/off switch and intensity control is a simple thumb-wheel and the whole is powered by a rechargeable 9-volt battery, giving it a running time of about 16 hours. A tinsel standard hearing-aid wire conveys the electrical stimulus to stainless steel electrodes with a 1.5-mm-diameter ball.

This ball is axially sprung, and the spring assembly is embedded into an ear mold. The mold itself is plastic and gold-plated so that it acts as the other electrode. The whole appearance is still that of a rather bulky hearing aid.

Results

The purpose of this paper is only to give a brief account of the clinical aspects of this new prosthesis. The details of the response to speech are given in the paper jointly published with Fourcin *et al.*[9] Nevertheless, from the point of view of the treating surgeon, certain features should be stressed. Of all the tested patients only one, an articulate and intelligent man deaf since early childhood (from meningitis), refused the system, stating after only 3 days' testing that it did not help him. A second patient, who responded well and showed a marked improvement in communication skills, has since rejected the prosthesis, stating in a kind and complimentary letter that ". . . I suppose I had got used to a silent world." Even here, by the nature of the prosthesis, he could change his mind at will and according to circumstances. Altogether four patients are now making use of our new technique, and the remaining tested patients are enthusiastically waiting their turn.

One patient, who had been bilaterally tested but has been issued only one prosthesis, remembers the bilateral tests with pleasure and claims that the sense of depth makes a considerable difference. Another patient, wearing two gold-plated ear molds, was stimulated across the head from one side to the other, which gave quite adequate results and which opens up striking possibilities even though these results have not yet been followed up.

Marked improvment in communication skills takes place and continues to take place many weeks after the initial stimulation of these patients.

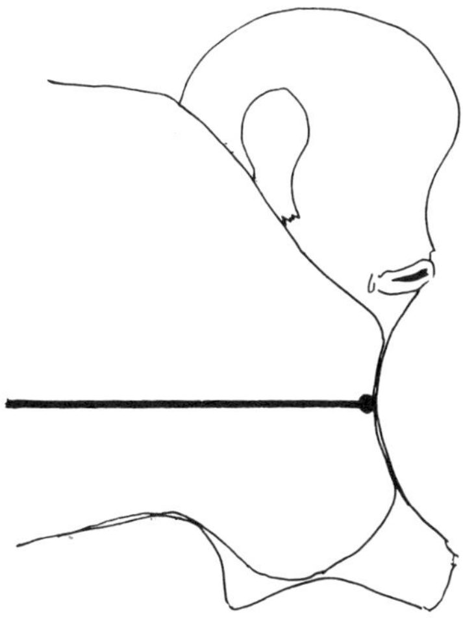

FIGURE 3. Tympanopexy showing tympanic membrane adherent to promontory with electrode placement.

Conclusions

1. There is no doubt now that electrical stimulation is of considerable advantage to the totally deaf lipreader and should be pursued.

2. The skills of communication are not limited to discrimination of words, but involve the understanding of speech as a whole, of which important features are the tone of voice and its rise and fall as well as the stressing of words and syllables. In this the effects of electrical stimulation are near-perfect.

3. The patient's own vocalization shows remarkable improvement.

4. There is no loss at all in communication skills when a totally external system is used as compared with those obtained with single-channel intracochlear stimulation.

5. The advantages of an external system that can be replaced as new developments progress are too obvious to enumerate.

References

1. Djourno, A. & C. Eyries. 1957. Prosthèse auditive par eratation électrique à distance du nerf sensoriel à l' aide d'un bobinage inclus à demeure. Presse Med. **65:** 1917.
2. Simmons, F. B. 1966. Electrical stimulation of the auditory nerve in man. Arch. Otolaryngol. **84:** 22–76.
3. Merzenich, M. M., R. P. Michelson, R. A. Schindler, C. R. Pettit & M. Reid. 1973. Neural encoding of sound sensation of the acoustic nerve. Ann. Otol. Rhinol. Laryngol. **82:** 486–503.
4. Chouard, C. H. & P. Macleoud. 1976. Implatation of multiple electrodes for rehabilitation of total deafness: Preliminary report. Laryngoscope **86:** 1743–1751.
5. Douek, E., A. M. Fourcin, B. C. J. Moore & G. P. Clarke. 1977. A new approach to the cochlear implant. Proc. Roy. Soc. Med. **70:** 379–383.
6. Fourcin, A. J., S. M. Rosen, B. C. J. Moore, E. E. Douek, G. P. Clarke, H. Dodson & L. Bannister. 1979. External electrical stimulation of the cochlea: Clinical, perceptual, psychophysical, speech-perceptual and histological findings. Br. J. Audiol. **13:** 85–107.
7. Douek, E. E., H. Dodson, L. H. Bannister, G. P. Clarke, S. M. Rosen, B. C. J. Moore & A. J. Fourcin. 1982. J. Laryngol. Otol. In press.
8. House, W. 1976. Cochlear implants. Ann. Otol. Rhinol. Laryngol. **85** (Suppl. 27).
9. Fourcin, A. J. *et al.* 1983. This volume.

AUDITORY RESULTS WITH SINGLE-CHANNEL IMPLANTS [a]

Robert C. Bilger

Department of Speech and Hearing Science
University of Illinois
Champaign, Illinois 61820

My task here is to evaluate the "auditory" perception provided to subjects fitted with single-channel cochlear implants and to contemplate the limits that such single-channel devices place on the individuals' perceptual experience. In the pursuance of this task, I will summarize briefly the "auditory" results obtained with such subjects, relying most heavily on my own work,[1] and will then try to relate these findings to current theories of auditory perception and of information processing.

From the standpoint of how the acoustic signals were coded electrically, it should be noted that we did not have experimental control of the encoding, but tested the subjects with the wearable stimulators as they used them routinely. Of the 12 subjects for whom data were obtained, 10 were patients of Dr. William F. House and used the Urban device, which amplitude modulated, nonlinearly, the signal voltage onto a 16-kHz carrier; while the other two were patients of Dr. Robin P. Michelson and used a device that delivered an analog voltage to the implanted electrode. This restriction was a condition of the contract with NINCDS under which the evaluation was conducted.[a] We were permitted, however, to conduct electroacoustic studies of the stimulators as the subjects wore them.[2]

Thus, in interpreting my remarks about psychoacoustic performance with single-channel implants, we must bear in mind that some of my results may be idiosyncratic to the coding built into the subjects' devices.

To establish a context for the summary of results to be presented here, the masking data we obtained should be dealt with first. For hearing subjects, the introduction of a second sound, the masker, either leaves the threshold for the test signal unaffected or raises threshold. The accepted explanations for masking data assume that the hearing subject is listening through a large number of auditory channels called "critical bands." If the hearing listener is forced experimentally to listen with a single critical band, then his data can best be explained in terms of intensive discrimination rather than masking.

The masking studies we conducted on subjects using single-channel cochlear implants (masking of signals at 250, 500, 1000, or 2000 Hz by a 500-Hz tone and by a white noise) gave results that can only be explained by assuming that the subjects were listening through a single "critical" band [1] (pp. 113–119). That is, the 500-Hz masker masked 250-, 500-, 1000-, and 2000-Hz signals equally well (in hearing subjects 250 Hz would not be masked at all by the 500-Hz masker). Further, the effect of our low-sensation level maskers was to improve threshold in most cases. If we must assume that the single-channel implant forces the subject to listen through a single "critical" band, then we must ask what the characteristics are of that band.

[a] Contract NO1–NS–5–2331 from the National Institute of Neurological and Communicative Disorders and Stroke.

0077–8923/83/0405–0337 $1.75/0 © 1983, NYAS

The results obtained by us [1] (pp. 105–113) and by others [3, 4] dealing with frequency discrimination are helpful in describing the band through which signals are processed. Our results are summarized in FIGURE 1, which shows ΔF as a function of frequency for each of seven implant subjects. Each letter is specific to a single subject. The crosshatched area represents expected results for naive subjects with normal hearing. As you can see, these implant subjects had essentially normal ΔFs at 125 Hz; but, as frequency of the signal increased, their ΔFs became larger and larger. (These are relative ΔFs, $\Delta F/F_c$, so that a value of 1.00 indicates a ΔF of one octave).

We can conclude that above about 500 Hz, subjects do not get information that will allow them to discriminate frequency. Further, we can conclude that the cutoff frequency of their band is somewhere between 125 and 250 Hz. The data in FIGURE 2 shed some light on the cutoff frequency. This subject had useable hearing in one ear and did frequency matching between his hearing and his electrically stimulated (an analog voltage) ear. As you can see, below about 160 Hz, this subject matched the acoustical and electrical frequencies quite well, but above 160 Hz, the matched electrical frequency becomes progressively lower.

If we accept the assumption that a single-channel implant provides a low-pass band that has a cutoff around 160 Hz and a gradual slope (3–6 dB per octave), then we must ask what can be done with this bandwidth. First, it will allow the subject to be aware of sounds at moderate levels throughout the audiometric frequencies (see Figure 1 in Bilger [1]). Second, signals that fall within that band can be scaled with respect to their intensity. That is, intensity discrimination is relatively normal for signals in or near the band (see Table 4 in Bilger [1]). Third, the frequency resolution within the band will support a

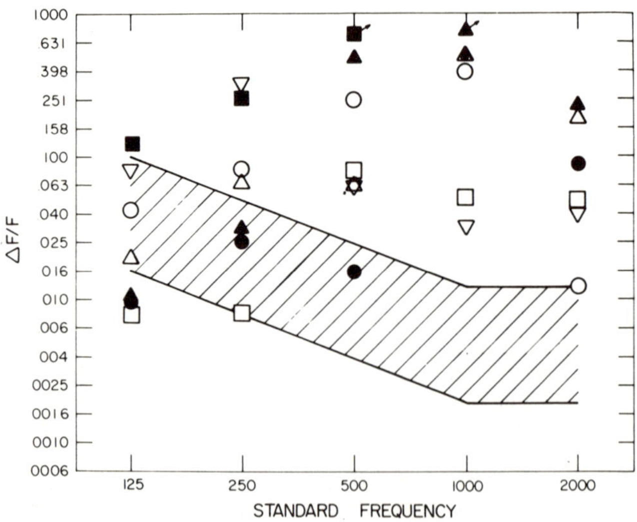

FIGURE 1. Relative frequency discrimination as a function of center frequency. The *crosshatched* area represents the range of frequency discrimination for listeners with normal hearing.

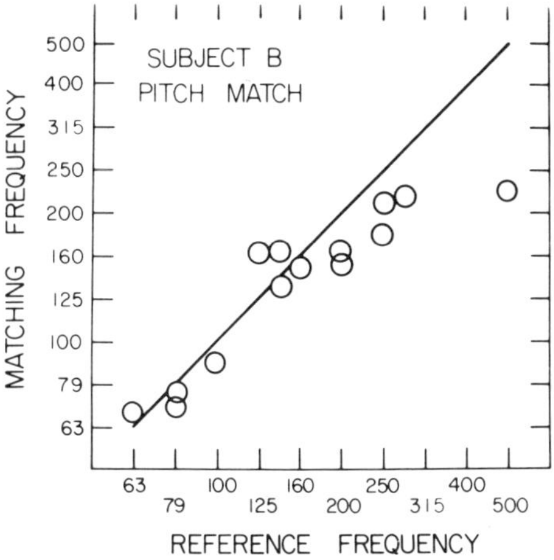

FIGURE 2. Pitch-matching data for a single subject. Subject had useable hearing in the reference ear (abscissa) and matched the reference pitch to the pitch of the electrical (analog) signal. (From Bilger.[1] Reprinted by permission.)

concept of pitch that may extend to signals slightly above 500 Hz. Fourth, the resolution of intensity will support the scaling of loudness (see Figures 3–5 in Bilger [1]). Finally, the electrical signals provided by a single-channel implant provide the subject with normal temporal discrimination, that is, the subjects can discriminate 10% changes in duration, even for signals well above the band, such as 2000 Hz (see Table 9 in Bilger [1]).

When we look at the subjects' ability to discriminate auditory and subsequent electrical patterns that vary along two of the three dimensions (frequency, intensity, and time) using nonspeech signals, the subjects fitted with single-channel implants were able to discriminate between patterns whose only differences were in the frequency of the pattern components, in the intensity of the components, in their duration, and in their rhythm. Except for intensity patterns which subjects could not discriminate when signals were outside the nominal 160-Hz low-pass band, these patterns were discriminable for even signals at 2000 Hz.

To deal adequately with discrimination of speech, we must first define discrimination of speech. Audiologists historically use the term "speech discrimination" to denote the ability to understand or label words, but discrimination should be defined generically as the ability to recognize that two things are different. In this latter context, we accumulated abundant evidence that subjects fitted with single-channel implants can make the necessary same–different discrimination when the signals are speech or speechlike sounds. This ability can be explained readily in terms of the temporal patterns of frequency and intensity into which one particular device converted speech. FIGURE 3 is taken from Wolf and Bilger [2] and illustrates three aspects of these "speech discrimination" experiments. The top line of this figure shows the electrical waveform delivered to a loudspeaker; the middle line shows the acoustic waveform delivered to the subject's stimulator; and the bottom line is the electrical waveform across the implanted electrodes (one electrode in the scala tympani and a reference electrode). The bottom lines here for /i/, /o/, and /u/ are not comparable to any aspect of the representation of speech in the nervous system of a normal-hearing listener; but these patterns are quite discriminable to the implanted listener. The listener using a single-channel implant may, under some circumstances, be able to recognize or label some *small* set of such complex stimuli. Such labeling, however, should be understood in an appropriate context.

On the basis of earlier work by Pollack, Miller [6] identified an important principle of information-processing by humans when he wrote of the "magic number seven plus or minus two." The typical human subject can label accurately between five and nine meaningless stimuli. One's digit span is an example of this limitation. (It is important to note, however, that special contexts can give special meaning to otherwise meaningless stimuli. For example, sitting in one's own living room in the evening sets a context for a variety of environmental sounds that would be meaningless in another context.) When subjects are asked to make a "same" or "different" judgment for a set of meaningless stimuli (for example, pure tones of varying frequency), their reaction times (RTs) are faster (by 40–60 msec) for a correct "different" than for a correct "same" judgment.[7] On the other hand, when subjects are asked to make a "same" or "different" judgment for meaningful stimuli (for example, printed letters), then their RTs for "same" is 40–60 msec faster than that for "different." This same–different experiment lets us know, for example, how hearing-impaired listeners are processing speech.

Reed [8] found that listeners who had difficulty in understanding speech (that is, identifying spoken words) behaved differently than normal subjects in the same–different reaction-time experiment. While her normal-hearing subjects [9] behaved in the expected manner (that is, correct "same" RTs were faster than correct "different" RTs, her moderately hearing-impaired subjects frequently responded to particular pairs of VC nonsense syllables as if they were meaningless stimuli (that is, their correct "different" RTs were faster than their correct "same" RTs). Of course, her severely impaired subjects could not even make most of the discriminations correctly.

The explanation for the reaction-time experiment is that in dealing with meaningless stimuli, the subject must process the entire waveforms that are stored in memory. As soon as there is a difference between memory traces, the subject can respond "different"; but he must process the entire memory trace before responding "same." [10] Meaningful stimuli, on the other hand, are processed differently in memory, in that "meaningfulness" means that the stimuli fall into categories established by experience and/or nature. In processing such meaningful stimuli, the subject has only to determine that two stimuli fall into the same category to respond "same" correctly; but if the stimuli are different, then the subject must search through all categories to respond "different" correctly.

The work of Plomp [11] and his associates would seem to suggest that for stimuli to sound natural and for them to be categorizable, of necessity they must enter the auditory system through several independent channels (critical bands). That is, although sounds that vary along a single dimension or are presented via a single-channel input can be categorized, this categorization is very different from the recognition and labeling of sounds generally associated with the perception of speech or music. That categorization of a single dimension is both too slow and too limited in extent to be considered a substitute for the perception of speech, which recognition derives its speed and extent from the many auditory channels devoted to it.

The great hope of those pursuing cochlear implants as a means of a rehabilitation for deafened individuals is that the patients will be able to under-

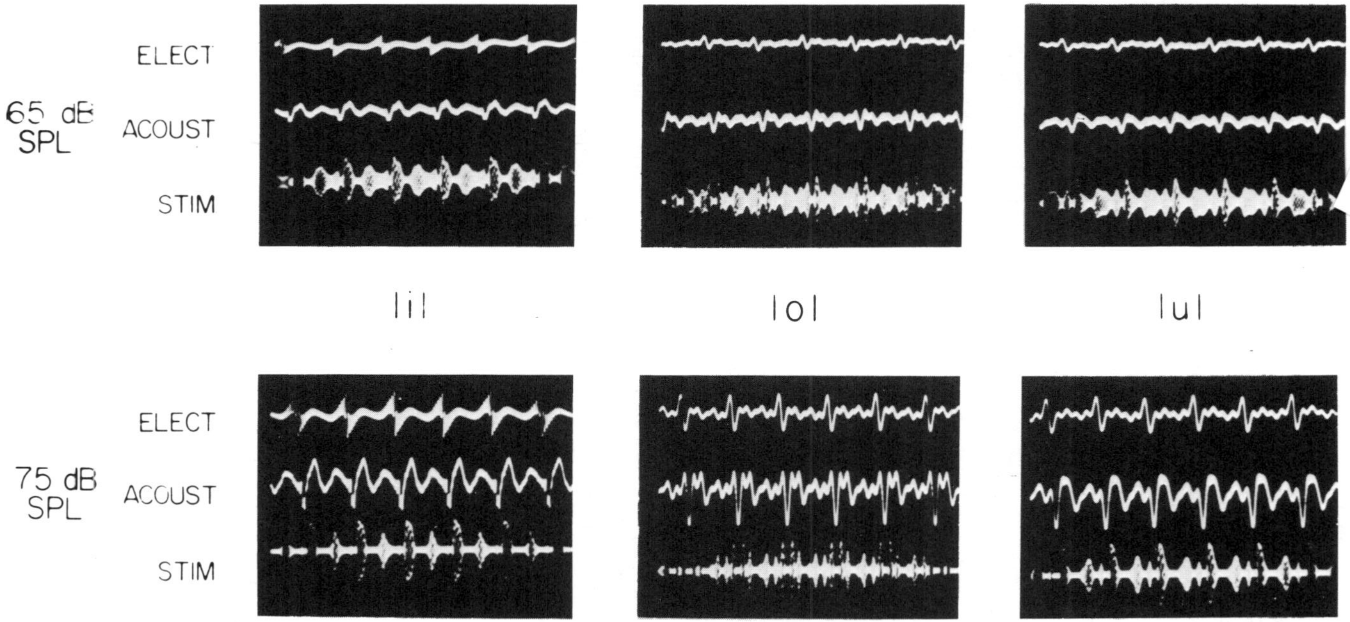

FIGURE 3. Output of amplitude-modulating stimulator for three synthetic vowels at two levels (65 and 75 dB SPL). The *top line* (ELECT) represents the electrical signal delivered to a loudspeaker; the *middle line* is the acoustic signal measured at the microphone port of the stimulator; and the *bottom line* of each row represents the voltage delivered to the implanted electrodes. (From Bilger.[1] Reprinted by permission.)

stand speech. It should be obvious to everyone that single-channel implants will not allow the wearer to understand speech on the basis of the single input channel described here. From our own work [1] it is also obvious that this single channel is of no real benefit to subjects who did not become deaf relatively late in life. That is, although the two prelingually deafened subjects whom we tested were excellent psychophysical observers, they were unable to use their implants to (a) enhance their lipreading scores, (b) improve the intelligibility of their speech, or (c) augment their ability to recognize common environmental sounds, all things that subjects deafened after the development of speech and language were able to achieve. On this basis, the trend of implanting prelingually deafened children with single-channeled prostheses should be reconsidered and alternate rehabilitative techniques pursued.

Finally, those investigators interested in multichannel implants should recognize that "meaningless" stimuli can be categorized in limited sample sets. In searching for coding schemes to achieve speech recognition (categorization) on a naturalistic basis, it behooves them to insure that their subjects are operating in the "speech mode" and not categorizing meaningless stimuli.

References

1. Bilger, R. C. 1977. Psychoacoustic evaluation of present prostheses. Ann. Otol. Rhinol. Laryngol. **86** (Suppl 38): 92–140.
2. Wolf, R. V. & R. C. Bilger. 1977. Electroacoustic measures of present prostheses. Ann. Otol. Rhinol. Laryngol. **86** (Suppl 38): 61–69).
3. Simmons, F. B., C. J. Monegeon, W. R. Lewis & D. Huntington. 1964. Electrical stimulation of the auditory nerve and inferior colliculus. Arch. Otolaryngol. **79:** 559–567.
4. Merzenich, M. M., R. P. Michelson, C. R. Petit, R. A. Schindler & M. Reid. 1973. Neural encoding of sound sensation evoked by electrical stimulation of the acoustic nerve. Ann. Otol. Rhinol. Laryngol. **82:** 483–503.
5. Pollack, I. 1952. The information of elementary auditory displays. J. Acoust. Soc. Am. **24:** 745–749.
6. Miller, G. A. 1956. The magical number seven, plus or minus two: Some limits on our capacity for processing information. Psychol. Rev. **63:** 81–97.
7. Bindra, D., D. C. Donderi & S. Nishisato. 1968. Decision latencies of "same" and "different" judgments. Percept. Psychophys. **3:** 121–130.
8. Reed, C. R. 1975. Identification and discrimination of vowel-consonant syllables in listeners with sensorineural hearing loss. J. Speech Hearing Res. **18:** 773–794.
9. Reed, C. R. 1975. Reaction times for a same–different discrimination of vowel–consonant syllables. Percept. Psychophys. **18:** 65–70.
10. Durlach, N. I. & L. D. Braida. 1969. Intensity perception. I. Preliminary theory of intensity resolution. J. Acoust. Soc. Am. **46:** 372–383.
11. Plomp, R. & A. M. Mimpen. 1968. The ear as a frequency analyzer. J. Acoust. Soc. Am. **43:** 764–767.

SURGICAL APPROACH FOR INSERTION OF MULTICHANNEL ELECTRODES INTO THE SCALA TYMPANI

Robin P. Michelson and Robert A. Schindler

Department of Otolaryngology
University of California
San Francisco, California 94143

In 1971 Michelson reported the results of electrical stimulation of the cochlea via the scala tympani. A single-channel form-fitting electrode was used.[1]

Four deaf volunteers received temporary implants through a tympanotomy approach. After a test procedure in the operating room, the electrodes were removed 6 months and 1 year later and two of these patients were implanted with a complete system with wearable devices. In both patients the round window was obliterated by new bone formation. In both patients a bony cast of the scala tympani was removed after freeing it from the margins of the round window.

The scala tympani is an ideal site for establishing electrode–tissue interface because it provides access, via the round window, to a linear display of auditory nerve fibers. Design of an optimal scala tympani electrode must allow for discrete excitation of preselected, restricted regions of auditory nerve. Additionally, the electrode must be fabricated of biocompatible materials to allow for the following requirements: (1) that the handling properties make the electrode safely implantable for sufficient distances into the scala tympani (23 to 25 mm); and (2) that the electrode be form-fitting to displace perilymph and, yet, small enough to account for variation in scala tympani size.

An electrode meeting all these requirements has been fabricated at the University of California, San Francicso (FIG. 1). The object of this report is to describe its characteristics and surgical implantation.

Due to the restricted access provided by the dimensions of the tapering scala tympani, the handling characteristics of the electrode are fundamental to successful implantation. In design of electrodes, stiffness, flexibility, and elasticity must be controlled in both the vertical and horizontal planes of the cochlear spiral. As the surgeon prepares to insert the electrode, the tip must be able to be straightened without damage to the electrode and must retain some of this straightening as the tip is positioned in the basal turn. At this point the electrode exhibits an "elastic memory," which allows the tip to curve inward as the array is gently inserted beyond the first cochlear spiral. Several observers have noted, both in cadaver temporal bones and in surgical cases, that some other electrode designs tend to veer upward as they are introduced past the first turn of the cochlea. This effect has frequently resulted either in rupture of the basilar membrane or fracture of the osseous spiral lamina at a point opposite the round window. To prevent this natural tendency to veer upward, this electrode must be stiffened in the vertical plane to reduce anterior bending while allowing full flexibility in the horizontal plane of the spiral (FIG. 2).

0077–8923/83/0405–0343 $1.75/0

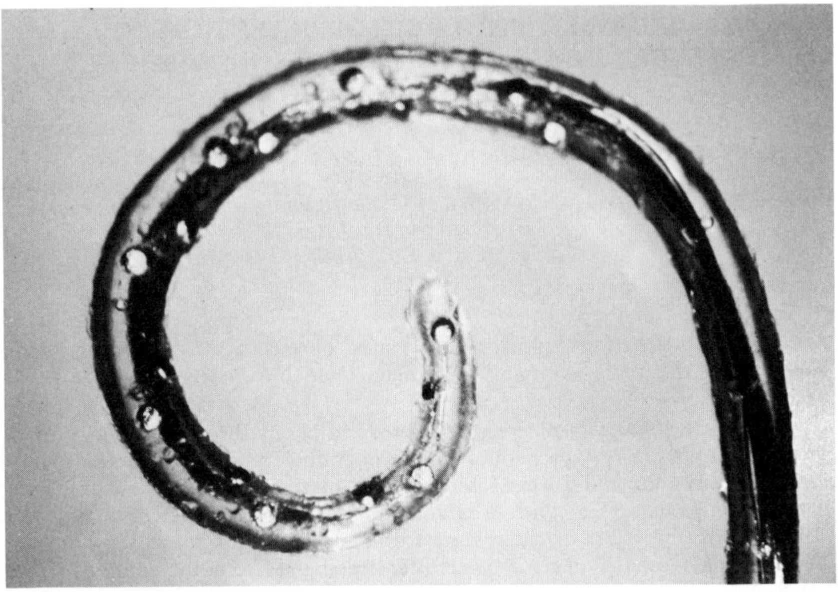

FIGURE 1. The University of California improved version of the original multichannel electrode. Note that contacts are larger and the array is slimmer, allowing insertion farther into the scala tympani than previously possible.

SURGICAL CONSIDERATIONS

However well-designed and fabricated, successful electrode implantation can only be achieved by surgeons adopting appropriate insertion strategies in the temporal bone laboratory and operating room. Initial observations must come from dissections in order to explain surgical approaches, insertion angles, and implantation forces which provide optimal chances for successful electrode placement.

The approach to the round window can be best achieved via the posterior canal wall tympanotomy. It provides a good view of the round-window niche, the round-window membrane, and basal scala tympani. The round-window niche varies considerably in normal and pathological temporal bones. It is frequently narrow and occasionally obliterated. Similar pathologic changes can occur with scala tympani. Fortunately, high-resolution CT scanning can preoperatively identify deaf patients with labyrinthitis ossificans, thereby selecting patients with a patent scala tympani. However, present high-resolution scans cannot accurately predict a narrowed scala tympani, and the implant surgeon should have alternative electrodes available to meet this challenge.

The incision used in approaching the posterior canal wall needs to be sufficiently large to cover the implanted electronic device. A large postauricular flap is elevated in continuity with a posterior tympanotomy to prevent any incision from crossing the implanted device. A groove is created in the posterior canal wall to improve exposure of the round-window niche and to seat electrode leads. A small cortical bone wedge supplemented with tissue adhesives may be used to prevent extrusion of the wires and invagination of ear-canal skin.

The round-window niche is removed with a fine diamond burr, exposing the round-window membrane. The outer wall of the basal scala tympani is removed to improve the insertion angle. Care must be taken to identify the basilar membrane and cochlear spiral. In order to prevent misapplication of a left electrode in the right ear, the surgeon must constantly maintain a visual image of the cochlear spiral. A left cochlea spirals to the right and a right cochlea spirals to the left when viewed through a posterior tympanotomy approach. When the surgeon's hand is held as though he or she is about to shake hands, the cochlea always turns in the direction of the finger of the right or left hand, respectively.

Insertion of the electrode may be assisted by gently straightening its tip. The enlargement of the round window and the basal scala tympani allows the surgeon to gain 3 to 4 mm of additional exposure of the cochlear spiral. Using plastic-coated instruments to prevent injury to the Silastic® carrier, electrode arrays may be inserted 18 to 25 mm. The tip of the electrode is controlled with a curved inserter, similar to an angled forceps. It must be placed in position near the first cochlear turn opposite the round window to prevent buckling of the flexible electrode tip. The electrode is then advanced, using a curved-forced probe and steadying the electrode with the inserter forceps.[2]

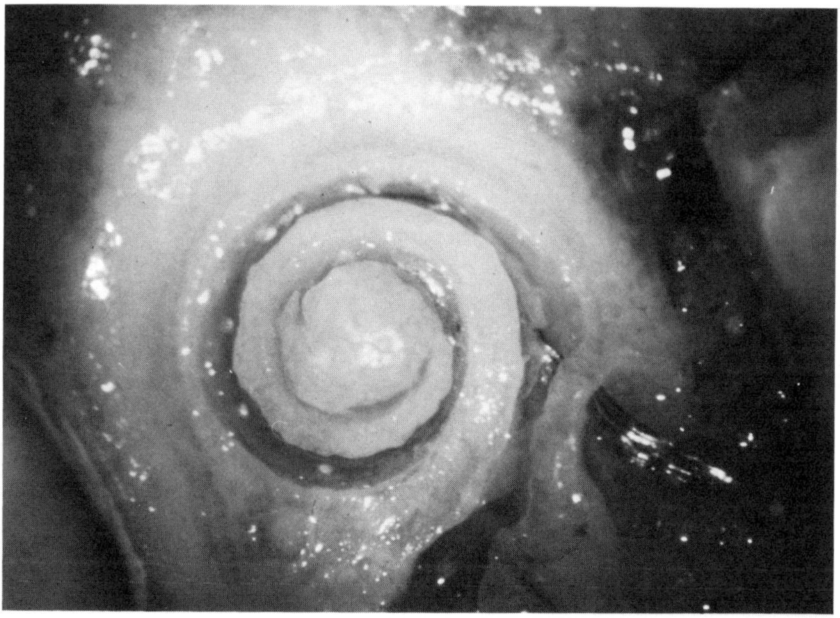

FIGURE 2. The electrode in place in a temporal bone. The array was first inserted and the dissection performed to reveal excellent placement.

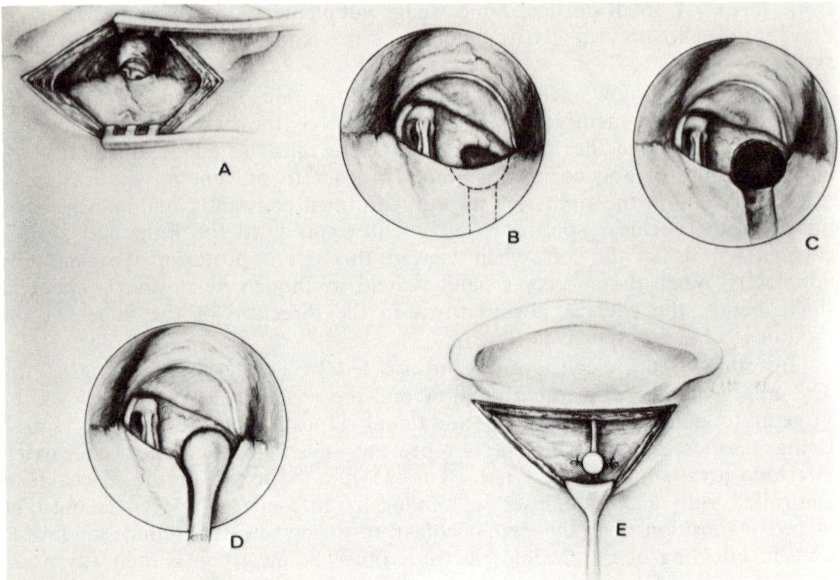

FIGURE 3. Artist's conception of the cochlear implant surgical procedure.

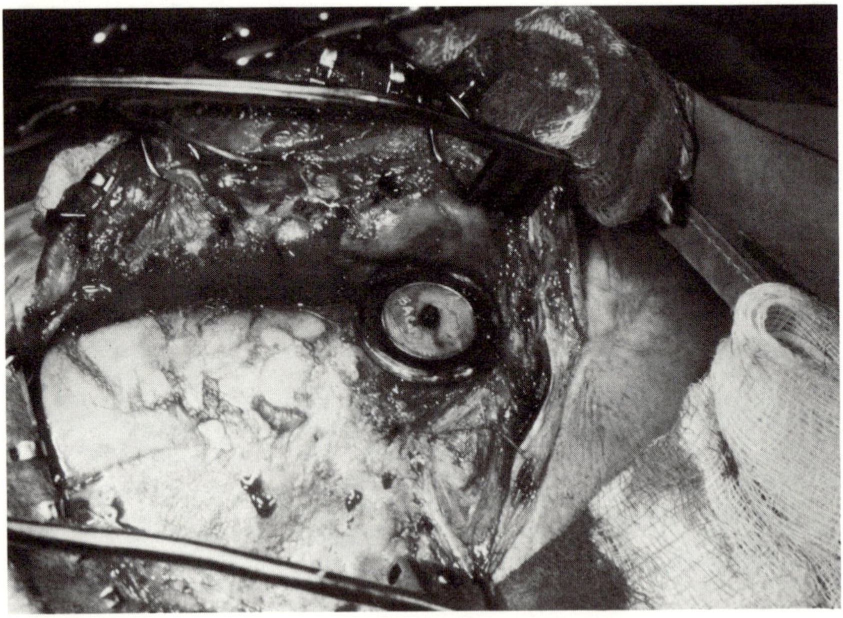

FIGURE 4. View of the UCSF device in place prior to final closure of the post-auricular skin flap.

After electrode insertion, the driving module and electrode leads are secured with tissue adhesives to the temporal bone. It should be noted that the proper orientation of the electrode and its leads can be achieved only if the driving module is free to move. One should not permanently affix the extracochlear elements of the implant until satisfactory electrode positioning is achieved. Instruments have been created to temporarily hold the driving module during electrode insertion, allowing the surgeon to more freely position the electrode (FIG. 3).[3]

Mishandling the delicately fabricated electrode will result in kinks and tears in the Silastic carrier complicated by disruption of the wire array. Wires may be broken or shorted and the basilar partition and osseous spiral lamina may be injured. Implantation of potentially multichannel cochlear electrodes requires consistent and precise placement in order to maximize the possibility of speech discrimination. Perforation of the basilar membrane and fracture of the osseous lamina, which have been noted in some single-channel implant systems, are not compatible with successful multichannel implants (FIG. 4).

CONCLUSION

The major risk of cochlear implantation is infection, either immediate or late. In totally implanted systems this complication has been minimal, but requires removal of the "foreign" body.

Transient postoperative vertigo has also resulted, but appears in our experience no worse than that associated with the commonly performed stapedectomy. Subliminal disturbance of balance is common.

Stimulation of the facial nerve has been occasionally observed under maximal stimulation levels, but is minimized with bipolar stimulation.

REFERENCES

1. MICHELSON, R. P. 1971. Electrical stimulation of the human cochlea. Arch. Otolaryngol. **93:** 317–323.
2. SCHINDLER, R. A. & B. BJORKROTH. 1979. Traumatic intracochlear electrode implantation. Laryngoscope **89:** 752–758.
3. SCHINDLER, R. A. & M. M. MERZENICH. 1974. Chronic intracochlear implantation: Cochlear pathology and acoustic nerve survival. Ann. Otol. **83:** 202–216.

FORMANT FREQUENCY DISCRIMINATION AND RECOGNITION IN SUBJECTS IMPLANTED WITH INTRACOCHLEAR STIMULATING ELECTRODES [a]

M. W. White

Coleman Laboratory
Department of Otolaryngology
University of California, San Francisco
San Francisco, California 94143

INTRODUCTION

Our group in the Coleman Laboratory has studied a subject implanted with 16 intracochlear scala tympani stimulating electrodes. A single-channel analog processor was tested. The processor consisted of a microphone, preamplifier, an instantaneous log compressor, and a linear filter, in that order. The linear filter reduced the low-frequency energy below 200 Hz and pre-emphasized the higher frequencies at about 6–12 dB/octave. Each of the two poles of the single-channel processor was attached to eight of the 16 wires of the electrode array. One pole was connected to the more medial eight electrodes and one pole was connected to the more lateral eight electrode contacts. The subject (L.Y.) was evaluated with standard speech intelligibility tests, basic psychophysical tests, and tests designed to determine what features of the speech signal were used by the subject to understand speech. The subject exhibited surprisingly good performance in understanding speech without the aid of lipreading. Without lipreading, the subject could recognize about 50% of the key words in CID (Central Institute for the Deaf) everyday sentences.[1] In a four-choice vowel-recognition task, the subject could consistently identify 50–60% of the monosyllabic words that were spoken ($n = 60$).

Experiments, reported here, were conducted to estimate which acoustic features were being utilized by this subject with a cochlear implant.

SYNTHETIC-VOWEL PAIRED COMPARISONS

Pairs of steady-state synthesized vowels were presented to the subject through an Electro-Voice E-V FIVE-C loudspeaker. The subject (L.Y.) was then asked to scale the difference between the two sounds on a scale of one ("identical") to seven ("very different"). The steady-state vowels were 300 msec in duration, with a fundamental frequency of 125 Hz. A digitally implemented, cascade speech synthesizer was implemented using infinite impulse response digital filters (FIG. 1). The formant frequencies were held constant throughout the 300-msec duration of the synthesized vowel. A 400-msec delay separated the first vowel from the second vowel in the pair.

[a] This work was supported by Grant NS–11804 and Contract NO 1–NS–7–2367 from the National Institutes of Health, and by Hearing Research, Inc., San Francisco, California.

0077–8923/83/0405–0348 $1.75/0 © 1983, NYAS

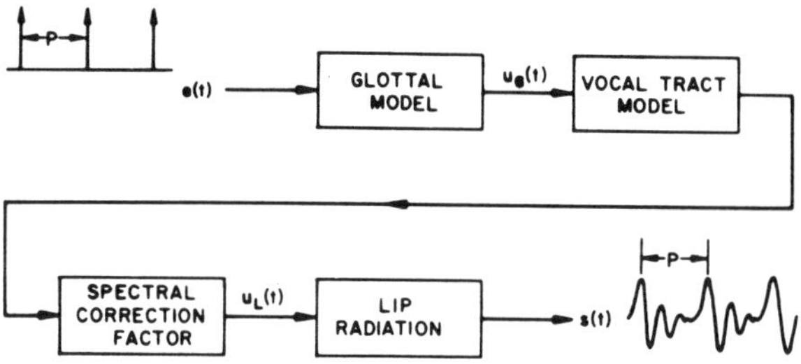

FIGURE 1. Block diagram of a cascade speech synthesizer. (From Markel and Gray.[6] Reprinted by permission.)

With synthetic speech, the experimenter can hold any or all speech variables constant. In this study, one variable in the vowel pair was changed and all the other variables were held constant. This is a considerable advantage in evaluating which speech features are discriminable by a subject. With natural speech, many parameters may co-vary and make interpretation more difficult. For example, vowel duration and the vowel's formant frequencies may co-vary.

Three pairs of synthetic vowels were generated in which the second formant frequency was significantly different in each pairing of the vowels, but the first formant frequency was held constant (TABLE 1). Two pairs of synthetic vowels were generated in which the first formant frequency was significantly different in each pairing of the vowels, but the second formant frequency was held constant within each pair (TABLE 2).

The five vowel pairs are listed in TABLE 3 with their respective formant frequencies. Each synthesized vowel was essentially identical in duration, fundamental frequency, third, fourth, and fifth formant frequencies (2500, 3400, and 3800 Hz, respectively), and the first through fifth formant bandwidths (100, 100, 170, 250, and 300 Hz, respectively).

When presented at the same RMS amplitude, each of the synthesized vowels was different in loudness to the subject. In order to determine whether the subject could discriminate between vowel pairs on the basis of spectral as opposed to gross amplitude information, an adaptive procedure was used to equalize the loudness of the two vowels within each vowel pairing.

TABLE 1

PERCEIVED DIFFERENCES BETWEEN TWO SYNTHESIZED STEADY-STATE VOWELS

	Phoneme:	
	/u/	/i/
Sounds like vowel in:	boot	beet
First formant frequency:	250 Hz	250 Hz
Second formant frequency:	900 Hz	2250 Hz
Subject's comments:	"oo's"	"oo's"
Subject's rating of the difference between the two sounds (scale 1–7, where 1 = no difference and 7 = very different)	1.25 (mean)	

TABLE 2

PERCEIVED DIFFERENCES BETWEEN TWO STEADY-STATE VOWELS

	Phoneme:	
	/i/	/æ/
Sounds like vowel in:	beet	bat
First formant frequency	250 Hz	1000 Hz
Second formant frequency	2250 Hz	2250 Hz
Subject's comments:	"oo's"	"ah's"
Subject's rating of the difference between the two sounds (scale 1–7, where 1 = no difference and 7 = very different)	7 (mean)	

One of the two vowels in a vowel pairing was held constant in level with what the subject considered a comfortable listening level. A 2I-2AFC adaptive procedure was used to equate the loudness of the other vowel in the vowel pair with that of the original vowel. In the adaptive procedure, the order of the two vowels was randomized in order to reduce temporal effects (for example, the first of two identical stimuli may sound louder). The subject was asked to press the button corresponding to the interval of the loudest sound. The adaptive procedure automatically adjusted the level in such a manner as to reduce the difference in loudness between the two vowels. In this manner, the difference in loudness between the two sounds was reduced until the subject was unable to differentiate between the two sounds on the basis of loudness.

After the vowels' loudnesses were equalized, pairs of vowels were presented to the subject. The subject was asked to "rate" or scale how different the two sounds were on a scale of one to seven, where "one" meant that the two stimuli sounded identical and "seven" meant that the two sounds were very different.

TABLE 3

FIVE SYNTHETIC VOWEL PAIRINGS USED IN THE SYNTHETIC VOWEL EXPERIMENT

	F1 (Hz) (1–7)	F2 (Hz)	Phonetic Symbol	Difference (Scaled)
Vowel pairing #1	700	1750	(ae)	2.0
	700	1100	(aa)	
Vowel pairing #2	550	800	(ao)	1.3
	550	1900	(eh)	
Vowel pairing #3	250	2250	(iy)	1.25
	250	900	(uw)	
Vowel pairing #4	250	2250	(iy)	7.0
	1000	2250	(ae)	
Vowel pairing #5	300	750	(uw)	6.0
	550	750	(ao)	

NOTE: The mean of the subject's response for each vowel pair is listed in the last column.

The five vowel pairings were presented in a pseudo-random order. Each one of the five vowel pairs was presented at least ten times during a test set. Two test sets were devoted to each of three different levels of high-frequency pre-emphasis of the second formant frequency region. The second formant frequency region was "emphasized" or amplified relative to the first formant frequency region in an effort to improve the subject's second formant discriminative ability.

FIGURE 2 and TABLE 3 present the averages of the subject's scaling of the differences between the synthetic vowels. If only the first formant frequencies (F1) of the two synthesized vowels were different, the subject rated the difference between the two sounds between 5.5 and 7 on the difference scale. Such vowel pairings sounded quite different to the subject. However, when only the second formant frequencies (F2) were different, the subject rated the difference between the two sounds between 1 and 2.5 on the difference scale. Many times such vowel pairings would sound "identical" or "almost identical."

When the subject was asked to describe the sounds that he heard, he would consistently describe the steady-state vowels with low first formant frequencies as /u/ (that is, an "oo" sound, as in boot), regardless of the second formant frequency (TABLE 4). Subject L.Y. would consistently describe the steady-state vowels with high first formant frequencies as /ɔ/ (that is an "ah" sound, as in law). The second-formant frequency did not appear to have any effect on L.Y.'s description of these steady-state vowels.

Similar results were obtained when the higher frequencies (that is, the second formant frequency region) of the synthesized vowels were amplified or "pre-emphasized" by an additional 6-dB/octave highpass filter. The third level of pre-emphasis involved the elimination of the first formant in the three vowel pairs in which only the second formant frequency was different. This was an attempt to reduce any "confounding" signals that might interfere with the second formant information. Unfortunately, the results were similar to those just reported. The subject could hear little, if any, difference between these vowels.

ERROR ANALYSIS OF A FOUR-CHOICE VOWEL TEST

The results of the synthetic vowel experiment prompted an analysis of the errors made in a natural-voice four-choice vowel test. In the test, one word was spoken and the subject was asked to choose which of the four words listed was the word spoken. For example, the subject might have to choose from the

FIGURE 2. Averages of the subject's scalings of the differences between vowel pairs. The vertical lines labeled F2 represent scalings in which only the second formant frequencies are different in the two vowels, while the vertical lines labeled F1 represent scalings in which only the first formant frequencies are different in the two vowels.

TABLE 4

PERCEIVED DIFFERENCES BETWEEN TWO SYNTHESIZED STEADY-STATE VOWELS

	Phoneme:	
	/u/	/ɔ/
Sounds like vowel in:	boot	law
First formant frequency:	300 Hz	550 Hz
Second formant frequency:	750 Hz	750 Hz
Subject's comments:	"oo's"	"ah's"
Subject's rating of the difference between the two sounds (scale 1–7, where 1 = no difference and 7 = very different)	6 (mean)	

following list of four words—*not, note, net, night*—in which only one of the four words was spoken. The subject consistently obtained scores of 50–60% correct in these four-choice, 60-trial tests.[2] When the subject made an error, the similarity between the features of the selected word and that of the spoken (that is, "target") word may be an indicator of which features are used by the subject in the recognition task.

For example, if the chosen vowel's first formant frequency was consistently similar to the target vowel's first formant frequency, one might conclude that the first formant frequency was either a perceptually significant feature or that it was correlated with such a perceptually significant feature.

The similarity between the target vowel's first and second formant frequencies and the selected (or "chosen") vowel's first and second formant frequencies was measured. The similarity was ranked by comparing the target vowel's formant frequency with each of the three possible vowel formant frequencies.

TABLE 5 illustrates the method by which distance ranks were calculated. In the four-choice vowel test, one word of the four was spoken. The subject was to pick which of the four was spoken. When the subject made an error in his choice, the error analysis determined whether the subject had chosen a word with characteristics similar to the spoken word's features. The spoken word's first formant frequency (F1) was compared with the chosen word's F1.

TABLE 5

METHOD BY WHICH DISTANCE RANKS WERE CALCULATED

Description	Word	First Formant Frequency (F1)	F1-(F1 of Target Word)	Distance Rank
Word spoken (that is, target word):	bean	270 Hz		
Word selected by subject:	boon	300 Hz	30 Hz	1 (nearest)
Word not selected:	burn	490 Hz	220 Hz	2
Word not selected:	ban	660 Hz	390 Hz	3 (farthest)

NOTE: The selected word's first formant distance rank therefore is 1.

The difference between the spoken word's F1 and the chosen word's F1 was calculated. Also, the differences between the spoken word's F1 and the F1 of the other two words were calculated. The three differences were ranked relative to each other. The word with the F1 farthest from the spoken word's F1 was ranked "3". Each trial in which an error was made was assigned a number equal to the rank of the word chosen within that trial. The average of these numbers (that is, distance or similarity ranks) was calculated and compared with the probability that such an average could be obtained if the words were chosen by chance. The same ranking procedure was used to rank the similarities between the spoken word's F2 and the chosen word's F2.

Two methods for ranking were used: In one case, the absolute value of the difference between the target vowel's formant frequency and that of the other three vowels' formant frequencies were used to determine the "distance rank" (as in TABLE 5). The second method was identical to the first, except that the logarithms of the vowels' formant frequencies were used instead of a linear scale, as in the first method. The second method, in effect, meant that the distance ranks were determined from the ratio of the target vowel's formant frequency and that of each of the three possible vowel formant frequencies. Interestingly enough, only in one of the 26 trials (in which the subject made an error) were the distance ranks different, as determined by the two methods. Because there was so little difference between the two methods, the ranks obtained from the linear frequency scaling method were arbitrarily chosen for the analysis.

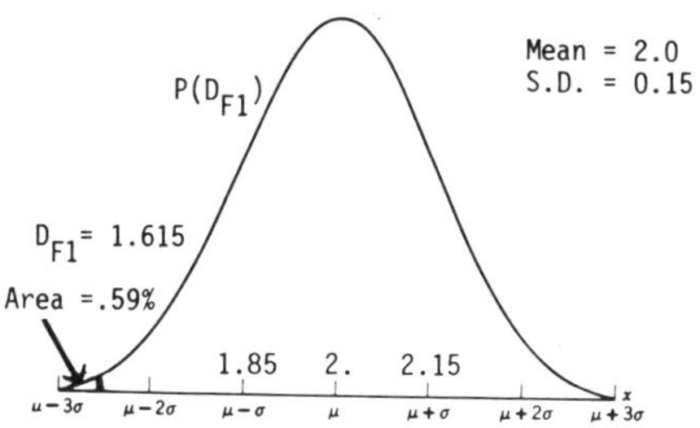

FIGURE 3. Probability of the average distance rank (n = 26), if F1 did not affect the subject's choice. DF 1 (= 1.615) was the actual average of the distance ranks for an average of 26 ranks. If F1 did not affect the subject's choice, a rank average of 1.615 or less would occur only in 0.59% of the averages.

The mean of the first formant distance ranks was 1.615 for the 26 error trials that were examined. If the subject's errors were not at all related to the similarity of the target and selected vowels' first formant frequencies, one would expect an average distance rank that was more nearly equal to "2.0". In fact, an average distance rank of 1.615 could only very rarely occur (approximately only 0.6% of the time) if the subject was not basing his decisions on some feature that was correlated with the vowel's first formant distance ranks (FIG. 3).

FIGURE 4 is a graph of the probabilities of second formant ranks, if the subject was not basing his decisions on some feature that was correlated with the vowel's second formant ranks. On this graph, a vertical line was drawn to illustrate the second formant distance rank average (DF 2 = 2.153) obtained for this sample of 26 trials. This average distance rank is only slightly greater than 1 standard deviation from the mean rank average calculated by assuming

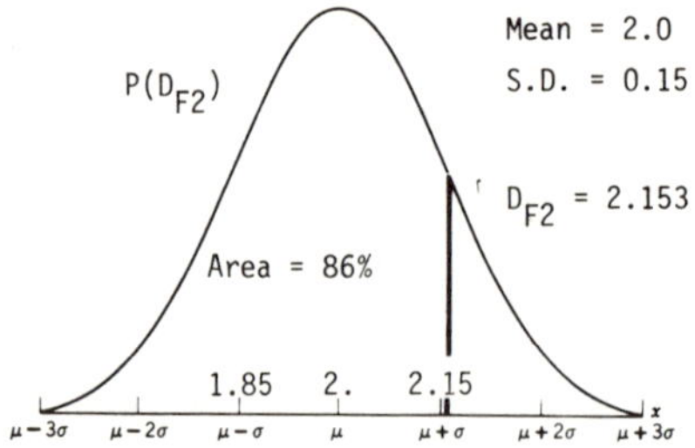

FIGURE 4. Probability of the average distance rank (n = 26), if F2 did not affect the subject's choice.

that F2 distance had no correlation with the subject's choice. The subject may not have used any second formant information. Or, if the subject did use second formant information, it is more likely that he used it in an inappropriate manner because he was more likely to choose a word containing a vowel with a second formant frequency farther from the spoken vowel's F2 than a word chosen by chance.

Another possibility exists. The second formant frequency distance ranks may be correlated (or negatively correlated) with the first formant frequency distance ranks. From the F1 error analysis described earlier, it seems likely that the subject's choices were correlated with the similarity between the first formant frequencies of the target and the selected vowel. If the F2 distance ranks are positively or negatively correlated with the F1 distance ranks, the second formant distance rank average could significantly deviate from what would be expected by chance—even if the similarity between the second formant frequencies of the target vowel and the selected vowel does not affect the subject's choice.

FIGURE 5 is a plot of the conditional probability of second formant frequency distance rank averages conditioned on a first formant distance rank average of 1.615. The second formant frequency's distance rank average of 2.153 is only about one-half a standard deviation from the "corrected" mean second formant distance rank average. This "corrected" or conditional probability distribution is a graph of the estimated probability of second formant distance rank averages if the subject did not use second formant frequency information. The "corrected" distribution function compensates for the *negative* correlation between the first and second formant distance ranks.

FIGURE 5 was obtained by fitting a continuous gaussian curve to the estimated discrete probability distribution. The fit was very good and simplifies the illustration. The discrete distribution was obtained by using a Monte Carlo

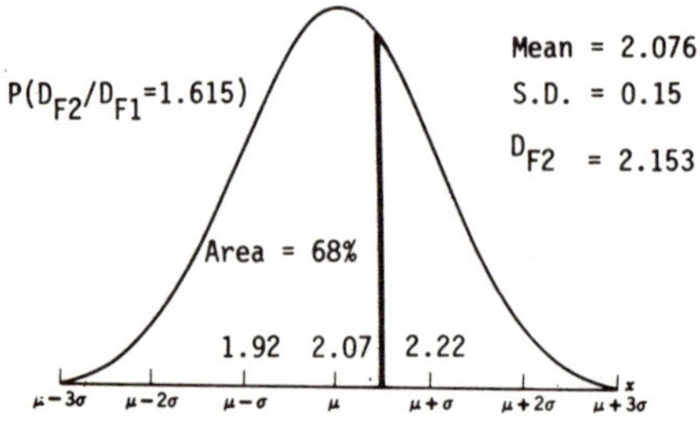

FIGURE 5. Probability of the average distance ranks of F2, if F2 did not affect the subject's choice of words, when DF1 was fixed at 1.615.

simulation technique. Ten thousand second formant distance rank averages were calculated. Each of the 10,000 second formant distance rank averages had a first formant distance rank average of 1.615. Otherwise, the vowel was randomly selected by the computer program in order to simulate a subject that was not using second formant information (but was using information that was correlated to first formant distance ranks). The 10,000 distance rank averages were used to generate a histogram that forms an estimate of the conditional probability distribution.

FIGURE 5 indicates that the subject's performance could be modeled as if he were not using second formant information, but only first formant information or information correlated with the first formants of the vowels.

SUMMARY OF RESULTS WITH SUBJECT L.Y.

It may be possible for some subjects with single-channel stimulation to use information that is carried in the frequency of the first formant. These experiments point strongly to the subject's ability to discriminate differences in steady-state vowels with significantly different first formant frequencies.

Can the subject use this discriminative ability in a natural speech-recognition task? The result just described was found to be consistent with the vowel identification task described earlier. The errors made by the subject in this four-choice vowel identification task were analyzed (error rate approximately 45%). When the subject made an error, he generally chose the word containing the vowel with a first formant frequency closest to the first formant frequency of the spoken word's vowel. The subject appeared to have no preference for vowels with a second formant frequency near the spoken vowel's second formant frequency.

One cochlear prosthesis group's [3] speech processor deletes any information pertaining to the first or the second formant frequency. Our data strongly imply that subject L.Y. was quite capable of using first formant frequency information.

In addition to first formant information, some voicing and nasality information may be obtained by some patients having implants.[2, 3] The Vienna group [4] has reported that some second formant information may be used by some of their patients.

MULTICHANEL SPEECH PROCESSORS

Recently we have tested a multichannel speech processor with another subject, C.B. The results have been encouraging. Both a single-channel speech processor (FIG. 6 and TABLE 6) and a three-channel speech processor (FIG. 7 and TABLE 7) were tested with this subject. The single-channel processor was similar to that used by subject L.Y.

Subject C.B. did not perform nearly as well as subject L.Y. did while using a single-channel processor. With her single-channel processor, C.B. performed in a manner similar to that of the majority of single-channel users who have been evaluated by Owens *et al.*[5]

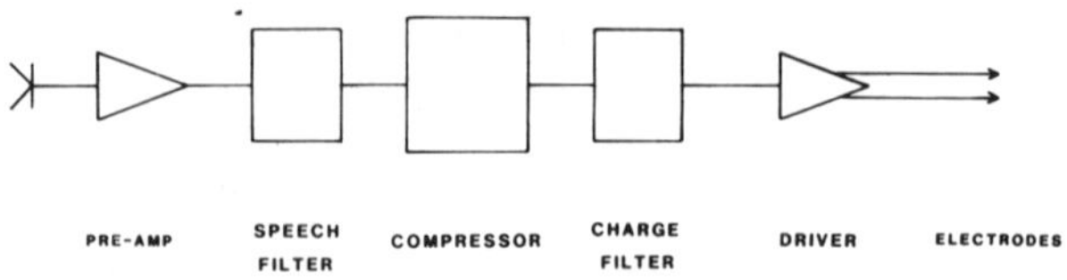

FIGURE 6. Block diagram of CB's single-channel speech-processor. TABLE 6 contains a list of the processor's specifications.

However, when the three-channel processor was utilized with subject C.B., her performance on a set of speech tests improved considerably (see Owens *et al.*[5]).

It is not safe to conclude that any given class (such as multichannel processors versus single-channel processors) of processors is optimal. It is very difficult even within individual subjects to ascertain which classes of speech-processors are optimal. It may be even more difficult to determine whether given classes of speech-processors are optimal for all, or groups, of implanted subjects. In subject C.B., a particular single-channel processor did not perform as well as a particular three-channel processor. However, additional adjustments of the single-channel processor variables may have improved her performance. Indeed, entirely different single-channel processors may have significantly improved her performance. The same can be said for the optimization of the three-channel processor.

In our processor adjustment and comparison procedure, we have used a vowel test and an initial consonant test to guide us in the optimization procedure. The tape-recorded tests are two-choice monosyllable word tests. These tests are designed to give us information relevant to processor design and adjustment. These natural speech tests evaluate to what degree the subject is able to utilize certain distinctive features (and/or other features correlated with these particular distinctive features). After many processor adjustments and quick evaluations (using the two speech tests described earlier and subject quality judgments), we then evaluate the subject for a much wider range of

TABLE 6

SINGLE-CHANNEL PROCESSOR SPECIFICATIONS FOR SUBJECT C.B.

Speech filter:	Single-pole highpass filter; —3 dB at 170 Hz.
Compressor:	Two-stage, cascaded compressors.
First stage:	150-μsec attack time. 300-μsec release time.
Second stage:	Instantaneous log compressor.
Compression ratio:	5:1 over the 60-dB input range. 10:1 over the upper 40 dB input range. The compression ratio increases dramatically at the higher input levels. The compressor clips at the higher input levels.
Charge filter:	Two-pole highpass filter; —3 dB at 300 Hz and —12 dB at 140 Hz.

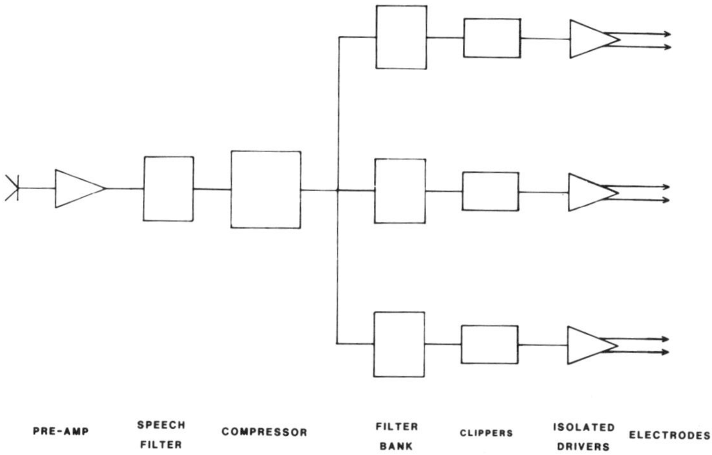

FIGURE 7. Block diagram of CB's three-channel speech-processor. TABLE 7 contains a list of the processor's specifications.

speech skills. The MAC battery [5] and several other speech tests have been developed for this purpose. This much larger and comprehensive test battery is our "benchmark" of performance for the implant subjects.

In the initial consonant test, subject C.B. was able to use voiced–unvoiced information (or information correlated with the voiced–unvoiced distinction) much more effectively with the three-channel processor than with the single-

TABLE 7

THREE-CHANNEL PROCESSOR SPECIFICATIONS FOR SUBJECT C.B.

Speech filter:	Single-pole highpass filter; —3 dB at 670 Hz.
Compressor:	Single stage, noninstantaneous compression. 0.5-msec attack time; 1.0 msec release time. 5–10 compression ratio over 60-dB input range. Compression greatly increases at the higher input levels.
Filter bank:	Three-pole highpass section; three-pole lowpass section. Both sections were designed for a filter function between a bessel and a butterworth characteristic. Low filter:[a] 200–800 Hz (—3dB intercepts). Mid filter: 850–1450 Hz. High filter: highpass filter; —3dB at 1450 Hz.
Limiters:	The bipolar clipping level is set approximately 0–20% above the maximal excursions of the speech signal.

[a] A "charge" filter was inserted immediately after the "low filter" to further reduce low-frequency components. The charge filter is a two-pole highpass filter (—3 dB at 300 Hz and —12 dB at 140 Hz).

channel processor. In the vowel test, C.B. was able to use first formant information (and/or information correlated with first formant frequency) more effectively with the three-channel processor than with the single-channel processor.

Initial measurements of an earlier version of the multichannel processor indicated that the subject was not using second formant information or information correlated with second formant frequency. Two changes were made to the multichannel processor to improve the subject's performance within this distinctive feature category. The upper 3-dB breakpoint of the "midrange filter" was adjusted from approximately 2000 Hz down to 1450 Hz and the lower 3-dB breakpoint of the "high filter" was adjusted from approximately 2000 Hz down to 1450 Hz. The purpose of this modification was to improve the separation of high-frequency second formants from low-frequency second formants. The second modification reduced the spectral distortion generated by the compressor that was located ahead of the filter bank. These modifications enhanced the capacity of the two upper channels to resolve differences in the second formant frequencies of speech segments. The improved resolution was measured by comparing the peak-to-peak output level of the two channels on a dual-trace oscilloscope for selected steady-state vowels. The vowels were chosen such that their second formant frequencies were considerably different. After these improvements, the subject C.B. performed significantly above chance on some of the tests used to measure her ability to use second formant information and/or information that was correlated with the second formant frequency. These tests do not give conclusive evidence that the subject was able to use the second formant frequency information in speech-recognition tasks. The subject may have used information that was correlated with second formant information. For example, the duration of vowel segments may have given a useful cue to the subject. However, the changes made in the processor that improved C.B.'s performance were primarily those that would affect only second formant resolution.

Summary

In a four-choice, vowel-identification task, the implanted subject (L.Y.) identified the spoken word in 50 to 60% of the trials (n = 60). Experiments were conducted to determine which acoustic features were being utilized by the implanted subject.

Pairs of steady-state synthesized vowels were presented to the subject. A difference-scaling procedure indicated that the subject could easily discriminate between synthetic vowels with different first formant frequencies. However, the subject had great difficulty in discriminating between synthetic vowels with different second formant frequencies when the first formant frequencies were identical.

This result was found to be consistent with an identification task using natural vowels in a single-word context. The errors made by the subject in a four-choice vowel-identification task were analyzed (error rate = 45%). When the subject made an error, he generally chose the word containing the vowel with a first formant frequency closest to the first formant frequency of the spoken vowel's first formant frequency. In contrast, when the subject made an error, he appeared to have no preference for vowels with a second formant frequency near the spoken vowel's second formant frequency. Consequently, speech processors that do not transmit first formant frequency information may be less useful to implanted subjects.

With another subject (C.B.), a single-channel and a three-channel speech-processor were evaluated. The subject's performance with the three-channel processor was considerably better than that obtained with the single-channel processor in a series of speech tests.[5]

ACKNOWLEDGMENTS

The entire staff of the Coleman Laboratory at the University of California, San Francisco, has contributed to this study. We wish to thank Pat Jones, Joe Molinari, Chuck Byers, Steve Rebscher, David Casey, Lindsay Vurek, Bob Shannon, Mike Merzenich, Robin Michelson, Bob Schindlar, Marcia Raggio, Dorcas Kessler, John Gardi, Earl Schubert, Elmer Owens, Chris Telleen, and Bill Garret for their valuable skills in helping us with our cochlear implant project.

REFERENCES

1. OWENS, E., D. KESSLER & E. SCHUBERT. 1982. Interim assessment of candidates for cochlear implants. Arch. Otolaryngol. **108:** 478–483.
2. OWENS, E. & C. C. TELLEEN. 1981. Speech perception with hearing aids and cochlear implants. Arch. Otolaryngol. **107:** 160–163.
3. FOURCIN, A. J., S. M. ROSEN, B. C. J. MOORE, E. E. DOUEK, G. P. CLARK, H. DODSON & L. H. BANNISTER. 1979. External electrical stimulation of the cochlea: Clinical, psychophysical, speech-perceptual, and histological findings. Br. J. Audiol. **13:** 85–107.
4. HOCHMAIR-DESOYER, I. J., E. S. HOCHMAIR, R. E. FISCHER & K. BURIAN. 1980. Cochlear prostheses in use: Recent speech comprehension results. Arch. Otorhinolaryngol. **229:** 81–98.
5. OWENS, E., D. KESSLER & M. RAGGIO. 1983. Results for some patients with cochlear implants on the minimal auditory capabilities (MAC) battery. This volume.
6. MARKEL, J. D. & A. H. GRAY. 1976. Linear Prediction of Speech. Springer-Verlag. Berlin.

COMPUTERIZED TESTING OF SIGNAL-ENCODING STRATEGIES WITH ROUND-WINDOW IMPLANTS[a]

N. Dillier, T. Spillmann, and J. Güntensperger

ENT Department
University Hospital
CH-8091 Zurich, Switzerland

Introduction

Our team has started work on cochlear implants in 1974. Our first implant operation was performed in 1977 in a 50-year-old patient deaf from meningitis since childhood. Two bipolar platinum electrodes, placed in the modiolus, could be directly accessed through a biocarbon percutaneous plug. Psychophysical testing during a 6-month period revealed frequency difference limens comparable to those of normal-hearing persons below 300 Hz.[3]

Because our experiences with the hard-wired percutaneous connectors had not been very convincing (the plug was inadvertently removed after 6 months), we decided to use only transcutaneous inductive coupling systems in the future. Results with temporarily placed removable electrodes at the round window in five patients in whom reproducible electroneural hearing sensations could be evoked as well as reports from other groups using round-window stimulation [1, 6] encouraged us, however, to try chronically implanted round-window electrodes. The results will be compared later with our modiolar electrode data and with other single-channel intracochlear stimulation data.

Materials and Methods

We consider these electrode implantations nevertheless to be experimental surgical procedures and therefore require informed consent and total bilateral peripheral hearing loss that cannot be treated by conventional surgical or prosthetic means. Our patients should also be willing to cooperate in our clinical evaluation experiments after implantation.

Since the time of the aforementioned single percutaneous two-channel modiolar implant experiment, another four totally deaf patients have been implanted. Pretests by ear-canal electrodes (reported elsewhere [3]) have shown positive results. Table 1 lists the clinical information. The patients had been informed about the experimental nature of this procedure several months before the operation. The first patient, R.G. (born in 1956), was congenitally deaf in both ears. The second patient, E.P. (born in 1950), had bilateral loss of cochleovestibular function after meningitis at the age of 9 months. The third patient, U.T. (born in 1941), experienced sudden hearing loss 2 years before implantation. The fourth patient, C.A. (born in 1961), also had bilateral loss of cochleovestibular function after meningitis at the age of 14. In all

[a] This work was supported by Grant 3.848.0.79 from the Swiss National Research Foundation.

0077–8923/83/0405–0360 $1.75/0 © 1983, NYAS

patients, no useful acoustic information was obtained by a conventional acoustic hearing aid. Data on only the first three patients are presented here since too little time has elapsed since the fourth was operated on.

The technical specifications of our implant have already been described elsewhere.[10] The active ball electrode (approximately 1 mm in diameter) and the reference electrode are made of platinum/iridium, and the receiver coil and demodulator circuit are encapsulated in medical-grade epoxy. The external part of our prosthesis consists of the microphone, preamplifier, and signal-processing circuits (all contained in a box measuring 10 × 6 × 3 cm) and the transmitting coil, which is placed behind the auricle, attached to an ear mold.

The surgical intervention consists of use of a typical access to the middle ear to perform mastoidectomy and electrode placement via facial recess and fixation with fibrin adhesive.

Testing is performed by means of a computerized system. Hearing and discomfort thresholds are determined in every test session. The responses to nonverbal frequency and amplitude differences, and pitch and intensity scaling, are systematically investigated and can be used to compare different electrode systems available in the future.

Speech material, such as numbers, monosyllables, spondees, and sentences, can be stored and analyzed with the same system. Analysis parameters (pitch, gain, formants, vocal-tract filter coefficients, and zero-crossing intervals) are used to generate on-line stimulation signals according to several processing algorithms. Stimulus parameters are fully programmable. Complex stimuli such as speech can also be processed and delivered by the computer.[4]

Results

The first measurements after the implantation were repeated determinations of the threshold of hearing and discomfort at several frequencies. Thresholds remained stable over the whole experimental period of 14 (R.G.), 10 (E.P.), or 3 (U.T.) months (Fig. 1). The threshold of discomfort was between 8 to 12 dB above the hearing threshold. Discomfort thresholds were measured as quickly as possible, and were therefore not as accurate as hearing threshold measurements.

Table 1

Summary of Information on Patients with Round-Window Implants

Patient	Age (yr) & Sex	Age at Onset of Deafness (yr)	Years Deaf:	Cause of Hearing Loss
R.G.	25, F	0	25	Congenital
E.P.	31, M	0	31	Meningitis
U.T.	41, F	39	2	Sudden deafness (left); congenital (right)
C.A.	20, F	14	6	Meningitis

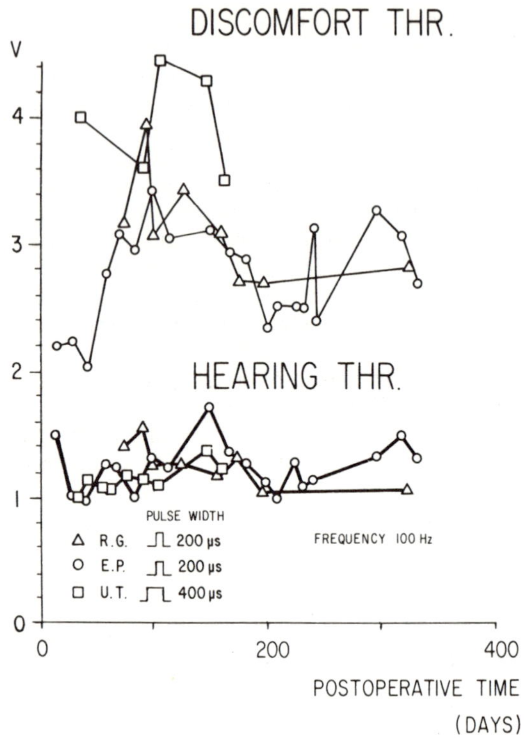

FIGURE 1. Thresholds of hearing and discomfort over time. THR, threshold; V, pulse amplitude (in volts) at transmitter-stage input of portable sound-processor.

Frequency difference limens could be determined up to 500 Hz. They were in the same range as the values of our first patient with modiolar electrodes.[4] FIGURE 2 shows two examples of pitch scaling. In the first experiment the patient was asked to scale frequencies between 20 and 100 Hz, in the second between 100 and 1000 Hz. Every experiment consisted of 100 trials with ten linearly spaced frequencies. Every frequency was repeated ten times in random order. The mean of these ten scalings is displayed in FIGURE 2 in logarithmic frequency scale. It can be seen that scaling is possible up to approximately 500 Hz. Frequencies below 100 Hz seem to be scaled slightly differently from frequencies above 100 Hz.

In a series of scaling experiments, the effect of training and feedback was investigated. FIGURE 3 shows normalized standard deviations plotted against the session numbers. Triangles denote experiments without feedback. Circles denote experiments with feedback, that is, the patient was shown the stimulated frequency value (in percent of chosen interval) after every trial. Training considerably improves the reproducibility in both conditions, and feedback will lead to even more consistent responses. All these experiments were carried out on one morning, with only short interruptions between each session. Considering the size of the scatter, it cannot be excluded that different feedback conditions

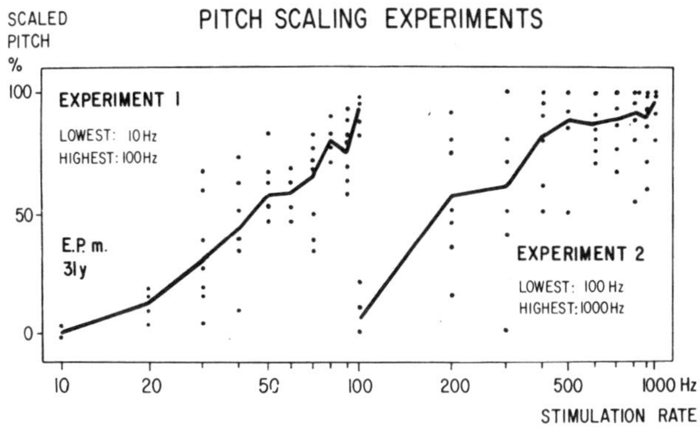

FIGURE 2. Pitch scaling examples in (1) low-frequency range and (2) high-frequency range.

(such as logarithmic instead of linear frequency scales) might have led to different shapes of the scaling function.

Amplitude difference limen results are shown in FIGURE 4. The values of patient E.P. were much lower and practically independent of stimulus level in contrast to the values of R.G. The dynamic range of E.P. was lower (only 8 dB or less) than that of R.G. (10 to 12 dB), which might explain this difference.

Numbers between 13 and 99 were used in identification tests. Every test comprised 40 randomly choosen numbers. FIGURE 5 shows the discrimination results over time for R.G. with the linear regression line (the correlation coefficient is statistically significant at $p < 0.001$). The tests were carried out with the portable speech-processor and the same speaker in all experiments. FIGURE 6 shows comparisons of speech test results in three conditions (S: stimulation alone, L: lipreading alone, SL: stimulation with lipreading). Again the

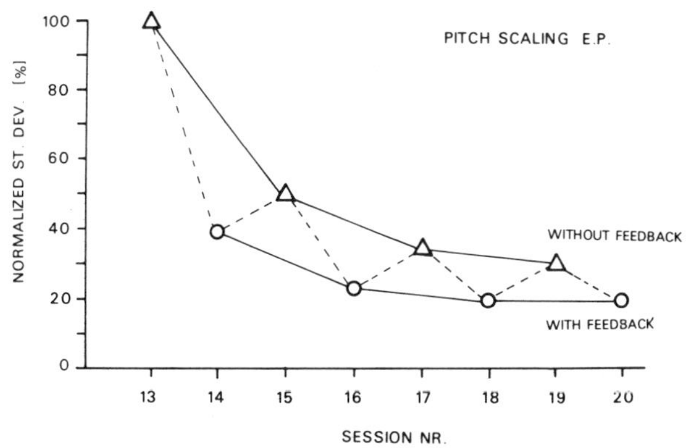

FIGURE 3. Effect of training and feedback in pitch scaling experiments in subject E.P. Every point represents 100 trials in the frequency range of 20 to 100 Hz.

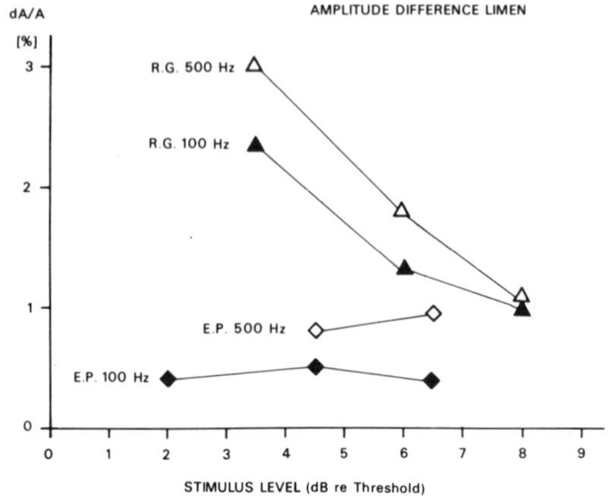

FIGURE 4. Amplitude difference limens. Intensities are referred to individual subjective thresholds.

stimulation tests were done with the portable stimulator and with the same speaker as in the lipreading or in the combined tests. The data were averaged over several sessions.

TABLE 2 lists the number of trials and the relative improvements in discrimination with lipreading compared to stimulation alone. The best effect of electrical stimulation is revealed in the speech-tracking test, where relative improvements of combined acoustic and visual input over visual input alone of 9–125% are obtained. Patient 3, with late-onset hearing loss, who is an excellent lipreader (because of pre-existing moderate to severe hearing loss and special-school education) scored best both with and without a prosthesis. She uses her prosthesis mostly in difficult communication situations where there are many competing speakers. The other verbal tests, voice (speaker sex) identification and the number recognition test, are less helpful in ascertaining specific

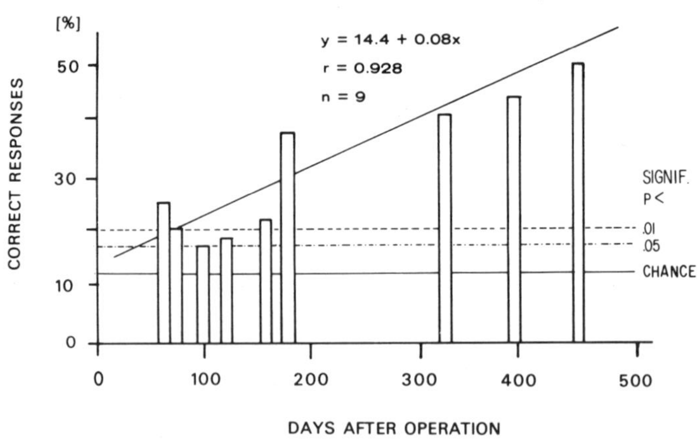

FIGURE 5. Improvement of number identification results with time in subject R.G. (closed test). Every column represents 40 responses to two-digit numbers (13–99) spoken by a male speaker via the portable sound-processor.

responses to the prosthesis either because these tests give extremely high values with electrical stimulation alone (in the voice identification test) or because lipreading alone is nearly perfect (in the numbers test). In the latter case, the addition of the acoustic input to the visual input alone does not provide a substantial gain. The failure of some tests to show a prosthetic gain does not agree with the real-life benefit and leads us to conclude that the choice of an appropriate test paradigm is crucial in electrode evaluation.

For vowel discrimination experiments, a closed set of digitally stored speech sounds has been used. Two amplitude coding options (lin, log) and three pulse-rate coding options (F0 = fundamental, F2 = second formant frequency

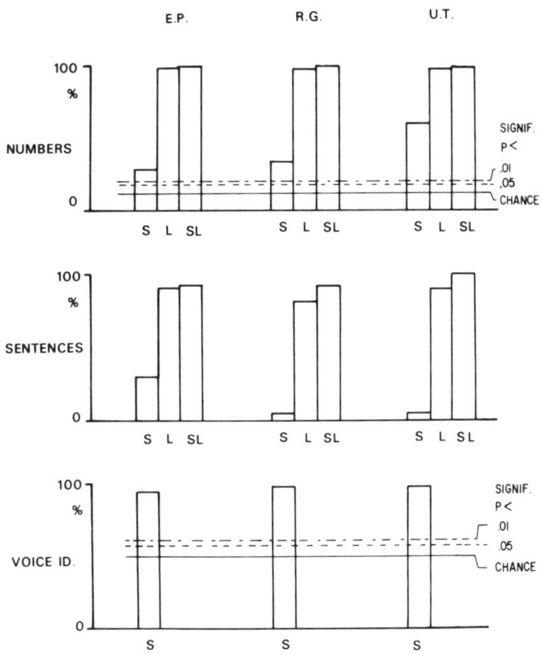

FIGURE 6. Speech-discrimination tests compared with lipreading. S = electrical stimulation alone; L = lipreading alone; SL = electrical stimulation plus lipreading.

divided by 18, ZC = zerocrossing intervals) are available with the laboratory speech-processor. The original fundamental and formant parameters of the half-second samples are listed in TABLE 3. Fundamental frequencies are similar for all five vowels, whereas F2 is low for ⟨A⟩, ⟨O⟩, ⟨U⟩ and high for ⟨E⟩ and ⟨I⟩.

Therefore, it can be expected that an F0 algorithm will not work well in separating these sounds, whereas an F2 algorithm should discriminate between the two groups of low (A, O, U) and high (E, I) second formant frequency. This is documented in TABLE 4, which shows confusion matrices for both stimulation algorithms. The contingency coefficient (which would be 1 if no confusions had occurred) is not significant at the 5% level for the F0 algorithm.

TABLE 2

OVERVIEW OF SPEECH-DISCRIMINATION RESULTS WITH ROUND-WINDOW ELECTRICAL STIMULATION

	Voice Identification	Number-Recognition Test			Speech Tracking		
Patient	SA (%)	SA (%)	LRA (%)	S + LR (%)	LRA (wpm)	S + LR (wpm)	Relative Improvement (%)
R.G.	98	33	97	99	12.1	13.2	9
E.P.	95	28	98	99	17.8	23.3	31
U.T.	98	60	97	98	19.2	43.2	125

ABBREVIATIONS: SA = discrimination by stimulation alone; LRA = discrimination by lipreading alone; S + LR = discrimination by combined stimulation plus lipreading; wpm = words per minute.

NOTE: Relative improvement $\frac{S + LR - LRA}{LRA} 100\%$.

The matrix for the F2 algorithm shows a contingency coefficient of 0.88 ($p < 0.001$). If only the two subgroups (A, O, U and E, I) are considered, this coefficient rises to 0.95.

However, vowel identification is probably not the main objective of a cochlear prosthesis. Acceptability and objective advantage may well depend on other factors. In a series of experiments, some speech-processing strategies were tried. FIGURE 7 shows a comparison of subjective scores and discrimination results in numbers tests. Only the four or five algorithms that scored best were tested systematically. Again substantial patient differences are apparent. Discrimination results and subjective scores correlate reasonably well for patients U.T. and R.G. It is interesting to note that in all patients results with the tests with the portable sound-processor (live speech) showed the best range, whereas the zerocrossing algorithm of the laboratory stimulator attained the same result as that of the portable stimulator only in patient E.P. The most probable explanation for this outcome seems to be the test situation. Another reason could be that the amplitude coding of the portable stimulator is neither linear nor fully logarithmic and is not exactly reproduced by the computer

TABLE 3

VOWEL IDENTIFICATION TESTS: STIMULATION PARAMETERS

Vowel	F0 (Hz)	F1 (Hz)	F2 (Hz)
A	153	724	1044
O	165	349	621
U	177	270	681
E	160	330	2467
I	183	198	2586

NOTE: Pulse-rate coding: F0, F2/18; amplitude coding: linear, logarithmic.

algorithms. From FIGURE 7 it also seems that pulse-rate coding by the fundamental frequency is superior to F2 coding. This might be even more true for longer speech samples, such as sentences. There is no conclusive evidence yet to allow us to decide whether coding of unvoiced (consonantal) speech sounds by high (over 200 Hz) or low (below 200 Hz) random pulse sequences is to be preferred.

TABLE 4

VOWEL CONFUSIONS IN PATIENT R.G. WITH TWO DIFFERENT ALGORITHMS [a]

	Response					
Stimulation	A	O	U	E	I	n
A	8	3	4	2	3	20
O	1	1	6	6	6	20
U	0	4	4	3	8	19
E	13	5	1	1	0	20
I	3	4	3	3	6	19
n	25	17	18	15	23	98

Rate: F0
Amplitude: linear
20.4% correct
Contingency coefficient = 0.44
NS

	Response					
Stimulation	A	O	U	E	I	n
A	16	1	1	0	0	18
O	4	11	4	0	1	20
U	6	3	10	0	1	20
E	0	0	0	18	2	20
I	2	0	0	6	12	20
n	28	15	15	24	16	98

Rate: F2
Amplitude: linear
68.4% correct
Contingency coefficient = 0.88
$p < 0.001$

[a] Pulse rate determined by fundamental frequency and pulse rate determined by second-formant frequency (divided by 18).

DISCUSSION

The results obtained with implanted electrodes at the round window are comparable to results with electrodes in the scala tympani or in the hearing nerve with respect to frequency resolution. Although the subjective quality of the perceived sounds is expected to vary depending on the stimulation site,[1, 2, 5, 9] it seems that timing effects of electrical stimulation are the principal factors of differential pitch perceptions.

The dynamic range with round-window stimulation seems to be somewhat lower than that with intracochlear stimulation, although the highest range (12 dB) is within the range obtained with scalar electrodes. Sinusoidal stimulation may give a slightly higher dynamic range, especially at lower frequencies, but we prefer to use pulsatile stimuli for safety as well as technical reasons.

Whether the differences in speech discrimination between our results and those of other groups [7, 8] using single-channel access can be explained by the place of stimulation remains to be shown in further studies. In contrast to the assertions of some authors using intracochlear single-channel electrodes, we could not achieve true open-word discrimination in any of our patients with any of the tested algorithms. Differences of testing methods and of the amount of training of implanted persons might play a substantial role in the variability

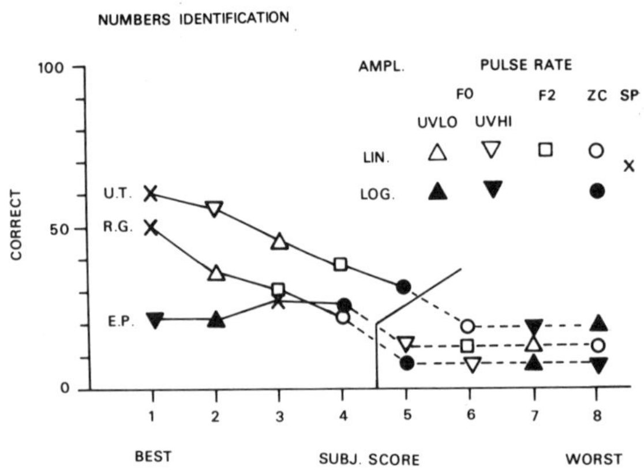

FIGURE 7. Speech-encoding algorithms: correlations between subjective scoring and discrimination results: two amplitude coding options (linear, logarithmic), pulse-rate coding by fundamental frequency (F0), second formant frequency (F2) divided by 18, and zerocrossing intervals (ZC). During unvoiced periods either a low (UVLO) or a high (UVHI) random pulse is generated. The portable sound-processor (SP) uses zerocrossings and automatic gain control as well as logarithmic compression, which is adjusted individually for every patient.

between implant centers. The small group of patients and too many clinical variables (cause, age at onset, and duration of deafness) prevents further speculation on preferred coding formulas at present. The patient with the best test results (U.T.) is postlingually deafened; the other two are prelingually deaf. Further improvement over time is still possible, as shown for results in number recognition for R.G. over 15 months (FIG. 5). The same might be the case for speech tracking, which in our experience is the best single test to obtain real-life benefit scores of electrical stimulation. Still, there remain other concepts of speech encoding not tested yet which may improve discrimination.

Our technique of electrical stimulation of hearing is a safe procedure involving only routine middle-ear surgery to place the induction coil within the mastoid bone and to put an electrode at the round-window margin. By an external stimulator, sounds are transformed to electrical stimuli suited to excite surviving fibers of the cochlear nerve. This helps the patient to communicate and provides some basic cues for speech discrimination. The ability to profit from these percepts can be considerably improved by accustomation and training, which are still in progress in all our patients.

Summary

After extensive testing of a patient with two bipolar modiolar electrodes connected to a percutaneous plug in 1977, we provided four patients with a single-channel monopolar round-window electrode connected to a tuned radiofrequency receiver coil. Loudness and pitch discrimination and results of psychophysical scaling experiments of extracochlear electrodes are comparable to those with intracochlear stimulation. Extensive testing with a computerized test system and with tape-recorded and live speech material showed that accurate vowel and speaker identification by stimulation alone is possible and that discrimination by lipreading is considerably improved. Interactive training sessions further improve discrimination results. Different signal-encoding algorithms can be used to generate in real time stimulation signals from prestored speech parameters (such as pitch, gain, formants, and zerocrossing intervals).

References

1. Chouard, C. H. & P. M. Macleod. 1976. Implantation of multiple intracochlear electrodes for rehabilitation of total deafness: Preliminary report. Laryngoscope **86:** 1743–1751.
2. Clark, G. M., Y. C. Tong, L. F. A. Martin & P. A. Busby. 1981. A multiple-channel cochlear implant. Acta Otolaryngol. **91:** 173–175.
3. Dillier, N., T. Spillmann, U. P. Fisch & L. J. Leifer. 1979. Encoding and decoding of auditory signals in relation to human speech and its application to human cochlear implants. Audiology **19:** 146–163.
4. Dillier, N., J. Güntensperger & T. Spillmann. 1980. A computer-controlled test system for electrical stimulation of the auditory nerve of deaf patients with implanted multielectrodes. Scand. Audiol. Suppl. **11:** 163–170.
5. Eddington, D. K. 1980. Speech discrimination in deaf subjects with cochlear implants. J. Acoust. Soc. Am. **68:** 885–891.
6. Fourcin, A. J., S. M. Rosen, B. C. J. Moore, E. E. Douek, G. P. Clark, H. Dodson & L. H. Bannister. 1979. External electrical stimulation of the cochlea: Clinical, psychological, speech-perceptual and histological findings. Br. J. Audiol. **13:** 85–107.
7. Hochmair, I. J., E. S. Hochmair, R. E. Fischer & K. Burian. 1980. Cochlear prostheses in use: Recent speech comprehension results. Arch. Oto-Rhino-Laryngol. **229**(2): 81–98.
8. House, W. F. 1976. Cochlear implants. Ann. Otol. 85 (Suppl. 27): 1–92.
9. Simmons, F. B. 1966. Electrical stimulation of the auditory nerve in man. Arch. Otolaryngol. **84:** 22–76.
10. Spillmann, T., N. Dillier & J. Güntensperger. 1982. Electrical stimulation of hearing by implanted cochlear electrodes in humans. Appl. Neurophysiol. **45:** 32–37.

CLINICAL RESULTS WITH A MULTICHANNEL PSEUDOBIPOLAR SYSTEM[a]

G. M. Clark, Y. C. Tong, and R. C. Dowell

Department of Otolaryngology
University of Melbourne
Victoria 3052, Australia

INTRODUCTION

A receiver–stimulator and multiple-electrode array were implanted in the scala tympani of a 46-year-old totally deaf man on August 1, 1978. This patient had lost all hearing after a head injury 18 months prior to surgery. Pure-tone Bekesy and speech audiometry showed no hearing in either ear at the maximum output levels of the audiometer, and no vibrotactile responses were elicited.

A second patient, a 63-year-old man, received an implant on July 17, 1979. This patient had a progressive sensorineural hearing loss extending over 30 years due to bomb blast and chronic infection. He had no help from a hearing aid for 13 years prior to surgery. Pure-tone Bekesy audiometry under headphones revealed no hearing in the left ear, and in the right he had thresholds of 125 dB SPL at 0.125 kHz; 115 dB at 0.25 kHz, and 117 dB at 0.5 kHz. There was no speech discrimination in either ear under headphones or in a monitored sound field. His right ear was fitted with a hearing aid (Calaid G12G) by the National Acoustics Laboratory, but at its maximum output level he received only a limited gain at 5.0 kHz and could not be aided.

The receiver–stimulator was implanted in a bed created in the mastoid region; an opening was made into the middle ear through a posterior tympanotomy; and the electrode arrays were passed through the round-window membrane into the scala tympani of the basal turn for a distance of 20–25 mm.

A series of psychophysical tests were then carried out over many months, and these helped to establish our present speech-processing strategy. With this strategy, the voicing frequency (F0) and energy, and the frequency and energy of the dominant spectral peak in the midfrequency range (F2) are extracted. The parameters for voicing determine the rate of stimulation at all electrodes. The parameters for the dominant spectral peak in the midfrequency range excite electrodes which convey appropriate spectral colors and loudness.[1-3]

The speech-processing strategy has been assessed using a number of audiological tests since no single test can provide all the necessary information about the help provided in understanding running speech. The audiological tests have been carried out in the following circumstances: live voice in an untreated room, live voice and prerecorded material presented in a sound-attenuated room with a one-way viewing mirror; and prerecorded material in a sound-attenuated anechoic room using a video monitor for lipreading tests.

[a] Financial assistance for this study was provided by the Department of Science and Technology of the Australian Government, the National Health and Medical Research Council of Australia, and the Deafness Foundation of Victoria.

0077–8923/83/0405–0370 $1.75/0 © 1983, NYAS

TABLE 1

VOWEL IDENTIFICATION MATRIX FOR PATIENT 1 WITH MULTIPLE-ELECTRODE STIMULATION ALONE [a]

	Stimulus					
Response	Heed	Hard	Hoard	Hid	Hud	Hod
Heed	18					
Hard		19	2			
Hoard		1	18			1
Hid	2			20		
Hud					20	15
Hod						4

[a] Percentage correct = 82%.

AUDIOLOGY

Phonemes

The patients were first evaluated at a phonemic and segmental level. The vowels were a closed set of the phonemes /i/, /a/, /ɔ/, /I/, /ʌ/, /ƀ/ in an H-vowel-D context. The results for patient 1 for electrical stimulation alone are shown in TABLE 1; these are the combined results for responses to male and female speakers. The patient obtained an 82% correct performance.[2] Notice that the main confusion was between *hod* and *hud*. The combined responses to male and female speakers for patient 2 are shown in TABLE 2; this patient obtained a 71% score.[2] In his case the main confusion was between both *hod* and *hud*, and *hard* and *hoard*. These results indicate that both patients were able to make use of the duration and second-formant frequency of the vowel nucleus as a cue for vowel identification. Confusions between the long vowels /ɔ/, /a/, /i/ and the short vowels /ƀ/, /ʌ/, /I/ were rare—three errors out of 200

TABLE 2

VOWEL IDENTIFICATION MATRIX FOR PATIENT 2 WITH MULTIPLE-ELECTRODE STIMULATION ALONE [a]

	Stimulus					
Response	Heed	Hard	Hoard	Hid	Hud	Hod
Heed	19					
Hard		11	4			1
Hoard		9	16			3
Hid				19	4	
Hud				1	14	9
Hod	1				2	7

[a] Percentage correct = 71%.

presentations for patients 1 and five errors for patient 2. The major confusions for both patients were between vowels with a relatively small difference in second-formant frequency.

In addition, we also compared the patients' performances in response to male and female voices. The results showed that patient 1 performed equally well for both male and female audiologists, but patient 2 had a poorer response for the male voice.

Our F0 and F2 laboratory-based speech-processor was also tested on the patients using a number of closed sets of consonants. The mean results for the two patients [4] are shown in Table 3.

For the ten consonants k, p, s, ʃ, tʃ, f, w, j, r, and n in a consonant–vowel context with the vowel /a/ there was a score of 35% for electrical stimulation alone.[2] For the eight consonants p, t, k, b, d, g, m, and n in a vowel–consonant–vowel context, there was a similar score for electrical stimulation alone and lipreading alone, but an increase to 62% for electrical stimulation combined with lipreading.[5] For the 12 consonants p, t, k, b, d, g, m, n, f, v, s, and z in a vowel–consonant–vowel context, the results were similar.[1]

TABLE 3

CONSONANT IDENTIFICATION IN PATIENTS 1 AND 2: MEAN PERCENTAGE SCORES

Test	EA	LA	E + L
10 Consonants -CV-/a/			
k, p, s, ʃ, tʃ, f, w, j, r, n	35%		
8 Consonants -VCV-/a/			
p, t, k, b, d, g, m, n	37%	36%	62%
12 Consonants-VCV-/a/			
p, t, k, b, d, g, m, n, f, v, s, z	36%	38%	64%

ABBREVIATIONS: EA = electrical stimulation alone; LA = lipreading alone; E + L = electrical stimulation plus lipreading.

An analysis of the identification of ten consonants for male and female speakers showed that patient 1 scored better for the female voice and patient 2 equally well for both voices. The identification of consonants was further analyzed in terms of the following features: voicing, nasality, affrication, duration, and place (see Miller and Nicely [6]). The results for the first patient, who used a wearable speech-processor, are shown in FIGURE 1, and are the average for male and female speakers. The 12 consonants studied were p, t, k, b, d, g, m, n, f, v, s, z. The overall percentage transfer was 47 for lipreading alone, 46 for electrical stimulation, and 72 for combined electrical stimulation plus lipreading. This indicated that electrical stimulation complements lipreading cues. FIGURE 1 shows that for voicing, nasality and duration, electrical stimulation alone gave a higher information transfer than did lipreading alone, and for all cues electrical stimulation combined with lipreading was significantly better than for lipreading alone.

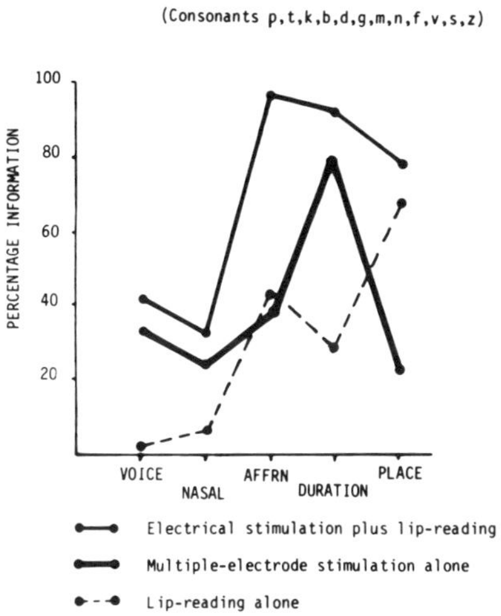

FIGURE 1. A graph of the percentage information transmitted for voicing, nasality, affrication, duration, and place for the following conditions: electrical stimulation alone, lipreading alone, and electrical stimulation plus lipreading.

A suprasegmental study was also carried out on the first patient to evaluate his ability to perceive prosody. He was presented with prerecorded sentences and asked whether the sentence was a question or a statement. With a question the sentence had a rising intonation, and with a statement a falling intonation. He was also asked to perform tasks requiring him to identify a one- or two-syllable word, a male or female speaker, the word in a sentence receiving the stress or accent, and the difference between spoken sentences and bursts of noise presented with the same rhythm as speech. The results are shown in TABLE 4, which shows the patient's scores to be as follows: for the question–statement determination, 19/20; the one- or two-syllable word, 45/45; the male–female speaker, 24/25; the accented word, 11/20; and noise versus voice, 36/40. These results were all significant at the 0.05 probability level and indicate that prosody was well perceived.

Words and Sentences

The performance of the F0, F2 speech-processor was assessed using a number of standard word and sentence tests. These tests were a closed-set of 16 spondee words and the modified rhyme test.[7] In addition, we used open-sets of

TABLE 4

PROSODY IN PATIENT 1 WITH MULTIPLE-ELECTRODE STIMULATION ALONE

Test	Items (n)	Score
Question–statement	20	19 [a]
One-syllable versus two-syllable	45	45 [a]
Male versus female speaker	25	24 [a]
Stressed word	20	11 [a]
Noise versus voice	40	36 [a]

[a] Significant at p = 0.05.

phonetically balanced (PB), easy vocabulary or WIPI words, open-sets of phonetically balanced AB (Arthur Boothroyd) words,[8] open sets of CID (Central Institute for the Deaf) everyday sentences,[9] open-set sentences of Kalikow, Stevens, and Elliott,[10] and a speech-tracking task.[11]

The average results for patients 1 and 2 for the phonetically balanced AB word test, the CID everyday sentence lists, and speech tracking as described by De Filippo and Scott [11] are shown in TABLE 5. These phonetically balanced word and sentence tests used open-set prerecorded material and were administered to both patients using a female voice. The tests were carried out in 1980 using a laboratory or computer-based speech-processor.

TABLE 5

MEAN PERCENTAGE SCORES ON WORD AND SENTENCE TESTS IN PATIENTS 1 AND 2: OPEN SET

Condition	AB Words		CID Sentences	Speech-tracking
	Phoneme	Word		
Multiple-electrode stimulation alone	20%	5%	11%	—
Lipreading alone	58%	20%	24%	9.0 words/min
Electrical stimulation plus lipreading	76%	50%	83%	24.8 words/min

The results showed that with the phonetically balanced word test, scored phonetically, the patients obtained 20% for electrical stimulation alone, 58% for lipreading alone, and 76% for electrical stimulation plus lipreading. When the test was scored on the basis of the words recognized, the patients achieved 5% for electrical stimulation alone, 20% for lipreading alone, and 50% for electrical stimulation plus lipreading.[12] For the CID sentence tests, the patients scored an average of 11% for electrical stimulation, 24% for lipreading alone, and 85% for electrical stimulation plus lipreading.[13] Finally, with speech-tracking the patients could repeat, at a rate of 9.0 words/minute, the passages read to them when using lipreading alone. With lipreading combined with electrical stimulation, their ability to understand connected discourse increased to 24.8 words/minute.[14]

These audiological findings indicate that the improvements obtained with multiple-channel electrical stimulation, as shown by the phoneme and feature scores, carry over to the perception of words, sentences, and connected discourse. They also show that multiple-channel electrical stimulation combined with lipreading produced very significant improvements in patients' abilities to communicate when compared to results with lipreading alone.

These improvements in speech perception were also confirmed with a closed-set modified rhyme and an open-set sentence test, as described by Kalikow, Stevens, and Elliott.[10]

Single-Channel versus Multiple-Channel Stimulation

After the audiological tests just described, a small wearable unit was designed that could be used by patients in their home environment. Our first patient received this unit in May 1980, and has been using it continuously ever since. During this time the speech-processor extracted and presented him with both fundamental frequency F0, and second formant F2 information. After the speech-processor was used in this way for some time, it was considered appropriate to compare the performance of the device for single-channel stimulation conveying F0 information, and multiple-channel stimulation providing both F0 and F2 information.

This comparison was undertaken during a 3-day-period in March 1982, using closed-sets of 16 spondee words, open-sets of phonetically balanced or PB words from the easy vocabulary of the WIPI list, and open-sets of CID everyday

Table 6

Single-Channel versus Multiple-Channel Stimulation in Patient 1

		Condition	Single Channel F0	Multiple Channel F0 + F2
Closed set	16 spondees	EA	28%	100%
	PB words			
Open set	Words	EA	0%	28%
	Phonemes	EA	8%	50%
		EA	0%	22%
Open set	CID sentences	LA	42%	36%
		E + L	60%	98%

Abbreviations: EA = electrical stimulation alone; LA = lipreading alone; E + L = electrical stimulation plus lipreading.

sentences. The tests were administered live by a male audiologist with experience in live-voice presentation. The patient was tested in a sound-attenuated room with the audiologist outside, and lipreading was assessed using a video monitor. The words and sentences were presented at an optimal loudness level determined on the basis of prior psychophysical findings. For the 16 spondees there was a total of 80 words presented.

The PB words were presented as lists of 25 words and separate lists were used for single- and multiple-channel assessments. The CID sentence lists contained 10 sentences and 50 score-words. Different lists were also used for single- and multiple-channel comparisons.

The results are shown in Table 6. The closed-set 16-spondee word-test scores for electrical stimulation alone were 28% for single- and 100% for multiple-channel stimulation. With open-set PB words the word score for electrical stimulation alone was 0% for single-channel and 28% for multiple-channel stimulation. When the test was scored phonetically, the patient obtained 8% for single-channel and 50% for multiple-channel stimulation. With open-set

CID sentences, the patient scored 0% for single-channel and 22% for multiple-channel electrical stimulation alone. He also scored 60% for single-channel and 98% for multiple-channel stimulation when electrical stimulation was combined with lipreading.

Conclusion

In conclusion, our audiological assessment shows that the F0, F2 multiple-channel speech-processor provides significant help with speech perception, and that the results for multiple-channel stimulation were very much better than those obtained for single-channel stimulation of the same patient.

References

1. Tong, Y. C. & G. M. Clark. 1980. Proc. Aust. Physiol. Pharmacol. Soc. **11:** 201P.
2. Tong, Y. C., J. B. Millar, G. M. Clark, L. F. Martin, P. A. Busby & J. F. Patrick. 1980. J. Laryngol. Otol. **94:** 1241–1256.
3. Tong, Y. C., G. M. Clark, P. M. Seligman & J. F. Patrick. 1980. J. Acoust. Soc. Am. **68:** 1897–1899.
4. Clark, G. M. & Y. C. Tong. Arch. Otolaryngol. **108:** 214–217.
5. Clark, G. M., Y. C. Tong & L. F. A. Martin. Ann. Otol. Rhinol. Laryngol. **90:** 227–230.
6. Miller, G. A. & P. E. Nicely. 1955. J. Acoust. Soc. Am. **27:** 338–351.
7. House, A. S., C. E. Williams, M. H. L. Hecker & K. D. Kryter. 1965. J. Acoust. Soc. Am. **37:** 158–166.
8. Boothroyd, A. 1968. Sound (Br. J. Audiol.) **2:** 3–10.
9. Hirsh, I. J., H. Davis, S. R. Silverman, E. G. Reynolds & E. Eldert. 1952. J. Speech Hear. Disord. **17:** 321–337.
10. Kalikow, D. N., K. N. Stevens & L. L. Elliott. 1977. J. Acoust. Soc. Am. **61:** 1337–1351.
11. De Filippo, C. L. & B. L. Scott. 1978. J. Acoust. Soc. Am. **63:** 1186–1192.
12. Clark, G. M., Y. C. Tong, L. F. A. Martin & P. A. Busby. 1981. Acta Otolaryngol. **91:** 173–175.
13. Clark, G. M., Y. C. Tong & L. F. A. Martin. 1981. Laryngoscope **91:** 628–634.
14. Martin, L. F. A., Y. C. Tong & G. M. Clark. 1981. Arch. Otolaryngol. **107:** 157–159.

RESULTS OF STIMULUS AND SPEECH-CODING SCHEMES APPLIED TO MULTICHANNEL ELECTRODES [a]

Les E. Atlas and Matt K. Herndon

AEL 132
Stanford Electronics Laboratory
Stanford, California 94305

F. Blair Simmons and Laurel J. Dent

Division of Otolaryngology
Stanford University School of Medicine
Stanford, California 94305

Robert L. White

Department of Electrical Engineering
Stanford University
Stanford, California 94305

INTRODUCTION

Most research in auditory implants is directed toward unaided speech comprehension for the profoundly deaf. Guided by past studies, the seemingly infinite number of possible electrical stimulation patterns for representing speech can be lessened, possibly resulting in speech-coding strategies that attain this goal. We hope to aid this convergence with this summary of the relative effectiveness of some speech-coding schemes we have appraised.

Since the summer of 1977, the Stanford Auditory Prosthesis Project has been evaluating the auditory perceptions of two subjects having four-wire modiolar electrode implants. The wire electrode array is connected to a five-terminal transcutaneous plug behind the implanted ear. Currently, only one volunteer subject, R.F., is undergoing testing; the other subject, J.M., underwent explantation in 1979 because of infection. R.F., who lives close to Stanford University, has been readily available for testing for the past 5 years. This testing has spanned the range from basic psychoacoustical studies to studies of performance with various speech-coding algorithms. These speech-coding schemes are the focus of this paper: we will present a summary of the rationale behind the coding schemes and data about the subjects' relative performance on them, and then we will conjecture on the reasons for the observed differences in relative performance.

BACKGROUND

One important, possibly principal, function of a speech-processing scheme is to match acoustic signals to known perceptual capabilities for electrical stimulation. These capabilities, as interpreted from psychoacoustical studies [1]

[b] The term "channel capacity" is used loosely here. Certainly the classical definition Institutes of Health.

0077–8923/83/0405–0377 $1.75/0 © 1983, NYAS

for the two implant subjects, are similar to those generally reported for auditory implants. FIGURE 1 depicts the effect of pulse rate and electrode stimulated on perceived pitch. These data show considerable difference in scaled pitch among the electrodes, as well as rising pitch with stimulation rate in the range 50–300 pulses per second (pps), but no change in pitch above 300 pps. We have also explored the relationship between stimulus intensity and perceived loudness. From this relationship we have developed a "map" that mimics the loudness growth in normal listeners. This map, a function relating acoustical sound power and charge delivered, implies a nonlinear compression of the acoustic power. Specifically,

$$Q = T + k(P)^{0.3}$$

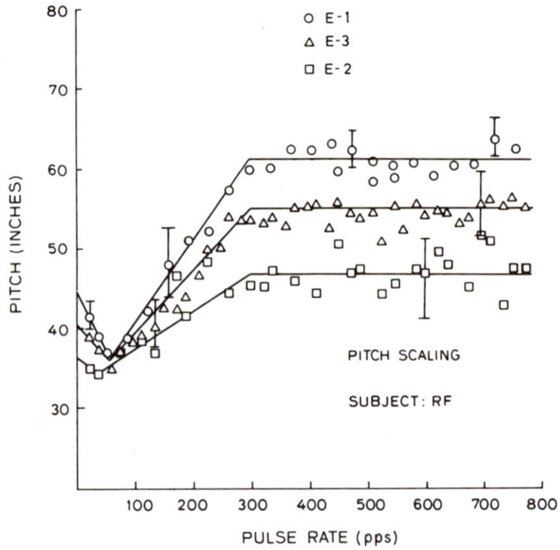

FIGURE 1. Pitch-scaling for three electrodes.

where Q = charge delivered, T = perceptual threshold, k = scaling constant, and P = acoustic power.

These observations imply that the parameters of perceived pitch and loudness are reduced relative to normal listeners. With the degradations in mind, we have considered some design philosophies for speech-processing schemes. One approach seeks to extract and present only that information that is most pertinent to conveying the phonetic informaion in speech. The second approach operates on the theory that the extraction of features is best left to the degraded, yet functional, natural auditory system (beyond the cochlea). Using the first approach, one attempts speech-processing strategies based on channel-capacity-reducing schemes, such as formant vocoders,[2] and tries to extract features and insert them in a manner matched to "channel capacity." [b] In the second approach one does not use feature extraction externally, but uses knowledge of the system degradations to "shape" the electrical stimulation patterns. An example of this is the map of normal-loudness growth onto the reduced dynamic range of electrical stimulation.

Another possible division of approaches rests on the mode of application of the speech-processing scheme. Here the dichotomy exists between research versus clinical uses. A research type of speech-processor may not be bound by the constraints inherent in a portable, real-time speech-processor intended for clinical use. The former processing scheme, with these relaxed constraints, can be designed to take advantage of the full memory and computational power of a large computer, allowing for such amenities as extensive and accurate feature extraction, arbitrarily close approximation of the perceptual maps derived from psychoacoustical data, and possibly future needs for phoneme recognition. On the other hand, for clinical applications, we wish to provide implanted subjects with a "wear-home" box. In this case computational facilities will be limited. Yet a wear-home box will allow monitoring of such developments as learning of speech cues with daily use of a given speech-processing scheme.

Methods

An assessment of a speech-coding strategy is intended as a prediction of performance in everyday use and as a guide to future strategy development. Anecdotal reports, while certainly valuable in assisting the adjustments of a speech-processing algorithm, do not provide any detailed quantitative information. Appropriate speech tests can provide this quantitative information. If the tests are grouped and analyzed on a task basis, the detailed information provided suggests the strong and weak points of a given strategy. Some tests are a measure of auditory discrimination, where the discrimination achieved provides a basic measure of information-transfer capability. Other tests measure speech identification, and focus more directly on speech understanding. The speech tests we have used are mainly measures of identification, thus serving as measures of speech understanding. We have assumed that these tests will predict speech comprehension performance in everyday use.

We have used two different batteries of standardized taped speech tests. The first of these batteries, the Minimal Auditory Capabilities (MAC) tests, was designed specifically for auditory implant subjects.[3] There are 13 tests in the MAC battery, but only 10 were used in these studies. For convenience, these tests may be divided into three levels of difficulty: "easy," "hard," and "intermediate."

The "easy" tests included tests that asked the subject to determine: (1) whether an utterance was a question or a statement; (2) whether an utterance was a voice or noise, where the noise amplitude followed the amplitude envelope of a voice; (3) which word in a sentence was accented; and (4) whether two spondees spoken in succession were the same word or two different words. Chance performance is nominally 50% on all items except item 3, where chance is nominally 25%.

[b] The term "channel capacity" is used loosely here. Certainly the classical definition of channel capacity is difficult to apply to auditory prostheses.

The two "hard" tests involved open-set material with no visual clues and no previous exposure to the material. There is an everyday sentences test, in which the subject is asked to repeat as much of a sentence as he understands and a spondee-recognition test, in which the subject is asked to repeat a spondee that is spoken.

The tests of intermediate difficulty provided the most useful information. In each of these tests the subject was asked to listen to a word spoken and then to select the word spoken from a set of four written choices. Each of the four choices was similar, being monosyllabic and differing by only one sound. For example, in the vowel test, the four choices differed only in their vowel, as in *leap, lap, lip,* and *loop*. There is also an initial consonant test and a final consonant test, in which the four choices differ only in those sounds. In the spondee test all four choices were spondees. Chance is nominally 25% in each of these tests.

The other test battery used with several of the speech-processing schemes was the Diagnostic Rhyme Test (DRT). This test was designed [4] to diagnose those acoustic features of initial consonants that are not perceived or discriminated well. Each item of the test involves two rhyming words, the initial consonants of which differ by a single phonemic attribute or feature. For example, the subject would choose between *nab* or *dab* when one of the two was spoken.

Results and Interpretation

Recalling the division between research and clinical uses that was made earlier, we will begin with discussion of the non-real-time research type of strategies, continue with the more clinical real-time schemes, and finish with the discussion of the effect of learning.

We have implemented four research-type strategies, non-real-time on a computer. The taped speech tests were digitized, processed by the algorithm, and then played back, real-time, to the subject. While the first three of these strategies stimulated one electrode (E1), the last strategy used three of the modiolar electrodes.

The first strategy is what we call the "zeroth-order algorithm." This algorithm purposely presented a limited amount of information in order to provide a baseline against which other algorithms may be compared. The algorithm put out a fixed-frequency 100 pps pulse train on electrode 1 (E1). The pulse train was amplitude-modulated according to the amount of power in the acoustic signal. Specifically, the amount of charge (Q) in a given pulse is a function of the amount of power (P) in the acoustic signal during the 10-msec period since the previous pulse. This functional relationship is based on the loudness map discussed earlier.

The second algorithm studied for research purposes was the "fundamental-frequency algorithm." This algorithm added fundamental-frequency information to the zeroth-order algorithm. Power level was mapped to charge level in the same fashion as in the zeroth-order algorithm, but the frequency of stimulation varied as a function of the fundamental frequency of the speech. Specifically, an electrical pulse was delivered to the electrode when (and only when) a glottal pulse was detected in the speech signal. The glottal pulses were detected using a linear-predictive algorithm developed by Lee.[5]

The third algorithm studied was the log-compressed analog algorithm. This algorithm presented an analog representation of the acoustic signal on E1. The signal was instantaneously log-compressed to compensate for the limited dynamic range of the prosthetic auditory system. When this electrical signal is amplified and fed to a speaker, the resulting sound is easily intelligible to the normal ear; thus, the signal presented to the subject's electrode is known to contain enough information for speech comprehension by normal listeners.

The fourth strategy tried, the formant-tracking algorithm, used three electrodes. The first two electrodes conveyed information about F1 and F2, and the third signaled whether the speech is voiced or unvoiced. This algorithm used a linear-predictive formant-tracker developed by Markel and Gray [6] to extract the F1 and F2 frequencies and amplitudes from the acoustic signal, and used the method of Knorr [7] to make a voiced/unvoiced decision.

TABLE 1

RESULTS OF SPEECH TESTS FOR FOUR RESEARCH-TYPE-ALGORITHMS

Test	Significance ($p < 0.05$)	Zeroth-Order		FO		Analog	Formant-Tracking	
		RF	NC	RF	NC	RF	RF	JM
Dates Administered		6/80	7/80	7/80	10/80	10/80	1/81	5/79
Question/statement	70%	50%	55%	65%	80%	50%	45%	56%
Noise/voice	65%	42%	60%	55%	52%	55%	68%	—
Accent	45%	45%	45%	60%	55%	60%	35%	—
Spondee same/different	70%	70%	75%	70%	80%	55%	45%	80%
Vowel	32%	32%	17%	33%	20%	32%	37%	33%
Initial consonant	35%	24%	30%	28%	25%	35%	44%	47%
Final consonant	35%	29%	27%	46%	40%	33%	44%	53%
4-choice spondee	45%	45%	20%	40%	35%	40%	40%	55%
Spondee recognition	5%	0%	0%	0%	0%	0%	0%	0%
Everyday sentences	5%	0%	0%	3%	1%	3%	1%	3%

When the speech was unvoiced, a high-frequency stimulus was delivered to E4. This stimulus consisted of a pair of pulses separated by 600 μsec and repeating every 2 msec; its amplitude was mapped as charge level, as in the zeroth-order algorithm. The formant frequencies were extracted and mapped onto the usable frequency range of the electrodes as inferred from FIGURE 1, that is, 50 to 325 Hz. For example, a formant at 200 Hz would cause a stimulus frequency of 66 pps and a formant of 2600 Hz would cause a stimulus at 325 pps. The amplitude of the formants was encoded as charge level, as in the zeroth-order algorithm (thresholds and maximum charge vary from electrode to electrode, however). F1 was placed on E3 and F2 was placed on E1.

The taped speech tests were processed by each of the four algorithms and presented to three subjects (TABLE 1). Subjects J.M. and R.F. are implant subjects, and subject N.C. is a normal-hearing subject. N.C. listened to the stimuli generated by these algorithms through a model that made them audible; this model was intended to make the stimuli sound approximately the same to N.C. as to the implant subjects. Subject J.M. was evaluated only on the formant-tracking algorithm. He actually had a less accurate but portable version of this algorithm and had about 6 months' experience using the portable device before he took the tests.

The "zeroth-order algorithm" provided a baseline against which the others may be compared. For example, some improvement is seen in the "fundamental-frequency algorithm" in the question/statement test and in the final consonant test. The improvement in final consonant identificaion may have resulted from improved performance in making the voiced/unvoiced distinction, possibly owing to the difference in direction of F0 before voiced versus unvoiced final consonants.

The "log-compressed analog algorithm" showed some improvement on the initial consonant test.

The "formant-tracking algorithm" showed the best overall performance. J.M. scored significantly above chance at the 5% level on all four of the intermediate tests. R.F. performed slightly better than for the other algorithms, although not as well as I.M.

Subsequent to the explantation of the electrode device in J.M., we decided to try five more speech-processing schemes with R.F. The goal of this study was to decide which scheme offered the best performance, to provide R.F. with a pocket-sized speech-processor embodying that algorithm, and then to study the effect of daily use of the processor on speech test performance over time. These algorithms are what was referred to earlier as the clinical types; the application is for a miniature, portable, real-time processor. The processor size dictates that computation is limited. Also, all algorithms were designed to use a single electrode (E1).

Speech tests with these algorithms were processed with real-time prototypes of the pocket-sized processor. The first processing strategy is depicted in FIGURE 2. This algorithm, called "compressed analog," is based on an instantaneous compressor that approximates the loudness map described earlier. As mathematically described by the loudness map, this compressor matches the wide power range of speech to the smaller range of charge necessary for the implant subject to perceive the continuum from threshold to quite loud. This algorithm also serves as the basic building block for the next four strategies that we tried. The automatic volume control (AVC) was used as an answer to the subject's complaints of sensitivity to microphone placement. His previous processor, which had no AVC, would only work well when the volume control was constantly adjusted to track differences in source to microphone distance.

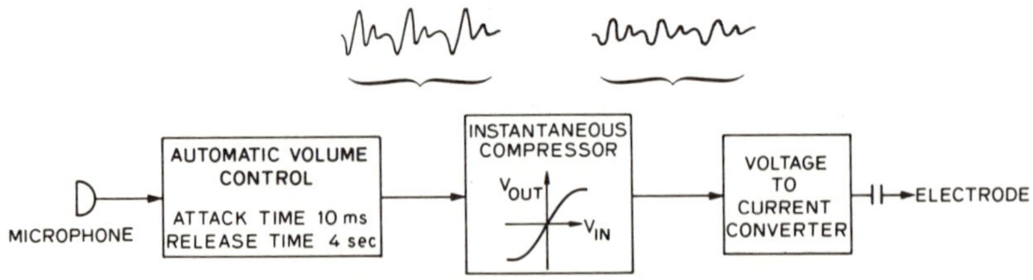

FIGURE 2. Compressed analog algorithm.

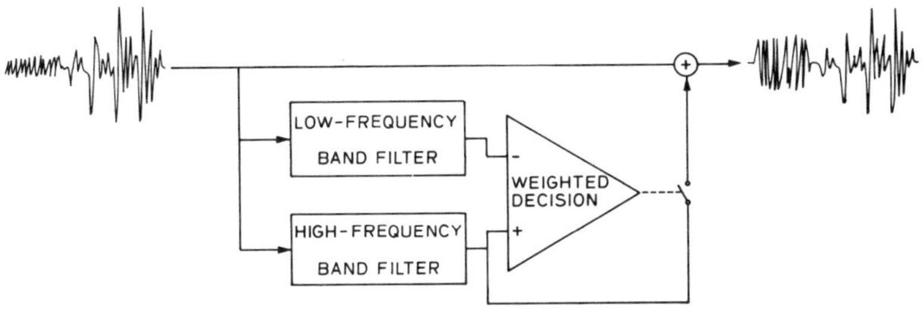

FIGURE 3. High-frequency cueing system.

The AVC is intended to automate these adjustments. The function of this AVC is best described by these remarks of Braida *et al.*[8]:

> . . . AVC is used to keep the long-term average presentation level (measured over time intervals corresponding to phrases or sentences) near that corresponding to maximum intelligibility. Since the action of automatic volume control should be slow compared to the sound variations that occur within syllables, it can be regarded as a slowly varying linear amplifier.

The sound variations within syllables are preserved as clues, where they are matched to the subject's loudness variation by the instantaneous compressor. The last block in the algorithm, the voltage-to-current converter, allows for the accurate metering of charge, independent of nonlinearities in electrode impedance.

FIGURE 3 illustrates the functional blocks that, when added to the "compressed analog algorithm," result in the strategy called "compressed analog with high-frequency cueing." Cueing is intended to emphasize the fricative and sibilant portions of speech, since these phonemes, while important, have less energy than in most voiced sounds. Since these low-energy sibilant and fricative phonemes tend to be dominant in high frequencies, a weighted comparison between high- and low-frequency bands can crudely recognize these features. Once recognized, the amplitude of these features can be boosted to energy levels closer to the voiced sounds. The phonemes with lower-frequency content will, in theory, pass through the cueing system unchanged. We experimented with various frequency bands for the decision, but found that this system sometimes identified vocalic /i/ as a fricative, regardless of the characteristics of the frequency bands.

FIGURE 4 depicts the basis for the "pulsatile" algorithm. These functional blocks, when integrated into the system seen in FIGURE 2, provide for a pulsatile representation of speech. The pulse-extraction scheme retains the zerocrossing and amplitude information in speech and uses this information to control the location and amplitude of biphasic stimulation pulses. These stimulation pulses, 250 μsec in width, follow the amplitude contour of speech, with a provision that pulses occur only when the speech amplitude is greater than a threshold. This "thresholding" reduces the sensitivity to noise. The input and output waveforms in FIGURE 4 illustrate how the pulses represent the amplitudes and locations of the peaks in the speech waveform. Note that the small peaks in the speech waveform are not represented; this is because of the thresholding.

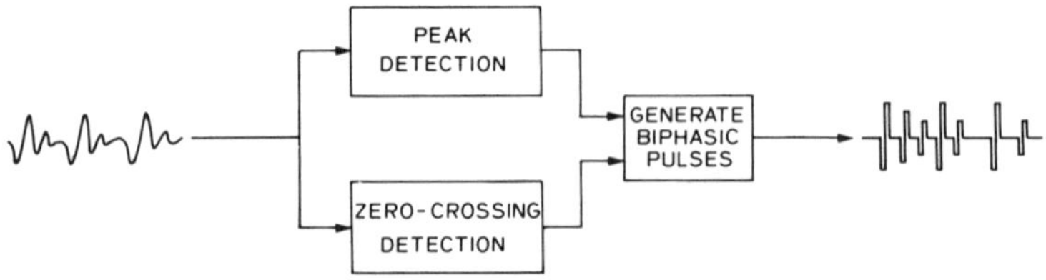

FIGURE 4. Pulse extraction.

The fourth algorithm, the "pulsatile with cueing" algorithm, is simply a combination of the last two algorithms mentioned. High-frequency cueing is used to emphasize the fricatives before the biphasic pulses are extracted.

The fifth, and last, scheme is called the "compressed analog followed by differentiation" algorithm. The intent here is to replace the on–off type of decision in the high-frequency cueing system with a smoother function. FIGURE 5 shows that, by having a stage of differentiation following the instantaneous compressor, the power of the high-frequency fricatives is boosted relative to that of the lower-frequency voiced portions of speech. The input and output waveforms in this figure illustrate that the higher-frequency content of the speech is boosted. Also, careful inspection reveals that the voiced portion of the speech is not unchanged: higher frequencies are boosted here also, emphasizing the zerocrossings (a possibly desirable effect).

The results of the comparison of these five candidate real-time strategies are summarized in TABLE 2. We used a battery of taped speech tests incorporating three of the MAC tests (question/statement, spondee same/different, and vowel identification) and four randomizations of the DRT (192 items). We tested these algorithms on one subject, R.F., thereby eliminating possible subject-to-subject variations. The results, while not revealing any marked differences between algorithms, show that some of these differences were significant.

The compressed analog algorithm (Ca.) resulted in performance significantly above chance for only the spondee same/different test. Possibly this algorithm provided enough information for the same/different discrimination task, but did not provide the information in a form recognizable enough to allow for the identifications necessary in the other three tasks.

Compressed analog with high-frequency cueing (Caq.) results show, again, performance significantly better than chance on the same/different task. The performance on the question/statement test improved, possibly owing to the more effective presentation of the duration of fricatives at the ends of sentences.

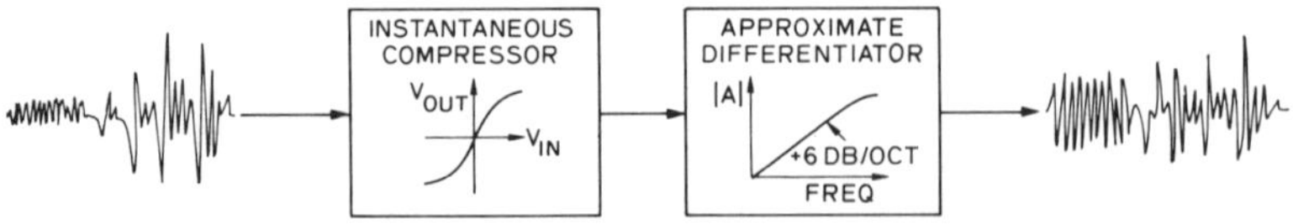

FIGURE 5. Post-compression differentiator.

The pulsatile algorithm (P.) performed like the Ca. algorithm; a result significantly greater than chance was seen only for the spondee same/different test.

The pulsatile with high-frequency cueing algorithm (Pq.) again demonstrated that the high-frequency cueing improves question/statement distinctions. Also, a drop in the result for the spondee same/different test was seen for Pq.

The final algorithm, the compressed analog followed by differentiation (Cad.), resulted in possibly the most pronounced improvement. Initial consonant identifications on the Diagnostic Rhyme Test were significantly above the chance level for only this Cad. algorithm. However, the performance on the spondee same/different test was not particularly good. Another interesting aspect of this Cad. algorithm was the unsolicited anecdotal report about the pitch of speech. The subject, R.F., initially reported that for this algorithm only, female voices sounded higher than male voices. R.F. also correctly ranked the nominal pitch of two male voices.

TABLE 2

RESULTS OF SPEECH TESTS FOR FIVE POSSIBLE PORTABLE ALGORITHMS

Test	Chance	Significance ($p < 0.05$)	Ca.	Caq.	P.	Pq.	Cad.
Question/statement	50%	70%	55%	75%	60%	80%	75%
Spondee same/different	50%	70%	80%	85%	75%	65%	65%
Vowel identification	25%	32%	31%	35%	27%	35%	27%
Diagnostic rhyme	50%	56%	44%	55%	45%	56%	63%

Of the five previously mentioned algorithms, one was chosen to be constructed as a pocket-sized processor and given to R.F. to take home. On the basis of the performance on the DRT and on the anecdote of accurate voice pitch, we decided to use the Cad. algorithm. Before giving R.F. the pocket-sized processor (the processor is named MSP-1: Miniature Speech Processor, version 1) to take home, we administered an almost complete battery of the MAC test using MSP-1. The DRT was also given. This series of tests was a prelude to a study of learning; after 4 months of everyday use, R.F. was again tested with the same taped speech tests played through MSP-1. The results of this study of 4 months' learning are listed in TABLE 3. This study demonstrated no definitive evidence of learning. While it is true that some test scores, such as the accent and vowel tests, improved, several other test scores dropped, indicating that any changes over the 4 months were mostly because of statistical variations and not reflections of any form of learning. Why was there no significant learning? The possibilities are: (1) Since the subject reports that what he hears does not sound speech-like, the clues presented cannot be well integrated into linguistic memory, hence, learning is difficult. Or (2), the number and types of speech clues available are not sufficient to provide for learning.

TABLE 3

RESULTS OF USE OF MSP–1 FOR 4 MONTHS

Test	Significance ($p < 0.05$)	Date Given: Oct. 15, 1981	Date Given: Feb. 16, 1982
Question/statement	70%	80%	60%
Noise/voice	65%	55%	60%
Accent	45%	45%	65%
Spondee same/different	70%	55%	60%
Vowel identification	32%	27%	35%
Initial consonant	35%	43%	32%
Final consonant	35%	33%	37%
Four choice spondee	45%	50%	30%
Diagnostic rhyme	56%	46%	52%

CONCLUSION

We have presented a summary of two implant subjects' performances on nine different speech-processing schemes. The formant-tracking algorithm, a multielectrode algorithm, performed slightly better than the single-electrode algorithms. High-frequency cueing of fricatives seemed to improve the question/statement distinctions, and differentiation following compression assisted initial consonant identifications. Our results suggest that different clues relevant to speech comprehension are optimized by each of the different modes of processing speech. There was no definitive evidence of learning after 4 months' use of a "wear-home" processor.

REFERENCES

1. HERNDON, M. K. 1981. Psychoacoustics and speech processing of a modiolar auditory prosthesis (Ph.D. dissertation). Technical Report No. G906–5. Integrated Circuits Laboratory. Stanford University. Stanford, CA.
2. MUNSON, W. A. & H. C. MONTGOMERY. 1950. A speech analyzer and synthesizer. J. Acoust. Soc. Am. **22**(A). 678.
3. OWENS, E., D. K. KESSLER, C. C. TELLEEN & E. D. SCHUBERT. 1980. The Minimal Auditory Capabilities Battery. Auditec. St. Louis, MO.
4. VOIRES, W. D., A. D. SHARPLEY & C. J. HEHMSOTH. 1973. Research on diagnostic evaluation of speech intelligibility. Final Report, Contract No. F19628–70–C–0182. Air Force Cambridge Research Laboratories. Bedford, MA.
5. LEE, D. T. L. & M. MORF. 1978. Fast algorithms for speech modeling. Technical Report No. M308–1. Information Systems Laboratory. Stanford University. Stanford, CA.
6. MARKEL, J. D. & A. H. GRAY. 1976. Linear Prediction of Speech. Springer Verlag. New York, NY.
7. KNORR, S. G. 1976. A hearing aid for subjects with extreme high-frequency losses. IEEE Trans. Acous., Speech, Sig. Proc. **24:** 473–480.
8. BRAIDA, L. D., N. I. DURLACH, R. P. LIPPMANN, B. L. HICKS, W. M. RABINOWITZ & C. M. REED. 1980. Hearing Aids: A Review of Past Research on Linear Amplification, Amplitude Compression, and Frequency Lowering. ASHA Monographs **19:** 52–53. American Speech-Language-Hearing Association. Rockville, MD.

LONG-TERM RESULTS OF THE MULTICHANNEL COCHLEAR IMPLANT [a]

C.-H. Chouard, C. Fugain, B. Meyer, and H. Lacombe

ENT Research Laboratory and ENT Department
Centre Hospitalo-Universitaire Paris-Saint-Antoine
75012 Paris, France

INTRODUCTION

Our studies, aimed at the restoration of hearing in patients with total deafness by means of a multichannel cochlear implant, were begun in 1973. Our first patients received implants that were connected by transcutaneous plugs to a portable apparatus. The phoniatric results that we obtained [1] allowed us to design a magnetic transcutaneous multichannel emitter that was delivered in 1976. To date we have implanted 48 patients with this device, and we are now reporting the long-term clinical results of this surgical technique of rehabilitation in patients who are totally deaf.

MATERIALS AND METHODS

Patient Selection

In every case the decision to provide a totally deaf patient with an implant depended on the following conditions: First, the patient must be totally deaf, with a blank audiogram and no response up to 250 Hz. Second, he must have a positive response to the electrical stimulation test through the round window of those cochlear nerve fibers still present. This test must be performed through a transmeatal approach by elevating the eardrum in order to obtain a good view of the round-window fossa, in which the tip of the stimulating electrode has to be placed. Thus, the risk of a false-negative response can be avoided. The electrical stimulus is a negative square wave, 0.1 msec in duration; its voltage may vary from 0 to 10 volts in constant intensity; its frequency rate varies from 0 to 1000 Hz.

The response to this test can be assessed subjectively. It necessitates local anesthesia because the patient has to describe the hearing sensation he perceives. This response may be objectively registered using the auditory brainstem responses evoked by the electrical stimulation of the cochlea; these responses can be also obtained with the patient under general anesthesia. This is especially useful in the case of children: these young, frightened patients would not easily accept local anesthesia.

This positive response merely signifies that at least a few auditory nerve fibers are present. Theoretically it does not say anything concerning the proportion of the fibers present or their distribution on the frequency map of

[a] This work was supported by the Institut National de la Santé et de la Recherche Médicale, the Caisses Nationale et Regionale d'Ile de France d'Assurance Maladie des Travailleurs Salariés, and the Ministère de la Recherche Scientifique de France.

0077-8923/83/0405-0387 $1.75/0 © 1983, NYAS

the cochlea, which would be useful to know in order to predict the quality of future rehabilitation. Nevertheless, as we shall see later, the value of this electrical threshold level seems to have some prognostic significance.

The clinical status of each patient is described in TABLE 1. The degree of socialization of each patient is determined with the help of five variables (social level, degree of intelligence, school level, language, and lipreading), the values of which, from 0 to 3, are summarized to obtain what we have called the patient's socialization coefficient, which may vary from 0 to 15.

Electrode Implantation Technique

The implanted electrodes are 90% platinum–10% iridium, 125 microns in bare diameter, and Teflon®-coated. The 12 electrodes are implanted one by one in the scala tympani through 12 fenestrations that are made in the cochlear bone. Each electrode must stimulate only the cochlear fibers that are just in front of its own bare tip. In order to obtain this selective stimulation, electrically insulated compartments are created by means of several pieces of Silastic® that are introduced through the fenestrations in the scala tympani. It must be emphasized that the functional location of these fenestrations does not correspond to the frequencies devoted to each electrode, which will explain the new sound-decoding system.

The surgical technique is simple: A large skin incision is necessary in order to keep the implanted receptor far from the scar. A middle-ear approach is sufficient to make the 12 fenestrations. A radical mastoidectomy allows the surgeon to visualize and make, as we have previously described,[2] five or six holes in the second turn and six or seven holes in the first turn of the cochlea (FIGURE 1). The impedance between electrodes is measured, and the efficacy of each of them is determined by means of brainstem-evoked responses, in order to be sure that enough, but not too much, Silastic was introduced. Because of bony chips, the electrodes are solidly attached with the help of cyano-acrylate-butyl; the eustachian tube is closed, sealing off the air-containing cavity of the middle ear and mastoid. The external auditory canal is carefully sewn shut near the meatus. Each electrode is connected to each channel of the receptor by means of a small connector that allows the device to be easily changed in case of failure.

Procedures for Placement of the Prosthesis

Our first twelve patients received an 8-channel implant. Then one year later we designed a 12-channel device, which has been implanted in all other patients. It is this 12-channel implant that we will now describe; it is now underwritten by the national health insurance companies of France.

The apparatus contains an outside emitter with batteries and an implanted receptor. The external device transforms the acoustic information into 12 series of signals formed so as to be transmitted in a coded fashion by means of an antenna to the implanted receptor, which consists of a receiving coil and a decoding system.

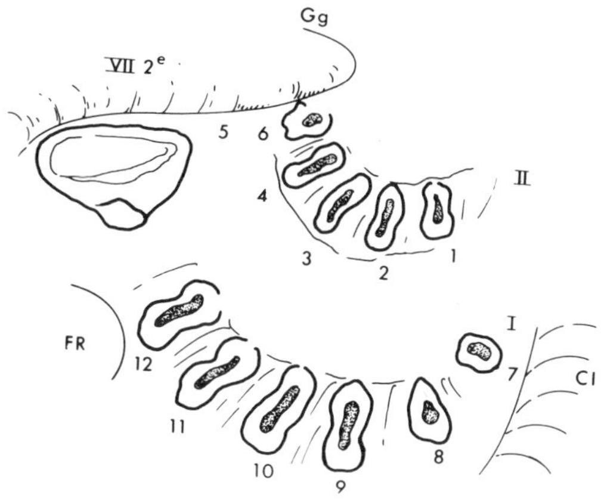

FIGURE 1. Location of the fenestrations on the promontory. Fenestrations 7 and 8 are sometimes difficult to make because the first turn dashes into the petrous bone, close to the internal carotid canal. The tip of each electrode is bent towards the apex unless only five fenestrations have been made in the second turn; in this case, electrodes 5 and 6 are implanted in the same hole, but electrode 6 is bent towards the basal turn. VII 2ᵉ = the second portion of the fallopian canal; Gg = the geniculate ganglion; I and II = the first and second turn; FR = the round window; and CI = internal carotid canal.

Outside Emitter

The emitter weighs 600 grams and is in the shape of a parallelepiped rectangle measuring 165 × 150 × 45 mm. The emitter may be worn on the shoulder or hidden in a bag. It is possible to connect it to an outside directional microphone.

The acoustic message is cut at 40 dB in order to favor speech understanding. Then it is divided into 12 channels by 12 filters. The different energies of each filter are selected one after the other with a multiplexer in 3-msec samples. Then a semilogarithmic conversion is made with a compression rate of 60 dB to adapt the electrical message to the characteristics of the ear. Each of these 12 energy levels is adjusted by a wheel ponderation system as a function of each electrode–nerve interface, which reflects differences resulting from the small variations of the surgical implantation procedure. Then these energy levels are converted to impulses of variable duration. In this way successive chains of impulses are produced, each chain having a start signal and an impulse of variable duration corresponding to each channel. The elementary impulse chaining cycle only functions when a signal must be sent, which greatly diminishes power consumption. All of these chains are modulated by a carrying wave of 3.2-MHz energy vector, which allows the cutaneous wall to be passed by means of an antenna.

Implanted Receptor

The implanted receptor is in the shape of a flattened, truncated cone 10 mm in thickness, with section slices of 25 and 30 mm in diameter, respectively. To

TABLE 1

CLINICAL STATUS OF THE 48 PATIENTS RECEIVING IMPLANTS

	Patient	Date of Operation	Age (yr) and Sex	Etiology	Specialization Coefficient: Variables	Specialization Coefficient: Total	Specialization Coefficient: SE	Remarks
1	(N.F.)	10/27/76	22,M	Tubal meningitis (SA)	1 1 2 2 2	8	25	
2	(B.J.-N.)	10/28/76	23,M	Meningitis; undetermined (SM)	1 1 2 2 1	7	10	
3	(L.P.)	11/3/76	18,M	Undetermined (SM)	3 2 3 2 1	11	15	
4	(R.J.-Y.)	6/23/77	19,M	Rnbella (SM)	3 3 3 3 3	15	15	
5	(L.M.)	7/5/77	30,F	Chronic otitis (SA)	3 3 3 3 3	15	25	
6	(C.A.)	8/3/77	15,F	Undetermined (SM)	3 2 3 3 2	13	10	
7	(T.E.)	8/10/77	11,M	Rubella (SM)	2 1 2 1 1	7	15	
8	(D.L.)	8/17/77	36,M	Tubal meningitis (SM)	2 1 2 1 1	7	30	Mute, no language
9	(P.C.)	10/13/77	27,M	Fracture (SA)	3 2 3 2 3	13	07	Foreign language
10	(L.G.)	10/19/77	37,F	Mumps (SA)	2 2 3 2 1	10	08	Foreign language
11	(A.M.)	11/9/77	45,F	Tubal meningitis (SA)	2 1 3 2 3	11	20	
12	(D.C.)	11/16/77	57,M	Otosclerosis (SA)	2 1 2 1 3	9	10	
13	(P.A.)	3/29/78	23,M	Meningitis; undetermined (SM)	1 1 2 1 1	6	05	
14	(Z.A.)	4/6/78	47,M	Chronic otititis (SA)	3 2 2 3 2	13	10	
15	(W.F.)	8/10/78	45,F	Otosclerosis (SA)	2 1 3 2 3	11	13	
16	(Q.J.)	8/10/78	22,F	Undetermined (SM)	2 1 1 1 1	6	10	Mute; no language
17	(A.A.)	8/16/78	16,M	Undetermined (SM)	3 2 3 2 2	12	10	Foreign language
18	(A.O.)	8/18/78	19,M	Undetermined (SM)	3 2 3 2 2	12	10	Foreign language
19	(A.E.)	8/21/78	18,F	Undetermined (SM)	2 2 2 1 1	8	07	Foreign language
20	(F.P.)	8/25/78	25,M	Fracture (SA)	3 2 3 2 3	13	10	Almost blind
21	(C.S.)	9/8/78	15,M	Undetermined (SM)	3 1 3 1 1	9	10	Foreign language
22	(L.J.)	9/15/78	27,F	Rubella (SM)	3 2 3 1 3	12	03	Blind (cataracts)
23	(H.J.)	10/25/79	30,M	Undetermined (SM)	1 1 1 1 1	5	10	Mute; no language
24	(P.E.)	5/2/79	56,M	Vascular (SA)	3 2 3 1 3	12	15	Blind (cataracts)
25	(L.R.)	5/9/79	42,M	Undetermined (SM)	2 1 1 1 1	6	03	Mute; no language
26	(G.T.)	6/13/79	42,F	Meningitis and streptococcal infection (SA)	3 2 3 3 3	14	20	

27	(B.J.-C.)	4/30/80	19,M	Undetermined (SM)	2	1	1	1	1	6	10	
28	(D.R.)	5/7/80	22,F	Undetermined (SM)	3	2	3	3	3	14	15	Mondini syndrome
29	(L.S.)	8/13/80	10,F	Undetermined (SM)	3	1	1	1	1	7	20	Autistic
30	(V.R.)	10/8/80	50,F	Chronic otitis (SA)	3	2	3	3	3	14	20	
31	(M.J.-D.)	10/15/80	32,M	Streptococcal infection (SM)	3	2	3	2	2	12	15	
32	(L.A.)	11/5/80	34,F	Rubella (SM)	1	1	2	1	1	6	15	Mute; no language
33	(N.J.)	1/28/81	25,M	Meningitis (meningococcal) (SM)	2	1	3	2	1	9	10	
34	(B.H.)	2/4/81	43,M	Undetermined (SM)	3	3	2	3	3	14	05	Foreign language
35	(W.J.)	2/25/81	41,M	Meningitis; undetermined (S)	3	3	3	3	2	14	07	Ossification of cochlear (5 electrodes)
36	(B.L.)	3/2/81	42,M	Undetermined (SA)	3	3	3	3	2	14	20	
37	(L.G.)	3/4/81	56,M	Chronic otitis (SA)	3	3	3	3	1	13	05	
38	(S.V.)	3/11/81	14,M	Rubella (SM)	2	2	1	1	1	7	15	Foreign language
39	(C.O.)	3/25/81	71,F	Otosclerosis (SA)	3	3	3	3	3	15	25	
40	(C.B.)	5/11/81	22,M	Undetermined (SM)	2	2	1	1	1	7	20	
41	(B.M.)	5/13/81	15,M	Undetermined (SM)	2	1	0	0	0	7	20	Autistic
42	(E.A.)	5/20/81	12,M	Undetermined (SM)	3	2	2	1	2	10	08	
43	(M.M.)	6/10/81	36,F	Pneumoccal meningitis (SA)	3	3	3	3	2	14	13	Aphasia
44	(L.M.)	2/17/82	28,F	Chronic otititis (SA)	2	3	2	3	1	11	15	
45	(M.M.)	2/24/82	46,F	Tubal meningitis (SA)	3	3	3	3	3	15	10	
46	(L.M.-A.)	3/8/82	28,F	Mumps (SA)	2	2	3	3	1	11	04	
47	(D.J.-F.)	3/10/82	28,M	Undetermined (SM)	2	1	1	1	1	6	15	Ossification of cochlear (6 electrodes)
48	(F.F.)	3/22/82	52,M	Undetermined (SA)	2	3	3	3	2	13	05	

ABBREVIATIONS: SA = postlingual deafness; SM = prelingual deafness; SE = value in decivolts of threshold level of round-window electric stimulation test.

avoid any variation in acoustic sensation from small changes in the antenna position, the receptor automatically keeps, up to a certain point, the same voltage-to-output signal. Below this limit, the receptor stops functioning. This tolerates a relative imprecision of the antenna position.

The multiplex message sent by the antenna furnishes each electrode with the appropriate information in the form of a train of impulses. The long-term risks of tissue electrolysis are practically nullified by an electric adaptation. The twelve channels of the receptor are peroperatively individually connected to the corresponding implanted electrodes.

Output Signal

In each electrode the output signal consists of positive square waves. Each positive square wave is immediately followed by a negative wave, longer than the positive one, but of the same energy, in order to avoid electrolytic damage. This square wave is defined by three parameters: frequency, voltage, and duration. Frequency is a constant parameter—it is equal to 300 Hz and is the same for all electrodes for each patient. The voltage for each electrode (between 2.5 and 6.5 volts) is selected the day after the surgical operation in order to compensate for the differences of threshold level of each electrode and then left constant. If necessary, a further change may be easily made in the emitter to compensate for progressive tissue scarring. The duration of the square wave pulses ranges from 0 to 200 μsec and is determined by means of either of two factors: (1) The first is a selection of pulse duration on a scale of 1 to 100 μsec as determined for each electrode by hand, using the coding wheel to calibrate threshold durations at the previously selected voltages for each electrode. This allows us to determine exactly the voltage-duration characteristics of each electrode. (2) Duration is automatically selected by the processor as a value between 1 and 2, proportional to the filtered input signal. This factor is multiplied times the previously determined threshold duration to obtain the duration of the pulse to be delivered to the electrode. This coding system adapts the quantity of energy delivered to each electrode to the electrodynamic range of the cochlea.

Only one electrode is stimulated at a time, and during this stimulation all the other electrodes are grounded. This bipolar system provides the cochlea with a stimulus current especially localized to each electrode. If the input signal necessitates a simultaneous stimulation of the twelve electrodes, this is effective in about 1 to 2.5 msec as a function of the intensity of the input signal and the threshold level of each electrode.

The quantity of energy delivered to each electrode depends on the value of the emitter filters. Two different configurations of filters are actually used as a function of the phoniatric performances of each patient (FIGURE 2). Thus, in some cases it is possible to partially overcome a disadvantageous distribution of remaining auditory nerve fibers on the cochlear keyboard that could not be preoperatively detected. Of course, any other filter configurations might be built if necessary.

The surface area of the bare tip of each electrode varies between 0.2 and 0.5 mm^2. Because of the tangential insertion of each electrode in the cochlear tube, the distance of its extremity to the nerve endings is always greater than 1 mm.

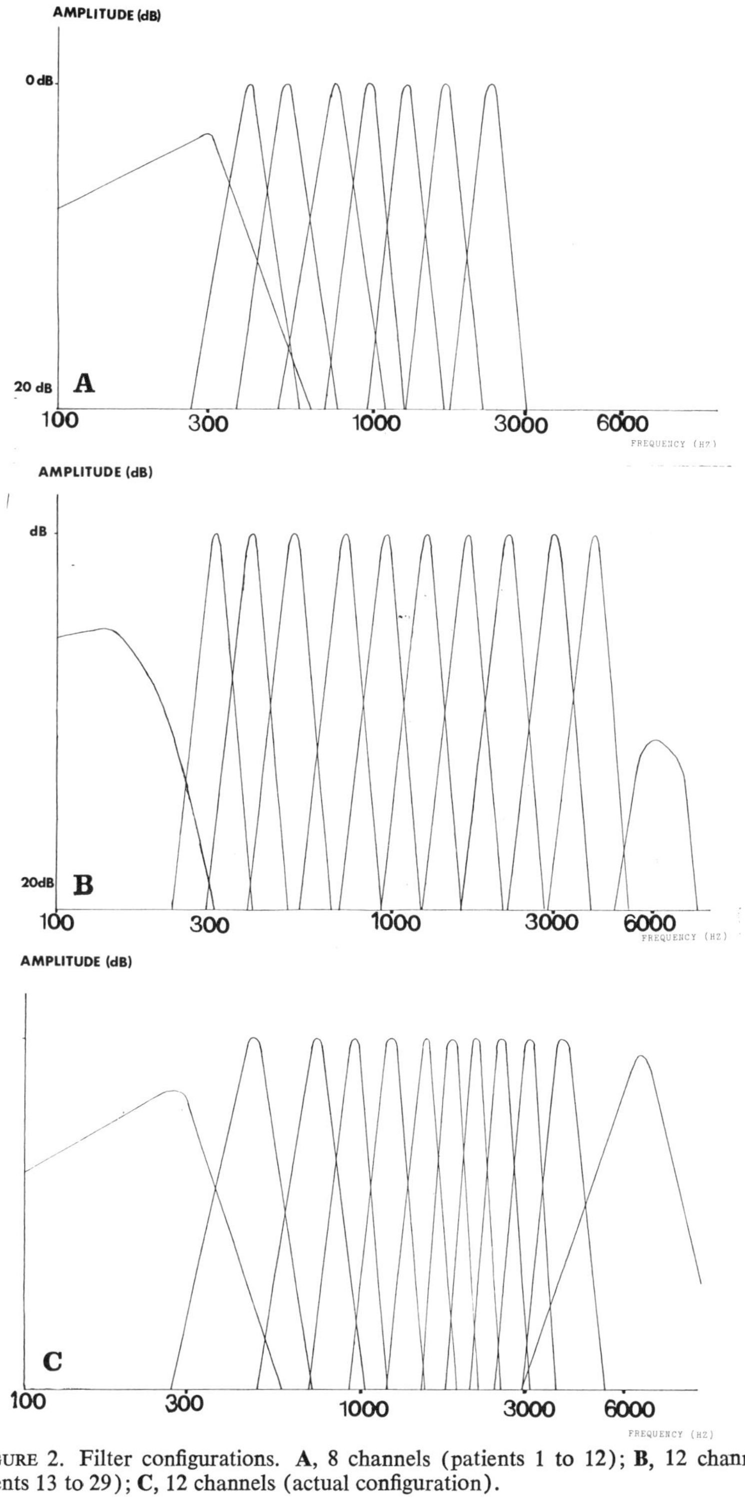

FIGURE 2. Filter configurations. **A**, 8 channels (patients 1 to 12); **B**, 12 channels (patients 13 to 29); **C**, 12 channels (actual configuration).

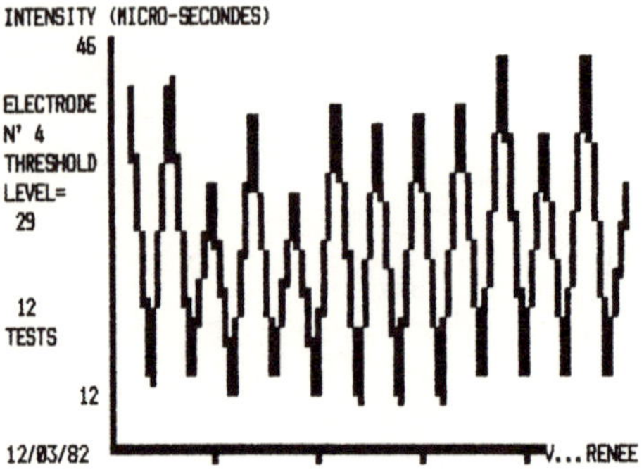

FIGURE 3. Determination of the threshold level of one electrode using a sort of electric Bekesy test. The variation of the duration (ordinate) of each square wave of the permanent electric stimulation corresponds to the variation of the intensity of the acoustic sensation.

Postoperative Electrophysiological Tests

During these tests the stimulation is artificial: the physician directly selects the electrical parameters of the stimulation by means of the coding wheels or a computerized device connected to the emitter. A few days after surgical implantation, the threshold level of each electrode is approximated by manual determination in order to find the starting value, that is, a voltage for each of the 12 channels, which allows an auditory response to be obtained stimulating each one of the 12 electrodes. Then, in the weeks afterward, the following tests are progressively performed with the help of a computerized command of the emitter: (1) The electrical threshold level of each electrode is determined precisely (FIGURE 3). (2) The frequency discrimination of two electrodes at different intensity levels is automatically determined. In these two electrodes, called A and B, for instance, two signals having the same intensity and the same duration are successively presented to the patient; these signals are selected randomly from the four possibilities AA, AB, BB, and BA. The patient must give one of the following responses: equal; different; or "please repeat the test, I am not sure of my sensation." The number of trials needed depends on the nature of the successive responses in order to have a statistically significant (5%) percentage of good or bad discrimination for each of the intensity levels of stimulation. (3) While two electrodes are successively stimulated, the patient is asked to determine which one of them corresponds to the highest and the lowest frequency that he perceives. Thus, for each patient it is possible to make a subjective frequency scale to verify the correct surgical implantation order of the different electrodes; errors may be rectified by changing the place of corresponding filters inside the emitter. Initially this test is impractical for prelingually deaf patients, who necessitate long training to understand the difference between high frequency and high intensity. (4) The patient may directly stimulate successively or simultaneously each of the twelve electrodes by pressing the keys of the computer keyboard like a piano. This distractive test allows the patient to better explain to his reeducator the phoniatric difficulties he may encounter.

Postoperative Training and Phoniatric Tests

During these tests the stimulus is an acoustic signal (noise, sound, speech) directly furnished to the emitter microphone. Phoniatric training consists of teaching the patient to recognize the different features of the new sounds that he is supplied with (rhythms, sounds of everyday life, and popular songs, then phonemes, words, and sentences). The patient's progressive performances are regularly measured by means of random bi- or polypropositional tests and percentages of word or sentence recognition. These tests are administered without the aid of lipreading in order to obtain an objective measurement of the efficacy of the prosthesis. In most cases words are selected in a random manner from a list that the patient can view; results are reported on a double-entry table (FIG. 4). In some cases words are selected without a reference list, but have some reference to the patient's vocabulary and general culture, which are frequently very poor in cases of prelingual deafness. Moreover, in such cases the progressive improvement of speech can be determined by means of successive sonagrams.

RESULTS

Surgical Complications

A few minor complications have been encountered. In eight of our first patients eardrum perforation occurred postoperatively, with intermittent discharge from the ear but without any change in the electrode threshold level. Furthermore, it must be emphasized that four of these patients suffered preoperatively from chronic otitis. This is not encountered any more, for we now fill the ear cavity with bony chips. We have had no complaints of other complications, especially no vertigo regardless of the preoperative vestibular status.[3]

Stimulus \ response		1	2	3	4	5	6	7	8	9	10	11	12	13	14	15	16	17	18	Total Correct	Total Stimuli
Repas	1	5																		5	5
Diner	2		3		2															3	5
Hangar	3			5																5	5
Salut	4		1		4															4	5
Prénom	5					5														5	5
Costume	6						5													5	5
	7																			27	30
	8																				
	9																				
Muguet	10										4				1					4	5
Bourgeon	11											4	1							4	5
Cadran	12											1	4							4	5
Lilas	13													5						5	5
Bijou	14										2				3					3	5
Réveil	15															5				5	5
	16																			25	30
	17																				
	18																				

FIGURE 4. Diagram of the results of recognition test of words of a list presented in a random manner (patient 3 [L.P.] one year after implantation [5/12/72]).

Tolerance for Implanted Materials

The quality of the electrode–nerve interface, indicated by the value of the threshold level of each electrode, is remarkably constant, even in the case of postoperative chronic ear discharge. Among the 515 electrodes that have been implanted (as we shall see later, patients 35 and 47 received only five and six electrodes, respectively), twelve did not function from the beginning for an unknown reason (perhaps excessive Silastic insulation). Among these 503 functioning electrodes, only 28 progressively lost their functional value for different reasons (receptor exchange, electrode traumatic fracture, unknown causes). It must be emphasized that our first three patients, implanted in 1976, have always had the same electrical threshold levels for more than 5 years. Electrical failure of the implanted receptor was encountered during our early trials and necessitated exchanging the device, but this is a very simple operation that can be performed with the patient under local anesthesia.

General Clinical Results

All preoperative cases of intense tinnitus (8 cases) due to chronic otitis (2 cases), otosclerosis (3 cases), skull fracture (2 cases) and undetermined cause (1 case) disappeared after implantation. In three patients with chronic otitis, vertigo, and nystagmus (occurring in two patients in the direction of the ear that was implanted), these symptoms also disappeared after implantation. We have never observed postoperative vestibular complications, and, as we have previously reported,[3] the preoperative vestibular status of each patient did not change after implantation.

All of our patients have been able to hear. The number of hours per day that the patient uses his prosthesis is an indicator of the patient's view of the value of the apparatus in his daily life (FIG. 5).

The psychologic and affective improvement of these patients with implants must be emphasized here, even though this type of progress is not as easily measurable as are other parameters especially phoniatric performance. From this point of view, the case of patient 29 is significant. Prior to implantation this autistic child had neither language nor any other kind of ability to communicate; now, 6 months after the operation, she is interested in persons and things, she has begun to speak and to write, and she is drawn into play with other children or members of her family. We must also report the cases of

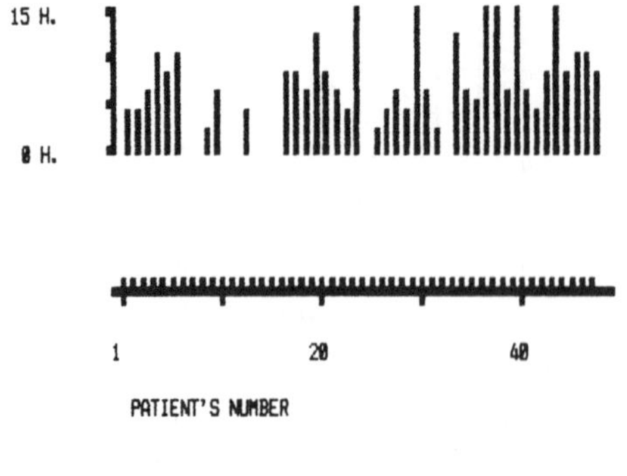

FIGURE 5. Approximate number of hours per day the patients activate the prosthesis. Despite their new hearing, patients 7, 14, 16 and 33 ceased to wear the device after several weeks or months of normal utilization; they are waiting for a more miniaturized emitter. Patients 8, 11, 12, 15 and 25 had electronic failure of the device and are waiting to exchange the defective receptor.

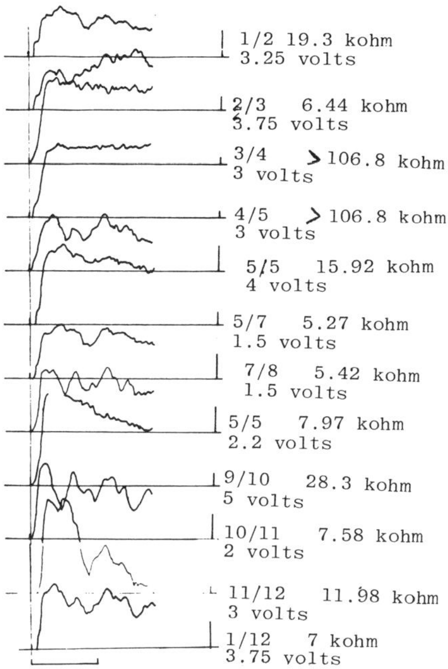

FIGURE 6. Registration of brainstem evoked responses elicited by peroperative electric stimulation of different pairs of implanted electrodes (patient 45). Changing the polarity of the stimulation does not change the response. For each curve are indicated on the right: the amplification (vertical bar = 10 μV), the relative pair of stimulated electrodes, the impedance at 300 Hz between these two electrodes, the voltage of the stimulation (square wave, 40 Hz, 0.3-msec duration). Horizontal bar = 5 msec.

patients 22 and 24, who suffered from total deafness as well as blindness due to an acquired or congenital cataract, and the case of patient 43, who suffered from total deafness and aphasia due to meningitis. In these dramatic situations, the psychoaffective effects of the implant have been even more marked than the improvement in speech discrimination.

Electrophysiological Data

The threshold level of the hearing sensation evoked by the round-window electrical stimulation test is described in TABLE 1. The impedance of each electrode and that between two electrodes varies between 5 to 20 kohm; it directly depends on the number and the size of Silastic pieces that are implanted through each fenestration (FIG. 6). The frequency discrimination between two electrodes depends on the intensity of the input signal, on the anatomic distance of these two electrodes (FIG. 1), on the quality of the surgical insulation of the cochlear compartments with Silastic pieces, and overall on the presence or absence of some auditory nerve fibers in the cochlear compartment considered (FIG. 7). At 30 dB up to the threshold level, 16 patients have shown no frequency confusion between each pair of neighboring electrodes, 10 confuse frequencies between two electrodes, 14 patients have this confusion for three to five electrodes; and 6 patients are only able to distinguish approximately low and high frequencies corresponding to the second turn and the basal turn electrodes (patients 8, 16, 23, 29, 32, and 41, who were deaf-mute and had practically no language preoperatively). The last three patients have undergone implantation too recently to be tested.

Hearing Rehabilitation

Sound Identification

All of our pâtients heard immediately after the operation. They were then asked to wear the device as often as possible. Within a few days they were able to recognize the familiar noises of everyday life. A classical tonal audiogram may objectively show the 40–60 dB dynamic range between threshold and the discomfort level due to emitter compression. All the patients are able to differentiate the intensity of several sounds. Frequency discrimination is easily done by postlingually deaf patients, provided that the two proposed frequencies are sufficiently different to involve two different electrodes and that the electrophysiological discrimination possibilities of these two electrodes that we have discussed earlier are sufficient. This discrimination necessitates progressive training, however, in cases of prelingual deafness.

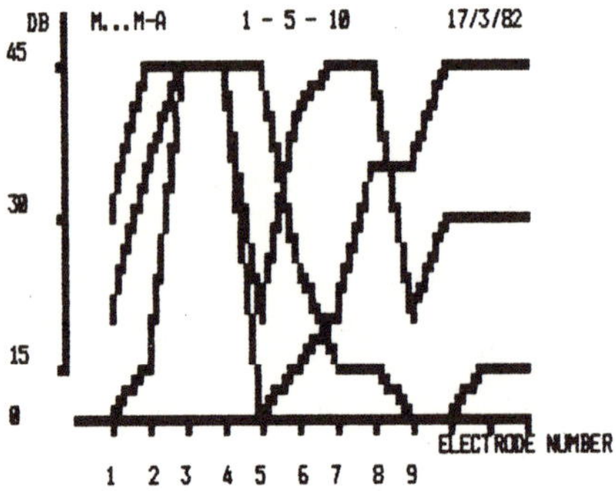

FIGURE 7. Diagram of frequency discrimination of electrodes number 1, 5 and 10 relative to the eleven other electrodes (patient 45). The ordinate is the maximum intensity (in dB up to the electric threshold level of each electrode) at which a statistically significant frequency discrimination (20 tests) remains between the tested electrode and the electrode whose number is indicated on the abscissa. The tests are generally not performed around 60 dB (discomfort level). In this case (see also FIGURE 6) there is probably too much Silastic around electrodes 3 and 4 and an absence of cochlear fibers in front of electrode 9.

Phonetic and Speech Discrimination without Help of Lipreading

Gradual training is necessary: the patient must learn to hear. Results depend principally on the phonetic items, even if these items vary from one patient to another. All the results we will now describe were obtained without the aid of lipreading.

Vowels. All of the patients present almost the same results, as described in TABLE 2. Important variations may only occur in prelingually deaf patients poorly reeducated prior to implantation. The most frequent confusions are observed between i and u, a and o, and a and e, but in some cases this confusion may now be lessened using another filter configuration.

Consonants. Voicing is perceived by almost 100% of 38 patients using the different propositions, but in eight of our first patients the differentiation score was only 30–70%. The details of discrimination results between two different sorts of consonants are described in TABLE 3.

Known words with a list. Among our 48 patients, 13 were excluded from this test for the following reasons: five patients received their implants too

TABLE 2

VOWEL IDENTIFICATION

Stimulus	First Filter Map Responses							Second Filter Map Responses						
	[a]	[ø]	[i]	[o]	[y]	[u]	[e]	[a]	[ø]	[i]	[o]	[y]	[u]	[e]
[a]	20							22						
[ø]	6	21						2	23					
[i]			22		5					24		4		
[o]	3	3		18				1	1		20			
[y]			9		16					5		20		
[u]	2					20							23	
[e]			8				11				3			15

NOTE: Each vowel is presented in a random manner; thus the total number of presentations is not the same for each vowel. These performances are practically similar for almost all the patients. The principal confusions are between i and u, a and o, and a and e. Compare the different performances of the two filter maps with FIGURES 2, 10, 11, and 12.

recently to be tested (cases 44 to 48); two patients had autistic deafness (cases 29 and 41); three patients had geographical difficulties in reeducation (cases 14, 20 and 33); one patient was a foreigner who did not stay long enough in Paris to demonstrate significant results (case 10); and two patients had early failure of the device (cases 16 and 25). These results are described in TABLES 4 and 5 and in FIGURE 8 (see also FIGURE 4).

TABLE 3

MEAN VALUE OF GOOD RESPONSES IN CONSONANT DISCRIMINATION AS FUNCTION OF ASSOCIATIONS IN 38 PATIENTS

	Voiced Explosive	Nonvoiced Explosive	Voiced Constrictive	Nonvoiced Constrictive
Voiced Explosive	ba–da = 20% ba–ga = 40%	ba–ka = 70%	za–ba = 65%	fa–ba = 90%
Nonvoiced Explosive	ba–pa = 75% ba–ta = 80%	pa–ta = 15%	ta–za = 80%	sa–da = 90%
Voiced Constrictive	ja–da = 60%	pa–za = 80%	za–ja = 5% va–ja = 25% va–za = 45%	va–fa = 80%
Nonvoiced Constrictive	fa–da = 80%	fa–ta = 65%	za–cha = 80% ja–cha = 80%	fa–sa = 5% fa–cha = 50% sa–cha = 55%

NOTE: One of the two phonemes of the studied pair was presented 20 times in a random manner so that the percentage of good responses could be appreciated (0% = random response). During the test the studied pair of phonemes was known by the patient. (Patients 46, 47 and 48 were not tested because they have too recently received their implants.)

TABLE 4

EVOLUTION OF PERCENTAGE OF GOOD IDENTIFICATION OF KNOWN WORDS WITH A LIST AS FUNCTION OF TIME: GENERAL RESULTS IN 35 CASES

	3 Months No. of Words			6 Months No. of Words			1 Year No. of Words			2 Years No. of Words		
Patient	2	4	8	2	4	8	2	4	8	2	4	8
1	60	20		70	40	20	70	40				
2	65	50	40	70	70	60	90	80	60			
3	10	80	70	90	90	80	90	90	80	90	90	80
4	90	100	80	100	97	97	100	100	97	100	100	97
5	90	100	90	100	97	97						
6	90	90	90	100	100	97	100	100	97	100	100	75
7	35	10	0	60	45	10	70	55	40			
8	70	10		80	35		90	52	52	95	75	60
9	80	80	70	97	97							
11	90	75	65	95	90		97	97	75			
12	90	90	25	100	90	62						
13	90	90		95	90	75						
15	80	45	10									
17	90	80	50	80	70	60	100	90	70	100	75	70
18	90	80	70									
19	60	50	20	80	50	50	90	60	60	90	65	60
21	90	80	5	87	80	75	90	87	65	9		
22	95	95	90	100	97	97	100	100	97	100	100	97
23	15	5		50	25		80	60	10			
24	95	95	90	97	97	97	100	100	98			
26	82	80	50	85	80	80	85	80	80			
27	90	50	45	95	85	80						
28	90	80	50	95	80	80						
30	95	90	80	100	95	92						
31	80	80	40	90	80	60						
32	30	5	0									
34	90	70	50	100	90	80	100	90	90			
35	90	60	40	95	70	60	95	80	75			
36	95	85	60	95	95	75	100	95	87			
37	90	70	50	90	80	60	95	85	65			
38	70	30	0									
39	90	60	40	95	75	50	100	90	80			
40	80	60	30	85	70	40						
42	90	80	60									
43	100	95	90	100	100	90						

NOTE: These lists of 2, 4 or 8 words contain words of identical length. Correlate these results with the data in TABLE 1.

Unknown words without a list. This test determines an important difference between prelingual deafness (bad discrimination) and postlingual deafness (good discrimination). Nevertheless, this difference may be reduced or increased by the mental and sociocultural status of each patient (TABLE 6).

Speech Discrimination with the Help of Lipreading

The percentages of recognition of 20 words presented to the patient 6 months after implantation with and without the help of lipreading are described in TABLE 7 for 24 patients. When preoperative lipreading was very poor, improvement with the prosthesis is low (4 patients). On the contrary, this improvement is significant when there is good preoperative ability to lipread; the ability to discriminate progressively increases in the subsequent months and years.

Voice Changes

Voice improvement depends on the kind of deafness. In patients with postlingual deafness normal timbre and melody are quickly recovered, but the voice speed remains slow for a long time, probably because the patient is distracted by hearing his own voice. In the case of prelingual deafness one may note on successive sonagrams (FIG. 9) a diminution of word duration and an

TABLE 5

PERCENTAGE OF GOOD IDENTIFICATION OF KNOWN WORDS WITH A LIST: PARTICULAR RESULTS IN 26 CASES (FROM 6 TO 12 MONTHS AFTER IMPLANTATION)

Patient	10 Words	20 Words	10 Sentences	20 Sentences
3	90%	75%	80%	50%
4	95%	95%	95%	95%
5	95%	90%	95%	95%
6	95%	95%	90%	90%
9	85%	80%	85%	75%
11	80%	78%	80%	80%
12	60%	45%	60%	45%
17	95%	75%	80%	75%
18	90%	75%	90%	75%
19	90%	60%	85%	57%
21	85%	80%	80%	58%
22	95%	95%	95%	95%
24	100%	97%	100%	100%
26	85%	62%	80%	55%
27	90%	50%	85%	48%
28	82%	72%	85%	72%
30	100%	85%	97%	85%
31	70%	52%	75%	52%
34	85%	65%	90%	65%
35	80%	60%	80%	60%
36	77%	55%	80%	60%
37	65%	40%	65%	45%
39	80%	55%	80%	50%
40	35%	20%	35%	20%
42	45%	25%	45%	25%
43	95%	90%	95%	90%

NOTE: The sentences are, insofar as possible, of the same rhythm and length (see TABLES 6, 7 and 9). Correlate these results with the data in TABLE 1.

Stimulus \ response		1	2	3	4	5	6	7	8	9	10	11	12	13	14	15	16	17	18	Total Correct	Total Stimuli
1	1	4									1									4	5
2	2		3					2												3	5
3	3			5																5	5
4	4				4						1									4	5
5	5					5														5	5
6	6						5													5	5
7	7		1					4												4	5
8	8								5											5	5
9	9									5										5	5
10	10	1									4									4	5
11	11											4	1							4	5
12	12												5							53	60
	13																				
	14																				
	15																				
	16																				
	17																				
	18																				

FIGURE 8. Diagram of the results of sentence recognition test (performed 7/5/80) with a known list presented in a random manner (patient 24 [P.E.]). The sentences were as follows: 1 = *il fait beau aujourd'hui;* 2 = *demain je vais au cinéma;* 3 = *quelle belle journée;* 4 = *prends ton petit dejèuner;* 5 = *je vais partir en vacances;* 6 = *j'ai trois enfants;* 7 = *il fait vraiment trop froid;* 8 = *je pars avec ma voiture;* 9 = *je vais chasser demain;* 10 = *la boulangerie est fermée;* 11 = *tu travailles trop;* 12 = *il est en colère.*

improvement in phonetic transitions; the formants become more separated from each other and there is a diminution of the background noises. These improvements are achieved quickly, but progress becomes very slow after a few months. Moreover, these voice changes vary from one patient to another without any detectable correlation with the clinical preoperative status.

Correlation between Clinical Results and Electrical Threshold Level of the Round-Window Stimulation Test

The value of the clinical results greatly depends on the patient's socialization coefficient. The more the patient is socialized, the better will be the results, even in the case of a very poor electrode–nerve interface. On the contrary, in the case of an adult deaf–mute patient with a very low intelligence coefficient, the clinical results will be feeble, even if the percentage of the cochlear nerve fibers that are still present is very high. Consequently, we may consider the correlation between the clinical results and the socialization coefficient to represent the approximate value of this electrode–nerve interface (TABLE 8). Therefore there is a significant correlation (degrees of freedom = 25; correla-

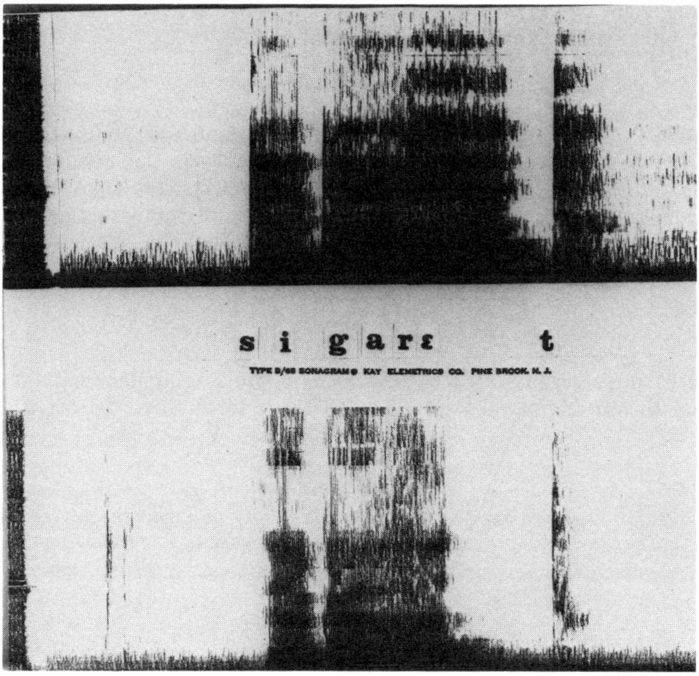

FIGURE 9. Sonagram of patient 3 before implantation (*top*) and 1 month after implantation (*bottom*).

TABLE 6

DISCRIMINATIONS AND CONFUSIONS OF PATIENT 24 IN RESPONSE TO UNKNOWN WORDS AND SENTENCES WITHOUT A REFERENCE LIST

Word	Response	Sentence	Response
Var	*Car*	*Bonjour Madame*	*Vénérable*
Seize	*Seine*	*Il fait chaud*	*Venez cachou*
Ponte	*Port*	*Il fait trés beau*	*Étibo*
Tard	*Bar*	*J'ai faim*	*J'ai faim*
Mille	*Midi*	*Ça va mieux*	*Ça va mieux*
Far	*Char*	*Viens manger*	*Moi manger*
Tonte	*Code*	*Je pars en vacances*	*Je pars en voyage*
Naine	*Béni*	*j'ai trois enfants*	*j'ai trois enfants*
Masse	*Race*	*J'aime le fromage*	*J'aime les promenades*
Lasse	*Hache*	*J'ai un chien*	*J'ai un chien*
Doigt	*Voix*	*Il parle beaucoup*	*Il parle beaucoup*
Toi	*Noix*	*Je chante toujours*	*Je chante toujours*
Gène	*Gène*	*J'aime lire*	*J'aime l'air*
Molle	*Meule*	*Viens ici*	*Bien si*
Chose	*Chone*	*Ce jardin est joli*	*Ce gendarme est joli*
Masse	*Lasse*	*Il a une belle voix*	*Il a une belle voix*
Loi	*Voix*	*Tais toi*	*De soi*
Rance	*Rond*	*Il fait froid*	*Il fait froid*

NOTE: This patient showed particularly excellent results.

tion coefficient = —0.381) between this interface and the electrical threshold level obtained during the round-window stimulation test.

Eight and Twelve Channels

Patients 1 to 12 received an 8-channel implant and all the others were implanted with a 12-channel device. As we can see in the various tables, the clinical results were generally better with 12 electrodes than with 8 electrodes. Nevertheless, these differences are not statistically significant because the number of the variables responsible is too high in relation to the low number of patients.

Comments

All of these results must be discussed in order to understand the mechanisms of this means of rehabilitation and to try to improve the efficacy of this

Table 7

Percentage of Word Recognition with Help of Lipreading with and without Implant Device

Patient	Without Implant	With Implant	Effects of Prosthesis on Discrimination with Lipreading
1	30	30	0
2	50	65	15
3	20	50	30
4	75	90	15
5	60	85	25
6	60	80	20
9	25	50	25
11	10	30	20
12	5	10	5
13	33	50	15
17	60	80	20
18	65	80	15
19	10	10	0
21	5	25	15
26	50	50	0
27	40	55	15
28	70	70	0
30	30	70	40
31	30	40	10
34	45	60	15
35	60	70	10
36	70	80	10
37	35	40	5
39	70	80	10
40	5	5	0
42	70	75	5
43	60	85	25

TABLE 8

ITEMS USED TO DETERMINE APPROXIMATELY THE EFFICACY OF THE ELECTRODE–NERVE INTERFACE

Patient [a]	A	B	T	K	T/K	SE
1	20	0	20	8	2.5	25
2	50	15	65	7	9.2	10
3	80	30	110	11	10	15
4	100	15	115	15	7	15
5	100	25	125	15	8.3	25
6	90	20	110	13	8.4	10
9	80	25	105	13	8	07
11	90	20	110	11	10	20
12	90	5	95	9	10.5	10
13	90	15	105	6	17.5	05
17	80	20	100	12	8.3	10
18	80	15	95	12	7.9	10
19	50	0	50	8	6.2	07
21	80	15	95	9	10.5	10
26	80	0	80	14	5.7	20
27	50	15	65	6	10.8	10
28	80	0	80	14	5.7	15
30	90	40	130	14	9.2	20
31	80	10	90	12	7.5	15
34	95	30	125	14	8.9	05
35	60	10	70	14	5	07
36	85	10	95	14	6.7	20
37	70	5	75	13	5.7	05
39	60	10	70	15	4.6	25
40	60	0	60	7	8.5	20
42	80	5	85	10	8.5	08
43	95	25	120	14	8.5	13

ABBREVIATIONS: A = percentage of discrimination of 4 known words with a list (with a prosthesis and without the help of lipreading) 3 months after the operation (see TABLES 4 and 5); B = effect of the prosthesis on speech discrimination with the help of lipreading; T = A + B (clinical results obtained due to the prosthesis); K = patient's socialization coefficient (see TABLE 1); T/K = approximate value of the electrode–nerve interface; value in decivolts of the threshold level of the round-window electric stimulation test.

[a] These variables have been clearly identified in only 27 patients.

12-channel implant in the future. The main points are the phoniatric results, the tolerance for the implanted materials, and the ability of the prosthesis to transmit the necessary information for speech understanding.

Phoniatric Results

The phoneme and word confusions that we observed when the patients did not have the aid of lipreading are the most interesting items for comment.

Vowels. If we consider the frequency localization of French formants

TABLE 9

FREQUENCY LOCALIZATIONS OF THE THREE FORMANTS OF THE FRENCH VOWELS

Vowel	First Formant	Second Formant	Third Formant
[a]	725	1300	2640
[ø]	510	1450	2450
[i]	260	2360	3050
[o]	350	865	2450
[y]	240	1850	2110
[o]	280	830	2230
[e]	350	2200	2500

(TABLE 9) and the first filter cutting map that we commonly used for the first 29 patients, one might think that all the formants of the different vowels were correctly transmitted (FIGS. 10 and 11); moreover, the temporal sampling of the device (3 msec) allows us to think that the characteristic frequency shifts of certain vowels are also transmitted. Nevertheless, it is also evident that there is too much information in channels 2 to 6 and proportionally not enough information in channels 7 to 12, which corresponds to the frequency location of the second and third formants. That is the reason for which we built a second filter battery, whose configuration is described in FIGURES 2 and 10.

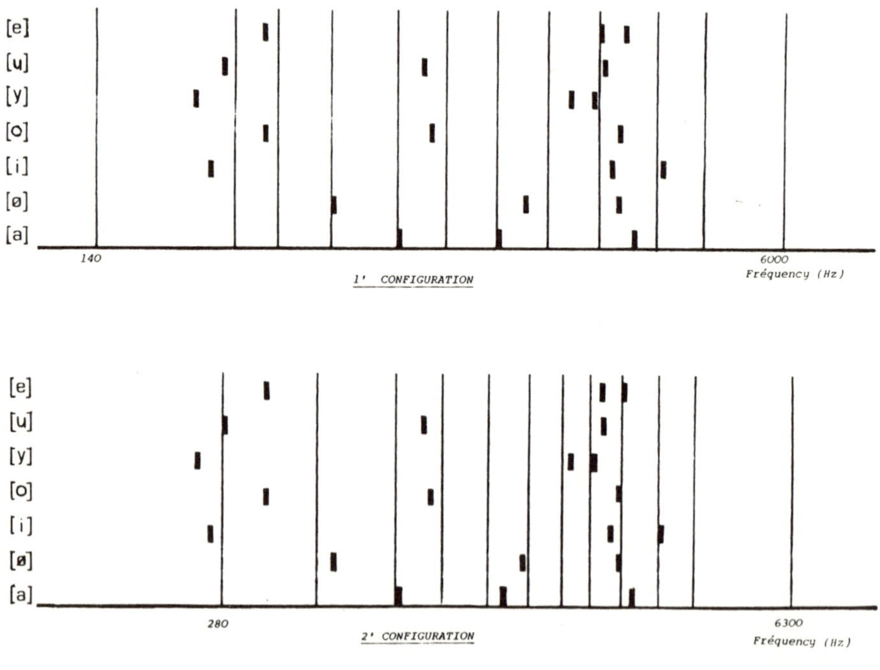

FIGURE 10. Comparison of the values of the three formants of the principal French phonemes and the values of the peaks of each filter of our second filter configuration.

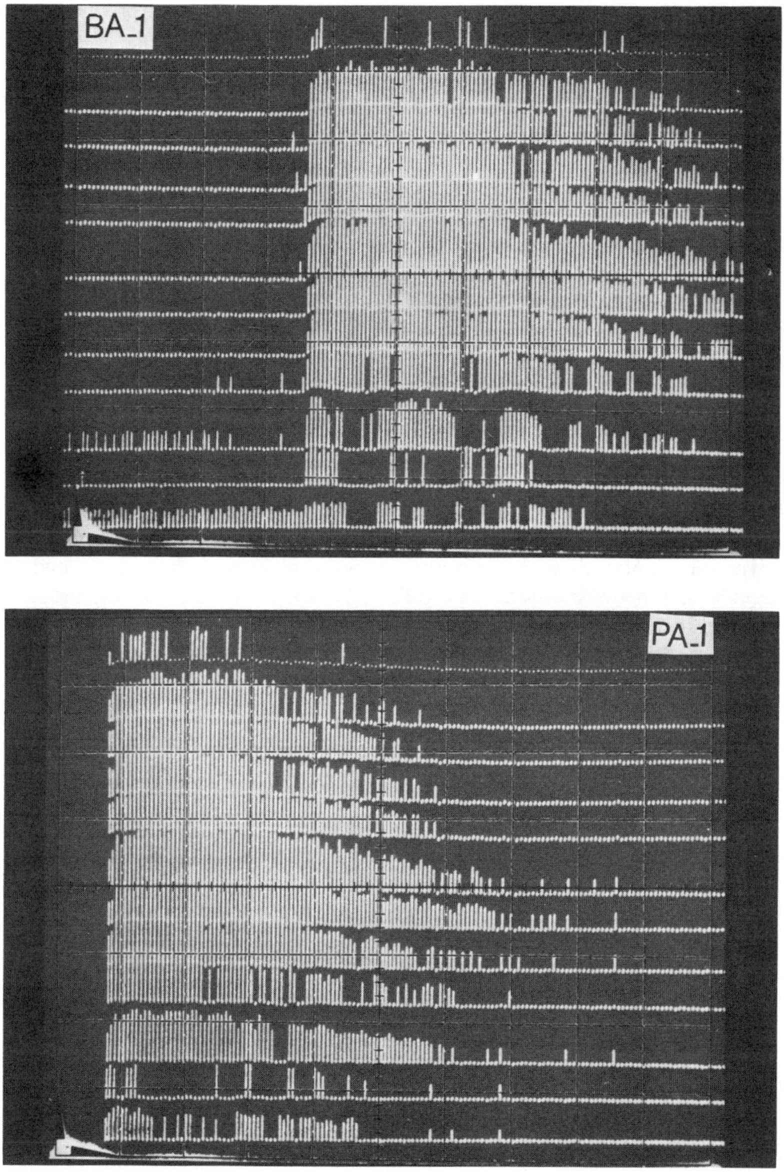

FIGURE 11. Oscilloscopic representation of the variations of the energy repartition in each of the 12 electrodes as a function of the input signal obtained with the first filter configuration (BA). (*Top*) electrode 12 (high pitch); (*bottom*) electrode 1 (low pitch). In this picture the variation of the energy is represented by a variation of the amplitude of each square wave (in fact, in our device it is represented by a variation of the duration of each pulse). The frequency of these square waves is constant (300 Hz). One division of the oscilloscope = 50 μsec. Note the voicing representation (about 100 Hz) on *bottom* (regular amplitude variation on each three pulses).

This second filter's configuration seems better: it stimulates fewer channels for one particular vowel and favors the formant bands to the detriment of low frequencies (FIG. 12). Nevertheless, it is not easy to be sure of this superiority; the number of our patients using this device is not sufficient to make a judgment yet. Furthermore, when we consider the difficulties in learning to use this device, it would be impossible to give the necessary tests to be sure that this second model is really better for all the patients. In fact it is possible that a particular model must be built for each patient that would take into account his different channel discrimination map and his own phoniatric difficulties.

Consonants. The good voicing discrimination that we obtain is due to our filter frequency map, which leads us to think that the glottic vibration or its first harmonic is well transmitted. This is demonstrated in FIGURES 11 and 12, in which this glottic vibration can be recognized. But all the consonant confusion that we observe (TABLES 4 and 5) may be explained by the fact that the highest filters take into account only one part of the energy of these consonants; besides the energy of the acoustic input signal is generally more feeble in these high frequencies than in the low-frequency bands (FIG. 2).

Known Words with a List. The different percentages for recognition of known words obtained with the multichannel implant must be appreciated with respect to phonetic features. The difficulties of phonemic discrimination described in TABLES 2 and 3 contribute to the difficulty of distinction of words containing these phonemes, the discrimination of which is already uncertain. Thus, one can understand the frequent confusions between two words containing the phonemes i and u, or ou and an (FIG. 4).

Unknown Words without a List of References. In the case of unknown words, the results directly depend on the number of references in the patient's memory, that is, the degree of socialization of the patient. This explains why these results are very poor in the case of deaf-mute patients. However, it must be emphasized that usually the patient is supplied with familiar sentences and is helped by lipreading.

Tolerance for Implanted Materials

In most cases, the threshold level of implanted electrodes does not vary with time, which probably means that the nerve endings are not injured by the intracochlear implanted material. The tangential introduction of each electrode in the osseous tube places the tip of each wire near the external wall of the coil far from the lamina spiralis. The electrical stimulation is not directly delivered to the nerve, but through the few millimeters of scar tissue that touches the cochlear tube.

In view of the fact that our first patients underwent implantation in 1976 and since then have had the same electrical threshold level and the same discrimination between each electrode, it can be seen that tolerance for implanted materials and electrode–nerve interface survival are no longer the main problems of the multichannel cochlear implant technique.

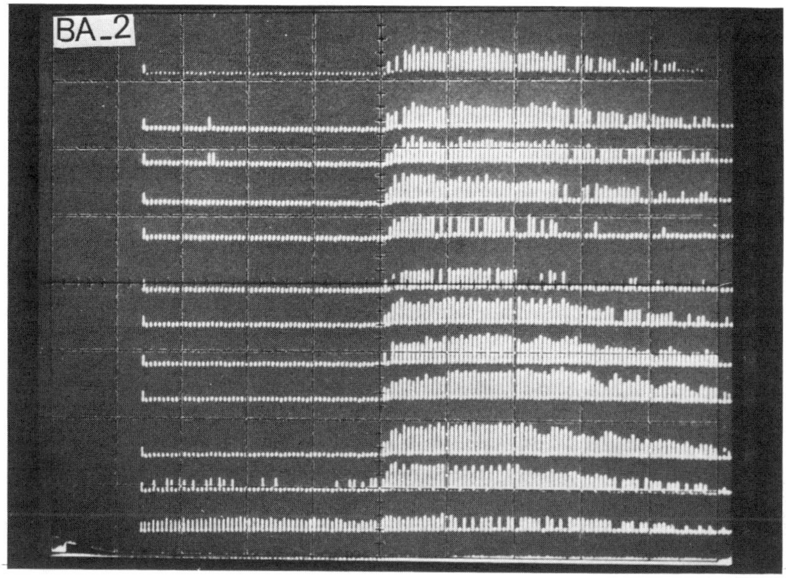

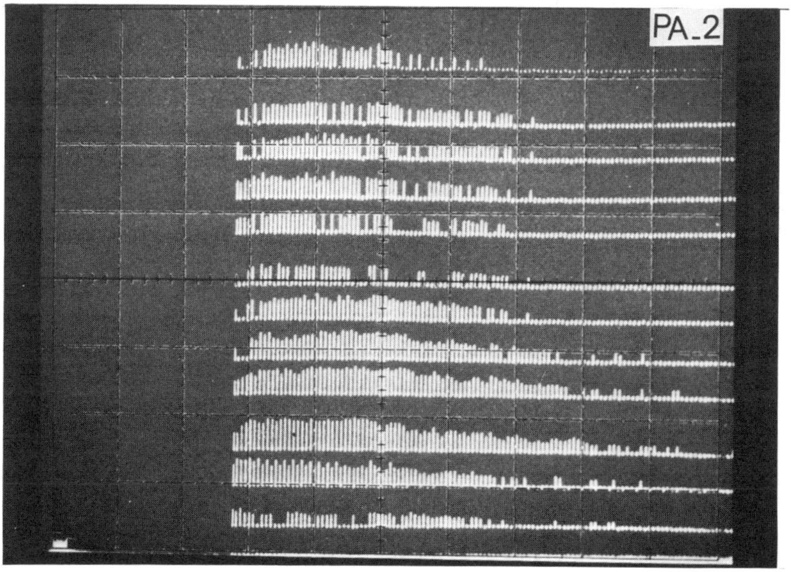

FIGURE 12. Second filter configuration. Data are same as in legend to FIGURE 11. Note the better formant representation in this second filter configuration as in the first one (FIG. 11). Note also the voicing representation in the lower electrode.

Prosthetic Performances

Even though the speech discrimination obtained is encouraging, it is still mostly insufficient. Thus we may ask whether it is either the prosthetic performance or the anatomopathologic features of each patient that is responsible for these mediocre results.

Let us consider the theoretical transmission of speech features the prosthesis has to generate at the suitable moment, the suitable number of spikes, and the suitable fiber of the cochlear nerve.

(1) Supplying the spikes at the suitable moment is definitely achieved by the apparatus, whose temporal sampling interval of 3 msec is more than enough as far as the propagation speed of the physiological basilar membrane vibration wave (2 to 5 msec) and the sampling capacity of the brain (about 20 msec) are concerned. Thus, timing and rhythm of speech are certainly transmitted to the patient's cochlea. This transmission is also evident concerning voicing and nonvoicing, as can be seen in FIGURES 11 and 12.

(2) Delivering the appropriate number of spikes is achieved if we consider the loudness of speech (40 to 100 dB). Because of compression rate of 60 dB of the device, the threshold level of each electrode, corresponding to acoustic information of 40 dB, is able to double when the acoustic energy passes from 40 to 100 dB.

(3) Directing the spikes to the suitable fiber is certainly imperfect, even if our filter configurations theoretically allow a good transmission of voicing and formants with only 12 channels. In fact, we are obliged to resort to a frequency transposition in order to place the 12 electrodes in the surgically available length of the cochlear tube. Moreover, as the contingent of fibers excited by one electrode is about one octave (that is, about 2 mm of the cochlea) the subjective tone is not a pure frequency but a noise band. When there is poor postoperative discrimination between two electrodes (see FIGURE 7), one might wrongly conclude that the peroperative electrical insulation of each cochlear compartment is insufficient; that is why measuring these electrode impedances during implantation is such an important part of the operation. In fact, the insulation is generally good enough. But the implanted cochlea is a pathologic cochlea, and when a nondiscriminative electrode is encountered we may conclude that in front of the electrode there are no cochlear fibers able to supply the patient with a sound sensation. This seems a good explanation for most of our poor clinical results.

We might hope to increase these performances in our patients by increasing the number of electrodes of the implant. Theoretically, our device is able to drive 14 channels, but at this point it seems difficult to implant two more electrodes without complicating the surgical procedure (a middle fossa approach would be necessary) or risking diminution of the electric insulation of each cochlear compartment.

CONCLUSION AND FUTURE PERSPECTIVES

The 12-channel cochlear implant device that we have designed with the help of the Bertin Society and have used for more than 5 years supplies totally deaf patients with a new hearing that is indeed imperfect, but that nevertheless allows words and sentences to be discriminated in all patients without the help of lipreading.

Still, we hope to improve these results. First, the computerized peroperative determination of electrode impedance and the verification of each electrode's value will allow electrical insulation of each cochlear compartment to be easily optimized. Theoretically, an electrode array will allow very easy resolution of this problem. We are now working with the Bertin Society on such a device, which will be able to prevent destruction of the nerve endings during introduction. However, we must emphasize that sometimes, especially when total deafness is due to meningitis, the cochlear tube is partially ossified. We have observed such a situation twice (in patients 35 and 47), when introducing an electrode array would have been impossible, and we were glad to have the opportunity to use the one-by-one electrode implantation technique (in these patients we could implant only five and six electrodes, respectively), even if it is a long and difficult method. In the coming months it is hoped that we will benefit from a miniaturized device with which it will be possible to supply each electrode with a particular voltage; this improvement will allow us to better discriminate small variations in intensity, which are surely important in speech discrimination.

On the other hand, in cases of prelingual deafness, implanting the patient with a cochlear device as early as possible seems to be useful in order to supply him or her with sound before central pathway atrophy becomes too great. Our youngest patient was 9 years old when he received an implant. We plan to progressively reduce this age limit in our indications for surgery.

Finally, we might ask whether a binary code instead of a frequency code would not be better to transmit the few hundred phonemes of speech, especially in prelingually deaf patients.

Summary

Clinical results obtained with the multichannel cochlear implant are described in 48 cases of total deafness (27 cases of prelingual and 21 cases of postlingual deafness). The tolerance for implanted material and the survival of the electrode–nerve interface have not yet been altered after more than 5 years. After some months of training the patients, the percentages of phoneme-, word-, and sentence-recognition vary from one patient to another, but depend approximately on the value of the threshold level of the round-window stimulation test, and the degree of socialization of each patient. These results suggest that the multichannel cochlear implant may now be considered as a useful tool in the rehabilitation of totally deaf persons.

References

1. Chouard, C. H. & P. MacLeod. 1976. Implantation of multiple intracochlear electrodes for rehabilitation of total deafness: Preliminary report. Laryngoscope **36:** 1743–1751.
2. Chouard, C. H. & B. Meyer. 1978. La mise en place intra-cochleaire de l'implant à électrodes multiples. Ann. Otolaryngol. **95**(9): 549–558.
3. Chouard, C. H., C. Fugain, B. Meyer & H. Lacombe. 1982. Résultats cliniques de l'implant cochleaire a multiélectrodes. Ann. Otolaryngol. **99**(3): 154–188.

COMPARISON OF PERCEPTS FOUND WITH COCHLEAR IMPLANT DEVICES

Carl G. Müller [a]

The Boys Town Institute for Communication Disorders of Children Omaha, Nebraska 68131

In this paper we first describe results of psychoacoustic tests of persons with cochlear implant devices (implanted listeners) and then point out aspects that are different from those found with normal listeners. Many of the findings on implanted listeners parallel those of hearing-impaired individuals with sensorineural loss of cochlear origin.[1] To some degree, this is expected because deafness of cochlear origin is normally a prerequisite for implantation. These parallels imply that implant stimulation and acoustic input cause similar responses at some level beyond the cochlea so that phenomena like incomplete temporal integration, Type II responses on Bekesy audiometry, and rapid loudness growth appear in both groups. This is presumably because the action of the basilar membrane or receptor cells is altered or missing in both hearing-impaired and implanted listeners.

The measures obtained most often from implanted listeners concern threshold, pitch, and loudness. These are psychological responses which can change as a result of stimulus parameters and psychological variables. Psychoacoustics has evolved to provide theories and techniques for the control and evaluation of these factors in order to obtain the most information from a test session.

Threshold

The threshold response with electrical stimulation depends on several stimulus parameters, among them: current, charge per half-wave pulse and its integral, frequency, pulse width, phase spectrum, and duration of presentation. Current has been the variable most often controlled. The impedance of an electrode is frequency-dependent [2] and decreases 3 to 5 decibels per octave. The level of current above which the impedance becomes nonlinear increases with frequency, independent of electrode material,[3] as has been demonstrated with a cochlear implant array.[4] Combined with the decreasing impedance function, the result is a fixed voltage limit between 0.2 and 0.5 volts, above which the system becomes nonlinear.

From work by Simmons [5] it was inferred that the charge per half-wave pulse would be constant at threshold.[6] A device built to control charge rather than current provided support for this concept with two implanted listeners,[7] until modifications to limit peak current were made for safety reasons. A recent report from the group at Stanford University [8] showed that threshold for some electrodes depended solely on charge, while for others, in the same patient, the

[a] Present address: Department of Speech Pathology and Audiology, University of Denver, University Park, Denver, Colorado 80208.

0077-8923/83/0405-0412 $1.75/0 © 1983, NYAS

charge required was rate-dependent. Most other implant groups [9–13] have found evidence for integration of charge per half-wave pulse over time. Thus, the charge per half-wave pulse needed for threshold will decrease as the rate of delivery of half-wave pulses increases.

The effect of sinusoidal frequency on threshold is not directly accounted for by either impedance changes or charge per half-wave pulse. The current required for threshold appears constant up to about 100 Hz, and then increases rapidly by as many as 20–30 dB until 750–1000 Hz, when it levels out again.[1] This threshold function occurs for signals with 50% duty cycle and may result from a mixture of the impedance function, charge per half-wave pulse, membrane-charging constants, and limitations on rate of neural following.

Pulse-width changes alter the charge per half-wave pulse and therefore can affect the threshold.[9, 10, 14–16] At very large pulse widths, threshold is determined by a constant current and is unchanged when pulse width is varied. At very short pulse widths, threshold requires constant charge per half-wave pulse, and this will increase as pulse width increases when constant current is maintained. The relationship between pulse width and threshold is not identical with the physiological "chronaxie" function (although this term is often used) because the thresholds of implanted listeners are perceptual, and not physiological, functions.

The distribution of a current or charge over one repetition period can influence the threshold. For signals of constant power spectrum, the waveform can be manipulated by changing the phase spectrum. Unpublished work by me at Stanford and Vienna showed that changes in the phase spectrum can produce changes in pitch, loudness, and threshold, even though the power spectrum remained unchanged. This occurs because of the dependence of threshold on both frequency and pulse width.

As the duration of a signal is increased (up to 100–300 milliseconds), the magnitude of the signal necessary for threshold decreases proportionately. For normal listeners a ten-fold increase in the duration of the signal causes the threshold to decrease by around 10 dB.[17] For implanted listeners [1, 9, 10] as well as the hearing-impaired with losses of cochlear origin,[18] the threshold does not decrease this rapidly.

The interstimulus interval (ISI) can also influence threshold. As the time between repeated tone-bursts is lengthened while the burst length and amplitude are maintained, there is a decrease in the power. However, for one patient (L.P.) tested in Vienna, when the ISI between 200-msec bursts was lengthened from 25 to 200 msec, a gradual 8-dB improvement in threshold occurred for a 2500-Hz sinusoid, but no change occurred for a 100-Hz sinusoid. Results for 500 Hz were intermediate between these two. This finding could be predicted from previous work [1, 19] which showed that Bekesy audiograms on implanted listeners are typically Type II,[20] that is, there is a difference in threshold between continuous and pulsed signals particularly at high frequencies. Therefore, threshold differences will occur as a function of the off-time between stimuli.[21]

Pitch Perception

The pitch associated with simple stimuli (sinusoids and pulse trains) is determined primarily by frequency or repetition rate for both normal and implanted listeners. Above some limiting rate, listeners scale the pitch as very high and little or no variation in percept is reported as the rate is changed. This limit, called pitch saturation, is found to occur at much lower rates (150 through 1000 Hz) for implanted listeners [22–25] than for normal listeners, although similar rates have been found for different electrodes of the same implant.[1, 8, 9]

It does not necessarily follow that spectral information is lost to the listener in regions where poor pitch-labeling occurs. When presented with complex signals comprising many harmonics (such as speech) a normal listener reports the pitch of the signal to be that associated with the pitch of the fundamental. Nevertheless, information about higher frequencies (such as formants) is processed. Implanted listeners also report the pitch of the fundamental when presented with speech, as well as with "missing fundamental" complexes in which the fundamental and other lower partials are not present. The absence of change in pitch at higher rates of stimulation does not rule out the processing of information above the saturation rate. Nor does the absence of lower-frequency components rule out the report of low pitch. Further tests are necessary to determine how much spectral information is available to implanted listeners.

From work at Stanford,[8] it is apparent that "time-separation pitch" [26] is perceived by implanted listeners. This pitch occurs, in addition to the pitch of the fundamental, when a pulse train of fixed rate consists of two pulses per repetition spaced a fixed distance apart in time. For Stanford's listener (R.F.), performance on a timing-discrimination task was better when the two trains were summed on the same electrode. With overall repetition rates of 100 per second, this subject could discriminate between signals that had pulse-pair separation differences of less than 1 msec.

The difference limen for frequency is similar for implanted listeners [1, 5, 13, 22–25, 27] and normal listeners [28] at rates up to 100 Hz. Above that, implanted listeners show progressively worse performance until at rates above 1000 Hz, a change of half an octave or more is necessary for 75% discrimination. Discrimination is possible at rates above the saturation of pitch perception. Changes in tonal quality or timbre may be responsible for this performance.

Loudness Perception

The parameters (described earlier) that influence threshold for implanted listeners also influence loudness. The interaction of these parameters is sometimes a function of sensation level, that is, the level of a signal above the threshold for that same signal. For example, in an experiment at Stanford University [29] it was found, as expected from measures of threshold as a function of pulse width, that a train of wide rectangular pulses required less current than a similar train of narrow pulses for equal loudness near threshold. However, at higher sensation levels, equal loudness was achieved when the narrower pulses had the same or even less current than the wider ones.

The dynamic range of electrical stimulation is limited both by the listener's threshold of discomfort and by the maximum voltage permitted before electrode nonlinearity. The range from audibility to discomfort in implanted listeners is between 8–20 dB and covers the entire normal perceptual range for loudness. That is, pain or discomfort does not occur while the stimulus is still at moderate loudness (although vestibular effects have been reported in midrange [32]). Loudness growth has been shown to be steeper in implanted than in normal listeners by a factor of six [1] or less.[30, 31] In one comparison of loudness functions, the stapedius reflex in an ear not operated on was elicited by electrical stimulation.[9] The reflex threshold occurred at about the same relative loudness (sones) above threshold in this patient (S.S.) as in normal listeners.[1]

The difference limen for amplitude in implanted listeners of 0.5 to 1.0 dB [1, 5, 7–10] is as good as or better than that of normal listeners.[33] This is consistent with the steeper loudness function. Averaged data from five implanted listeners in Vienna showed no clear effect of sensation level on the intensity difference limen. However, one listener (S.S.), carefully tested for this, showed a reduction in the difference limen from 0.5 dB to less than 0.2 dB as sensation level was raised. A similar pattern is observed in data from normal listeners.

Electrode Effects and Pitch

When different electrodes in a multichannel array are stimulated with identical signals, listeners are able to distinguish differences among them and to apply consistent labels to them. When subjective ordering of these percepts is compared to the physical ordering of electrodes, there is usually very good correspondence [5, 22, 34, 35] (although difficulties exist with modiolar electrodes [8, 36]). The stimuli used to obtain these clearly differentiable percepts are usually pulses delivered at very low rates. As soon as the repetition rate rises sufficiently, the pitch associated with repetition rate overwhelms these electrode-specific percepts. Although the original hope of many researchers was to utilize the "place pitch" concept through multichannel stimulation, the dominance of rate-pitch caused some to conclude that no "place pitch" was present.[24]

The fact that perceptual ordering agrees with cochlear order is not sufficient evidence for "place pitch," regardless of the stimuli used. It is necessary to show that "pitch" is the right term for this percept. One way to do this might be to demonstrate that melody could be conveyed by switching across the electrodes without altering the stimulus. Another point in its favor would be if pitch matching of electrode "place" pitch were shown to correlate with the cochlear map. In normal listeners, frequencies of several thousand hertz stimulate the basal turn. Therefore, we would expect that electrical stimulation of the basal turn would produce a pitch associated with very-high-frequency stimuli. There is, however, little evidence [10] for such a direct relationship. Nearly all pitch-matching and -scaling experiments show that very high pitches are not perceived.

In normal listeners, when the overall perception of a stimulus changes, while pitch and loudness remain unchanged, we generally refer to that percept as timbre. The most reliable verbal attribute of timbre is the contrast "sharp–dull," which has been shown to be highly associated with the frequency position of the energy concentration of the spectrum.[37] Moreover, this contrast can be both scaled and matched, as pitch can, and is not strongly affected by the spectral fine structure.[38] A recent study [27] with implanted listeners employed this contrast in labeling of electrode position. These investigators found that subjects could use these labels consistently and that rapid changes across electrodes can be accurately distinguished.

The difficulty of assigning pitches to stimuli that contain both "volley" and "place" pitches can be seen in a study of normal listeners [39] in which rectangular pulses (at rates of 90 to 150 times per second) were used to ring filters tuned to 2000 Hz. Some listeners would match the pitch to that of the filter ("place" pitch), while others would match it to the rate of the pulse train ("volley" pitch). All were able to hear either pitch as soon as it was varied. Thus, a signal may contain more than one pitch, although only one is evident to the listener at a given moment. It may also be true that the percept "pitch" is best associated with the perception of movement across a psychological space, rather than a fixed position within it. The knowledge about pitch perception in normal listeners is still rudimentary.

Perceptual changes associated with different electrodes may interfere with attempts to play melodies through implants using rate-pitch,[5, 13, 22] which has proven quite difficult. One observation [22] was that a melody played using normal musical ratios only produces the correct pitches for one electrode out of many. This implies that the effects of electrode position could influence not only the absolute pitch assigned, but also the relative pitch of musical ratios. More investigation is required to determine the influence of electrode position on rate-pitch.

Unusual Aspects of Pitch Perception

Exceptions to a monotonic mapping of rate to pitch have been found by two groups.[8, 9] In these cases, low pitches cannot be elicited. That is, at very low rates the pitch is perceived as higher than at slightly greater rates. This may occur because of interference from the electrode-specific percept as rates become too low to maintain rate-pitch perception.

Several studies have reported strong order effects in pitch judgments. Two of these [5, 8] report that (for some pairs of stimuli) when the first stimulus is perceived as much lower in pitch than the second (with good discrimination shown by test scores), reversal of the order results in a "same" judgment (and poor discrimination scores). Thus "low–high" is more easily perceived than "high–low" for the same pair of stimuli. Other reports [36, 40] point to greater difficulty or inconsistent test results when order is permuted.

Pitch matching may also be influenced by order effects.[5, 24, 35] In recent attempts in Vienna to obtain pitch matches, an implanted listener was asked to adjust the frequency of one tone-burst to match the pitch of another on the same electrode while the tones repeated in a pattern of two tone-bursts followed by silence. Her decision on pitch matching was easily altered by changing the order of the two tone-bursts relative to the silent interval.

In experiments with modiolar (Stanford) and scala tympani (Vienna) implants in which the relative phase of components was altered, listeners reported that the pitch of a signal could change. This occurred for both two- and seven-component complexes of sequential harmonics including the fundamental. The largest pitch shift (more than one octave) occurred for listener R.F. at Stanford with a seven-component complex when the phase of the second harmonic was shifted 180 degrees from the cosine phase of the other harmonics. Smaller, but reliable, pitch shifts were reported for many, but not all, phase shifts. It appears that the fine structure of the waveform within repetition periods has an influence on the perceived pitch.

In the course of phase experiments, it was often seen that the sensation level of the stimulus had a strong effect on pitch. Large pitch differences between two signals could be completely lost by raising the level of both signals as little as 1 decibel. In nearly all cases of phase-influenced pitch, increasing the level produced less clear perceptual differences once both signals were above threshold. It has been observed previously [5, 41] that increasing the sensation level of some signals moves pitch upwards. We believe that the interaction of pitch and sensation level is a major problem both in the collection of psychophysical data and in its interpretation for the design of speech-processors.

Unusual Aspects of Loudness Perception

It was mentioned in the section on threshold that the impedance of an electrode can become nonlinear at sufficiently high levels. Above this level, there is a sudden drop in impedance which is accompanied by a paradoxical increase in loudness.[5] We assume that the sudden impedance drop represents a point at which either the waveform itself is altered, causing an increase in loudness, or that the production of distortion products distributes the energy over a broader frequency range, bringing more energy into the lower (and more sensitive) frequency region.

If this point occurs within the dynamic range of the listener, then we would expect a break in the loudness-scaling function. This has been found in two listeners.[1, 42] For both subjects, loudness increased at one rate below some level and then showed a transition to a much steeper rate above this. In both subjects, thresholds rose over time. One (L.Y.) underwent explantation and the other (C.K.) has little use of her device because of the very high thresholds. Perhaps the presence of the loudness nonlinearity hints at unexplained phenomena causing threshold loss.

In normal listeners, constant signal power is required for constant loudness until energy falls within more than one critical band. Then signal power must be reduced for constant loudness, presumably because integration across critical bands is taking place. In a cursory check of this with one implanted listener (S.O.) in Vienna, noise with bandwidths from 0.1 to 3.0 octaves (centered at 100, 250, 500, and 1000 Hz) was presented and the listener was asked to adjust signal power until the noise reached a specified comfortable loudness. The noise was electronically equalized to compensate for the form of her sensitivity curve at threshold. Results were similar at all center frequencies and showed a gradual increase in the power necessary for equal loudness as bandwidth increased, reaching 3–4 dB by a width of three octaves. This result is opposite to the effect in normal listeners and shows that neither average signal power, power within a restricted band, nor integration across different bands is solely responsible for loudness in implanted listeners. It is likely that statistics of the waveform also play a role.

As was mentioned in the section on threshold, a small increase in loudness is produced as repetition rate increases.[5, 10, 35] This is commonly found for pulsatile signals and probably represents integration of charge per half-wave pulse. Other researchers [43, 44] have shown data that support different loudness growth functions for different rates of stimulation. However, when loudness-scaling functions are regraphed as the logarithm of loudness versus sensation level (dB), different slopes are not evident.[1] The effect of sinusoidal stimulation frequency on loudness is nearly the same as on threshold in that, for the same current, low frequencies are much louder than high frequencies. Thus, equal-loudness contours follow a course parallel to the threshold curve.

Loudness is also affected by the phase of complex signals. For example, for one listener in Vienna, waveform inversion of a particular suprathreshold seven-component signal could make it inaudible. Loudness differences were often reported as the primary cue when phase-shifted signal pairs were discriminated with 90–100% accuracy. In the majority of phase experiments, loudness and pitch were inversely related: given equal power, the lower-pitched sound was usually louder. Both pitch and loudness could be affected by sensation level, with higher levels producing greater similarity of the two signals.

Summary

Much of what has been observed in psychoacoustic testing of implanted listeners is similar to that seen in normal or hearing-impaired listeners with only parametric modification. What is lacking is evidence for critical band phenomena and for frequency selectivity. The unique interaction of waveform and sensation level with pitch, loudness, and threshold appears only in implanted listeners. Direct waveform processing, without spectral decomposition, appears to be the means by which information is brought to the nervous system through electrical stimulation. The operations by which this is coded to create percepts of pitch and loudness remain to be elucidated.

Acknowledgments

I am indebted to the many implanted listeners who have volunteered their time in this research. Colleagues at Stanford University and at the Technische Universität in Vienna provided invaluable discussion and support, but responsibility for the opinions and interpretations expressed here must fall on me. I thank especially Dr. Richard Fischer for his collaboration and assistance in data collection.

References

1. Müller, C. G. 1981. Survey of cochlear implant work. J. Acoust. Soc. Am. **70:** S52.
2. Fricke, H. 1932. The theory of electrolytic polarization. Phil. Mag. (Series 7). **14:** 310–318.
3. Jaron, D., S. A. Briller, H. P. Schwan & D. B. Geselowitz. 1969. Nonlinearity of cardiac pacemaker electrodes. IEEE Trans. Bio-Med. Eng. BME–**16:** 132–138.
4. Hochmair-Desoyer, I. & E. S. Hochmair. 1980. An eight-channel scala tympani electrode for auditory prostheses. IEEE Trans. Bio-Med. Eng. BME–**27:** 44–50.
5. Simmons, F. B. 1966. Electrical stimulation of the auditory nerve in man. Arch. Otolaryngol. **84:** 2–54.
6. Gheewala, T. R. 1976. A CMOS implantable auditory prosthesis using integrated circuits technology. Technical Report No. 5306–1. Stanford Electronics Laboratories. Stanford, CA.

7. MATHEWS, R. G. 1978. Sound processing for an auditory prosthesis. Technical Report No. 5306–3. Stanford Electronics Laboratories. Stanford, CA.
8. HERNDON, M. K. 1981. Psychoacoustics and speech processing for a modiolar auditory prosthesis. Technical Report No. G906–5. Stanford Electronics Laboratories. Stanford, CA.
9. FISCHER, R. 1981. Methodik und Experimente zur psychoakustischen Evaluation des durch Cochlearprothesen wiedererlangbaren Hörvermögens in sensorineural Ertaubten. Doctoral dissertation. Technical University of Vienna. Vienna, Austria.
10. EDDINGTON, D. K., W. H. DOBELLE, D. E. BRACKMANN, M. G. MLADEJOVSKY & J. L. PARKIN. 1978. Auditory prostheses research with multiple channel intracochlear stimulation in man. Ann. Otol. Rhinol. Laryngol. **87** (Suppl. 53): 1–39.
11. TONG, Y. C., R. C. BLACK, G. M. CLARK, I. C. FORSTER, J. B. MILLAR, B. J. O'LOUGHLIN & J. F. PATRICK. 1979. A preliminary report on a multiple-channel cochlear implant operation. J. Laryngol. Otol. **93:** 679–695.
12. SHANNON, R. 1980. Personal communication.
13. FOURCIN, A. J., S. M. ROSEN, B. C. J. MOORE, E. E. DOUEK, G. P. CLARKE, H. DODSON & L. H. BANNISTER. 1979. External electrical stimulation of the cochlea: Clinical, psychophysical, speech-perceptual and histological findings. Br. J. Audiol. **13:** 85–107.
14. CLARK, G. M., Y. C. TONG, R. BLACK, I. C. FORSTER, J. F. PATRICK & D. J. DEWHURST. 1977. A multiple electrode cochlear implant. J. Laryngol. Otol. **91:** 935–945.
15. MERZENICH, M. M. & M. W. WHITE. 1977. Cochlear implant: The interface problem. *In* Functional Electrical Stimulation: Applications in Neural Prostheses. F. Hambrecht, Ed.: 321–340. Marcel Dekker. New York, NY.
16. DILLIER, N. 1978. Entwicklung und klinische Evaluation einer Gehörsprothese für sensorisch taube Patienten basierend auf der elektrischen Stimulation des achten Nervs. Doctoral dissertation. Technical University. Zürich, Switzerland.
17. SCHARF, B. 1978. Loudness. *In* Handbook of Perception. E. C. Carterette and M. P. Friedman, Eds., Vol. **4:** 187–242. Academic Press. New York, NY.
18. WRIGHT, H. N. 1968. The effect of sensori-neural hearing loss on threshold-duration functions. J. Speech Hear. Res. **11:** 842–852.
19. MÜLLER, C. G. 1981. Psychoacoustics in auditory implant research. *In* Proceedings of XII World Congress of Oto-rhino-laryngology, Budapest, Hungary, June 21–27. L. Surján & Gy. Bodó, Eds.: 531–535. Akadémiai Kiadó. Budapest, Hungary.
20. JERGER, J. 1960. Bekesy audiometry in analysis of auditory disorders. J. Speech Hear. Res. **3:** 275–287.
21. JERGER, J. & S. JERGER. 1967. Psychoacoustic comparison of cochlear and VIIIth nerve disorders. J. Speech Hear. Res. **10:** 659–688.
22. EDDINGTON, D. K., W. H. DOBELLE, D. E. BRACKMANN, M. G. MLADEJOVSKY & J. PARKIN. 1978. Place and periodicity pitch by stimulation of multiple scala tympani electrodes in deaf volunteers. Tr. Am. Soc. Artif. Int. Organs **24:** 1–5.
23. SIMMONS, F. B., C. J. MONGEON, W. R. LEWIS & D. A. HUNTINGTON. 1964. Electrical stimulation of acoustical nerve and inferior colliculus. Arch. Otolaryngol. **79:** 559–567.
24. MERZENICH, M. M., R. P. MICHELSON, R. A. SCHINDLER, C. R. PETTIT & M. REID. 1973. Neural encoding of sound sensation evoked by electrical stimulation of the acoustic nerve. Ann. Otol. Rhinol. Laryngol. **82:** 486–503.
25. HELMERICH, L. 1981. Psychoacoustic results on cochlear implant patients. Paper presented at the 4th Annual West Coast Cochlear Prosthesis Workshop, Pacific Grove, California, August 2–4.

26. THURLOW, W. R. & A. M. SMALL. 1955. Pitch perception for certain periodic auditory stimuli. J. Acoust. Soc. Am. **27:** 132–137.
27. TONG, Y. C., G. M. CLARK, P. J. BLAMEY, P. A. BUSBY & R. C. DOWELL. 1982. Psychophysical studies for two multiple-channel cochlear implant patients. J. Acoust. Soc. Am. **71:** 153–160.
28. WIER, C. C., W. JESTEADT & D. M. GREEN. 1977. Frequency discrimination as a function of frequency and sensation level. J. Acoust. Soc. Am. **61:** 178–184.
29. ATLAS, L., M. HERNDON, C. MÜLLER, F. B. SIMMONS & R. L. WHITE. 1980. Psychoacoustical characterization of an auditory prosthesis. Paper presented at the 3rd Annual West Coast Cochlear Prosthesis Workshop, Seattle, Washington, July 24–25.
30. MICHELSON, R. P., M. M. MERZENICH, C. R. PETTIT & R. A. SCHINDLER. 1973. A cochlear prosthesis: Further clinical observations; preliminary results of physiological studies. Laryngoscope **83:** 1116–1122.
31. HOUSE, W. F. & B. J. EDGERTON. 1980. A multiple-electrode cochlear implant: Preliminary tests results. Paper presented at the 3rd Annual West Coast Cochlear Prosthesis Workshop, Seattle, Washington, July 24–25.
32. BLACK, F. O., F. B. SIMMONS & C. WALL, III. 1980. Human vestibulo-spinal responses to direct electrical eighth nerve stimulation. Acta Otolaryngol. **90:** 86–92.
33. JESTEADT, W., C. C. WIER & D. M. GREEN. 1977. Intensity discrimination as a function of frequency and sensation level. J. Acoust. Soc. Am. **61:** 169–177.
34. MICHELSON, R. P. & R. A. SCHINDLER. 1981. Multichannel cochlear implant. Preliminary results in man. Laryngoscope **91:** 38–42.
35. SIMMONS, F. B., J. M. EPLEY, R. C. LUMMIS, N. GUTTMAN, L. S. FRISHKOPF, L. D. HARMON & E. ZWICKER. 1965. Auditory nerve: Electrical stimulation in man. Science **148:** 104–106.
36. DENT, L. J., F. B. SIMMONS, M. K. HERNDON, L. E. ATLAS & R. L. WHITE. 1981. Two experiments in frequency modulation: Pulse-rate modulation and "place quality" modulation. Paper presented at the 4th Annual West Coast Cochlear Prosthesis Workshop, Pacific Grove, California, August 2–4.
37. BISMARCK, G. VON. 1974. Timbre of steady sounds: A factorial investigation of its verbal attributes. Acustica **30:** 146–159.
38. BISMARCK, G. VON. 1974. Sharpness as an attribute of the timbre of steady sounds. Acustica **30:** 159–172.
39. DAVIS, H., R. SILVERMAN & D. R. MCAULIFFE. 1951. Some observations on pitch and frequency. J. Acoust. Soc. Am. **23:** 40–42.
40. MLADEJOVSKY, M. G., D. K. EDDINGTON, W. H. DOBELLE & D. E. BRACKMANN. Artificial hearing for the deaf by cochlear stimulation: Pitch modulation and some parametric thresholds. Tr. Am. Soc. Artif. Int. Organs **21:** 1–7.
41. SIMMONS, F. B., R. L. WHITE, M. G. WALKER & R. G. MATHEWS. 1981. Pitch correlates of direct auditory nerve electrical stimulation. Ann. Otol. Rhinol. Laryngol. **90** (Suppl. 82): 15–18.
42. SHANNON, R. V., E. OWENS & D. KESSLER. 1980. Human psychophysical results of electrical stimulation: Effects of waveform and electrical configuration. Paper presented at the 3rd Annual West Coast Cochlear Prosthesis Workshop, Seattle, Washington, July 24–25.
43. HOCHMAIR-DESOYER, I. J., E. S. HOCHMAIR, R. E. FISCHER & K. BURIAN. 1981. Preliminary speech perception results through a cochlear prosthesis. *In* Neuronal Mechanisms of Hearing. J. Syka & L. Aitkin, Eds. Plenum Press. New York, NY.
44. SHANNON, R. V. 1981. Growth of loudness for sinusoidal and pulsatile electrical stimulation. Ann. Otol. Rhinol. Laryngol. **90** (Suppl. 82): 13–14.

Part VIII. Pre- and Postoperative Evaluation of Patients

INTRODUCTION

Robert A. Houde

Center for Communications Research
Rochester, New York 14621

Evaluation of approaches to the design of a cochlear implant is entirely determined by pre- and postoperative evaluation of the implanted patient, the effectiveness of the implant being determined by the improved performance of the individual on standard audiological tests of auditory perception and processing. In addition to standard auditory testing, there is, in the case of the cochlear implant, the need to evaluate the degree to which neural function is possible both pre- and postoperatively. Particular care must be taken to separate the signal-processing characteristics of the device from the auditory processing of the electrical stimuli by the patient.

ESTIMATING NERVE SURVIVAL BY ELECTRICAL ABR [a]

F. Blair Simmons and Lee Smith

Division of Otolaryngology/Head and Neck Surgery
Stanford University School of Medicine
Stanford, California 94305

There is now a considerable body of evidence that some persons are more effective users of implants than others, even with the same coding schemes and electrodes; some of this evidence appears elsewhere in this volume. One of several possible reasons for this variability is probably the numbers of surviving nerve fibers or ganglion cells. This paper describes a method by which it may be possible to know, either before or after implantation, the relative proportion of viable neurons in the auditory nerve.

Materials and Methods

We damaged the cochleas of 17 cat ears to produce varying degrees of nerve degeneration by surgical trauma, aminoglycoside perfusion, and by liquid-nitrogen freezing. Three to six months later these animals were reanesthetized and a monopolar electrode was placed just inside the round-window membrane by no more than a millimeter. We then electrically stimulated this electrode with 10/sec, 0.25 msec/phase charge-balanced pulses and recorded brainstem electrical activity by computer averaging—the ABR responses. This electrically induced ABR (EABR) was recorded differentially between an electrode in the frontal sinus and the opposite scala tympani. Typically, 256 samples were obtained and stored on tape for 50- to 100-μA increments in the electrical stimulus between threshold and a maximum where the seventh nerve stimulus artifact interfered with the eighth nerve brainstem response. Six presumed-normal control ears were also used.

The cats were then killed and the cochleas removed and immediately perfused with iced phenol. After decalcification, the bones were cut in half in the midmodiolar plane, paraffin-embedded, and sectioned by conventional methods. Each 100-μ slice was stained with hematoxylin and eosin and mounted for estimates of ganglion cell survival. The surviving cells were estimated in quartiles by two independent readings for the lower basal, upper basal, lower middle, upper middle, and apical turns. These survival estimates were then compared with the EABR input–output functions, threshold-to-maximum amplitude of the most consistent and prominent wave at 2.7 ($\pm$ 0.3) msec.

FIGURE 1 shows these EABR input–output functions for 20 of these 24 ears. The functions are sorted into four groups according to surviving ganglion cells. Four ears (all with aminoglycoside perfusion) had no surviving cells and no measurable EABRs. The vertical bars show the full range of response amplitudes for ears in each category. Except for the control group, there were about equal numbers of ears in each category.

[a] This work was supported by Grant NS 10532 from the National Institutes of Health.

The correlations in FIGURE 1 show that threshold is a very poor predictor of neuron survival. Cochleas with as few as 25% surviving cells had EABR thresholds that were not strikingly different from those with 100% survival. On the other hand, the slopes and peak amplitudes of the suprathreshold EABR showed a strikingly good correlation with neuron survival. In fact, there was no overlap whatsoever in these functions among the four groups of ears.

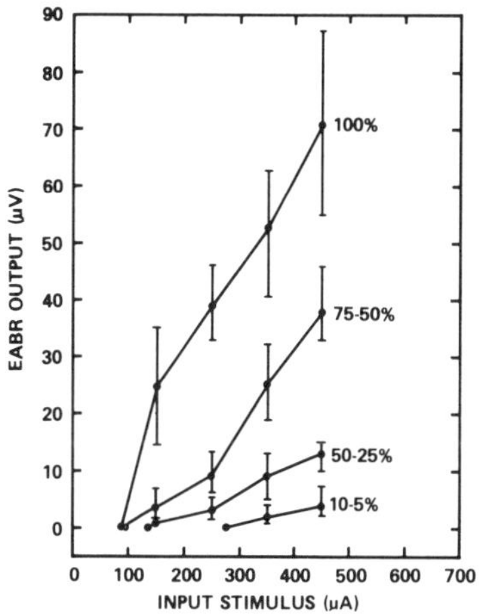

FIGURE 1. Input–output functions for electrically induced ABR's from cat cochleas with varying numbers of surviving ganglion cells. The vertical bars show the total ranges within each group. (From Smith and Simmons.[1] Reprinted by permission.)

DISCUSSION

Our goal with these data is the development of the method for use in human subjects. The techniques are simple and it is a low-risk procedure to temporarily place a comparable electrode in the same location and apply these same stimuli. Readout by EABR and by perceptual reports (threshold, maximum loudness, and some scaling for loudness difference limens) can be done with little trouble. It is critically important to do these studies, even when the surgeon placing the implant has already made up his mind for placement of single or multiple electrodes in the patients' ear. The truth now is that no one is really able to predict "successful" results from probable "failures." This is likely to continue unless we develop better methods of decision-making.

We find it interesting, for example, that essentially all ears that have received implants to date have heard something by electrical stimulation, unless there was so much osteoneogenesis present in the cochlea that no space remained for an electrode. While 5% residual nerve fibers may be sufficient for hearing some electrically induced sounds, it makes no sense whatsoever to place a multielectrode in such an ear and expect speech recognition.

REFERENCE

1. SMITH, L. & F. B. SIMMONS. 1982. Estimating eighth nerve survival by electrical stimulation. Ann. Otol. Rhinol. Laryngol. In press.

THEORETICAL CONSIDERATIONS IN TESTING SPEECH PERCEPTION THROUGH ELECTROAUDITORY STIMULATION [a]

J. M. Pickett

Sensory Communication Research Laboratory and Rehabilitation Engineering Center
Gallaudet College
Washington, D. C. 20002

In this paper I briefly characterize some of the basic phonetic features of speech that are necessary for its communication and relate the features to some problems in implant testing. A section on speech-reception testing methods is also included.

There is a strong trend in current theories of speech perception to take a developmental approach, so I have used a similar theoretical approach here. However, this is simply to provide an interesting up-to-date framework for discussing speech perception, and is not to be used for theoretically oriented studies.

Prosody and Phoneme in Perception

The phonetic features are usually classified as prosodic versus phonemic, and this distinction is very useful for our purposes as well as for theories of speech perception in general. Prosodic information in speech consists of certain patterns of variation of the voice pitch (fundamental frequency), the intensity, and the temporal patterns. The variations forming the prosodic patterns usually take place over a span of one or more syllables; thus they are called "suprasegmental," as opposed to variations related to the smaller segments that form the individual vowels and consonants (phonemes).

At the end of the babbling stage, the utterances of young children often embody the prosodic features of the home-language. The child of 18 to 24 months often speaks with good prosody; the melodic contours (intonation) and the rhythmic patterns of the child's speech sound like conversation, for example, as if the child is asking questions and making statements; vowels and consonants alternate properly, forming syllables, but in these "conversations" the child does not necessarily use any words of the language; this behavior appears early before the child knows very many words. In other words the child seems to communicate with prosodic patterns before using phonemic word structure to any significant extent.

The developmental primacy of prosody is necessary to support basic functions in both production and perception. In production the phonation of vowels and the constrictions of the consonants must be produced in proper timing relationships before intelligible words can be uttered. The pitch intonation

[a] This work was supported by the Gallaudet Research Institute and by the National Institute of Handicapped Research under Grant G008103979 for the Rehabilitation Engineering Center for the Deaf and Hearing-Impaired at Gallaudet College.

0077–8923/83/0405–0424 $1.75/0 © 1983, NYAS

"contours" serve to demarcate larger units of meaning, such as phrases and sentences. It is well known that syllables and words are not well demarcated by the visible articulations of lips and tongue. Therefore, a person can be helped greatly in lipreading if he perceives only the prosody.[1] This gives cues for the syllable- and word-boundaries, and also for the larger meaning units such as sentences and changes of topic (paragraphs).

Prosody through Implants

Fourcin and his colleagues were the first to recognize the importance of providing prosodic information through an implant. In a recent study with profoundly deaf subjects who had had normal hearing until shortly before the experiment, the pitch of the speaker, that is, the fundamental frequency alone, was impressed on the cochlea through an electrode placed on the round-window area. The subjects reported that they could perceive the "voice" of the speaker. They were tested for their ability to label upward pitch-tracks as "questions" and downward pitch-tracks as "statements." They were reasonably accurate in this task. This indicated that prosodic cues might be provided electrically.[2] Another test involving perception of prosody is the story-tracking test of aided lipreading developed by De Filippo and Scott.[3] A description of the tracking method is in the last section of this paper.

There are no standardized materials for these tests. In fact, the tracking test would seem nearly impossible to standardize because it involves interaction between the patient and the test speaker. However, the value of the electrical stimulation can be tested by turning it off, continuing the story, and measuring the rate of progress of lipreading alone. A procedure like this was demonstrated at this conference in a videotape shown by Fourcin and Rosen to demonstrate the effect of adding only the voice-pitch/amplitude signal to lipreading by a normal listener. When this procedure was formally tested, the correct word-reception rate increased by nearly a factor of two. Thus, it appears that provision of only limited prosodic information for the newly but profoundly deafened person, through electrical stimulation, would improve lipreading success considerably.[1]

Phonemic Information

The phonemic information of speech is built onto the prosody; the phonemes are the consonants and vowels; technically they are the sequential subunits of syllables that differentiate words. A given phoneme is not a single acoustic pattern, but a class of patterns produced by similar, but not identical, articulations. The variations of the members of a phoneme class are called allophones. Consider the *s*-sounds at the beginnings of the words *sill, still,* and *spill*; these three *s*'s differ from one another in articulation because of the tongue's articulatory positions needed to produce the different following sounds, *i*, *t*, and *p*. These must be anticipated for timely attainment and the anticipation begins during the *s*-articulation. The resulting differences in *s*-articulation cause differences in the sound pattern of *s*. These illustrate three allophones of the phoneme /s/; it has been estimated that /s/ consists of at least 100 allophones.

The phonemes are known to be basic units in speech production and perception. Some theorists believe that phoneme perception is carried out by a process that derives the differential production features of the phonemes. (For a review of these "motor" theories of speech perception, see Pickett,[4] pp. 189–206). These theories presently seem to be peripheral to implant testing, but are mentioned here for the interest of the reader.

In any case, the phonemes of speech occur at a rate of 8 to 10 per second, and there are about 40 different phonemes in English. Thus, for the speech perceiver, instead of having to choose among 40 different possibilities about 10 times per second, it seems more feasible to perceive the presence or absence of only the seven known articulatory features of each consonant phoneme: voicing, obstruent (stop), nasality, glide, and three places of constriction and, for the vowels, openness, place of constriction, and duration. Indeed, these features are known to structure the phoneme perception of both normal and deafened listeners.[5–7]

During speech development, hearing children very early seem to perceive features that distinguish phonemes, even before they produce them differentially to distinguish intelligible words. At this stage of perceiving speech, the child is probably merely learning to associate very salient acoustic–phonetic features, produced repeatedly by the child's caretakers, to specific situations.

However, the acoustic patterns of a feature differ, depending on context and speaker. How does the child's perception eventually become organized to classify the variant allophones into phonemes? An attractive theoretical scenario for the child's learning of the proper grouping of the allophones into phoneme classes is that the child's successful experiences in imitating the various acoustic patterns heard for a given phoneme enables the child eventually to hear the variants in terms of the successful articulation, and finally in terms of the abstract phoneme classes that differentiate among meanings (see Pickett,[4] pp. 199–201, and the references there).

An aid to this process is the fact that the acoustic patterns reflecting the articulation features are already very salient to the auditory system, almost immediately after birth (1 to 4 months). For example, the infant's discrimination of the voicing feature of consonants shows the same discrimination of the relevant acoustic pattern difference, between voiced and unvoiced stops, as that of adults.[8, 9] This difference resolves to a difference in time between the onsets of low-frequency versus high-frequency sound in the release pattern of the stop. This onset difference is called voice onset-time (VOT). If the onsets are close to simultaneous, it is a voiced stop. If the low onset lags the high onset by 30 msec or more, it is an unvoiced stop. These two patterns are very salient to the auditory system, apparently almost from birth. It is probably built-in saliences of audition, like this one, and the tendency of languages to use them for phoneme distinctions, that support the rather rapid acquisition by the normal child of communication by spoken language.

Thus, the most effective way to compensate for profound hearing loss would be to provide the naturally salient auditory patterns, because the central auditory system seems well designed to work these patterns into a generalized abstract system for perceiving language messages, as described by Studdert-Kennedy.[10]

Implant Cues to Voicing

To transmit the stop-voicing VOT cue most naturally, implant stimulation would have to be localizable separately at low-frequency and high-frequency places in the cochlea. Multiple-channel devices may be designed to do this, as for example in the experimental "Australian system" of Clarke and his colleagues. In tests of this system, the transmission of the voicing feature was modestly aided (transmitted at 30% correct).[11] Thus, multiple channels cannot guarantee consonant voicing transmission, but this can be tested using feature-oriented tests and response analysis, as did Tong *et al.*[11]

There may also be some cues to consonant voicing in the voice pitch. In some contexts there is a low-frequency voicing during the constriction intervals of voiced consonants that is absent from the constrictions of unvoiced consonants. The Australian system may also transmit this cue to the patient.

Place Cues

The "place" features of phonemes are related to the different places of constriction and shape configurations of the vocal tract which are associated with the movements and states attained by articulation to produce the vowels and consonants. Acoustically these features are realized in changing patterns of the speech spectrum, often called the formant structure. In particular, the first three resonances of the vocal tract, formants one, two, and three, occurring in the frequency range up to about 3000 Hz, define the perceived spectra of the different vowels and of some of the consonants. The acoustic features of the bursts of stop consonants and of the fricative noises also show spectral patterns that are important for their auditory discrimination. These are described by Stevens in this volume.[12]

Implant Cues to Place

An implant system, in order to transmit the place features, would need to simulate at least the overall auditory representation of the gross shape of the input spectrum. With present simultaneous stimulation on multiple electrodes, we probably do not have sufficiently discrete stimulation of the array of cochlear nerve fibers to adequately represent the spectrum shape. However, a multiple system with only a single electrode in action at any time, such as the Australian nine-point experimental system, may be able to provide discriminable high-frequency pitch sensations to represent the general frequency-weighting of the power spectrum viewed as a whole. In the tests of this system by Tong *et al.*[11] word reception depending on discriminating place features was analyzed from the patient's responses. However, the place perception was not found to be very good (14% correct transmission).

The remaining features of consonants are the so-called manner features: glide, nasal, stop, fricative. These can be considered to be normally cued by certain combinations of fundamental frequency (pitch), spectral patterns, and temporal patterns. The distinctions of stop (duration), nasal, and fricative were tested on the system of Tong *et al.*; these discriminations were achieved at a level of about 30% correct transmission.

Cue- and Feature-Testing versus Overall Performance Testing

If we take the feature approach to implant testing, we are theoretically close to the basic units of speech perception. The acoustic–perceptual cues to the features are fairly well understood.[4] Thus, the pattern of feature perception seen through the implant can provide some indications of what auditory speech information is achieved by the combined implant–auditory system processing. It should be noted, though, that this interpretation has limitations due to redundancies between features in defining the phonemes. The best recent treatment of this approach with hearing-impaired listeners is by Bilger and Wang.[13] Specific acoustic speech cues to feature discrimination by the hearing-impaired have also been tested using computer-processed natural speech and discrimination tests with synthetic cues.[14] These methods may turn out to be useful for fine-tuning of the signal processing in implant systems. For general assessment of performance, sentence tests, word tests, and phoneme confusion analysis to examine features transmission would be sufficient.

Potential of Synthetic Speech Cues for Listening Training

Classical auditory training methods employ natural speech stimuli that are not well controlled as to embodiment of essential cues. However, implant patients often will vary greatly in discrimination for the various cues in natural speech. This would indicate that the use of carefully coordinated, individually tailored training materials and procedures could improve the efficiency and outcomes of the patients' training. This may be accomplished by using synthetic speech.

In our own studies of synthetic formant transition-discrimination by partially deaf listeners we often found that a listener improved in discrimination performance, presumably because of the clearly isolated formant cue and the procedure of answer-feedback. How might this improvement in synthetic cue discrimination be made to carry over to speech perception? In the case of isolated formant transitions, cue discrimination might be trained with other formants suppressed at first and then increased progressively. Another cue parameter that can be controlled using synthesis is the rate of formant transition. Slow transition rates might first be presented in isolation for training. When faster, speech-like rates could be perceived, gradually the isolated transition would be imbedded in contexts.

Real-speech context, because of the overlapping of speech movements, changes the extents of formant transition and sometimes the directions and rates. These changes may cause some cues to be ambiguous. However, these interactions are important because they provide serial pattern information about the adjacent phoneme articulations. In other words, the transition patterns between two or three adjacent phonemes contain cues to the perception of all of the phonemes of that group. All of these complex interactions must be accommodated and used for completely normal decoding of speech messages.[15]

Speech synthesis with natural variations can provide training material that is systematically programmed and adapted for individualized auditory training. Hand-held and desk-size synthesizers could be developed for practice at home and for training in the clinic.

Methods of Testing Speech Communication Systems

The following section is a summary of various techniques and problems in testing the speech communication performance of aids for the deaf. The main topics covered are the choice of speech units, methods of sentence testing, and choice of performance measures. Under each topic, specific methods are referred to and briefly discussed in terms of advantages and disadvantages for goals of system testing. No attempt is made to describe all the tests available. The emphasis is on problems in testing systems as aids to speech communication. Specific aids, however, are not discussed; these are described elsewhere in this volume, and in Levitt *et al.*,[16] where a discussion of classical methods will also be found (pp. 35–38).

Choice of Speech Units for Test Presentation

Fundamental speech units, such as phonemes, need to be tested for systems where it is possible and important to be able to cause changes in transmission of basic speech units by changes in the system. For example, changes in phoneme confusion patterns may indicate specifically how the system-processing *really* works, as opposed to predictions from a model of the system, be the model implicit or explicit.

Larger speech units, at least of sentence length, often need to be tested for one or more reasons: to test general validity, to take into account any important concerns about the memory, or language-knowledge of the listeners, and to obtain important signal variations in input that would affect performance. Villchur [17] pointed out that the advantages of input signal compression would be greatest when there is a large variation in speaking intensities. Therefore, the possible advantages of compression should be tested on sentences.

Methods of Test Presentation and Response to Sentences

Classical method. In this method the subject is asked to listen to and then write the presented sentence or answer a question about the content of the sentence. The advantages of this method are: (1) its face validity; and (2) that it is easy to find or construct. The disadvantages are: (1) it is language-dependent and memory-dependent; (2) it cannot be repeated very many times unless there are several hundreds of different sentences available; and (3) there is poor homogeneity of any relatively small set of sentences.

Pollack–Pickett method. This method was used both with read sentences and natural recorded conversation in an experiment to demonstrate auditory versus structural context effects.[18] Only part of a test sentence is presented. The amount of the sentence presented (in terms of number of successive words) is varied. Presentation may be in two ways: (1) on paper (no memory problem, but takes temporal processing factors out of the picture) or (2) by sound (includes temporal processing factors). The listener identifies all he can or the part missing from the given printed partial sentence.[19]

This method was used successfully by Pollack and Pickett, on conversation, and thus can have high face validity.

The SPIN method. In this test sentences are presented with a test word at the end. The test words have precalibrated predictability on the basis of the sentence context. Two types of sentence frames provide either a low predictability or a high predictability of the same words.[20]

The method seems somewhat stilted, that is, it lacks high face validity, but it is the only standard test aimed at systematic assessment of the listener's use of internal language. If the sentence frame is displayed, there would be no auditory memory problem for the listener. Variations could be designed with the test word or words at sentence positions other than at the end.

Foust-Gengel repetition method. In this method the listener is given three sets of word-response blanks (one blank for each word) for each test sentence. Three successive presentation trials are given; after each presentation trial, the listener fills in a set of the word-response blanks. The test is scored according to essential correctness of the meaning-bearing words.

This is an interesting method for low-level of perceived input information, such as in tactile devices or auditory implant, and with severe-to-profound deafness. Foust and Gengel [21] found an increase in scores over the three presentations.

Live variations might be designed that would incorporate the speaker's adjustments to not being understood by the listener on the first presentation.

Adaptive sentence method.[22] This method is designed for rapid determination of the level of noise or of required signal level for a selected level of correct sentence reception. The procedure presents a series of very simple three-word statements that are to be answered by the listener as either true or false. An example is the sentence "Water is dry." If the listener answers correctly a criterion number of sentences, say two out of the first three, the signal level is reduced for the next three sentences; if still correct at criterion, the signal level is again reduced, and so on until a lower level is reached at which a criterion number of sentences, two of three, are answered incorrectly. Then the procedure is reversed: the level is increased successively until the criterion correct number has been reached. Again the level is reduced, and so on, until the sequence of levels at which the reversals have occurred is sufficiently stable to define a mean level. The criterion proportions used may be chosen to yield either a high level of correct reception or a moderate one. The criterion cited here defines a signal level that would produce 50% correct reception if the level were kept constant over a sufficient number of trials. Other levels of correct reception can be determined by using different critical proportions for the up-and-down changes of signal level.[23]

NTID method. This method is used primarily in training of speech-reading at the National Technical Institute for the Deaf.[24] Information is presented on the topic: for example, "The test sentence is spoken by a man talking to a clothes salesman." Then the test sentence might be: "I'm afraid this suit will be too small."

An alternative method would first present the sentence, get the response, then give the topic of the sentence and present it again, and then get a new response: compare for assessing a patient's ability to use a context and to break his set, which can cause him to assume an erroneous context. The problem of assumed erroneous context by lipreaders was originally noted by James D. Miller and his colleagues De Filippo and Scott, at Central Institute for the Deaf.

Levitt [22] noted that this method might profitably be used with graduated "obstruction" of the test material.

Possible new methods using computer-displayed sentences. In this method a sentence, or part of a sentence, is displayed after or while some versions of the sentence are presented by sound to the listener; then the listener is asked questions about what was heard with regard to the displayed sentence, such as:

(1) Was the speaker a man, woman, or child? (2) Was the sentence spoken as a question or a statement? (3) Was the first word as shown (target word flagged with underline by computer)? (4) Was the second word as shown (target word flagged with underline by computer)? The target word could be flagged before or after presentation if a memory variable is pertinent.

If the answer to the targeted word is *no*, then the listener could be asked to give the actual word, or to choose it from a displayed list of alternatives. Or, successive displays with a word blank could be given with more and more context added, either by sound or by display.

All responses could be supplemented by a confidence rating. The part displayed could be varied, depending on the content of an undisplayed part, as a test of use of context.

This method would lend itself to experiments measuring effects of amount of context. For example, one would compare scores on early, middle, and late flagged words in each sentence. Also, the listener could be asked to rate each word as to emphasis expressed by the speaker.

Sims *et al.*[25] have used techniques similar to some of the ones just described in testing and training deaf persons for improved everyday communication at the National Technical Institute for the Deaf.

In tests of lipreading factors, comparison of scores under a condition of preutterance partial display versus no predisplay would be a measure of the development of memory capacity for using new cues.

Reaction-time or response-time methods. Some British workers have recently used "reaction time" (RT) as a method of assessing hearing.[26] They report, for example, that hearing-impaired subjects, with scores higher than 90% correct in word discrimination, have much longer RTs than do normal subjects at similar performance levels. They believe that with use of RT measures, test lists can be shortened considerably for a given desired level of reliability of score differences (sensitivity).

In general, reaction time indicates the complexity of the perceptual process and thus it may be used to study the use of word context by the listener [27] and even the process of acoustic cue-decoding in perception of phonemes.[28]

It would seem that RTs might be derived in all types of speech testing. Obviously, though, RT would be easiest to collect on single-word responses.

Tracking method.[3] This method measures the rate of successful word transmission for a speaker–listener pair using meaningful fluently spoken material, usually some relatively simple text, such as a story or novel. The speaker speaks the first phrase and the lipreader (or listener) then speaks the phrase back to the speaker. If the listener is wrong, the speaker repeats the phrase, receives another response, and so on, until the listener is correct. As the story proceeds and thus the context is built up, the overall rate of progress becomes dependent on the efficiency of perception of the signal information. De Filippo and Scott developed the method to compare lipreading performance with and without a tactile speech aid.

The absolute rate of progress, of course, is highly dependent on the material and the individuals. Variations of the method might make it more independent of talker–listener strategies. The method might be under better control if each utterance could be stored, on video or audio, for identical playback.

Levitt [22] suggested that "sticking points" in the tracking could be defined, so that the lengths of "stuck" periods would reflect the listener's skill at selecting new alternatives. The word rate in the relatively successful passages between "stuck" periods would reflect system variables.

Describe-an-object method. This method, developed by Richards,[29] tests fluent speech communication by having the speaker cause the listener to identify an object or picture by listening to a describer over the test system. The time to identify is the index of transmission.

Performance Measures

It might be very beneficial to stand aside from the classical "transmission index" procedure of matching the listener's output against input, word-for-word, for percent-correct scoring. Some new procedures that do not score for the percentage of words correct are the tracking test of De Filippo and Scott,[3] the quality rating procedures of Studebaker *et al.*,[30] and some tests of heard prosodics.

A problem with sentences is that they tend to be heard "all-or-none." Thus, sentence comprehension over a system may not be a very sensitive, continuously valued measure, as a function of system variables. However, this may not be important if only an approximate value of the variable needs to be determined.

Scores, whether they be percentage correct, ratings, or rate of story progression in the tracking procedure, can be compared between systems in various well-known standard ways.

An interesting new procedure may be especially useful when a very large number of systems is under study. Rabiner *et al.*[31] developed a rating-tournament method to try to avoid having to transmission-test all the systems. Four systems are first "preference-compared" by the listener, by paired rating judgments, System A with System B, and System C with System D. If A is rated by the listener as better than B, and C is rated better than D, then A and C are compared; the better of A versus C is then chosen to advance for comparison with the winner from another set of four systems. The two winners are then "comparison-rated" and also transmission-tested for percent words correct to confirm the rating-tournament outcome. Of course, the risk exists that a highly intelligible system was eliminated in the rating tournament for reasons unrelated to performance, for example, because it did not sound or feel very pleasant.

Learning Problems in Speech Testing

We would like to have test performance differences predict the outcome of long-term experience with communication systems, yet we have only a limited amount of time for training and testing. How can long-term listening experience be shortcut? Some training feedback methods have been suggested: Engelmann and Rosov[32] first reported what might be called the comparison-feedback method, in research on a tactile vocoder for the deaf. If a subject responded with an error, for example, saying "now" for "how," the speaker said, "No, not *now* but *how*."

Variations of this method might be advantageous. For example, all or selected alternative words of the set under test might be given after an error.

A key problem in identification learning is normalization for variations in acoustic patterns due to different styles and rates of utterance and different speakers. Sparks *et al.*[33] found a decrease in tactile vowel identification when the number of talkers increased. These factors need to be introduced during training, and their effects measured, and normalization criteria described. Aside from normalization problems in learning to use a special speech aid, it might also be expected that long-term severely deaf listeners would differ greatly in their ability to normalize acoustically received speech.

References

1. Rosen, S., A. Fourcin & B. Moore. 1981. Voice pitch as an aid to lip-reading. Nature **291:** 150–152.
2. Fourcin, A. J., S. M. Rosen, B. C. Moore, E. E. Douek, G. P. Clarke, H. Dodson & L. H. Bannister. 1979. External electrical stimulation of the cochlea: Clinical, psychophysical, speech-perceptual and histological findings. Br. J. Audiol. **13:** 85–107.
3. De Filippo, C. L. & B. L. Scott. 1978. A method for training and evaluating the reception of ongoing speech. J. Acoust. Soc. Am. **63:** 1186–1192.
4. Pickett, J. M. 1980. The Sounds of Speech Communication. University Park Press. Baltimore, MD.
5. Shepard, R. 1972. Psychological representation of speech sounds. *In* Human Communication: A Unified View, chapt. 4. E. David and P. Denes, Eds. McGraw-Hill. New York, NY.
6. Walden, B. & A. Montgomery. 1975. Dimensions of consonant perception in normal and hearing-impaired listeners. J. Speech Hear. Res. **18:** 444–455.
7. Pickett, J. M. 1979. Perception of speech features by persons with hearing impairment. *In* Current Issues in the Phonetic Sciences, Vol. 9 (H. & P. Hollien, Eds.), Part 2 of Current Issues in Linguistic Theory. E. Koerner, Ed. John Benjamins. Amsterdam.
8. Eimas, P. 1974. Linguistic processing of speech by young infants. *In* Language Perspectives—Acquisition, Retardation, and Intervention. R. Schiefelbusch and L. Lloyd, Eds. University Park Press. Baltimore, MD.
9. Kuhl, P. K. 1979. The perception of speech in early infancy. *In* Speech and Language: Advances in Basic Research and Practice, Vol. 1. N. Lass, Ed. Academic Press. New York, NY.
10. Studdert-Kennedy, M. This volume.
11. Tong, Y. C., G. M. Clark, P. M. Seligman & J. P. Patrick. 1980. Speech processing for a multiple-electrode cochlear implant hearing prosthesis. J. Acoust. Soc. Am. **68:** 1897–1899.
12. Stevens, K. This volume.
13. Bilger, R. & M. Wang. 1976. Consonant confusions in sensorineural hearing loss. J. Speech Hear. Res. **19:** 718–748.
14. Pickett, J. M., S. G. Revoile & E. M. Danaher. 1983. Speech-cue tests of hearing. *In* Hearing Research and Theory, Vol. 2. J. Tobias and E. Schubert, Eds. Academic Press. New York, NY.
15. Liberman, A. & M. Studdert-Kennedy. 1978. Phonetic perception. *In* Handbook of Sensory Physiology, Vol. 8: Perception. R. Held *et al.*, Eds. Springer Verlag. Berlin.
16. Levitt, H., J. Pickett & R. Houde, Eds. 1980. Sensory Aids for the Hearing-Impaired. IEEE Press. New York, NY.
17. Villchur, E. 1978. *In* Proceedings of the 8th Danavox Symposium on Sensori-Neural Hearing Impairment and Hearing Aids. C. Ludvigsen and J. Barford, Eds. Suppl. 6 Scand. Audiol.
18. Pollack, I. & J. Pickett. 1964. Intelligibility of excerpts from fluent speech: Auditory *vs* structural context. J. Verb. Learn. Verb. Behav. **3:** 79–84.

19. Morrison, H. M. & J. W. Black. 1957. Prediction of missing words in sentences. J. Speech Hear. Dis. **22:** 236–240.
20. Kalikow, D., K. Stevens & L. Elliott. 1977. Development of a test of speech intelligibility in noise using sentence materials with controlled word predictability. J. Acoust. Soc. Am. **61:** 1337–1351.
21. Foust, K. O. & R. Gengel. 1974. Personal communication. Sensory Communication Research Laboratory, Gallaudet College.
22. Levitt, H. 1982. Unpublished comments at Advisory Meetings of the Rehabilitation Engineering Center, Gallaudet College, Washington, DC.
23. Levitt, H. 1971. Transformed up-down methods in psychoacoustics. J. Acoust. Soc. Am. **49:** 467–477.
24. Sims, D. 1980. Personal communication. Communication Department, National Technical Institute for the Deaf, Rochester, NY.
25. Sims, D., J. Von Feldt, F. Dorvaliby, K. Hutchinson & T. Myers. 1979. A pilot experiment in computer-assisted speechreading instruction utilizing the Data Analysis Video Interactive Device (DAVID). Am. Ann. Deaf **124:** 618–623.
26. Wright, R., M. Spanner & M. Martin. 1981. Pilot experiments with a reaction time audiometer. Br. J. Audiol. **15:** 275–281.
27. Pollack, I. 1963. Reaction times to unknown word sets in noise. Lang. Speech **6:** 189–195.
28. Kozhevnikov, V. & L. Chistovich. 1965. The original translated report of this work is not readily readable, even if available. I have provided a detailed summary in Ref. 4: 194–197.
29. Richards, D. L. 1973. Telecommunication by Speech. Halstead Press. Wiley. New York, NY.
30. Studebaker, G. A., J. D. Bisset, D. M. Van Ort & S. Hoffnung. 1982. Paired comparison judgments of relative intelligibility in noise. J. Acoust. Soc. Am. **72:** 80–92.
31. Rabiner, L., H. Levitt & A. Rosenberg. 1969. Investigation of stress patterns for speech synthesis by rule. J. Acoust. Soc. Am. **45:** 92–101.
32. Englemann, S. & R. Rosov. 1975. Tactile hearing experiment with deaf and hearing subjects. J. Except. Children **41:** 243–253.
33. Sparks, D., P. Kuhl, A. Edmonds & G. Gray. 1978. Investigating the MESA (Multipoint Electrotactile Speech Aid): The transmission of segmental features of speech. J. Acoust. Soc. Am. **63:** 246–257.

AUDITORY ASSESSMENT STRATEGY AND MATERIALS FOR ADULT AND CHILD CANDIDATES FOR COCHLEAR IMPLANTATION

Brad J. Edgerton, Laurie S. Eisenberg, and Margaret A. Thielemeir

House Ear Institute
Los Angeles, California 90057

In this paper we will deal with some of the issues involved in the auditory assessment of the severe to profoundly hearing-impaired. Clinically, audiologic assessment frequently has the dual purpose of providing information that is used in the medical diagnosis and to indicate potential avenues of rehabilitation. There are few clinical tests, however, that will meet this need for the severe to profoundly hearing-impaired patient. Standard suprathreshold tests, such as the CID-W22 [1] or the Modified Rhyme Test,[2] are too difficult for these patients to perform, and therefore this group has generally been excluded from an in-depth appraisal of its auditory perceptual abilities.

The tests and strategies used by the clinician should be determined on the basis of the decisions that the clinician must make with respect to patient or project management. Specific patient management issues include: (1) selection and fitting of a "best" prosthesis; (2) establishing a specific rehabilitation plan; (3) monitoring patient progress; and (4) providing information for improved prosthesis design. Because of the limitations of space, this paper will deal principally with the auditory testing issues involved in prosthesis selection and development of the rehabilitation plan for deafened adults and children. One of the first management decisions that should be made is what type, if any, of auditory prosthesis is most appropriate for a given patient. For this population the term prosthesis refers to hearing aids or cochlear implants. To evaluate what kind of prosthesis is the most beneficial, threshold and suprathreshold testing using pure-tone (or noise), speech, and environmental sound stimuli is required. Testing should be done with and without hearing aids when possible. At the House Ear Institute (HEI) the basic protocol includes the following tests:

Unaided Earphone

(1) Pure-tone thresholds
(2) Pure-tone uncomfortable loudness levels (ULL)
(3) Speech-detection threshold
(4) Most comfortable level for speech
(5) Monosyllable–Trochee–Spondee test (MTS) [3]

Aided-Sound Field

(1) Warble-tone thresholds
(2) Speech-detection threshold
(3) MTS test
(4) Environmental sounds test [4]
(5) Subjective evaluation

The pure-tone threshold and ULL data are collected to make appropriate hearing-aid selections for evaluation and trial. Speech and environmental sounds

0077–8923/83/0405–0435 $1.75/0 © 1983, NYAS

tests are included to evaluate more thoroughly the patient's ability to discriminate more complex and meaningful stimuli. Speech and environmental sounds tests are included throughout the evaluation since we have found that it is difficult to estimate patients' performance on these measures from their auditory thresholds.

For example, in FIGURE 1, patient performance scores on a four-alternative forced-choice consonant–vowel–consonant rhyme test [5, 6] are plotted as a function of their speech detection thresholds. From the figure it can be seen that speech discrimination scores have a tendency to get poorer as threshold gets poorer, although clearly there are some patients who do not follow this pattern. It is likely that different prostheses will be recommended for those patients showing better speech and environmental sound discrimination than for those who do not.

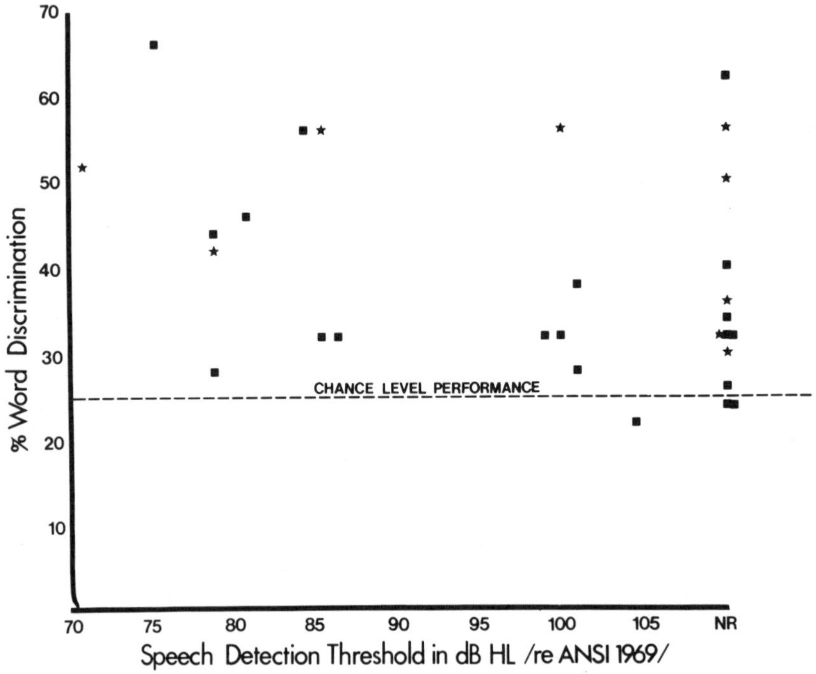

FIGURE 1. Norton rhyme test scores plotted as a function of speech detection threshold.

The protocol that we are recommending for use during these early stages of evaluation includes only the MTS and Environmental Sounds tests as suprathreshold indicators. We believe, however, that these two measures provide very representative patient profiles. Previously our test battery included a more extensive environmental sounds test, a six-item closed-set spondee test, and a 50-item four-alternative forced-choice rhyme test. The time required for test administration, however, is not justified on the basis of the information that is derived for use in making decisions regarding prostheses fittings.

The MTS test was developed by Erber and Alencewicz [3] and consists of 12 words, four in each of the three stress categories—monosyllable, trochee, and spondee. The word list is presented in TABLE 1. The MTS test is clinically efficient in that it provides information about two levels of perception, stress discrimination, and word identification, without requiring two separate tests. This test utilizes a forced-choice format with the patient selecting a response from a 12-item list. Each test condition consists of each word from the 12-item list repeated twice in a pseudorandom order. The patient is always familiarized with the test stimuli before test administration and a "ready light" is used during the test to indicate when each stimulus will occur. The patients' responses are recorded on a matrix, and the number of correct word and stress identifications is determined. Errors in the patients' perceptions of stress can be analyzed with respect to their severity, with the poorest indicator being the monosyllable for spondee confusion.

The Environmental Sounds test [4] is a 20-item five-alternative forced-choice test. The sounds have been recorded so as to be uniform in overall intensity and duration; there are four randomizations of the test. Patients are instructed to read the five answer-choices from a response sheet and then to circle the sound they hear. Sounds are repeated once if necessary; guessing is encouraged. A ready light is used to signal the presence of a test item and numbered cards are held up by the tester so that the patient does not lose his place on the response form.

When evaluating the performance of severe to profoundly hearing–impaired listeners with amplification we follow several guidelines: (1) we ensure that prior to evaluation an ear mold is obtained that allows the maximum benefit of the hearing aid to be attained; (2) we limit the output of the hearing aid to 130 dB SPL or less, as estimated at the eardrum; (3) we evaluate at least two "appropriate" hearing aids; and (4) we present speech and environmental sound stimuli at 70 dB SPL, a reasonable sound level, with the prosthesis adjusted to a comfortable level.

The need for special consideration with regard to the ear-mold fitting became obvious as we encountered a large number of patients who were not wearing hearing aids or who were not benefitting optimally from the aids they were wearing because of acoustic feedback. Because of the magnitude of this problem a research project was begun to develop improved techniques for ear-mold fabrication. At the present time, custom ear molds are fabricated in our own laboratory prior to the hearing-aid evaluation.

TABLE 1

MONOSYLLABLE—TROCHEE—SPONDEE TEST ITEMS

	Monosyllable	Trochee	Spondee
1.	Bed	Button	Baseball
2.	Cat	Chicken	Birdhouse
3.	Duck	Doctor	Popcorn
4.	Pig	Turtle	Toothpaste

TABLE 2

MEAN AND RANGES OF RAW SCORES FOR THE ENVIRONMENTAL SOUNDS TEST AND THE MONOSYLLABLE—TROCHEE—SPONDEE TEST (STRESS AND WORD) OBTAINED FROM 86 COCHLEAR IMPLANT PATIENTS

	Raw Scores		
Test	$\overline{X}$	Low	High
Environmental sounds	11	0	19
Monosyllable—trochee—spondee			
Stress	18	4	24
Word	8	0	19

The decision to limit the output of the hearing aid to 130 dB SPL or less was made for two reasons. On the basis of our experience, patients who functionally need amplification above this level do not typically do well with amplification, and in cases where there is residual hearing, and amplification is beneficial, we do not want to jeopardize that hearing with overamplification.

Two "appropriate" hearing aids are usually evaluated because we believe that relatively minor differences in hearing-aid performance may make substantial differences in perception when operating at the upper limits of the auditory system. Evaluating two hearing aids also reduces the chance that an unusually poor performance, spuriously achieved, will serve as the only basis for important decisions regarding prosthesis selection.

Decisions regarding which of several hearing aids is the most appropriate for a patient are usually based on the traditional comparison of test scores and the patients' subjective ratings. The most difficult decision, however, occurs for those patients who perform marginally with hearing aids; in these cases we mostly determined whether a cochlear implant is a suitable alternative. This *a priori* decision has become particularly important because our clinical and research findings indicate that if there is useful residual hearing, frequency discrimination will be better with an appropriately fit hearing aid than with the cochlear implant. As a tool for the clinician we have provided basic descriptive information, as shown in TABLE 2, for the Environment Sounds and MTS tests. To use this information in the decision-making process the clinician compares the patients best aided performance with the range of scores obtained from the patients with cochlear implants (CI). Although many additional factors must be considered, patients wearing hearing aids who perform at or above the average for CI patients would probably not be considered good candidates for the cochlear implant. On the other hand, patients wearing hearing aids who perform more poorly than do patients with cochlear implants would be counseled that they probably would benefit from the implant. TABLE 3 provides Environmental Sounds and MTS test scores for two patients who are typical of the patients being evaluated for the cochlear implant. In the table it is apparent that patient 1 would not be a good candidate because of his high level of performance with a hearing aid, while patient 2 could benefit from the implant.

Generally the development of the rehabilitative plan is based on a much more extensive evaluation than is provided for prosthesis selection. Recently,

Owens and Telleen[7] have developed a test battery, the Minimal Auditory Capabilities (MAC) battery, which offers a wide spectrum of test materials and can be used to provide a more comprehensive assessment of the auditory capabilities of the severe to profoundly hearing impaired. (A more detailed description of the MAC battery by Dr. Owens appears in this volume.) We would, however, like to summarize some of the recent experience that we have had using the MAC battery to evaluate cochlear implant patients. The MAC test has been administered to nine postlingually deafened adults using CIs. In general, performance on the subtests with open-response formats (spondee recognition, CID sentences, words in context and NU 6) has been extremely poor; these tests were beyond the capabilities of the patients evaluated. The tests that were within the abilities of most of the patients were: question/statement, vowel, noise/voice, accent, initial consonant, spondee same/different, everyday sounds, four-choice spondee, final consonant, and visual enhancement.

In terms of the specific results obtained, the question/statement and accent subtests revealed above-chance performance for five of nine and six of eight patients, respectively. These results are consistent with other prosodic experiments done at the HEI with CI patients. Vowel discrimination was extremely poor among these patients; above-chance performance was obtained for only one patient. This was a little surprising when we consider our pilot studies of vowel perception among CI patients.[8] Noise/voice discrimination was above chance in all but one patient; voice identification was above chance in all cases.

Spondee identification from a closed set was above chance for six of eight patients. These results were consistent with those obtained using the HEI spondee test. In the evaluation of initial consonants, above-chance performance was obtained from only five of nine patients. This is in contrast to the results obtained from the final consonant subtest, in which all subjects performed above the chance level. For both the initial and final consonant subtests the correct identification of the voicing feature reached significance more frequently than either the gliding feature or the nasality feature. The results obtained on the consonant subtests are in agreement with previous clinical and research findings.[6]

Of the six patients given the environmental sounds test, all were able to identify the following items: telephone busy signal, person talking, and a person laughing. No patients could identify a rooster crowing, person coughing, or crowd/party noise. The items patients found easiest to identify on the MAC

Table 3

Raw Scores for Two Patients for the Environmental Sounds Test and the Monosyllable—Trochee—Spondee Test (Stress and Word)

Patient	Environmental Sounds	MTS	
		Stress	Word
1	16	23	14
2	4	12	4

Note: Patient 1 is a poor candidate for cochlear implantation. Patient 2 could be considered for a cochlear implant.

environmental sounds subtest are in some cases the same items that are easiest to discriminate on the HEI environmental sounds test.

The improvements in speechreading resulting from auditory cues via the cochlear implant varied among patients. The patient demonstrating the least benefit was the only patient scoring above chance on all of the other subtests. The patient with the second best overall performance on the MAC battery demonstrated the most improvement in speechreading ability with auditory cues (45%). The patient demonstrating the poorest overall performance on the MAC battery also was the poorest speechreader with auditory cues.

Performance on the different MAC subtests demonstrates a varied discrimination profile across patients. Useful information about prosody, word discrimination, and segmental features as well as for speechreading was obtainable. At the present time we are continuing our evaluation of the MAC battery with the goal of developing individual patient profiles, which will be useful in the long-term rehabilitation process.

Evaluation of Children for Implantation

Auditory assessment of children for a cochlear implant presents a special set of considerations for the implant team. The primary consideration is the confirmation of profound hearing loss. Behavioral audiometry is often very accurate in diagnosing the loss in the older child, but it is very inaccurate for diagnosing hearing loss in the infant or very young child. Auditory brainstem response (ABR) testing is the most effective clinical tool to date for assessing hearing in the very young population, but it is limited in that it cannot measure the true profoundness of loss. For example, ABR test results are the same for a total loss as for a loss in which a small amount of residual hearing is present in the very low frequencies. This residual hearing greatly influences the child's ability to make use of amplified sound. The second major consideration in the assessment of children is how much benefit can be derived from hearing aids. The definition of "benefit" for the profoundly deaf child is extremely difficult because of age-related testing obstacles, cognitive factors, and a lack of experience with sound.

Educators of the deaf, particularly advocates of the auditory/oral approach, maintain that almost all deaf children have some usable residual hearing which can be aided by amplification. Hearing aids, in conjunction with an early interventive program of intense auditory training, can enable the child to develop a listening function as a prelude to learning speech and language.[9–11] Human and animal studies indicate that extensive organ of Corti damage results in some further, but not total, retrograde degeneration over time of spiral ganglion cells, cochlear nerve fibers, and cells within the cochlear nucleus.[12–16] Findings of Webster and Webster[17,18] suggest that congenital deafness (or any early deprivation of sound) causes an incomplete maturation of cells in the cochlear nucleus; this development takes place postnatally and apparently requires auditory stimulation. These studies lend support to the belief that early detection and remediation are crucial.

There are children, however, who do not respond successfully to oral education or who show no progress with hearing aids.[19] Histopathologic findings on temporal bones which compare different causes of profound sensorineural hearing loss indicate that in some patients whose deafness is caused by such things as meningitis (bacterial labyrinthitis) and some cases of congenital deafness there are very few remaining cochlear neurons. It is interesting to note that even among the implant subjects, those whose deafness is congenital or caused by meningitis show the poorest neural functioning, as revealed on tone-decay testing [20] and auditory brainstem response (HEI study in progress). These findings may help to explain why some children are not responsive to acoustic amplification. However, it is impressive that subjects (adults and children) with these causes of deafness are able to respond to the electrical stimulation delivered by the implant.

It is important to judge the child's ability to use a hearing aid. Aided and unaided thresholds are not always predictive of hearing-aid success or failure. For example, we have seen patients at the House Ear Institute who demonstrate an almost total loss on an audiogram, but who score significantly above chance on closed-set discrimination tests when tested with high-powered hearing aids. On the other hand, there are those patients who may show aided responses out to 2000 Hz or 3000 Hz, yet cannot perform even very simple discrimination tasks, or cannot tolerate the sound at these levels. Standard speech discrimination tests are too difficult for patients with this extent of loss. It was essential to find tests that assess discrimination of simple speech or speech components, in order to project how well a profoundly deaf child may learn to use the minimal cues available through a hearing aid. Two measures are currently being used for evaluating the discrimination abilities of the children. One measure is the Test of Auditory Comprehension. This test was standardized on children between the ages of 4 through 12 years old with varying degrees of hearing loss (moderate to profound in severity). The test is designed to evaluate auditory comprehension in a sequenced hierarchy of difficulty. Unfortunately, we are finding that this test gives very limited information, as children with profound losses score very poorly on the test. For that reason a new test has been developed at HEI which is specifically designed for the profoundly deaf child. The test is entitled the Discrimination after Training (DAT) test. The DAT is based on the monosyllable–trochee–spondee test (used with our adult subjects), but is broken down into much simpler discriminations. The test progresses in a hierarchy of difficulty beginning with tactile and visual discriminations and proceeding to auditory-only. It uses nonspeech and speech stimuli. The speech consists of syllables and words of differing stress patterns. If the child cannot initially perform a task, then training is initiated in specific steps. Results are based on the different levels within the hierarchy that can be achieved with competency. If the child is performing better with hearing aids than would be expected with the implant, then cochlear implantation would not be recommended.

Equally important to objective test data is observation over time. This is based on academic records, audiologic reports, and parent/teacher observations as to the child's progress with aids. Questionnaires are also currently being devised as checklists for teachers and parents to fill out. This would particularly be geared for the very young child, whom we would want to observe at least up to the age of 2 years to see if a listening function is being developed.

We strongly believe that children be given an adequate trial with hearing aids. However, if no progress is seen (that is, no awareness to sound and no speech development), then the cochlear implant would be considered as the appropriate next step in trying to bring sound to the deaf child.

REFERENCES

1. HIRSH, I. J., H. DAVIS, S. R. SILVERMAN, E. G. REYNOLDS, E. ELDERT & R. W. BENSEN. 1952. Development of materials for speech audiometry. J. Speech Hear. Dis. **17:** 321–337.
2. HOUSE, A. S., C. E. WILLIAMS, M. L. HECHNER & K. D. KRYTER. 1965. Articulation testing methods: Consonantal differentiation with a closed response set. J. Acoust. Soc. Am. **37:** 158–166.
3. ERBER, N. & C. ALENCEWICZ. 1976. Audiologic evaluation of deaf children. J. Speech Hear. Dis. **41:** 256–267.
4. NORTON, N. B. & K. I. BERLINER. 1977. Environmental sounds: Test and training program for the hearing impaired. Paper presented at American Speech and Hearing Association, Chicago, 1977.
5. EISENBERG, L. S., R. LUCKEY, N. B. NORTON & K. I. BERLINER. 1977. A discrimination task for profoundly deafened adults: HRRC Rhyme Test. Paper presented at American Speech and Hearing Association, Chicago, 1977.
6. NORTON, N. B. & B. J. EDGERTON. The Norton rhyme test for the profoundly deafened adult. In preparation.
7. OWENS, E. & C. TELLEEN. 1981. Speech perception with hearing aids and cochlear implants. Arch. Otolaryngol. **107:** 160–163.
8. DENT, L. Vowel discrimination with the single-electrode cochlear implant: A pilot study. *In* Cochlear Implants: Progress and Perspectives. W. House and K. Berliner, Eds. Ann. Otol. Rhinol. Laryngol. **91** (Suppl. 91): 41–46.
9. GRIFFITHS, C. 1967. Conquering Childhood Deafness. Exposition Press, Inc. New York, NY.
10. POLLACK, D. 1970. Educational Audiology for the Limited Hearing Infant. Charles C Thomas. Springfield, IL.
11. SILVERMAN, S. R., H. S. LANE & D. R. CALVERT. 1977. Early and elementary education. *In* Hearing and Deafness, 4th ed. H. Davis and S. R. Silverman, Eds. Holt, Rinehart and Winston. New York, NY.
12. KERR, A. & H. F. SCHUKNECHT. 1968. The spiral ganglion in profound deafness. Acta Otolaryngol. **65:** 586–598.
13. OTTE, J., H. F. SCHUKNECHT & A. G. KERR. 1978. Ganglion cell populations in normal and pathological human cochlea. Implications for cochlear implantation. Laryngoscope **88:** 1231–1246.
14. WEBSTER, D. B. & M. WEBSTER. 1978. Cochlear nerve projections following organ of Corti destruction. Otolaryngology **86:** ORL-342–353.
15. YLIKOSKI, J., Y. COLLAN & T. PALVA. 1978. Pathologic features of the cochlear nerve in profound deafness. Arch. Otolaryngol. **104:** 202–207.
16. GHORAYER, B., A. SARWAT & F. H. LINTHICUM, JR. 1980. Viable spiral ganglion cells in congenital and acquired hearing loss. J. Laryngol. Otol. **94:** 367–376.
17. WEBSTER, D. B. & M. WEBSTER. 1977. Neonatal sound deprivation affects brain stem auditory nuclei. Arch. Otolaryngol. **103:** 392–396.
18. WEBSTER, D. B. & M. WEBSTER. 1979. Effects of neonatal conductive hearing loss on brain stem auditory nuclei. Ann. Otol. Rhinol. Laryngol. **88:** 684–688.
19. NORTHERN, J. L. & M. P. DOWNS. 1978. Hearing in Children, 2nd ed. Williams & Wilkins. Baltimore, MD.
20. BRIMACOMBE, J. A. & L. S. EISENBERG. 1981. Auditory fatigue in subjects with the cochlear implant. Paper presented at the annual meeting of the American Speech, Hearing, and Language Association, Los Angeles, CA.

RESULTS FOR SOME PATIENTS WITH COCHLEAR IMPLANTS ON THE MINIMAL AUDITORY CAPABILITIES (MAC) BATTERY [a]

Elmer Owens, Dorcas Kessler, and Marcia Raggio

Department of Otolaryngology
University of California, San Francisco
San Francisco, California 94143

Three major types of cochlear implant systems are in use at present: a single-channel stimulator with a single electrode,[1,2] a single-channel stimulator with a multielectrode,[3-7] and a multichannel stimulator with a multielectrode.[8-10] The purpose of this study is to observe differences among patients using these three systems.

Subjects and Implant Systems

All subjects were adults with postlingual hearing loss who had received a cochlear implant. Electrode placement in each case was in the scala tympani. In four subjects, designated Implant I, the implant system was a single electrode with a single-channel stimulator; in another group of six subjects, Implant II, the system was an eight-bipolar electrode array (16 wires) with a single-channel stimulator; and in one subject, Implant III, an eight-bipolar electrode array was connected alternately to a three-channel or a single-channel stimulator.

Of the four Implant I subjects, one used a Michelson-type of stimulator [11,12] developed about 10 years ago, and the remaining three used a House-type of stimulator.[1] Diagnoses were ototoxic deafness in two instances and unknown in two others.

Subjects in Implant II constituted a succession of patients who received a prosthesis at the University of California (UCSF) between May 1979 and May 1981. Michelson and Schindler [5,6] have provided descriptions of the prosthesis and the surgical approach. Three patients in this group had a progressive hearing loss (two familial and one due to otosclerosis). The other three losses were attributed to meningitis, ototoxic drugs, and Cogan's syndrome.

The Implant III patient, a 61-year-old woman who experienced a progressive loss, is presently a research subject at UCSF. Her implant system permits activation of the eight-bipolar electrode array directly through a temporary cable that encases the 16 leads from the electrode. For daily use she has received a wearable single-channel stimulator that is essentially the same as the Implant II stimulator. It is connected to all 16 wires of the electrode array by means of a 16-pin connector attached to the percutaneous cable. The same connector accommodates a three-channel stimulator (desk model) as well as computer-controlled stimuli. The three-channel stimulator, which contains adjustable amplification, compression, and filtering controls, can activate any

[a] This work was supported by Grant NS12998 from the National Institute of Neurological and Communicative Disorders and Stroke, Bethesda, Maryland.

0077-8923/83/0405-0443 $1.75/0 © 1983, NYAS

one, two or three of the eight-bipolar electrodes at a time. In a process involving an extensive exploration of electrode combinations and settings of the three-channel stimulator, efforts were made to find the three "best" electrode pairs and the most appropriate settings for maximum speech recognition. A recorded narration was used to obtain subjective judgments on the quality of the speech by the subject, and objective measurements of vowel and consonant recognition were obtained with some consonant–vowel–consonant (CVC) word lists. The Minimal Auditory Capabilities (MAC) battery [7,13] was administered when the most propitious electrode pairs and stimulator settings had been selected. The temporary cable and connector will be replaced in a secondary surgical procedure by a permanent (wearable) three-channel stimulator employing inductive coupling in which these favorable electrode locations and settings of the desk-model stimulator will be duplicated.

PROCEDURE

The MAC battery was given to each subject in the sound field of an audiometric test suite, materials being presented over a speaker system at individual most-comfortable-loudness levels. Except for three of the four subjects in the single-electrode group, who were tested at different audiology clinics, all testing was conducted at UCSF. All testers were qualified audiologists and subjects were not familiarized with the test materials.

RESULTS AND DISCUSSION

Among the eight closed-set tests of the MAC, the vowel and initial consonant tests have been selected for detailed comparisons because of their relative importance for speech recognition. A sample of each kind of item is shown as follows:

heat	tip
hit	zip
hate	pip
hat	chip

One of the alternatives in each item on the response form is the stimulus presented on tape. The subject listens and checks the word he thinks he heard. All words are of the consonant–vowel–consonant (CVC) form; only the vowel varies in the vowel items and only the initial consonant varies in the consonant items.

FIGURE 1 shows individual raw scores for both the consonant and vowel tests. The bars of the graphs in the figures were arranged so that specific subjects can be followed individually—for example, bar 1 in each group is always the same subject. The Implant II scores are noticeably higher than those of the Implant I group; the means are 30.8 and 20.8, respectively, for the consonants, and 19.7 and 15.0 for the vowels. For the consonants, the Implant II mean is above the 0.05 confidence level, that is, the score that would be obtained by chance only 5 times in 100. The Implant I mean is under the 0.05 level, but well above chance. For the vowels, the Implant I

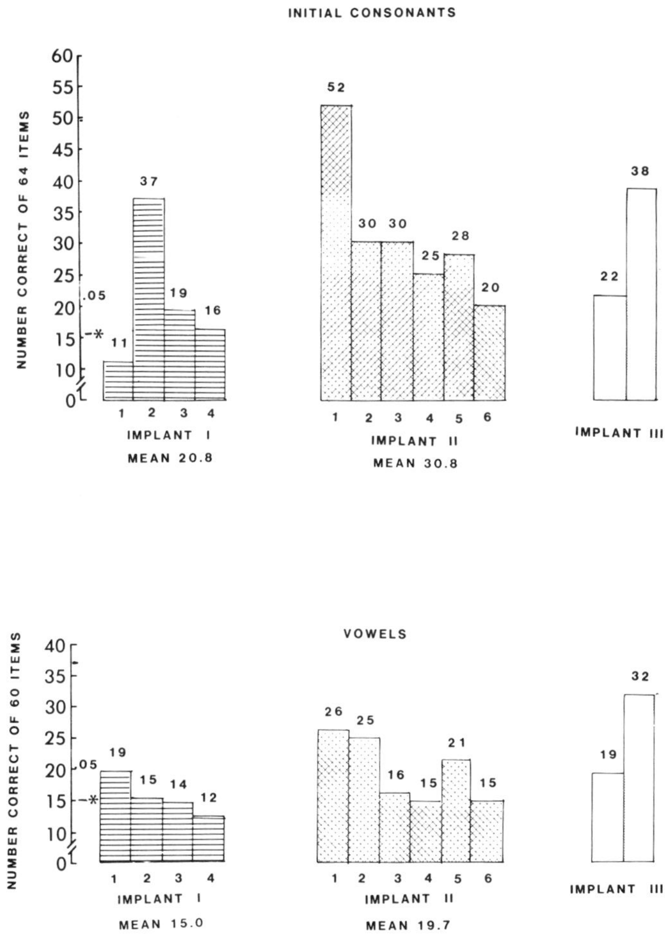

FIGURE 1. Individual raw scores for the vowel and initial consonant tests of the Minimal Auditory Capabilities battery. Each bar within a group refers to the same subject—for example, bar 1 of Implant I for the initial consonants represents the same subject as bar 1 of Implant I for the vowels.

subjects scored at around chance and the Implant II subjects scored just short of the 0.05 level. It would therefore appear that Implant I subjects tend not to recognize vowels in this format.

Of special interest is subject 1 in the Implant II group, who consistently achieved the highest scores of the subjects with Implants I and II. He had experienced a progressive familial hearing loss and was 59 years old at the time of testing. His superior performance is not explainable at present. In the Implant I group, subject 1 is unique in that he has used his implant regularly for 11 years.

The subject of Implant III, using the one-channel stimulator, scored close to the mean of the Implant I group on the consonants and well below the mean for Implant II; on the vowels, her score was above the Implant I mean and close to the Implant II mean. With the three-channel stimulator, her scores on both tests showed an immediate and striking improvement that was consistent with her subjective impression and that could not be attributed to experiential or learning activities. Actually, any effects of learning would have accrued mainly with the single-channel stimulator. The MAC test had been given at 2 weeks, 5 weeks, and 11 weeks post surgery to the subject while she was using the single-channel stimulator. These three protocols were averaged to arrive at the scores in FIGURE 1. Scores on the second and third test administrations corresponded closely, and both of these protocols were somewhat better than the first. Daily training sessions averaging 1 hour had been provided between the first and third MAC test administrations. In addition, incidental learning probably occurred in the subject's daily use of her single-channel stimulator outside the clinic environment. With respect to the three-channel condition, the MAC test was administered twice, each time with a different set of stimulator adjustments. Scores were generally the same in each instance and were averaged for use in FIGURE 1. Undoubtedly, the subject had gained some listening experience with her three-channel stimulator in the course of the work leading to the most appropriate stimulus parameters, but it amounted to only a small percentage of her total listening experience as compared with the single-channel stimulator. Despite the preponderance of training with the single-channel stimulator and regardless of when the MAC Battery was administered, scores on all tests were consistently better in the three-channel condition.

For the remaining six closed-set tests and an open-set test for recognition of everyday sounds, the mean scores for Implant I and II groups were generally equivalent, as shown in TABLE 1. For the Implant III subject, however, the scores for the three-channel condition were higher than for the single-channel condition on all of these tests.

TABLE 1

MEAN SCORES FOR THREE IMPLANT GROUPS ON THE OPEN-SET EVERYDAY SOUNDS TEST AND ON CLOSED-SET TESTS EXCLUDING THOSE FOR VOWELS AND INITIAL CONSONANTS

					Implant III	
Tests	Chance	0.05	Implant I	Implant II	One-Channel	Three-Channel
Question/statement	10	14	13.5	16.5	11.3	14.5
Noise/voice	20	25	26.3	28.0	36.3	37.0
Accent	5	8	12.0	13.3	4.7	8.0
Spondee same/different	10	14	17.8	16.8	12.3	18.5
Four-choice spondee	5	8	12.5	10.5	9.0	16.5
Final consonants	13	18	29.0	29.5	24.7	34.5
Everyday sounds	—	—	5	5	2	5

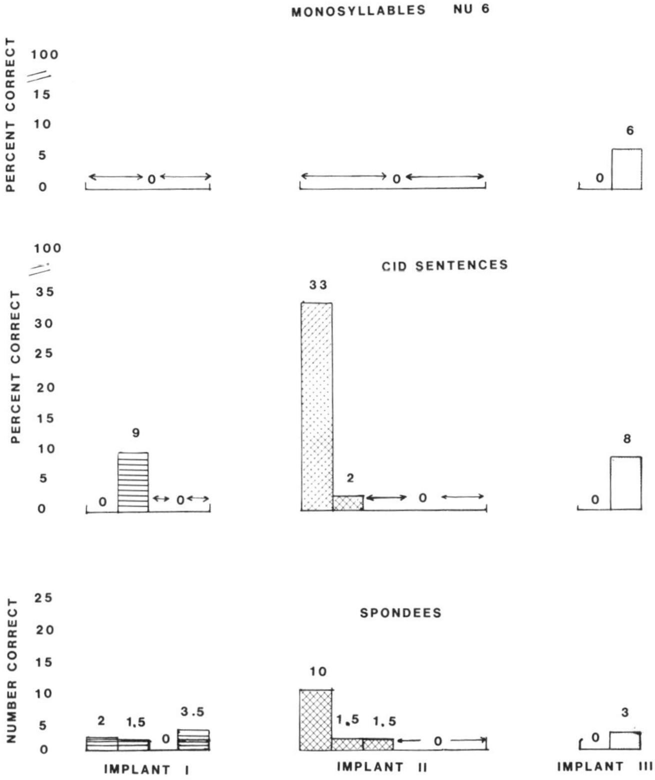

FIGURE 2. The results on open-set speech recognition tests for individual subjects.

OPEN-SET TESTS OF SPEECH RECOGNITION

FIGURE 2 shows the results for three of the four open-set speech tests of the MAC battery, in which a stimulus is given and the subject's task is simply to repeat it. The fourth open-set speech test was omitted because results for these subjects were almost identical to those for the Northwestern University (NU 6) 50-item monosyllable test included in FIGURE 2. The sentence test is composed of four sets (10 sentences each) of the Central Institute for the Deaf (CID) everyday sentences. The percentage score is based on a total of 200 key words among the four sets. The spondee test is composed of 25 two-syllable words.

On the spondee words, a half-point was given for correct repetition of half the word, for example, "football" for "baseball." One subject with Implant I, three with Implant II, and the subject of Implant III in the single-channel mode scored zero in spondee recognition. The remaining three subjects with Implant I, two of the Implant II subjects, and the subject of Implant III in the three-channel mode recognized 1.5 to 3.5 of the 25 spondees. Subject number 1 of the Implant II was again outstanding with a score of 10. This subject's high performance continued on the CID sentences test with a score of 33%. Only one subject with Implant I could recognize any words in sentences; subject 2 with Implant II scored 2%, and the subject of Implant III (three-channel condition) scored 8% On the NU 6, the most difficult test of the MAC battery, the only success was a score of 6%, achieved by the subject of Implant III in the three-channel condition.

Except for the outstanding results attained by subject 1 with Implant II, the open-set scores revealed no marked differences between Implants I and II. Only half of the Implant I and Implant II subjects were able to recognize even these simple speech materials in an open-set format. Moreover, there was no way to predict which of the subjects would be the successful ones. For example, expectations had been that subject 4 with Implant II would be superior to subject 1 in that group. Subject 4's hearing loss stemmed from ototoxic drugs (which presumably would leave the auditory nerve fibers largely intact), and he was twenty-five years younger than subject 1.

Because of this unpredictability, the results shown for the subject of Implant III are of great import at the present time. The consistently higher performance by this subject with the three-channel stimulator compared with the single-channel condition indicates the need not only for multichannel stimulation, but also for a means of determining the most appropriate patterns or configurations of electrode activation. Had treatment of this subject been completed with a single-channel stimulator, her improvement in hearing with a prosthesis would have been generally on a par with the poorer scores of the other two groups, and her real potential would not have been known. The exploration undertaken with the three-channel stimulator enabled her to achieve a much higher performance on the MAC test to the extent that she became the first patient in our series to recognize some monosyllable words in a standard open-set test condition.

Visual Cues

Even the best performance among these implant subjects indicates a severe residual hearing handicap when it is realized that NU 6 monosyllable-word scores as high as 50 or 60% in the routine clinic population are nevertheless considered to reveal seriously debilitated hearing capacity. Thus, the most successful implant patients to date are still extremely handicapped communicatively. Consequently, the contribution of visual cues, mainly from lipreading, must be stressed.

The lipreading scores of the subjects in each group are shown in FIGURE 3. CID sentences, other than those used in auditory testing, were given in a "live," face-to-face situation. First, 20 sentences were administered with the prosthesis "off," followed immediately by 20 sentences with it "on." Scores were based on the number of key words correct. Lipreading ability with the prosthesis "off" varies considerably (bar on left of the pair for each subject). The bar on the right of each pair shows the score for the prosthesis "on" condition. The mean amounts of improvement from the "off" to the "on" condition are 26.0, 13.1, and 29.0% for Implants I, II and III, respectively. The range of improvement with activation of the prosthesis is from minus 7 to plus 44, one subject showing no improvement and two showing a slight decrease. Accordingly, improvement in lipreading with a cochlear implant cannot be predicted with certainty. Not surprisingly, the poorer lipreaders have been notably appreciative of the auditory cues provided by an implant. Subject 1 with Implant I and subject 2 with Implant II were unusually poor lipreaders before receiving their implants, and the immediate lipreading improvement (with no training) was instrumental in their satisfaction with their devices. Investigation into the lipreading aspects of cochlear implant prostheses is of primary concern.

Despite its importance, lipreading is of limited aid because it is not consistently available—for example, in poorly lit conditions, in using the telephone, in watching TV, and in trying to understand persons who use poor articulation or minimal lip movements. Actually, conditions conducive to lipreading are tenuous outside of a one-to-one, face-to-face communicative situation. The emphasis in research at the UCSF continues to be focused on auditory speech perception. The most promising approach at present seems to be through multichannel stimulation of a multielectrode array.

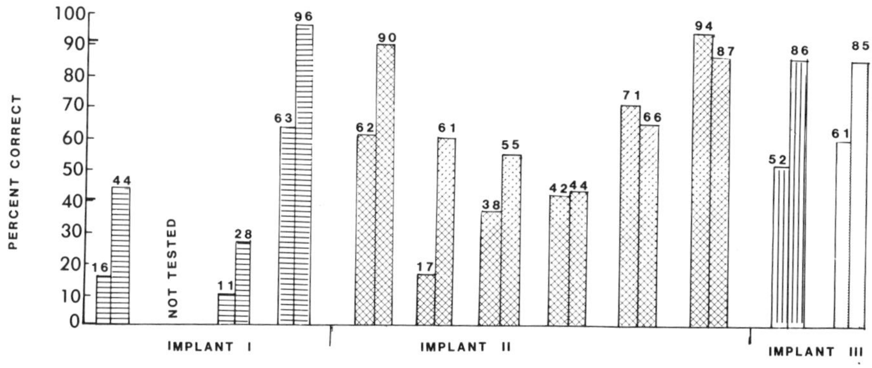

FIGURE 3. Lipreading scores for individual subjects. The bar on the *left* for each subject shows the score with the prosthesis "off"; the bar on the *right* shows the prosthesis "on" score. Test materials were CID sentences scored on the basis of key words correct.

CONCLUSIONS

On the basis of results of the Minimal Auditory Capabilities battery for the subjects of this study, the following conclusions are offered:

1. Subjects with an eight-bipolar electrode array in the scala tympani and a single-channel stimulator (Implant II) scored better, on the average, in vowel and initial-consonant recognition than did subjects with a single electrode and a single-channel stimulator (Implant I). One subject in the former group was consistently superior to all other subjects in the two groups. With the exception of this subject, scores on open-set speech recognition tests were generally equivalent for the two groups.

2. One subject (Implant III) with an eight-bipolar electrode array, who was tested with both a three-channel desk stimulator and a single-channel wearable stimulator, scored markedly higher in the three-channel mode on the vowel, initial consonant, and speech recognition tests.

3. On the other tests of the MAC battery, scores for the Implant I and II subjects were generally the same; scores on these same tests for the three-channel condition of Implant III were consistently higher than those for the single-channel condition.

4. Intra- and intersubject scores were unpredictable.

5. The results for Implant III indicated the advantages of multichannel stimulation (in this case, three channels), but only after the most appropriate electrode combinations and stimulator settings had been established through exploration with the use of a temporary direct connector to the electrodes. Had no such interim exploration been undertaken, the potential of this subject in speech recognition would not have been revealed.

6. The residual postimplant auditory deficit necessitates attention to visual cues in communication. Lipreading scores improved immediately for most subjects when the prosthesis was activated compared with results with the prosthesis in the "off" condition. Improvement cannot be predicted in all instances, however. Although the importance of lipreading to cochlear implant subjects seems to have been established, its tenuous utility in real-life situations must be recognized.

7. Multichannel stimulation of a multielectrode array is shown to be a promising approach to the achievement of speech recognition with a cochlear implant.

References

1. House, W. F., D. L. Bode & K. I. Berliner. 1981. The cochlear implant: Performance of deaf patients. Hearing Instruments **32:** 13–18.
2. Douek, E., A. T. Fourcin, B. C. J. Moore & G. P. Clark. 1979. A new approach to the cochlear implant. Proc. Roy. Soc. Med. **70:** 379–383.
3. Hochmair, I. J., E. S. Hochmair, R. E. Fischer & K. Burian. 1980. Cochlear prostheses in use: Recent speech comprehension results. Arch. Otorhinolaryngol. **229:** 81–98.
4. Hochmair-Desoyer, I. J., E. S. Hochmair, K. Burian & R. E. Fischer. 1981. Four years of experience with cochlear prostheses. Med. Progr. Technol. **8:** 107–119.
5. Michelson, R. P. & R. A. Schindler. 1981. Multichannel cochlear implant: Preliminary results in man. Laryngoscope **91:** 38–42.
6. Michelson, R. P. & R. A. Schindler. 1981. Multichannel cochlear implants: Current status and future developments. Laryngoscope **91:** 886–888.
7. Owens, E., D. K. Kessler & E. D. Schubert. 1982. Interim assessment of candidates for cochlear implants. Arch. Otolaryngol. **108:** 478–483.
8. Chouard, C. H. 1980. The surgical rehabilitation of total deafness with the multichannel cochlear implant. Audiology **19:** 137–145.
9. Clark, G. M., Y. C. Tong & L. F. A. Martin. 1981. A multiple-channel cochlear implant: An evaluation using open-set CID sentences. Laryngoscope **91:** 1981.
10. Eddington, D. K. 1980. Speech discrimination in deaf subjects with cochlear implants. J. Acoust. Soc. Am. **8:** 885–891.
11. Michelson, R. P. 1971. Electrical stimulation of the human cochlea. Arch. Otolaryngol. **93:** 317–323.
12. Merzenich, M. M., R. P. Michelson, C. R. Pettit, R. A. Schindler & M. Reid. 1973. Neural encoding of sound sensation evoked by electrical stimulation of the acoustic nerve. Ann. Otol. **82:** 486–503.
13. Owens, E., D. K. Kessler, C. C. Telleen & E. D. Schubert. 1981. The Minimal Auditory Capabilities (MAC) Battery. Hearing Aid J. **34:** 9.

IMPACT OF FDA REGULATIONS ON THE COCHLEAR IMPLANT FIELD

Harry R. Sauberman

Bureau of Medical Devices
Food and Drug Administration
Silver Spring, Maryland 20910

Introduction

This paper will discuss the nature and impact of the FDA regulations that govern the field of cochlear implants.

The Food and Drug Administration was granted authority in this area by Congress on May 28, 1976, when the Medical Device Amendments to the Federal Food, Drug and Cosmetic Act were signed into law. These amendments are designed to provide a balanced approach towards the regulation of medical devices. The intent is to protect the patient from unsafe or ineffective devices, to instill a degree of confidence in devices that are prescribed by physicians and other health professionals, and to see that advances in the application of technology to medicine are not hampered or otherwise stifled with unnecessary restrictions.

The Bureau of Medical Devices, with which I am associated, is charged with the implementation of these amendments. Basically, the regulations state that a medical device sold in interstate commerce has to be safe and effective for its intended use. The law does not permit the marketing of a new device, such as the cochlear implant, until safety and efficacy studies have been completed and a premarket approval application has been filed and approved.

As a way of gaining an understanding of the FDA's regulations as they apply to the cochlear implant, this paper proceeds to:

(1) give an overview of the amendments with an historical perspective;
(2) review the chronological sequence the agency (the FDA) went through in drafting regulations for medical device investigations;
(3) highlight the key participants and factors in a cochlear implant investigational study; and
(4) review the elements that should be contained in an application for a cochlear implant study, including a discussion of items that have to be explained to a patient to obtain informed consent.

The discussion of these latter items underlines the data base that is needed for marketing approval when the data from an investigational study are organized, analyzed, and summarized in a premarket approval application.

Historical Background

Before the Medical Device Amendments were signed, there was no direct requirement for a device manufacturer to validate safety and efficacy. A medical device could be developed and manufactured and could go directly

0077–8923/83/0405–0451 $1.75/0 © 1983, NYAS

to a patient without this assurance. The writers of the amendments recognized the importance of this need for testing and filled the void by requiring all medical devices that are intended for human use to be placed in a regulatory category that would assure their safety and efficacy. This procedure, known as classification, stipulated that all medical devices in interstate commerce at the time of enactment had to be classified into one of three regulatory categories.

The classification for a particular device has to be consistent with the potential risks or hazards that accompany the use of that device. Class I requirements represent the lowest level of regulation to which all devices are subject. These requirements consist of general controls, such as manufacturer registration, keeping of records and reports, and following good manufacturing practices. If a device has been specified as being only in Class I, then it has been established that Class I requirements are sufficient to assure safety and efficacy. Class II, the next level of regulation, is designated for devices for which general controls are not sufficient and performance standards are necessary. For a device to be in Class II there must be medical and scientific information currently available from which a standard can be developed. Devices in Class III are the most highly regulated. They must undergo a comprehensive medical and scientific evaluation known as premarket approval. Certain implants, such as the cochlear implant, for which safety and efficacy standards cannot be written at this time because of lack of available information, are typical of the types of devices one would find in Class III.

The amendments required that the FDA establish advisory committees of experts to assist in the classification of devices and in the review of premarket approval applications. One of these committees is the Ear, Nose and Throat Advisory Section of the Ophthalmic, ENT and Dental Devices Panel. Included in the amendments is the mandate given to the FDA under Section 520(g) of the act to regulate the clinical investigation of new postenactment medical devices such as the cochlear implant.

With the enactment of the amendments, the FDA has worked conscientiously to formulate regulations for adequately protecting human subjects who are involved as participants in medical device investigations. The first draft of a proposed regulation was published in August 1976. After considerable comments were received, a modified regulation was later proposed in May 1978. Additional comments were received and reviewed. A final regulation was published in the *Federal Register* on January 18, 1980, which became effective on July 16, 1980. Its official or formal name is "Procedures for Investigational Device Exemptions." Known as the IDE regulation, it sets forth the procedures and conditions under which investigations of medical devices may be conducted while exempting a device from certain requirements of the Amendments.

The IDE regulation was slightly revised on January 27, 1981 to provide more specific information on the responsibilities of institutional review boards (IRBs) and to delineate the type of information to be contained in a patient consent form. Copies of the regulation and its revision document are available from the FDA.

In a manner similar to that of classification, the FDA regulates clinical investigations of medical devices according to the severity of risk involved. The agency has defined a significant risk device as one intended to be either an implant or a life-supporting or life-sustaining device and which, in addition, presents a potential for risk to the health and safety of a patient. It may also be a device that is of substantial importance in diagnosing, mitigating, or treating a disease, but which carries with these benefits a potential for serious risk.

The cochlear implant, by virtue of its design and by virtue of the placement of wire electrodes into the area of the cochlea has been determined to be a device with significant risk. As such, it is subject to all of the provisions of the IDE regulation. This includes the provision that states that before any investigation of a significant risk device can begin, the FDA must approve an IDE application submitted by the sponsor of a study.

Key Participants and Factors in IDE Studies

In any IDE study there are four principal participants: sponsors, who are responsible for initiating the study; investigators, who carry out the study; institutional review boards (IRBs), who approve and monitor the study; and patients, who agree to participate in the study. The roles and responsibilities of the sponsor, investigator, and IRB are critical to the success of a cochlear implant study. An investigational plan must be approved by an IRB before a study can begin. FDA approval is necessary and requires a complete IDE application. Of special concern are the items of informed consent that are designed for patient protection. It is important to take a close look at these specific areas.

Responsibilities of the Sponsor

Consider the sponsor of a cochlear implant study. He is the person or company in charge of the overall course or direction of the study and he will be ultimately responsible for its success or failure. If successful, the accolades will go to the sponsor.

The sponsor is responsible for developing the investigational plan and for completing the IDE application. This application has to be reviewed and approved by an IRB and the FDA before the investigation may begin. In this undertaking the sponsor is responsible for making an initial assessment of patient risk. He is responsible for submitting all pertinent information concerning reports of earlier investigations and for selecting qualified investigators. He must obtain IRB review and approval.

Once the study has begun, the sponsor is responsible for seeing that the investigation is properly monitored and that proper notifications are sent to the IRB and to the FDA. It is the sponsor's responsibility to maintain a compendium of all pertinent records and reports, and to insure that the device is not promoted, advertised, or commercialized.

Responsibilities of the Investigator

An investigator is the individual who actually conducts a clinical investigation. It is under his immediate supervision and direction that a cochlear stimulator is implanted.

In accordance with the IDE regulation, an investigator must have a signed agreement with his sponsor indicating that he will follow a specific investigational plan and stating that he will abide with all applicable FDA and IRB requirements. An investigator may not begin a cochlear implant study at an institution without first receiving IRB and FDA approval.

The investigator is responsible for the surgical management and care of the cochlear implant patient and for his postoperative care and audiometric rehabilitation. He must ensure that the implant device is used only as stated in the investigational plan.

The investigator must obtain the informed consent of the patient as an integral item of his responsibility. He must be assured that the patient fully understands the nature of the implantation procedure and, furthermore, that the patient has an assessment of the potential risks and benefits from the procedure.

Often, a clinical investigator may wish to modify the investigational plan in order to accommodate a particular patient's needs or his own way of doing things. Changes such as these should be made only after appropriate justification and review by the sponsor, the IRB, and the FDA. Such a change can alter the initial conditions for analysis of the clinical data, thereby making evaluation very difficult when different procedures are used. Consequently, the FDA's position regarding changes is that adherence to the protocol should be maintained whenever possible. FDA approval is required if it is believed that the change will affect the scientific soundness of the study or the safety, health, and well-being of the patient. In the case of an emergency, where an investigator has to deviate, this deviation must be reported to the sponsor and to the IRB.

Like the sponsor, the investigator is also charged with record-keeping and reporting requirements. He is additionally responsible for noting any and all unanticipated or adverse effects as a result of the implant surgery.

Responsibilities of the Institutional Review Board

The IRB represents an institutional review committee that has been formally designated, under delegation of authority, to evaluate the risks and benefits of an investigational procedure and to monitor the progress of a study. Institutional review boards generally apply ethical standards as part of their review and are sensitive to local community attitudes in their evaluations. For the case of a cochlear implant study, an IRB would review the scientific soundness of the investigational plan and would recommend either approval, modification, or disapproval.

In terms of composition and structure, an IRB must have at least five members, all of whom must have a diversity of background and the professional competence to review a cochlear implant procedure. Their role is to ascertain the acceptability of a proposed study at their institution in terms of institutional commitments and regulations, applicable law, and local standards of professional conduct.

One of the important responsibilities of an IRB is the role it plays with respect to protection of the patient. IRBs are responsible for seeing that information that is given to a patient is in accordance with the required elements of informed consent. An IRB may require that additional information be given to a patient when, in the IRB's judgment, this information would add meaningfully to the patient's welfare.

If an IRB decides to disapprove a cochlear implant study, it must notify the investigator in writing of the reasons for disapproval. In this situation, the investigator must be given an opportunity to respond either in person or in writing.

An IRB is responsible for monitoring the progress of an investigational study. The frequency of these reviews should be consistent with the estimated risk of the surgical procedure, but must occur at least on an annual basis. In this role, IRBs have the opportunity to observe the patient-consent process as well as aspects of the clinical study.

Items to be Contained in a Cochlear Implant IDE Application

What types of information should be contained in an IDE application from a sponsor who is seeking to conduct a cochlear implant study? The application should contain the name and address of the sponsor, a report on all prior cochlear implant investigations, and a complete investigational plan. The plan should describe what the device is supposed to accomplish, how it functions, its principal mode of operation, and its critical components. The plan should further provide a risk–benefit analysis and should discuss the scientific basis for the investigation. The clinical procedures should be delineated, including procedures and methods for evaluating the performance of the device postoperatively.

Other items that should be contained in the IDE application include a copy of the patient consent form, a copy of the investigator agreement form, and an identification of the investigators who will be participating in the study and their respective IRBs. The name, address, and chairman of each IRB that reviewed the investigation should be provided along with a statement certifying IRB approval. A certification must also be provided indicating that all investigators chosen to participate in the study have signed the agreement form, or that they will sign the agreement form before they are added to the study.

The IDE application should contain a description of the methods, safeguards, and quality controls used in the manufacturing, packaging, and storage of the device. For example, there should be microbiological and toxicological data indicating biocompatability and sterilization assurance with respect to the implantable components. Information on electrical safety should be provided as well as information on leakage currents in the event of failure of the device.

Complete labeling for the device should be provided in the IDE application. If the sponsor is planning to charge for the device, then a statement should be provided explaining why this charge does not constitute commercialization.

Patient Protection: Items of Informed Consent

The informed consent of a patient is a necessary and essential item in any clinical study. It is considered by the FDA as an integral item of the investigational plan. Informed consent, however, can only be judged to be adequate and sufficient if certain information is first given to a prospective patient.

The patient must be told that the study involves the use of an investigational device that is expected to produce auditory stimulation in response to sound. He should be told about the benefits, size, and scope of the study and its expected length. The patient should be given a full explanation of the operation of the device, its expected longevity and reliability, and the procedure by which it will be implanted. There should be an identification of specific medical and surgical procedures that are considered experimental. In addition, procedures for postoperative care and audiometric rehabilitation should be explained. The patient should also be told of any discomfort he may expect from the device, and he should be apprised of possible complications and risks that may arise from the surgical procedure.

It is important that the patient receive a full disclosure of alternative procedures or other courses of therapy that are available. The patient should be made aware of his right to withdraw from participation in the study at any time. The patient must also be told the identity of a person who will be able to answer any questions about the study or about his rights.

The patient must be informed of the extent of confidentiality of records identifying himself and he must be informed that the FDA may inspect these records. The patient must also be informed as to whether or not medical treatment or compensation will be provided in the event of injury; if so, what it consists of, or where further information may be obtained.

Because the cochlear implant has been designated as a significant risk device, these elements of informed consent have to be presented in a written format and have to be signed by the patient before his participation in the study.

Summary

An overview of the impact of the FDA's investigational device regulation on the field of the cochlear implants has been presented. It can be seen that the regulation has been established to provide a legal framework for conducting clinical investigations with medical devices. The regulation incorporates the concepts of institutional review and the informed consent of the patient. These concepts are not new; they have existed for a long time as part of medical research in the United States.

We believe that the institutional review board will serve to effectively review and monitor the clinical course of patients receiving cochlear implants. We also believe that we have developed a regulation that maximizes patient safety, while encouraging investigation of the device. We understand and appreciate that IRB monitoring is far more efficient and effective than having FDA personnel on hand at various institutions around the country to monitor investigational studies. We know full well the added complexity that a bureaucratic monitoring process can bring to a clinical investigation. We think that the IRB approach is the most direct, straightforward, protective, and cost-effective approach that can be taken.

We appreciate the benefit that a patient receives in having a competent and expert investigator. The regulations were written to rely on these investigators for expertise in their particular specialty in conducting and evaluating the clinical studies.

We recognize the role of the sponsor, who has made a commitment to the improvement of health care through advancement in technology, and who seeks to restore or to produce some degree of hearing for the totally deaf. Without a sponsor, these studies would not be possible.

And last, but not least, we recognize the all-important role of the patient, who provides the clinical data base. The patient's welfare and safety must be considered in any clinical study.

The IDE regulation has been in effect since July 1980. It provides the opportunity for the FDA and the medical and scientific communities to work together for the success of medical-device investigations. We can all pride ourselves on our high standard of medical excellence. When we can work together, this standard will rise even higher.

Part IX. Potential Coding Solutions for Electroneural Speech Discrimination

INTRODUCTION

Donald K. Eddington

Institute for Biomedical Engineering
University of Utah
Salt Lake City, Utah 84112

The four papers in this session deal with issues relevant to encoding speech as electrical stimuli for intra- and extracochlear electrodes. One working hypothesis that most investigators use when thinking about speech-encoding for cochlear implants is that the auditory nerve is the neural tissue excited by these stimuli. The viability of this tissue in the sensorineural deaf is therefore an important issue and is addressed in the paper by Raúl Hinojosa.

The remaining three papers deal directly with encoding speech and demonstrate two fundamental approaches to this task. The strategy exemplified by Remez and Rubin consists of identifying one or more characteristics of the speech signal and specifically encoding those characteristics in the stimulation waveform. One hopes that a restricted number of speech characteristics, properly encoded, will provide intelligible speech or improved lipreading when combined with the current state of electrode and processing technologies. The speech characteristics that Remez and Rubin encoded as three tones were the amplitude and frequency of the first three formants. The fact that normal listeners perceive the phonetic content of the utterances encoded may direct more attention to the property of coherent spectrum variation as an important speech characteristic to be considered.

The last two papers are both directed toward the encoding strategy that attempts to elicit activity patterns on the auditory nerve fibers that mimic those found in the normally hearing individual. If the normal patterns of neural activity could be reproduced, a postlingually deafened individual should, theoretically, be able to spontaneously recognize and understand speech. Unfortunately the ability to mimic these patterns is severely limited by electrode technology, processing techniques, and the imperfect understanding of the normal activity patterns themselves. One hopes, therefore, that mimicking a restricted number of the features of these activity patterns will result in better speech communication for the deaf. C. W. Parkins proposes a speech-encoding system that is based on a model designed to simulate several response properties of auditory neurons. M. M. Merzenich describes a multielectrode system for scala tympani implantation that may make the coding considerations he discusses practical.

HISTOPATHOLOGY OF PROFOUND SENSORINEURAL DEAFNESS [a]

Raúl Hinojosa

Section of Otolaryngology
Pritzker School of Medicine
University of Chicago
Chicago, Illinois 60637

Mitchell Marion

Department of Otolaryngology
Indiana University
Indianapolis, Indiana 46223

Cochlear implants should theoretically function best in profoundly deaf ears that have a sufficient number of peripheral auditory neural elements capable of receiving and transmitting electrical impulses to central nuclei. Recent observations [1] suggest that the neural elements most likely to be stimulated by cochlear electrodes are the spiral ganglion cells. Serial sections of the entire cochlea are well suited for detailed observations on these cells and their peripheral fibers as well as the sensory epithelium along the organ of Corti.

In 1980, Hinojosa and Lindsay [2] correlated the state of the acoustic ganglion with that of the organ of Corti and of the peripheral fibers in eight patients with profound deafness. Ganglion cell counts were obtained and compared with average counts in five normal temporal bones. These investigators found that the state of survival of the ganglion cells and the organ of Corti varied widely in the cases examined.

We now provide additional information on this topic. From the temporal bone collection at The University of Chicago, which consists of more than 1000 specimens, we identified a group of 65 ears from 40 patients, all of whom were totally deaf (TABLE 1), and another group of 14 ears from 8 patients with profound hearing loss only above 2000 Hz (TABLE 2). From both groups, we selected 16 representative cases for histopathologic study, which included cochlea and spiral ganglion reconstruction. The state of the organ of Corti and the presence or absence of peripheral cochlear nerve fibers were also noted. The ganglion cell counts were compared with average counts obtained for 12 normal adult temporal bones (TABLE 3).

The 16 cases selected included only those in which stimulation of the eighth nerve would have been practical. Therefore, we excluded cases in which the cause of profound deafness was an acoustic neuroma, temporal bone malignancy, or a congenital lesion associated with a severely limited life expectancy. Of the 16 ears selected for study, 15 came from patients who were totally deaf and included cases of bacterial labyrinthitis (two patients) and viral labyrinthitis (two), otosclerosis (two), trauma (one), ototoxicity

[a] This study was supported in part by Grants NS–03358 and NS–07038 from the National Institute of Neurological and Communicative Disorders and Stroke and by the Research Fund of the American Otological Society, Inc.

0077–8923/83/0405–0459 $1.75/0 © 1983, NYAS

TABLE 1

CAUSES OF PROFOUND SENSORINEURAL DEAFNESS (PTA[a] > 90 dB) IN 65 EARS

Cause of Deafness	Number
Congenital	
Scheibe type of dysplasia	7
Mondini type of dysplasia	4
Aplasia of the organ of Corti	2
Kearns–Sayre syndrome	2
Alport's syndrome	2
Congenital hypoxia	2
Subtotal	19 (29%)
Acquired	
Otosclerosis	12
Bacterial labyrinthitis	10
Viral labyrinthitis	7
Ototoxicity	5
Paget's disease	4
Trauma	3
Metastatic cancer	2
Ménière's disease	2
Acoustic neuroma	1
Subtotal	46 (71%)
Total	65 ears

[a] PTA stands for pure-tone average and is defined as the average of hearing threshold levels for 500, 1000, and 2000 Hz.

(one), Paget's disease (one), and several varieties of congenital deafness (six). The other case (presbycusis) was selected from the group of patients with profound high-tone sensorineural deafness (TABLE 4).

MATERIAL AND METHODS

Our observations were made on histologic preparations consisting of horizontal sections of human temporal bones cut at 20 μm. Every tenth section was stained with hematoxylin and eosin and used for study. The organ of

TABLE 2

CAUSES OF PROFOUND HIGH-TONE SENSORINEURAL DEAFNESS[a]

Cause of Deafness	Number
Presbycusis	6
Ototoxicity	6
Ménière's disease	1
Otosclerosis	1
Total	14 ears

[a] Profound high-tone deafness is defined as an average loss of 90 dB or greater for the hearing threshold levels at 2000, 4000, and 8000 Hz.

TABLE 3

GANGLION CELL COUNT AND LENGTH OF COCHLEA IN TWELVE HISTOLOGICALLY NORMAL TEMPORAL BONES FROM INDIVIDUALS WITH NORMAL AUDIOGRAMS

	Age (yr)	Ganglion Cell Count	Length of Cochlea (mm)
	23	35,796	29.34
	23	35,074	29.60
	26	31,768	31.88
	26	31,901	31.24
	27	29,978	37.25
	32	32,311	30.42
	32	35,826	33.46
	39	32,935	34.20
	42	29,802	30.80
	50	34,741	32.34
	53	39,520	33.60
	53	37,325	32.62
Average	35.5	33,915	32.25

Corti was reconstructed according to the method of Guild *et al.*,[3, 4] as modified by Schuknecht.[5] Inner and outer hair cells and supporting cells were charted along the organ of Corti, and estimates were made on the number of remaining peripheral fibers in the osseous spiral lamina of each section (FIG. 5A).

Reconstruction of the spiral ganglion was modified from previous techniques.[4, 5] The borders of the spiral ganglion, and not of Rosenthal's canal,

TABLE 4

SUMMARY OF CASES PRESENTED

Patient	Age (yr) & Sex	Diagnosis	Ganglion Cell Count
1	73, M	Viral meningogenic labyrinthitis	7,305
2	6, M	Viral endolymphatic labyrinthitis	19,826
3	46, F	Bacterial labyrinthitis	Zero
4	57, M	Bacterial labyrinthitis	22,125
5	80, F	Head trauma	13,110
6	60, F	Otosclerosis	10,127
7	68, F	Otosclerosis	13,139
8	67, M	Streptomycin ototoxicity	19,608
9	79, M	Paget's disease	18,117
10[a]	77, M	Presbycusis	25,783
11	6, M	Scheibe type of dysplasia	23,912
12	73, F	Scheibe type of dysplasia	9,471
13	19, F	Kearns–Sayrc syndrome	10,849
14	31, F	Alport's syndrome	18,687
15	18, M	Mondini type of dysplasia	16,055
16	53, F	Congenital aplasia (organ of Corti)	16,663

[a] Patient 10 had profound high-tone sensorineural deafness (see TABLE 2).

were measured in each section. The first coil of the organ of Corti served as the reference point for reconstruction of the first coil of the spiral ganglion; this, in turn, became the reference point for the second and third coils. With tracing paper, the spiral ganglion was reconstructed in two dimensions and superimposed on the organ of Corti. All ganglion cells that showed a nucleolus were counted by the same investigator, who used an ocular grid. Since ganglion cells from each tenth section were counted, the count was multiplied by ten to yield the total number of cells for that group. We applied a correction factor of 0.95 to eliminate the error of counting nucleoli located at the interfaces between sections.

The organ of Corti was then divided arbitrarily into 5-mm segments, starting at the basal turn. The most distal portion of the apical turn represented the segment of the organ of Corti past 30 mm. At each 5-mm division, a radially directed line was drawn from the organ of Corti to the spiral ganglion. The lines thus divided the spiral ganglion and the organ of Corti into corresponding segments (FIG. 1). Ganglion cell counts from each of these segments were totaled and expressed as a percentage of the normal average count for that segment as determined from the reconstruction of 12 normal temporal bones.

RESULTS

Acquired diseases were the most common cause (71%) of total sensorineural deafness in the entire group of 65 ears (TABLE 1): otosclerosis, bacterial labyrinthitis, and viral labyrinthitis were the most frequent disorders. Congenital anomalies accounted for 29% of the cases, with the Scheibe type of anomaly predominating (TABLE 1). In the group of cases in which deafness

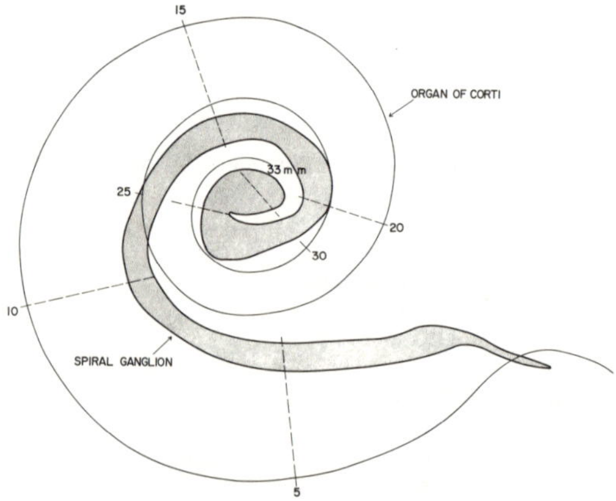

FIGURE 1. Graphic reconstruction of both the spiral ganglion and the organ of Corti. The organ of Corti is divided into 5-mm segments, starting at the basal end. The most apical segment is that portion of the organ of Corti past 30 mm. Lines drawn radially from the organ of Corti to the spiral ganglion divide the ganglion into corresponding segments.

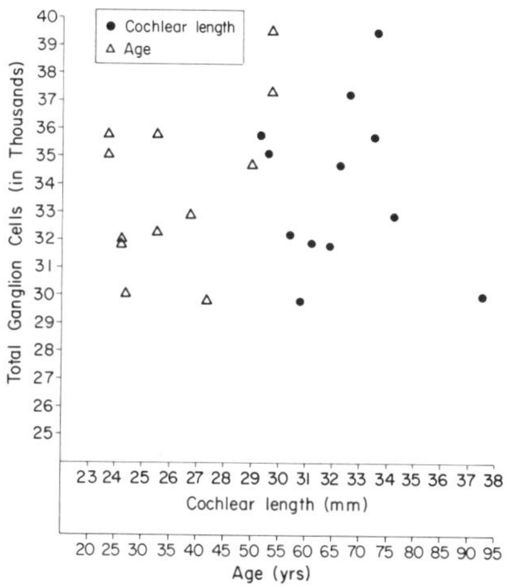

FIGURE 2. For each of 12 normal temporal bones studied, total ganglion cell counts are plotted against the age of the patient and the length of the cochlea. No correlations are seen.

was profound only above 2000 Hz, presbycusis and ototoxicity were the most common causes (TABLE 2).

As shown in TABLE 3, total ganglion cell counts in 12 normal adult temporal bones ranged from 29,802 to 39,520. In this group, total cell counts did not seem to be correlated with either the age of the patient or the length of the cochlea (FIG. 2). However, in a report on 100 hearing ears from subjects whose ages spanned 9 decades, ganglion cell populations were found to be inversely related to age.[6]

Total ganglion cell counts from the profoundly deaf ears (TABLE 4) ranged from 7,305 in an ear from a patient diagnosed as having viral labyrinthitis to 25,783 in an ear with presbycusis. However, one patient who had suffered from bacterial labyrinthitis developed severe labyrinthitis ossificans involving the entire cochlea, and in this case no ganglion cells were seen. The difference in total number of ganglion cells between the normal and pathologic ears is clearly evident (FIG. 3).

Viral Labyrinthitis

Viral infections of the labyrinth may produce pathologic changes which demonstrate varying degrees of degeneration, ranging from a mild loss of hair cells in the basal turn to total destruction of the organ of Corti, spiral ganglion, stria vascularis, and vestibular sense organs. Viral labyrinthitis may accompany specific viral syndromes such as measles, mumps, or rubella. However, several types of viruses, all of which can produce upper respiratory tract illnesses, can also cause labyrinthitis and hearing loss.[7] New bone formation at the level of the round window has not been found to be characteristic of viral infections.

Viral Meningogenic Labyrinthitis

Profound deafness may occur as an infrequent complication of viral meningoencephalitis. Often the virus is not identified in these cases, but invades the inner ear from the meninges and characteristically produces endolymphatic

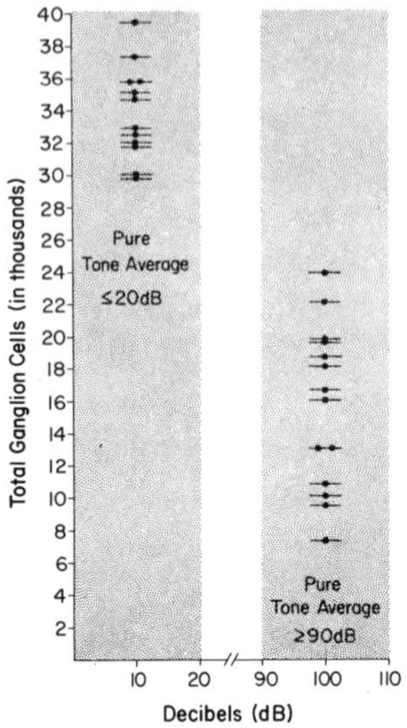

FIGURE 3. Total ganglion cell counts are plotted with respect to pure-tone averages for the group with normal hearing (*left*) and for the group with profound deafness (*right*). (The pure-tone average is the average hearing loss at frequencies of 500, 1000, and 2000 Hz.)

hydrops. In this type of infection, the spiral ganglion cells are exposed directly to the inflammatory process and are likely to undergo advanced degeneration.[8] Patient 1 had profound deafness as a result of viral meningogenic labyrinthitis. Histopathologic study of the cochlea demonstrated total destruction of the organ of Corti, with complete absence of peripheral fibers. Ganglion cells

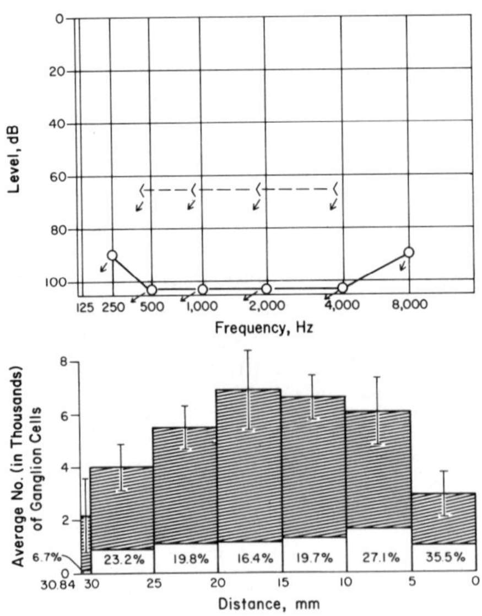

FIGURE 4. In this figure and in subsequent ones, the histogram shows the number of ganglion cells counted in each 5-mm section along the organ of Corti. Each entire block represents the normal average cell count for that segment, as determined from the reconstruction of 12 normal temporal bones. Standard deviations are indicated by vertical markers. The *clear area* in each block represents the surviving ganglion cells expressed as a percentage of the normal count for that section. Frequencies on the audiogram correspond roughly to the position along the organ of Corti indicated below on the histogram.

This histogram is for the right ear of patient 1 (73 years of age), who had viral meningogenic labyrinthitis. The audiogram shows total deafness. The percentage of ganglion cells remaining shows marked depletion in all segments.

were severely reduced in all turns (FIG. 4), and the stria vascularis had degenerated throughout.

Viral Endolymphatic Labyrinthitis

The pathologic changes in this type of infection include degeneration or destruction limited mainly to the endolymphatic system, along with the tendency to reduce the volume of the endolymph in the cochlear duct and saccule.[9] The utricle may occasionally be involved in this process as well. Patient 2 was a 6-year-old child who became profoundly deaf after having mumps at the age of 24 months. Reconstruction of the cochlea revealed a total loss of the organ of Corti throughout the basal turn and up to the 25-mm mark. Peripheral fibers, however, were present (10 to 20%) in the basal turn, with the number of axons progressively increasing into the middle and apical turns (FIG. 5A). Ganglion cells showed a moderate reduction in number with approximately 50–70% of the cells remaining in all coils (FIG. 5B). The stria vascularis had degenerated.

Bacterial Labyrinthitis

In the preantibiotic era, profound deafness caused by labyrinthitis of bacterial origin was commonly due to meningococci. Survivors of meningococcal meningitis frequently were deaf in one or both ears. Histopathologic observations made during the acute inflammatory stage of this disease revealed that the main portal of entry into the inner ear was the internal auditory meatus.[10–13] Temporal bones from these patients examined several years after the infection characteristically demonstrate new bone formation.[14] The new bone can vary in extent, but typically occurs in the region of the round window and the basal coil of the cochlea. With the use of antibiotics, complete recovery from bacterial infections of the nervous system is the rule. Occasionally, however, either unilateral or bilateral profound hearing loss can occur.

Profound deafness associated with fibrosis and ossification of the labyrinth has also resulted from severe otitis media. In such cases, the infection spreads through either the round window or the oval window into the inner ear; that is, it is otogenic rather than meningogenic.[15] Adult patients often do not recall the insult that resulted in their deafness; however, radiographic examination of the inner ear in these cases may reveal evidence of ossification in the labyrinthine spaces.

We selected two cases of total deafness that occcurred after meningococcal meningitis from a group of 10 such cases to illustrate the great variability in the pathologic findings. The cochlea from patient 3 demonstrates the result of a severe bacterial invasion of the inner ear. There is total destruction of all neural elements, which are completely replaced by new bone formation (FIG. 6).

Reconstruction of the cochlea from patient 4 revealed that the sensory cells of the organ of Corti were absent throughout all turns, with new bone formation at the round window. Peripheral fibers were absent in all sections, and the stria vascularis had degenerated throughout. The number of ganglion cells, however, was only moderately reduced in the basal turn; the second and apical turns were affected most, with an average reduction in number to about 50% (FIG. 7).

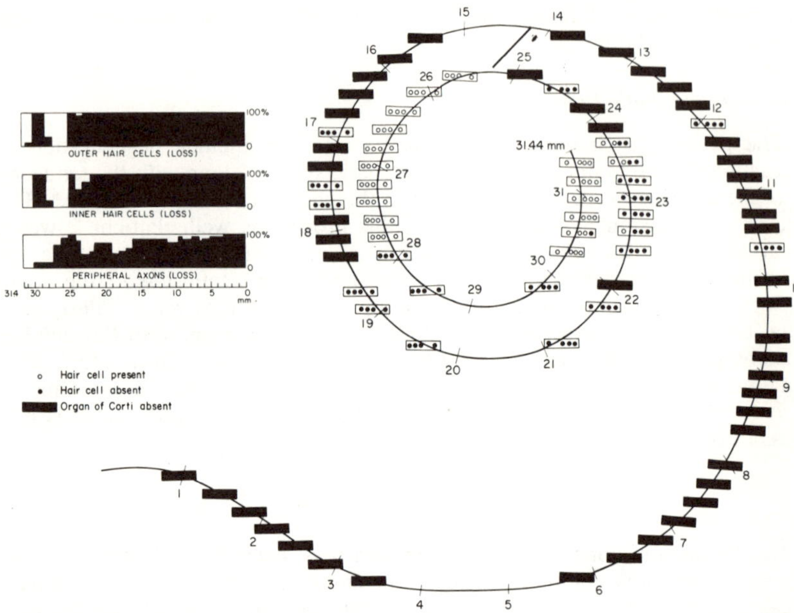

FIGURE 5A. In the reconstructions of the organ of Corti, 1-mm divisions are marked from base to apex. Each *small rectangle* depicts the state of the organ of Corti in that location, including the presence or absence of hair cells. Also illustrated are three bar graphs, which demonstrate the percentage of remaining outer hair cells, inner hair cells, and peripheral fibers along the organ of Corti (*clear areas*). The case shown is that of patient 2, aged 6 years, who had viral endolymphatic labyrinthitis due to mumps at the age of 2. The organ of Corti demonstrates an almost total loss of hair cells and supporting cells throughout the basal turn. Peripheral fibers are present in the basal turn (10–20%) and increase progressively into the middle and apical turns.

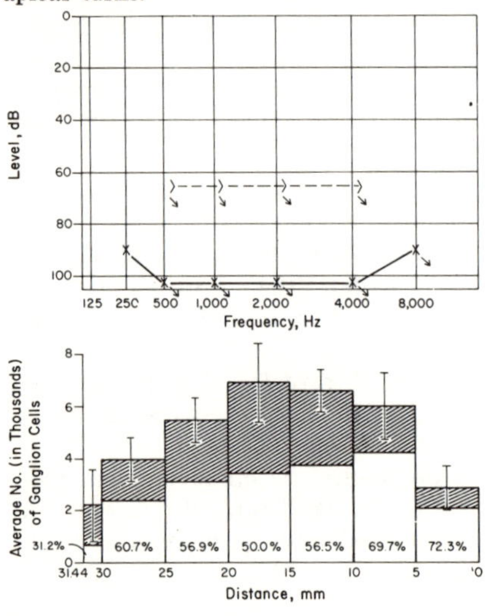

FIGURE 5B. The audiogram of same patient as in FIGURE 5A indicates a profound sensorineural hearing loss in the left ear. The number of ganglion cells is only moderately reduced in all turns, with 50–70% of cells remaining.

Trauma to the Head

Profound deafness, either unilateral or bilateral, can result from a severe blow to the head. Injury may cause a temporal bone fracture or generalized concussion, and both may result in deafness. Transverse fractures of the temporal bone occur perpendicular to the long axis of the petrous pyramid and across the inner ear, resulting in acute and profound deafness. Healing of the fracture line tends to be incomplete, with extension of the middle-ear mucosa into the inner ear.[16] A severe concussion with hemorrhage into the inner ear

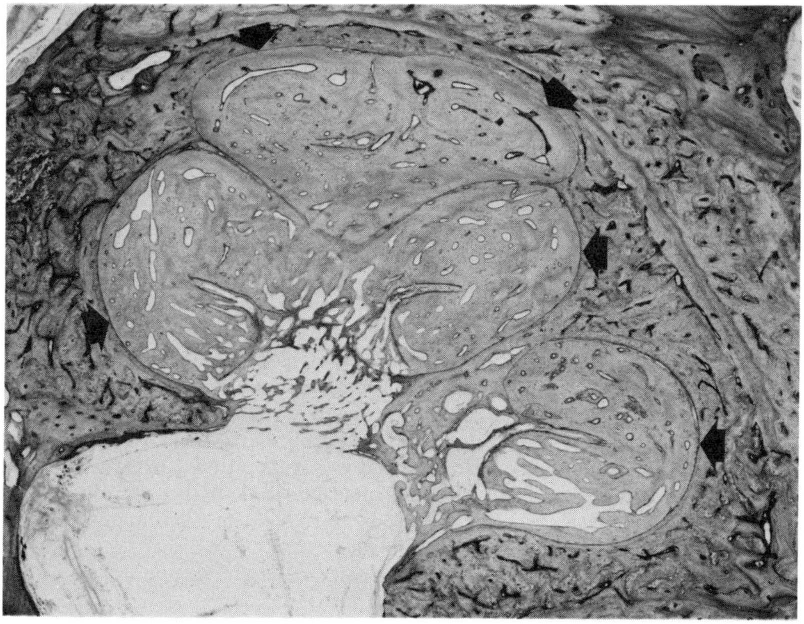

FIGURE 6. Photomicrograph of section of temporal bone in patient 3, aged 46 years, who suffered from a severe bilateral bacterial meningogenic labyrinthitis in childhood. All soft tissue of the cochlea (*arrows*) has been destroyed and has been completely replaced by new bone. (Hematoxylin and eosin stain; magnification $\times 11$).

may cause profound deafness, without an identifiable fracture through the pyramid. Patient 5 represents such a case. Reconstruction of the cochlea revealed partial preservation of outer hair cells of the organ of Corti. These were located only in the midportion of the basal turn. The remainder of the sensory epithelium had degenerated. Peripheral fibers were almost totally absent, and ganglion cell counts were drastically reduced throughout all turns, with the middle and apical coils the most severely affected (FIG. 8). The stria vascularis was present in the lower basal turn, was partly present in the upper basal turn, and had totally degenerated in the middle and apical turns.

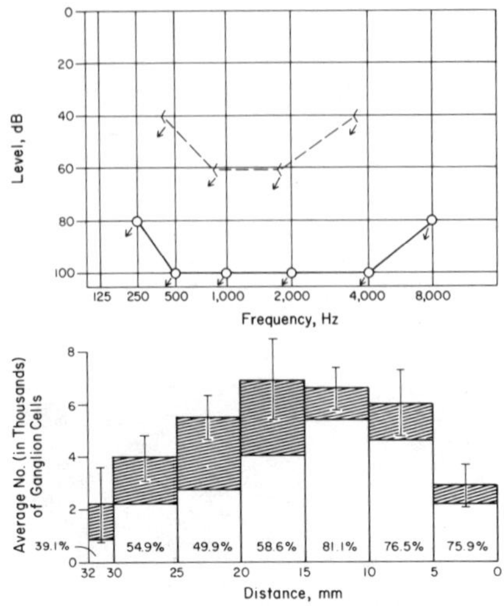

FIGURE 7. Patient 4, aged 57 years, had bilateral bacterial meningogenic labyrinthitis at the age of 15. The audiogram shows no response for either air or bone conduction in the right ear. Ganglion cell populations are only moderately reduced, with the basal coil (0–15 mm) being the least affected.

Otosclerosis

Although the extent of development of otosclerosis varies greatly in adults, two types can be distinguished on the basis of its distribution in the otic capsule.[17] In the first type, the otosclerotic focus is limited to specific areas (the oval and round windows and the internal auditory meatus), and the disease typically remains a conductive disturbance. In some instances, this type of otosclerosis can be associated with a progressive degeneration of the acoustic ganglion later in life. However, this degeneration corresponds closely to that observed in a type of presbycusis characterized by threshold loss for all frequencies, and a cause-and-effect relationship to otosclerosis remains unclear.[18]

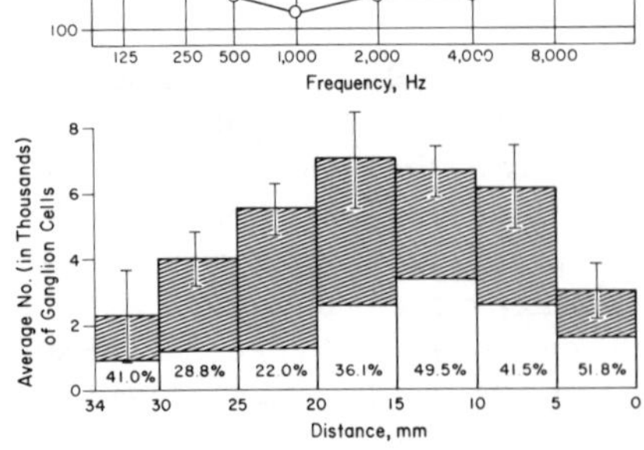

FIGURE 8. Patient 5, aged 80 years, suffered a bilateral hearing loss after trauma to the head at the age of 40. The audiogram of the right ear demonstrates a profound sensorineural hearing loss. Ganglion cells are markedly reduced in the middle and apical turns; in the basal coil, approximately 50% of cells remain.

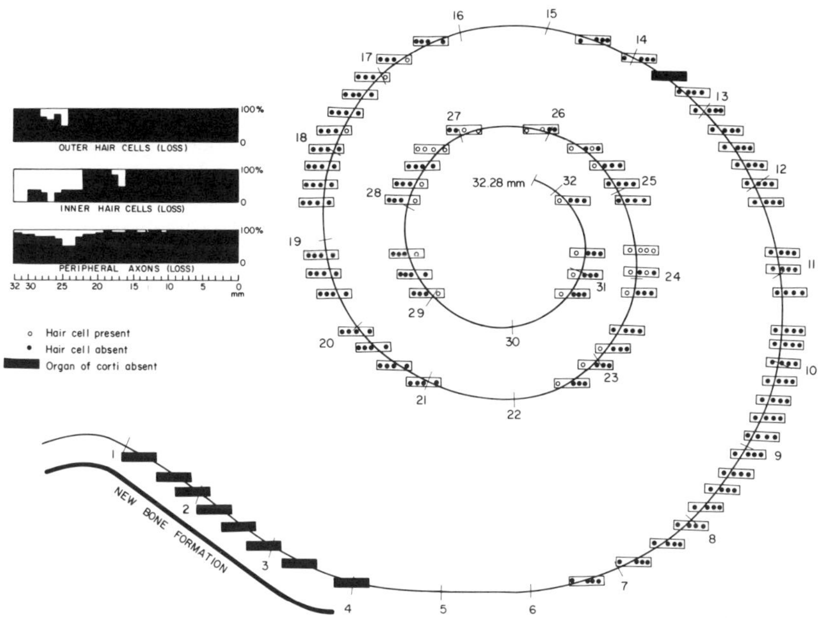

FIGURE 9A. Patient 6, aged 60 years, had extensive otosclerosis. The organ of Corti was severely degenerated in the basal and lower middle turns. Inner hair cells are present only in the upper middle and apical coils. Peripheral axons are depleted throughout. New bone had formed in the first 4 mm of the cochlea.

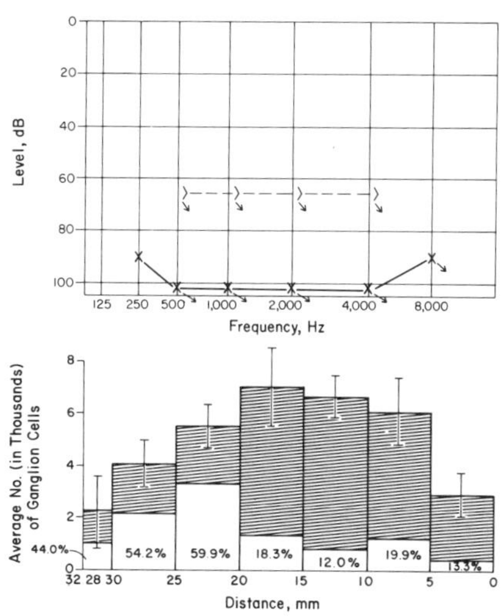

FIGURE 9B. Audiogram of same patient as in FIGURE 9A shows almost total loss of hearing. Ganglion cell counts are severely reduced in the basal and lower middle coils; reduction is less past 20 mm.

The second type of otosclerosis is much more active, with multiple foci of disease in both the cochlear and vestibular parts of the otic capsule. Stapes fixation typically occurs early. With continued progression of the disease, the otosclerotic foci fuse and occupy a major portion of the otic capsule, including the endosteal layer. Next, a sensorineural hearing loss becomes superimposed on a conductive loss. Labyrinthitis ossificans at the level of the round window is a relatively frequent finding in this type of advanced otosclerosis. Two cases of this type, associated with profound sensorineural hearing loss, were reviewed.

Patient 6 had extensive, severe otosclerosis. The cochlear reconstruction demonstrated inner hair cells in the middle and apical turns, with severe atrophy of almost all peripheral axons (FIG. 9A). Ganglion cell counts were less than 20% of normal in the basal and lower middle coils, with only moderate reduction in the upper, middle, and apical coils (FIG. 9B). The stria vascularis had degenerated in the basal and apical coils and was preserved in the middle coil. New bone formation was found in the first 4 mm of the cochlea at the level of the round window (FIG. 9A).

Patient 7 was a 68-year-old woman with several foci of otosclerosis involving the footplate, round-window niche, and the ampullary wall of the posterior canal. The organ of Corti was completely destroyed in the first 8 mm of the cochlea, with spotty persistence of inner hair cells throughout the remaining turns. Outer hair cells were partially present only in the second and apical turns. Peripheral fibers were severely reduced throughout (FIG. 10A). Ganglion cell counts revealed a significant reduction in all coils (FIG. 10B). Furthermore, there was a partial degeneration of the stria vascularis, especially in the second and apical turns.

Ototoxicity

Patient 8 developed bilateral profound deafness of rather acute onset while taking streptomycin for acute pulmonary tuberculosis. In a pathologic study of the right temporal bone which was carried out 9 years after the onset of deafness, the cochlea revealed total degeneration of the organ of Corti. The peripheral fibers were absent up to the 19-mm mark, with 5% remaining in the middle turn and up to 30% in the apical turn. Ganglion cell counts showed that about 50% of cells remained in the basal turn, increasing to approximately 70% in the middle and apical turns (FIG. 11). The stria vascularis was present throughout all turns.

Paget's Disease

In most instances, patients are diagnosed as having Paget's disease only incidentally on routine radiographs. Hearing impairment and vertigo are among the common symptoms when this disorder affects the inner ear. The hearing loss is usually bilateral and sensorineural and involves only the high frequencies. Occasionally, however, the hearing loss may be profound.[19] The cause of the sensorineural degeneration of the inner ear in Paget's disease is unknown.

Patient 9 represents a case of Paget's disease in which sensorineural deafness progressed to total deafness over several years. Reconstruction of the right cochlea revealed an almost total degeneration of the sensory cells of the organ of Corti in all turns (FIG. 12A). The stria vascularis had mildly degenerated, mainly in the basal and middle coils. Seventy to 100% of the peripheral

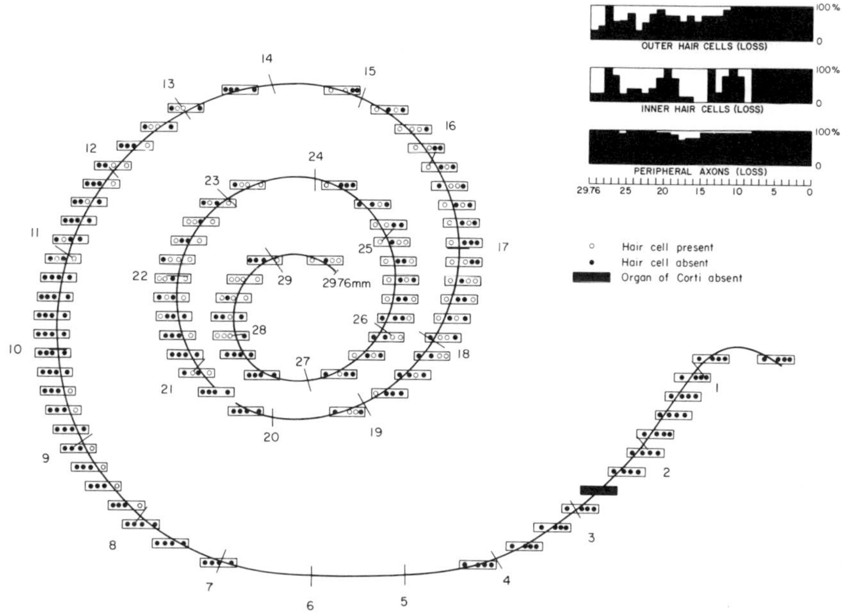

FIGURE 10A. Patient 7, aged 68 years, had otosclerosis with multiple foci involving the otic capsule. The organ of Corti is completely degenerated in the first 8 mm. The inner hair cells persist in several areas of the remaining turns. The outer hair cells are present in about 30–50% in the second and apical turns. The peripheral axons are severely reduced throughout.

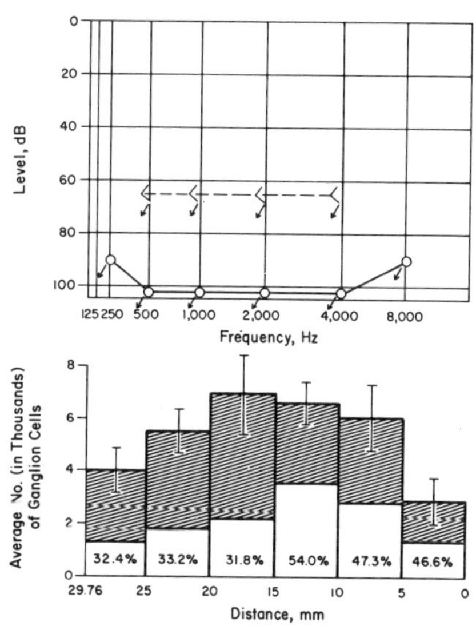

FIGURE 10B. The audiogram of same patient as in FIGURE 10A shows no response to either air or bone conduction in the right ear. The ganglion cell population is reduced to 60–70% of normal in all coils.

axons were present (FIG. 12A). Ganglion cells, which were severely reduced in the basal coil, increased progressively in number into the middle and apical turns (FIG. 12B).

Presbycusis

Presbycusis is a progressive sensorineural hearing impairment that begins during or after middle age. Profound bilateral deafness at all speech frequencies is rare in this group, but can occur in individuals who live beyond the average life span.

Patient 10 was a 77-year-old man who had suffered a progressive sensorineural hearing loss since the age of 54 years. At the age of 69, the hearing in his right ear rapidly deteriorated. An audiogram revealed a pure-tone threshold of 70 dB with a total loss of hearing above 2000 Hz (FIG. 13B).

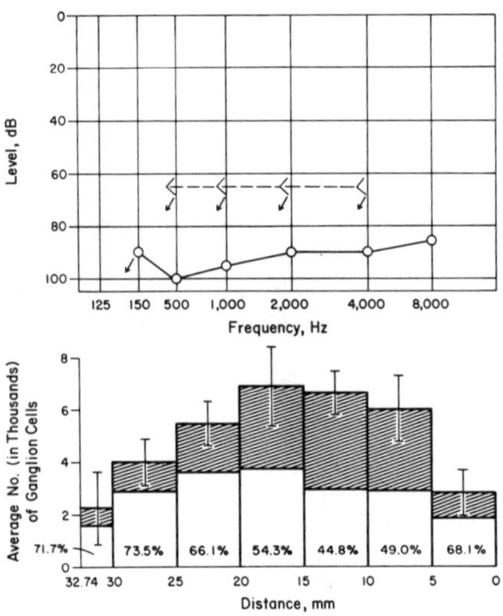

FIGURE 11. Patient 8, aged 67 years, eveloped bilateral profound deafness at he age of 58 after streptomycin adminstration. The audiogram of the right ear emonstrates a profound sensorineural earing loss. Ganglion cells are moderately reduced in the basal coil, with cells ncreasing in number toward the apex.

Cochlear reconstruction of the right ear demonstrated total loss of the organ of Corti in the first 11 mm of the basal coil, with variable preservation of the hair cells throughout the remainder of the cochlea. Peripheral cochlear nerve fibers were also absent in the basal turn, but increased steadily into the apex (FIG. 13A). Extreme degeneration of the stria vascularis was observed throughout the upper and middle coils. Ganglion cell counts were mildly reduced in all turns (FIG. 13B).

Congenital Deafness

A detailed discussion of the histopathologic findings in profound childhood or congenital deafness is beyond the scope of this paper. A detailed monograph on this topic has been published.[20]

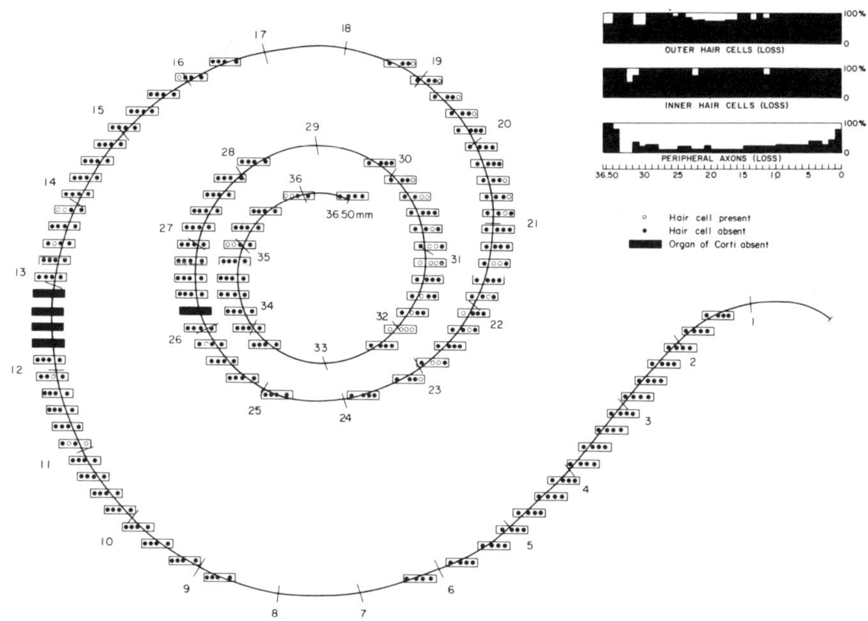

FIGURE 12A. Patient 9, aged 79 years, with Paget's disease, developed a progressive sensorineural deafness. The organ of Corti demonstrates an almost complete absence of inner and outer hair cells in all turns. Peripheral fibers, however, are only mildly reduced in number.

In a high percentage of cases, deafness at birth is associated with other congenital abnormalities. Often, such patients have a dysplasia of the inner ear that is due to either a sporadic mutation or inherited anomaly, or the result of a chromosomal aberration. Typically, the deafness that results is

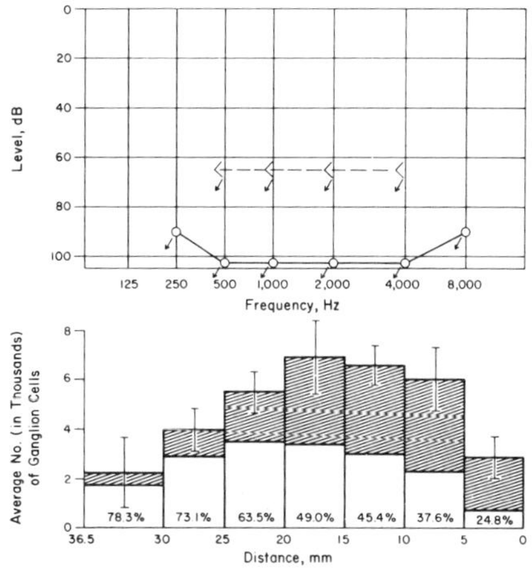

FIGURE 12B. The audiogram of same patient as in FIGURE 12A shows total hearing loss in the right ear. The number of remaining cells increases progressively from the base (25%) toward the apex, where only a minor reduction of cells is seen.

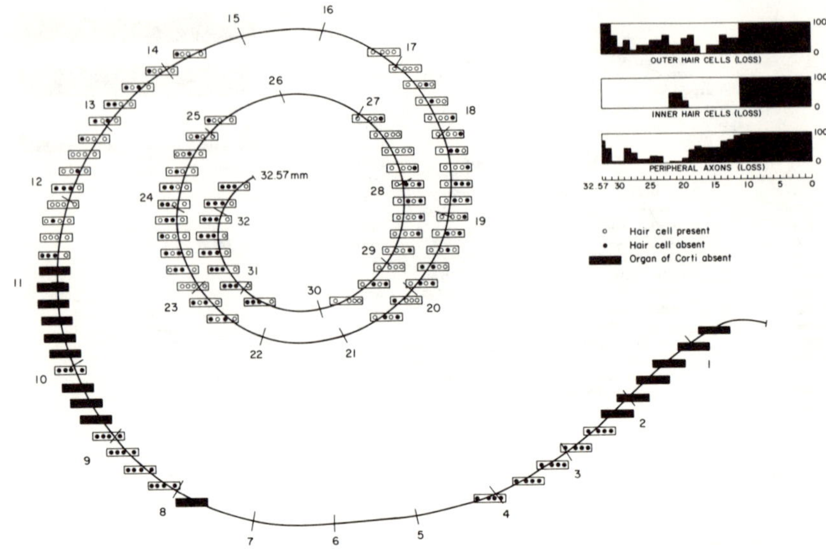

FIGURE 13A. Patient 10, aged 77 years, with presbycusis, is the only case selected from the group with profound high-tone sensorineural deafness. The organ of Corti demonstrates a total loss of sensory elements in the lower basal coil, with variable persistence of hair cells throughout the rest of the cochlea. Peripheral fibers are also absent at the base, but increase toward the apex.

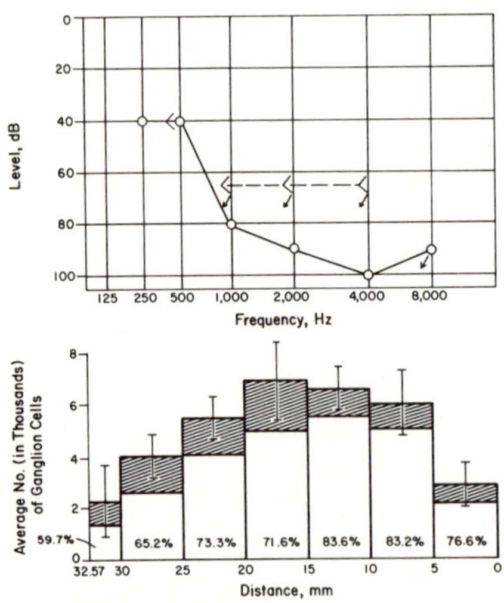

FIGURE 13B. The audiogram of the right ear of same patient as in FIGURE 13A shows a profound sensorineural loss at 2000, 4000, and 8000 Hz. Ganglion cell counts are mildy reduced in all turns.

bilateral, but it may also be unilateral. The Scheibe type of congenital dysplasia, which is the most common, is characterized by degeneration of the cochlea and saccule, leaving the utricle and semicircular canals functionally intact.

Both patients 11 and 12 represent cases of congenital dysplasia of the Scheibe type in which deafness had been diagnosed in infancy, but the cause had not been determined. Patient 11 was a 6-year-old girl who suffered a lethal head injury from an automobile accident. Histopathologic findings in the temporal bone were limited to the cochlea and saccule. The organ of Corti was absent in all coils, whereas about 25% of the nerve fibers persisted in the basal turn, 50–70% were found in the second turn, and 30% existed in the apical turn. Approximately 70% of the ganglion cells were preserved throughout most of the cochlea, with the exception of the apical turn (FIG. 14). The stria vascularis was absent in most areas.

Patient 12, who had been profoundly deaf since infancy, died at the age of 73 years from carcinoma of the kidney. The pathologic findings showed cochleosaccular degeneration. The atrophy of sensory structures within the cochlear duct and saccule was extreme, along with hydrops of the cochlear duct. The peripheral axons had totally degenerated. Ganglion cell counts were severely reduced throughout all turns (FIG. 15). The stria vascularis had degenerated.

Kearns–Sayre Syndrome

The combination of retinitis pigmentosa, external ophthalmoplegia, and heart block was originally reported in two cases by Kearns and Sayre.[21] Sensorineural deafness of varying degrees has occurred in patients with this syndrome. Occasionally, the deafness progresses to the profound stage. In one case (patient 13), sensory cells of the organ of Corti demonstrated severe degeneration throughout, with only 5% of the normal number of peripheral fibers remaining. The cochlear ganglion revealed a severe loss of cells throughout all turns, except in the lower basal coil (FIG. 16). The stria vascularis was also absent in all turns.

Alport's Syndrome

The combination of sensorineural deafness and hemorrhagic nephritis occurring as a familial disorder was first pointed out by Alport.[22] The precise

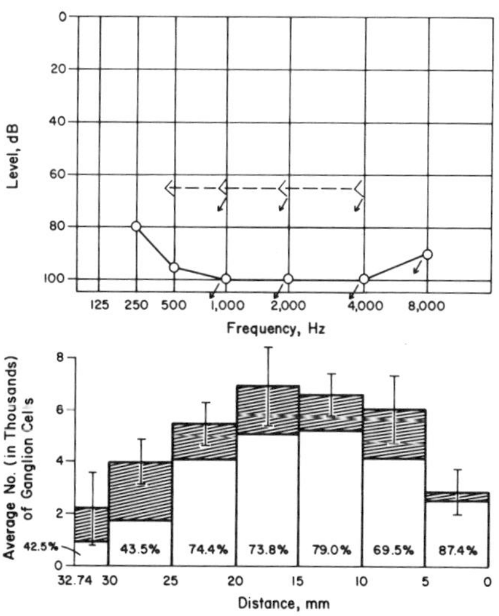

FIGURE 14. Patient 11, aged 6 years, with the Scheibe type of anomaly. The audiogram of the right ear demonstrates a profound hearing loss. Ganglion cells are well preserved in most coils, except in the apical turn, where a moderate reduction is seen.

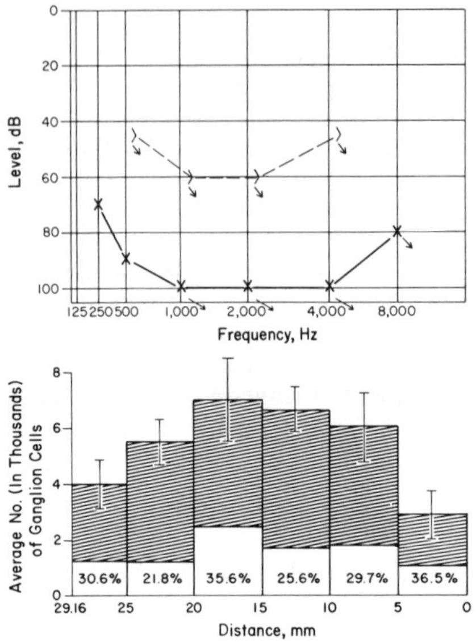

FIGURE 15. Patient 12, aged 73 years, with the Scheibe type of anomaly. The audiogram reveals a profound sensorineural loss. Ganglion cell counts are severely reduced in all turns.

mode of inheritance is still controversial; females seem to be affected more often than males, but the syndrome tends to be much more severe in the latter. Hearing loss is usually bilateral and progressive and is often first noted at about the age of 10 years.

Patient 14 represents a probable case of Alport's syndrome. Cochlear reconstruction showed that the organ of Corti was absent, with total absence of peripheral fibers. The stria vascularis showed marked degeneration except in the middle part of the basal turn. The cochlear ganglion revealed only a moderate reduction of cells throughout all turns (FIG. 17).

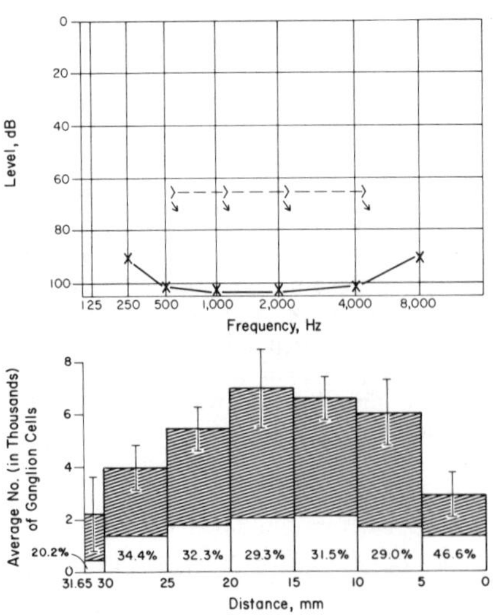

FIGURE 16. Patient 13, aged 19 years, with Kearns–Sayre syndrome. The audiogram shows a profound loss in the left ear. The histogram demonstrates a diffuse loss of ganglion cells throughout all turns, with the lower basal turn being the least affected.

Mondini Dysplasia

The Mondini type of anomaly has been redefined in recent years as representing varying degrees of dysplasia, all having in common an underdeveloped cochlear capsule.[23] The extent of the changes in the sensory epithelium and ganglion cells may vary from case to case, and apparently, even with the loss of one cochlear turn, hearing can be normal.[24] In patient 15, cochlear reconstruction demonstrated total atrophy of the organ of Corti in the basal turn, with patchy persistence of sensory cells in the middle and apical turns. The peripheral axons were absent in the first 10 mm, but increased steadily toward the apex (FIG. 18A). The stria vascularis appeared to be normal in most areas. The spiral ganglion had a unique shape in a two-dimensional reconstruction, and ganglion cell populations were reduced to approximately 50% of normal throughout (FIG. 18B).

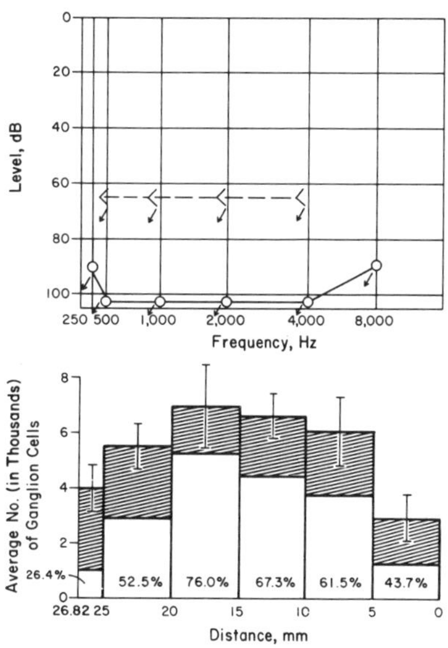

FIGURE 17. Patient 14, aged 31 years, with probable Alport's syndrome. The audiogram shows a total loss of hearing. The histogram reveals a mild reduction of cells in the upper basal and second turns.

Aplasia of the Organ of Corti

Patient 16 was a 53-year old, mentally retarded woman who had been deaf since infancy. Associated abnormalities included a convergent strabismus of the right eye, a high narrow palate, and an asymmetric face. Microscopic examination demonstrated that the organ of Corti was poorly developed in all coils. Pillar cells, hair cells, and Hensen's cells appeared rudimentary in the basal and lower middle coils, but became recognizable in the apical regions. The peripheral fibers were absent in the first 16 mm, but progressively increased in number toward the apex (FIG. 19A). Ganglion cells were reduced in all coils, the upper middle and apical turns being affected least (FIG. 19B). The stria vascularis was fairly well developed throughout.

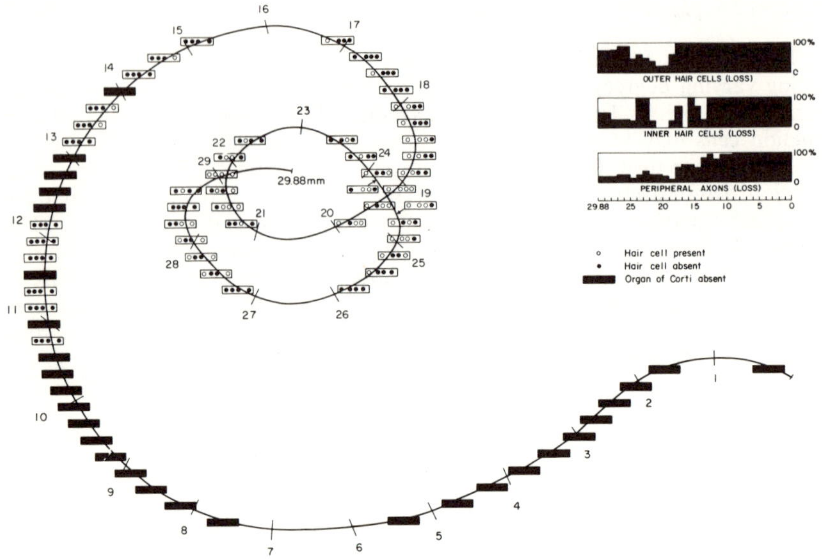

FIGURE 18A. Patient 15, aged 18 years, with congenital deafness caused by the Mondini anomaly. The organ of Corti is completely absent in the basal turn, with variable persistence of cells in the middle and apical coils. The shape of the organ of Corti is abnormal, with the middle turn positioned above the apical turn. Peripheral fibers are also absent in the basal coil, but are present in increasing numbers toward the apex.

In this case, the combination of mental retardation, deafness, and skeletal stigmata may have been caused either by a genetic or an acquired defect. As is quite often the case, the classification of a childhood deafness is not always possible, even on the basis of the pathologic findings.

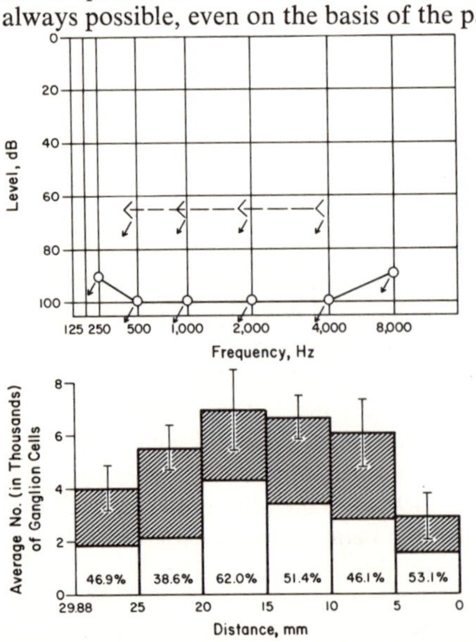

FIGURE 18B. Audiogram taken on the right side in same patient as in FIGURE 18A demonstrates a total loss of hearing. Ganglion cell counts are only moderately reduced in all turns.

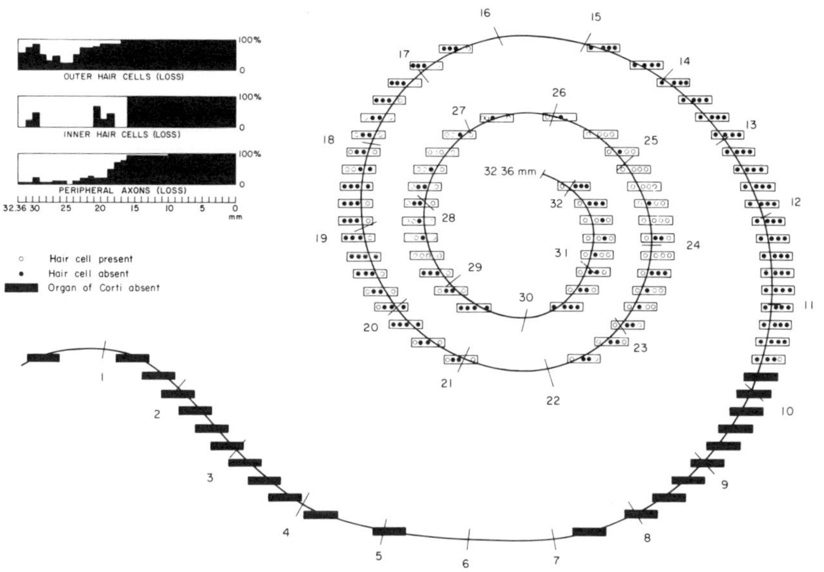

FIGURE 19A. Patient 16, aged 53 years and mentally retarded, with aplasia of the organ of Corti. The peripheral fibers and inner hair cells are absent in the basal coil, but are present in the middle and apical coils.

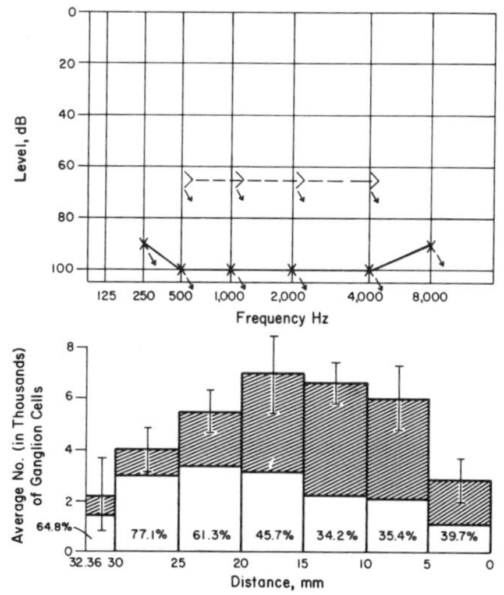

FIGURE 19B. Audiogram of the left ear of same patient as in FIGURE 19A shows total deafness. Ganglion cells are severely reduced in the base, but are more numerous past 15 mm.

DISCUSSION

A consistent pathologic correlate of profound sensorineural deafness, observed in this report as well as in others,[2, 25] is a severe and often total destruction of the organ of Corti. If the original injury to the cochlea, whether traumatic, infectious, metabolic, or genetic in nature, is severe enough, the organ of Corti will be destroyed. A prospective cure for patients who suffer from total hearing loss is the recent development of devices that can stimulate the cochlear nerve directly. These cochlear implants should theoretically function best in those patients in whom an adequate number of cochlear neurons is available for stimulation. Therefore, the cases presented in this report were selected primarily to illustrate the degree to which the spiral ganglion had degenerated in the presence of profound sensorineural deafness.

Of particular importance to the understanding of profound sensorineural deafness is the question of what constitutes an adequate or minimum supply of ganglion cells needed for hearing. The answer to this question remains unknown. We do know that normal cell counts are estimated to be around 30,000.[4, 26] The counts obtained from 12 normal temporal bones presented in this report revealed an average cell count of 33,915, with a range of 29,978 to 39,520 (TABLE 3).

Injury to the organ of Corti, with a subsequent loss of ganglion cells, is thought to result from retrograde degeneration of peripheral cochlear nerve fibers. However, the precise relationship between the loss of hair cells and supporting cells along the basilar membrane and the effect of this loss on the spiral ganglion remains controversial. Otte, Schuknecht, and Kerr[6] have stated that, in acquired lesions, ". . . the extent of loss of the spiral ganglion cells seems to parallel the extent of injury to the supporting cells of the organ of Corti (particularly Deiters' cells and pillar cells) rather than to hair cells." This suggests that, if the pillar cells and Deiters' cells remain, there may be little or no loss of spiral ganglion cells. According to Spoendlin,[27] however, the specific loss of the inner hair cells, regardless of the presence or absence of the outer hair cells, is followed by massive retrograde degeneration of the cochlear neurons. Thus, as long as the majority of inner hair cells remain, there is no appreciable effect on the spiral ganglion.

Neither of these theories is supported by the material presented in this report. In eight temporal bones (from patients 1, 4, 5, 8, 11, 12, 13 and 14) we found complete degeneration of the organ of Corti, including all hair cells and supporting cells. Nevertheless, ganglion cell populations ranged from 7,305 to 23,912 and therefore did not necessarily correspond to the severe degeneration along the basilar membrane. Furthermore, in four of these temporal bones (patients 1, 4, 5, and 14), no peripheral cochlear nerve fibers could be identified. Even in this subgroup of cases which demonstrated a complete destruction of all peripheral auditory sensorineural elements, cell counts ranged from 7,305 to 22,125.

In seven of our cases, there was less than total destruction of the organ of Corti. In four of these (patients 2, 10, 15, and 16), segments along the organ of Corti where inner hair cells were present correlated well with the presence of peripheral fibers. Ganglion cell counts in these four temporal bones were only moderately reduced, ranging from 16,000 to 25,000. However, in both patients suffering from extensive otosclerosis (patients 6 and 7), there was an almost total loss of peripheral nerve fibers in segments where inner hair cells were present. Finally, there was one case (patient 9) with a near-normal population of peripheral fibers, 18,117 ganglion cells, and a total loss of inner hair cells.

The material presented suggests that in patients afflicted with profound sensorineural deafness, the degree of degeneration of the organ of Corti, including the supporting cells, does not necessarily correlate with either the number of remaining peripheral cochlear nerve fibers or the number of remaining spiral ganglion cells. Furthermore, the loss of peripheral cochlear nerve fibers is associated with a variable reduction in the number of ganglion cells. Therefore, it seems reasonable to assume that factors other than the state of the organ of Corti, supporting cells, and peripheral fibers have an effect on the extent of ganglion cell loss.

Injury to the spiral ganglion can occur directly as part of a more generalized cochlear lesion. A severe blow to the head may cause extensive hemorrhage into Rosenthal's canal, causing injury to the spiral ganglion cells. Similarly, bacterial labyrinthitis may result not only in inflammation of the eighth nerve, but also in a subsequent labyrinthitis ossificans in which the entire cochlea, including the spiral ganglion, can be replaced by new bone formation. Therefore, in some cases, the state of the ganglion can be expected to correspond to the degree of injury caused by the original cochlear lesion. However, since the inner ear cannot be examined directly, the extent and degree of injury caused by the original cochlear lesion are unknown. In two patients (3 and 4), both of whom became profoundly deaf as a result of bacterial labyrinthitis, cochlear reconstruction demonstrated a complete loss of the organ of Corti and supporting cells. Although one of these patients had no cells remaining in the spiral ganglion, which was completely destroyed and replaced by new bone (FIG. 6), the other still had 22,125 cells remaining in Rosenthal's canal (FIG. 7).

In cases of viral labyrinthitis (patients 1 and 2), the degree of cochlear injury varies. In a study by Otte *et al.*,[6] an individual with bilateral deafness due to mumps had more than two-thirds of the normal number of ganglion cells remaining; however, in eight ears deafened by measles and six ears with sudden sensorineural deafness, ganglion cell estimates varied considerably. A further complication is the fact that, in cases of viral labyrinthitis, the specific virus is often not identified.

The two cases of otosclerosis presented in this report (patients 6 and 7) were selected because of the profound sensorineural deafness that was superimposed on a previous conductive deafness. The mechanism by which otosclerosis may produce sensorineural deafness is not known, although it is most often seen when the lesion involves the endosteal layer of the otic capsule.[28] Reconstruction of temporal bones from these two patients demonstrated similar sensorineural injuries. An almost complete loss of peripheral nerve fibers was associated with a severe reduction of ganglion cells. Inner hair cells, however, were present in varying numbers.

Most human temporal bones from patients with ototoxicity have been studied in the acute stage, shortly after administration of the drug, and possibly before a significant degeneration of acoustic ganglion cells had taken place. In a report on neomycin ototoxicity,[29] temporal bones were examined 17 days after drug administration. The organ of Corti had degenerated; however, the spiral ganglion demonstrated an excellent population of cells. Temporal bones from another patient,[25] who received 12 grams of kanamycin over an 8-day period, were examined 3 months after drug administration, and in this case, also, both ears had an excellent population of ganglion cells. In this report, we have presented a case of ototoxicity in which the temporal bones were obtained and examined 9 years after drug administration (patient 8). The organ of Corti was absent throughout, but the spiral ganglion again demonstrated a relatively abundant population of cells in all turns.

The number of cells remaining in the spiral ganglion may also be influenced by the continuous loss of these cells over time produced either by the original cochlear lesion or by the process of aging. The variable loss of sensorineural elements over time thought to be due to aging is called presbycusis. Although presbycusis is probably the most common type of deafness in late adult life, we could not find any case in our collection that had a profound sensorineural loss defined as a pure-tone average greater than 90 dB. The patient included here had a 70-dB loss for the speech frequencies and a profound loss only above 2000 Hz (patient 10). Cochlear reconstruction demonstrated the least amount of sensorineural injury among all bones examined, with the highest number of cells remaining in the spiral ganglion.

In two patients (11 and 12), congenital deafness was the result of cochlear dysplasia involving the organ of Corti and saccule, known as the Scheibe type of anomaly. In both cases, histopathologic findings in the sensory epithelium and the saccule were identical. However, ganglion cell counts were 23,912 in a 6-year-old child and 9,417 in a 73-year-old person. Although the interplay of factors that cause spiral ganglion cell injury is not always evident, these two cases indicate that the capacity of the original cochlear lesion to produce a continued loss of cells over time may be significant.

A previous study by Otte *et al.*[6] included the analysis of two ears from patients whose deafness was the result of trauma to the head and transverse temporal bone fractures. One, who died just 4 months after the injury, had a good population of ganglion cells; however, the other patient, who died 30 years after injury, had a poor population of cells in all turns. Similarly, a patient included in this report, an 80-year-old woman who had become deaf at the age of 40 after a severe blow to the head, had a severe reduction of ganglion cells in all turns (patient 5).

Summary

In all the cases of profound deafness that we examined, the sensory epithelium along the basilar membrane had severely degenerated. However, ganglion cell counts and peripheral fiber estimates demonstrated a high degree of variability when analyzed with respect to the state of the organ of Corti or the etiology of the original cochlear disorder. We conclude that a complex interplay of factors determines the number of cells remaining in the spiral ganglion at a given time. It appears impossible at present to predict which diseases or toxic states produce primarily a sensory loss while leaving a uniform and adequate number of cochlear neurons functionally intact. We would like to emphasize that although the ganglion cell counts were consistently reduced in all our cases of profound sensorineural deafness, it has always been a surprise to us to find that the actual numbers of surviving cells are considerable. Of 15 patients, all of whom were totally deaf, only 3 had ganglion cell counts less than 10,000, whereas the majority had counts well above 15,000. Observations of this kind are possible only if accurate ganglion cell counts are carried out. Estimating the number of spiral ganglion cells by only looking at microscopic sections usually results in estimates of greater cell loss than is actually present.

References

1. Clopton, B. M., F. A. Spelman & J. M. Miller. 1980. Estimates of essential neural elements for stimulation through cochlear prosthesis. Ann. Otol. Rhinol. Laryngol. **89** (2 Pt. 2, Suppl. 66): 5–7.

2. Hinojosa, R. & J. R. Lindsay. 1980. Profound deafness: Associated sensory and neural degeneration. Arch. Otolaryngol. **106:** 193–209.
3. Guild, S. R. 1921. A graphic reconstruction method for the study of the organ of Corti. Anat. Rec. **22:** 141–157.
4. Guild, S. R., S. J. Crowe, C. C. Bunch, *et al.* 1931. Correlations of differences in the density of innervation of the organ of Corti with differences in the acuity of hearing, including evidence as to the location in the human cochlea of the receptors for certain tones. Acta Otolaryngol. **15:** 269–308.
5. Schuknecht, H. F. 1953. Techniques for study of cochlear function and pathology in experimental animals: Development of the anatomical frequency scale for the cat. Arch. Otolaryngol. **58:** 377–397.
6. Otte, J., H. F. Schuknecht & A. G. Kerr. 1978. Ganglion cell populations in normal and pathological human cochlea: Implications for cochlear implantation. Laryngoscope **88:** 1231–1246.
7. Lindsay, J. R. 1959. Sudden deafness due to virus infection. Arch. Otolaryngol. **69:** 13–18.
8. Cohn, A. M., H. P. House & J. R. Lindsay. 1970. Deafness in early childhood. Laryngoscope **70:** 1665–1679.
9. Lindsay, J. R. & W. G. Hemenway. 1954. Inner ear pathology due to measles. Ann. Otol. Rhinol. Laryngol. **63:** 754–771.
10. Perlman, H. B. & J. R. Lindsay. 1939. Relation of the internal ear spaces to the meninges. Arch. Otolaryngol. **29:** 12–23.
11. Hagens, E. W. 1940. Pathology of the inner ear in a case of deafness from epidemic cerebrospinal meningitis. Ann. Otol. Rhinol. Laryngol. **49:** 168–176.
12. Henneford, G. E. & J. R. Lindsay. 1968. Deaf-mutism due to meningogenic labyrinthitis. Laryngoscope **78:** 251–261.
13. Matz, G. J., H. B. Lockhart & J. R. Lindsay. 1968. Meningitis following stapedectomy. Laryngoscope **78:** 56–63.
14. Suga, F. & J. R. Lindsay. 1977. Labyrinthitis ossificans. Ann. Otol. Rhinol. Laryngol. **86:** 17–30.
15. Suga, F. & J. R. Lindsay. 1975. Labyrinthitis ossificans due to chronic otitis media. Ann. Otol. Rhinol. Laryngol. **84:** 37–45.
16. Fredrickson, J. M., A. W. Griffith & J. R. Lindsay. 1963. Transverse fracture of the temporal bone: A clinical and histopathological study. Arch. Otolaryngol. **78:** 770–784.
17. Lindsay, J. R. 1973. Histopathology of otosclerosis. Arch. Otolaryngol. **97:** 24–29.
18. Suga, F. & J. R. Lindsay. 1976. Histopathological observations on presbycusis. Ann. Otol. Rhinol. Laryngol. **85:** 169–175.
19. Lindsay, J. R. & F. Suga. 1976. Paget's disease and sensori-neural deafness: Temporal bone histopathology of Paget's disease. Laryngoscope **86:** 1029–1042.
20. Lindsay, J. R. 1973. Profound childhood deafness: Inner ear pathology. Ann. Otol. Rhinol. Laryngol. **82** (Suppl. 5): 1–121.
21. Kearns, T. P. & G. P. Sayre. 1958. Retinitis pigmentosa, external ophthalmoplegia and complete heart block. Arch. Ophthalmol. **60:** 280–289.
22. Alport, A. C. 1927. Hereditary familial congenital haemorrhagic nephritis. Br. Med. J. **1:** 504–506.
23. Beal, D. D., P. R. Davey & J. R. Lindsay. 1967. Inner ear pathology of congenital deafness. Arch. Otolaryngol. **85:** 134–142.
24. Polvogt, L. M. & S. J. Crowe. 1937. Anomalies of the cochlea in patients with normal hearing. Ann. Otol. Rhinol. Laryngol. **46:** 577–581.
25. Kerr, A. & H. F. Schuknecht. 1968. The spiral ganglion in profound deafness. Acta Otolaryngol. **65:** 586–598.

26. Rasmussen, A. T. 1940. Studies of the VIII cranial nerve of man. Laryngoscope **50:** 67–86.
27. Spoendlin, H. 1975. Retrograde degeneration of the cochlear nerve. Acta Otolaryngol. **79:** 266–275.
28. Lindsay, J. R. 1980. Otosclerosis. *In* Otolaryngology, vol. II, 2nd ed. M. M. Paparella and D. A. Shumrick, Eds. Saunders. Philadelphia, PA.
29. Lowry, M. D., M. May & P. Pastore. 1973. Acute histopathologic inner ear changes in deafness due to neomycin: A case report. Ann. Otol. Rhinol. Laryngol. **82:** 876–880.

CODING OF THE SPEECH SPECTRUM IN THREE TIME-VARYING SINUSOIDS [a]

Robert E. Remez

Department of Psychology
Barnard College
Columbia University
New York, New York 10027

Philip E. Rubin

Haskins Laboratories
New Haven, Connecticut 06510

David B. Pisoni

Department of Psychology
Indiana University
Bloomington, Indiana 47405

INTRODUCTION

A range of alternatives now exists for coding the rich spectrum of speech signals. Some techniques create highly intelligible speech by producing signals from digital records of sampled natural utterances. Other techniques, like those used in formant synthesizers and LPC-vocoders, may generate intelligible though less natural-sounding speech from schematic representations of the essential correspondences between acoustic structure and phonetic properties. Perceptual experiments have found that some acoustic impostors of speech are intelligible, while others are not. Intelligible synthesis has been said to retain those acoustic properties of natural speech that are necessary for perception, and those that are unintelligible are said to discard at least some of them. This characterization of intelligibility stated in perceptual terms seems to mean that the identification of phonetic sequences is based just on those acoustic elements, or cues, that bear phonetic information. In practice, however, the cues prove elusive to define. The phonetic value of any particular extract of the natural signal may vary widely, depending on contextual factors. Except by hindsight, it becomes difficult to state precisely which elements in a given signal possess phonetic value and which do not. Overall, then, it seems self-evident that the intelligible simplifications of the signal incorporate the acoustic properties of natural speech upon which perception relies. But the definition of those essential acoustic properties remains a wholly empirical matter.

A number of classic experiments [1] show that successful recodings of the speech signal need not contain every acoustic detail of natural utterances. Nevertheless, our practice of describing the apparently relevant acoustic details as particular short-time spectra or as particular transitions of formants in

[a] This work was supported by Grant HD 15672 (to R.E.R.) and Grant HD 01944 (to Haskins Laboratories) from the National Institute of Child Health and Human Development, and by Grant MH 24027 (to D.B.P.) from the National Institute of Mental Health.

0077–8923/83/0405–0485 $1.75/0 © 1983, NYAS

regions of the spectrum has led us to overlook the potential contribution of phonetic information from *coherent* spectrum *variation.* Our recent experiments with sinusoidal replicas of speech signals address this topic, and the results of these tests indicate that coherent variation of acoustic patterns can provide sufficient phonetic information for the linguistically competent listener. Moreover, these studies revealed that speech perception can be reliable given a stimulus possessing none of the first-order properties of natural speech. The implications for the development of coding schemes to use in intelligent prostheses are quite explicit, or so it would seem: the time-varying coherence of the spectrum bears phonetic information, apparently independent of the elements that compose the dynamic patterns.

Perception of Sinusoidal Signals

In our studies [2–5] we have used signals consisting of three time-varying sinusoids, each of which varies in a formant-like manner. We fabricate each sinusoidal pattern by computing the resonant center-frequencies of a natural utterance, using the analysis technique of linear prediction.[6] The table of values produced through this analysis is used to set frequency and amplitude parameters of a sinewave synthesizer. Typically, three tones are synthesized, each imitating the frequency and amplitude changes of one of the first three formants. Sinusoidal tone-complexes lack fundamental frequency, harmonic spectrum, and broadband formants (the short-time characteristics of natural speech), although there *is* energy, albeit infinitely narrowband, at the computed resonance peaks throughout the duration of each pattern. In consequence, the time-varying properties of the sinewave pattern, specifically the coherence of the *changes* of the energy peaks over time, replicate the natural case.

The perceptual effects of sinewave stimuli were easy to predict. Because the short-time spectra of three-tone signals differ drastically from natural and even synthetic speech; because no talker is capable of producing three simultaneous "whistles" with these bandwidths, in this frequency range;[7] and because the frequency and amplitude changes of the tones are not synchronized, the perceiver should hear three independent streams, one for each sinusoid. The perceiver should hear no phonetic qualities.

However obvious this prediction seemed, there was an equally plausible, though contrasting, prediction. Suppose that the listener was able to disregard the short-time differences between sinusoidal signals and speech, and could attend, instead, to the overall pattern of change of the three tones. The pattern of change of the frequency peaks resembles the resonance changes produced by the vocal tract when articulating speech. If the listener can apprehend this coherence in the time-varying properties of the nonspeech signal, then he should hear a phonetic message spoken by an impossible voice.

Given nonspeech stimuli whose time-varying properties are analogous to vocal signals, listeners perceived the signals in *both* of the ways we predicted. Those listeners who were told nothing about the stimuli heard science-fiction-like sounds, electronic music, sirens, computer bleeps, and radio interference. Those listeners who instead were instructed to transcribe a "strangely synthesized English sentence" did exactly that—they identified the unnatural "voice" quality of the patterns, but transcribed the patterns as they would have the original utterances upon which we based the sinewave stimuli.[2]

In addition to this manipulation of instructions, we also varied the particular stimulus between the groups of listeners. Seven stimulus conditions were used in all, in which subjects heard either three tones, or tones in pairs, or the individual tones. The results of this manipulation indicated that the subjects demanded very specific stimulus structure to detect the phonetic message. Only the three-tone combination and the pair of T1 and T2 (matched respectively to the first and second formants) were transcribed correctly. None of the single-tone patterns was judged to contain any of the words, even when listeners knew which words to expect. We might conclude from this that single formants do not possess sufficient information for phonetic perception.

These studies indicate that speech perception is possible despite drastic departures from the short-time spectra of natural speech—despite absence of broadband formants, harmonic spectrum, and fundamental frequency—insofar as the time-varying properties of speech signals are preserved; and, insofar as the listener is able to attend to the coherent time-variation of the acoustic pattern. Evidently, both of these general qualifications must be met for phonetic perception of sinusoids to occur, for listeners who were not warned to expect speech did not for the most part hear phonetic sequences in tones.

Effects of Phone Class, Amplitude Variation, and Temporal Variation on Intelligibility

Although we have found that sinusoidal replicas of naturally produced utterances are less intelligible, overall, than is speech produced by a conventional terminal analog process, this differential effect does not appear to depend on the recalcitrance of particular phone classes. We might have initially suspected that voiceless stops and fricatives would be unproducible by this technique. On the contrary, we found that those kinds of segments are recognized without benefit of semantic or contextual constraints, as in the sentence "Will Do*c*tor Bron*s*tein meet *Th*orn*t*on in Winni*p*e*s*au*k*ee." Note that nasals, liquids, stops, voiced consonants and vowels are all susceptible to this kind of exclusively time-varying code.

It seems, too, that listeners do not glean much information from the amplitude variation of the tones, nor do they particularly mind grossly inappropriate amplitude values. If the sinusoidal sentences were characterized as "impoverished" stimuli, then we would have expected that inappropriate amplitude values would degrade perception. The absence of other acoustic elements resembling the natural-signal constituents should have forced listeners to rely on whatever other acoustic structure was available, and relative amplitude has been correlated not only with syllable structure, but with vowel and consonant identity as well. However, coherent frequency variation appeared to be sufficient. In fact, with sinusoidal signals the rate of variation is crucial for perception. In a study in which the rate of frequency variation of three tones was manipulated, sinewave sentences were not intelligible at rates of frequency change that departed more than a factor of two from the natural rate of variation. These effects indicate, first, that the normal listener may ordinarily make extensive use of time-varying information during ordinary speech perception. Second, the sufficiency of the complex three-tone carrier holds the prospect for a device that conveys the set of phonetic segments without the necessity of reproducing the entire rich spectrum of natural signals.

Problems with the Technique

Despite the evidence we have discussed in favor of the view that phonetic information is adequately conveyed by the time-varing spectrum, we should point out several potential drawbacks with this method. Because no tone component follows the fundamental frequency contour (our tests show that a fourth tone tracking FØ does not fuse with the phonetic percept), this acoustic aspect is simply omitted from transmission. In consequence, listeners do not experience the sinusoidal voice pitch to be modulated in the same way a natural voice is, and our tests show that Tone 1 is doubling as acoustic information for manner and intonation. Prosodically, sinusoidal speech is unusual, and distractingly so to the listener.

Additionally, sinusoidal replicas of speech are not uniformly highly intelligible, as our tests have shown. Typically, we present a series of sentences, each one repeated three or four times. Listeners then transcribe what they hear. Perhaps because of the strangeness of the sinusoidal voice, at least 30% of our typical, normal adult subjects hear no phonetic segments. Eliminating them from the group improves intelligibility statistically, but only to about 65% correctly identified words. Clearly, we must determine the effect of familiarity with sinusoidal signals on transcription, if there is any effect to speak of. Research by Grunke and Pisoni [8] is encouraging on this score. In their study, naive listeners learned to classify sinusoidal "syllables" composed of tones. Subjects labeled the tone patterns either with acoustic symbols that referred to the tone properties of spectrum changes (for example, rising, falling, steady) or with phonetic labels appropriate for the phonetic value each pattern was thought to have (for example, ba, da). Acoustic labeling was more reliable for the single tones and for double-tone patterns analogous to the second and third formants. Essentially, when conditions for phonetic perception of tones were not satisfied, acoustic labels were easier to learn. However, three-tone patterns were more reliably classified with the phonetic rather than acoustic terms. This indicates that the stimulus properties themselves facilitate the subject's attention to phonetic information. The effect of familiarity with three-tone signals on phonetic perception of sinusoids deserves further attention.

To conclude, our studies of speech signals replicated with tonal patterns has revealed that time-varying structure alone can convey phonetic information. While we particularly hope that our pursuit of this issue will resolve the paradoxes of isolated-cue conceptualizations of the information in speech signals, it is not uninteresting to speculate whether this coded simplification of the rich spectrum of speech might not present a possible technique for use in cochlear implants. Even in view of the basic questions that remain for us, we contribute the results to our tests with the normal listener to this end.

Summary

Recent perceptual experiments with normal adult listeners show that phonetic information can readily be conveyed by sinewave replicas of speech signals. These tonal patterns are made of three sinusoids set equal in frequency and amplitude to the respective peaks of the first three formants of natural-speech utterances. Unlike natural and most synthetic speech, the spectrum of sinusoidal patterns contains neither harmonics nor broadband formants, and is indentified as grossly unnatural in voice timbre. Despite this drastic recoding of the short-time speech spectrum, listeners perceive the phonetic content if the temporal properties of spectrum variation are preserved. These observations suggest that phonetic perception may depend on properties of coherent spectrum variation, a second-order property of the acoustic signal, rather than any particular set of acoustic elements present in speech signals.

Acknowledgments

We wish to thank Louis Goldstein and Michael Studdert-Kennedy for their helpful, relentless criticism.

References

1. Liberman, A. M. & M. Studdert-Kennedy. 1978. Phonetic perception. *In* Handbook of Sensory Physiology. Vol. VIII: Perception. R. Held, H. Leibowitz, and H.-L. Teuber, Eds.: 143–178. Springer Verlag. New York, NY.
2. Remez, R. E., P. E. Rubin, D. B. Pisoni & T. D. Carrell. 1981. Speech perception without traditional speech cues. Science **212:** 947–950.
3. Remez, R. E., P. E. Rubin & T. D. Carrell. 1981. Phonetic perception of sinusoidal signals: Effects of amplitude variation. J. Acoust. Soc. Am. **69:** S114.
4. Remez, R. E. & P. E. Rubin. Phonetic perception of sinusoidal signals: Effects of temporal variation. Paper presented at the Twenty-Second Annual Meeting of the Psychonomic Society, November 14, 1981.
5. Remez, R. E. & P. E. Rubin. 1982. Perception of voice pitch in sinusoidal imitations of speech. J. Acoust. Soc. Am. **71:** S96.
6. Markel, J. D. & A. H. Gray, Jr. 1976. Linear Prediction of Speech. Springer Verlag. New York, NY.
7. Busnel, R. G. & A. Classe. 1976. Whistled Languages. Springer Verlag. New York, NY.
8. Grunke, M. E. & D. B. Pisoni. 1982. Perceptual learning of mirror-image acoustic patterns. Percept. Psychophys., **31:** 210–218.

A FIBER SUM MODULATION CODE FOR A COCHLEAR PROSTHESIS

Charles W. Parkins, Robert Houde,
and
John Bancroft

Division of Otolaryngology
University of Rochester
School of Medicine and Dentistry
Rochester, New York 14642

One approach to developing a stimulation code for a cochlear prosthesis is to attempt to mimic the normal physiologic neural responses to acoustic stimulation. FIGURE 1 demonstrates a simplistic view of the sensory deafness problem. Normally, the basilar membrane with its traveling wave acts as a series of mechanical bandpass filters. The movement of each frequency-specific location is detected by the transducers of the system, representing the hair cells of the organ of Corti. This analog information is then converted to a digital pulse code which is sent out on a number of transmission lines representing single neurons in the auditory nerve. In the pathologic situation in which the transducers are damaged (sensory deafness), the cochlear prosthesis attempts to bypass the defective transducers and directly stimulate the neural transmission lines. Since the information transmitted over the transmission lines is normally in a digital code, it makes little sense to try to stimulate them in an analog manner. We must therefore devise a signal processor that will convert the original analog acoustic signal into a digital pulse code which will maximize the ability of the central auditory nervous system to process this input in a normal manner, resulting in pitch, loudness and, most importantly, speech discrimination.

The characteristics of single auditory neuron responses to acoustic stimulation have been well documented earlier in this volume. FIGURE 2 demonstrates some of these characteristics in a 538-Hz neuron's response to a tone-burst at its characteristic frequency (CF). The top trace is the analog signal representing the acoustic stimulus. The next 16 traces represent the single auditory neuron's response to each of sixteen consecutive repetitions of the stimulus. In this digital response, the only information delivered is whether or not a response has occurred at a specific point in time. This figure also illustrates the probabilistic nature of the response. The bottom trace represents the summed responses to 200 stimulus presentations, the poststimulus time (PST) histogram. When the response is compared with the stimulus, a time lag is found in the response due largely to the traveling wave of the basilar membrane. There are also more responses at the onset of the stimulus than at the end, even though the stimulus is of constant amplitude. This is the well-documented adaptation effect.[1, 2]

THE SIGNAL PROCESSOR

On the basis of the large volume of eighth nerve single-neuron data available in the literature, a number of models have been proposed [3] to relate

0077–8923/83/0405–0490 $01.75/0 © 1983, NYAS

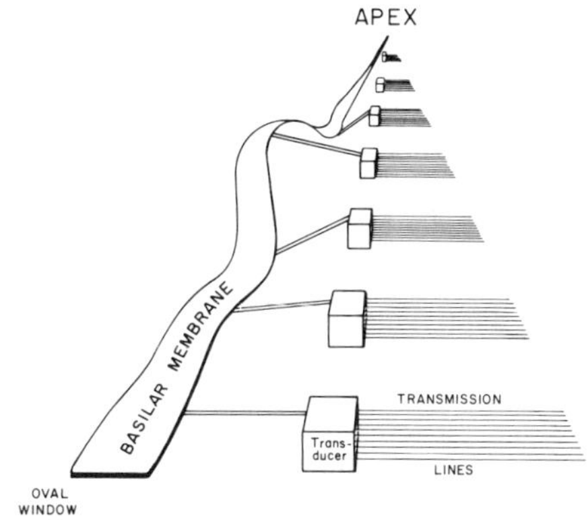

FIGURE 1. Mechanical model of cochlear function.

the acoustic signal input to the neural output. The model we have proposed [4] is shown in FIGURE 3. The incoming signal, I_t, is separated into its frequency components by the mechanical bandpass filter function of the basilar membrane and its interaction with the hair cell. This produces a phase lag between F_t and I_t greatest at the low-frequency end of the spectrum. The bandpass signal, F_t, is halfwave-rectified by the hair cell's stimulatory displacement phase and lowpass-filtered by the 1-msec refractory period of the hair cell or hair-cell neuron transmission.[5]

The final hair-cell/neuron processing stage may be modeled as an adaption processor including a logarithmic compression. The lowpass signal, K_t, is first logarithmically compressed to a decibel scale normalized at neural thresh-

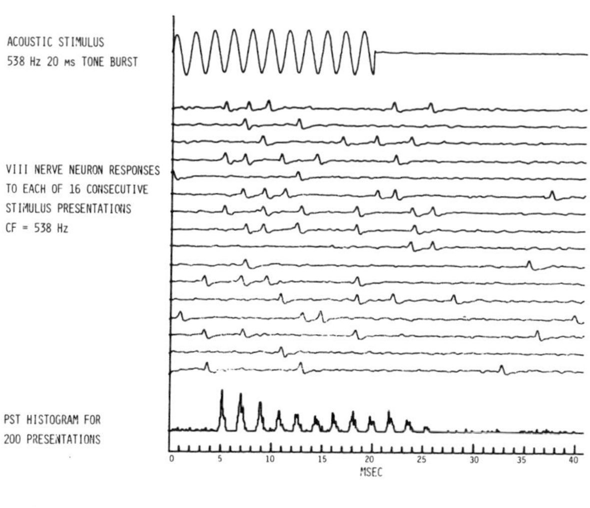

FIGURE 2. Single auditory nerve neuron response. The neuron characteristic frequency (CF) = 538 Hz; the stimulus frequency = 538 Hz.

old. The dynamic range is limited to 30 dB, above which it saturates. The adaptation algorithm was partially modeled after Smith's results and fit to single-neuron data from our laboratory. A phenomenologic model was used in which a finite number of transmitter sites (50) was assumed for the transducer (hair cell). The number of transmitter sites active at any point in time is proportional to the logarithmically compressed signal. The output signal, representing the probability of neural response, is proportional to the number of active sites plus the volume of transmitter available at the sites, delineating an additive adaptation similar to that described by Smith.[1] Each transmitter site was modeled as recovering when not stimulated or being depleted when stimulated, both as exponential functions. Two depletion (adapting) time constants (1 msec and 21 msec of weighted importance of 9.5:1) and two recovery time constants (5 msec and 50 msec) were used. The resulting signal, H_t, serves as the input signal into a number of individual neuron spike generators that are probabilistic in nature, producing discharge rates in the transmission lines (neurons) that are both proportional to the amplitude of the probability signal, H_t, and also to the time since the last neural response occurred.

The result of each of these processing stages is compared with real data from a 538-Hz CF eighth nerve neuron in FIGURE 4. The first trace is the acoustic stimulus, a sharp rise/fall time toneburst at the neuron's CF. The second trace, F_t, demonstrates the result of the bandpass filter shaped to the neuron's frequency threshold curve (tuning curve). The filter and basilar membrane latency shifts account for the latency of the neuron's response. The

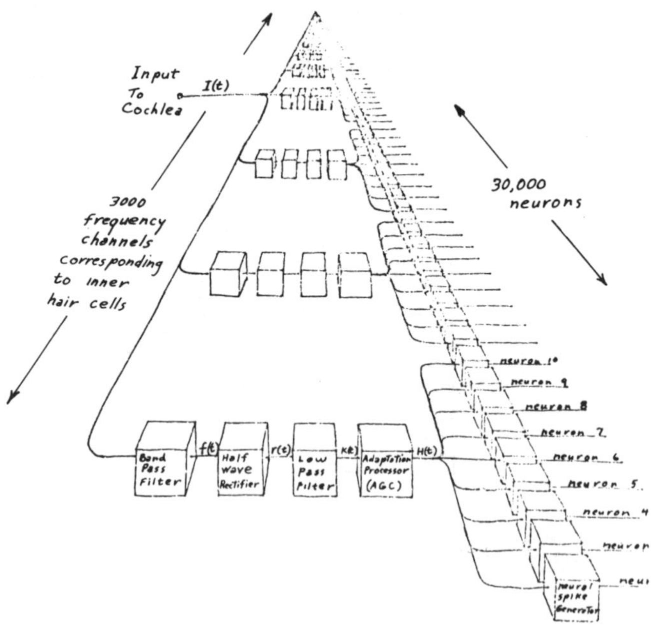

FIGURE 3. Peripheral auditory processor model.

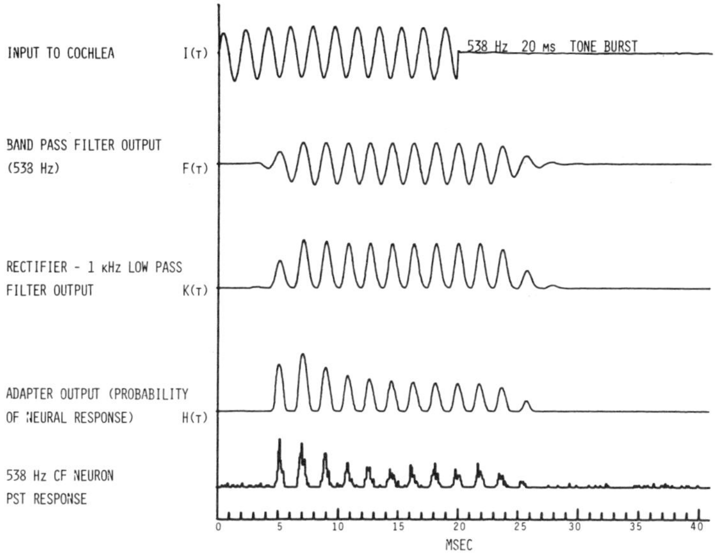

FIGURE 4. Processing model results at 538 Hz. I(t) is the acoustic stimulus used to produce the PST histogram response from a 538-Hz CF neuron shown in the last trace of the figure. F(t), K(t), and H(t) represent the results of processing the initial acoustic stimulus I(t) as diagrammed in the processing model seen in FIGURE 3.

filter effect also produces a more gradual rise/fall time with some post-stimulus ringing. The 1-kHz lowpass filter has little effect on this 538-Hz waveform in K_t. The adaptation effect seen in H_t emphasizes the onset of the toneburst and improves the fit of the processed analog signal with the last trace, which is the neuron's actual response to the stimulus plotted as a PST histogram. This processing model also predicts the responses of high-frequency neurons as seen in FIGURE 5, which illustrates a neuron with a characteristic frequency of 2045 Hz. Here the lowpass filter has a much more prominent effect seen in the third trace. It produces a DC shift following the toneburst envelope with an AC ripple representing phase-locking. The closer the stimulus is to the 1000-Hz lowpass filter, the greater the ripple and the greater the phase-locking. Again, the adaptation effect is necessary to match the processed signal to the neuron's PST response.

FIGURE 6 demonstrates the effect of this processing scheme on a more complex stimulus, speech. The top trace is the first 70 msec of the word "boot." The importance of the adaptation effect is seen in the difference between the third and fourth traces. The adaptation effect strongly emphasizes the burst of the "b" and the timing of the onset of voicing at the beginning of the "u." The emphasis of this timing is also seen in the PST histogram in the bottom trace. This timing is very important in the differentation between voiced and nonvoiced consonants in speech and may be very important in the design of the cochlear implant processor. FIGURE 7 demonstrates the difference between low-frequency (535 Hz CF) and high-frequency (3045 Hz CF) processing. The 1,000-Hz lowpass filter has a much more noticeable effect in high-frequency processing. At the 3045-Hz frequency, the processor output shows little phase-locking and mainly an envelope following of the glottic pulses. Again, the adaptation effect is necessary to maximize the fit between processor output and neural response.

Besides retaining the phase-locked features necessary to produce the volley code for pitch perception and the multichannel configuration necessary for tonotopic pitch coding, this theoretical processor also retains the phase relationships of neurons responding to stimuli at non-CF frequencies. The resulting phase shifts reproduce the timing results of the traveling wave effect of the basilar membrane. The processor therefore maintains the time and phase differences between neural frequency populations, which will allow the function of more sophisticated pitch-decoding schemes, such as that proposed by Mundie.[6] Mundie demonstrated that the nonlinear propagation velocity of the basilar membrane resulted in the storage within the basilar membrane of 1.75 cycles of any stimulus frequency at any point in time. This results in two stimulatory phase basilar membrane displacements for each stimulus frequency, with the location and spacing of these stimulatory displacements (and, therefore, responding neural populations) specific for each stimulus frequency. Mundie then postulated a coincidence or cross-correlation pitch detector based on the phase-locked responses of these two population groups.

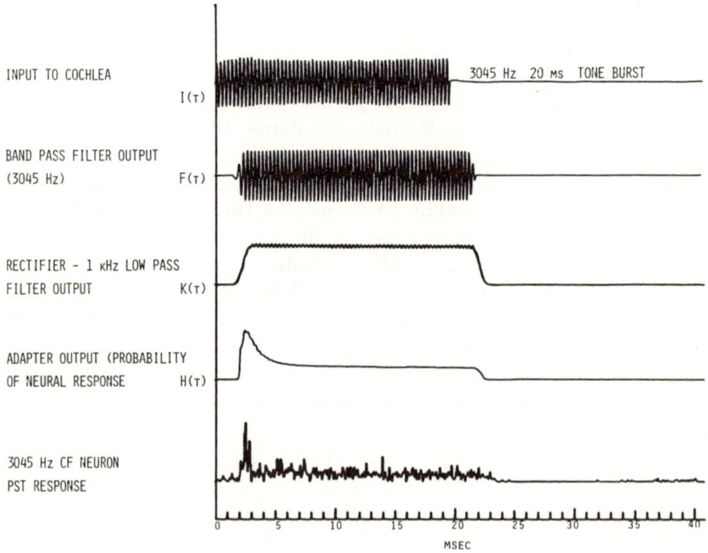

FIGURE 5. Processing model results at 3,045 Hz. I(t) is the acoustic stimulus used to produce the PST histogram response from a 3,045-Hz CF neuron shown in the last trace of the figure. F(t), K(t), and H(t) represent the results of processing the initial acoustic stimulus I(t) as diagrammed in the processing model in FIGURE 3.

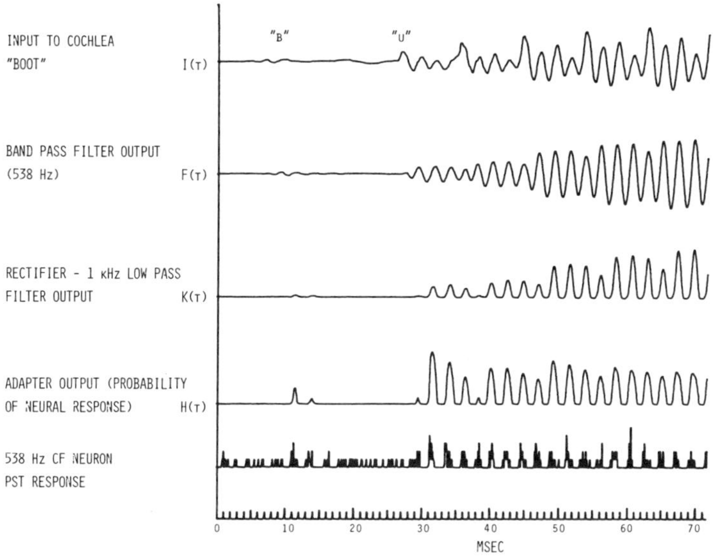

FIGURE 6. Processing model results for speech at 538 Hz. The first trace, I(t), is the first 72 msec of the word "boot," which was used to obtain the PST histogram shown in the last trace from a 538-Hz CF neuron. F(t), K(t), and H(t) represent sequential processing stage outputs of the processor model (FIG. 3) processed at a center frequency of 538 Hz.

THE STIMULUS GENERATOR

The PST histogram used to demonstrate the relationship between the neural response and the stimulus is constructed by adding the responses of one neuron to many repetitions of the same stimulus (see FIGURE 2). The auditory neurologic system probably does not function in this fashion since it must decode one isolated presentation of the stimulus. Because of the probabilistic nature of the neural response and because adjacent neurons vary minimally in frequency selectivity and latency, one can assume that sampling the responses of 100 adjacent neurons to one stimulus presentation will produce a very similar PST histogram to that produced from 100 responses from one neuron. It would, however, be a "simultaneous" histogram rather than the usual "sequential" PST histogram. We could therefore consider each of the individual eighth nerve responses shown in FIGURE 2 as coming from adjacent neurons. This assumption would be more pertinent to the topic of auditory coding since it is much more likely that the central auditory system "listens" to the "simultaneous histogram" from a population group, rather than being involved in a lengthy temporal integration necessary for a sequential analysis of individual neurons (although the temporal integration of loudness over a 200-msec period is a well-documented phenomenon). The goal for electrical stimulation, therefore, should be to produce an instantaneously responding fiber sum which is proportional to the output of the signal processing model, H_t, at any point in time.

It is fairly well agreed that a multichannel electrode system will be necessary to utilize the tonotopic code for pitch perception. We have chosen a 15-channel device utilizing bipolar stimulation to limit the spread of neural excitation from any one channel. For the purpose of this paper, assume that such a device can be atraumatically implanted in the scala tympani of the cochlea to reach the second turn, encompassing the pitch locations for 200 to 6000 Hz. Also assume that the pathologic disorder is purely sensory and that there is a full complement of functional neurons. The electrode placement for one channel is diagrammed in FIGURE 8 for a pair of electrodes 80 μ^2 spaced 60 μ apart.

A number of constraints must be considered in developing the stimulus generator for these electrodes. To avoid injury, the stimulus current must be limited to less than 38 microcoulombs per square centimeter of real electrode surface and per phase [7]; the electrical fields produced by various stimulus levels must be determined; and the 500-μsec absolute refractory period of the neuron to electrical stimulation must be considered. We have constructed a three-dimensional computer model of the electrical fields generated by such an idealized electrode pair. The model assumes an infinite volume of uniform conductance and does not take into consideration the relative resistances of perilymph, soft tissue, and bone. The increased resistance of the bony spiral lamina will act as an attenuator of the current refracting the current contours where they intersect those impedance changes, but will not alter the basic principles, as demonstrated by the model. A sectional view of the bipolar

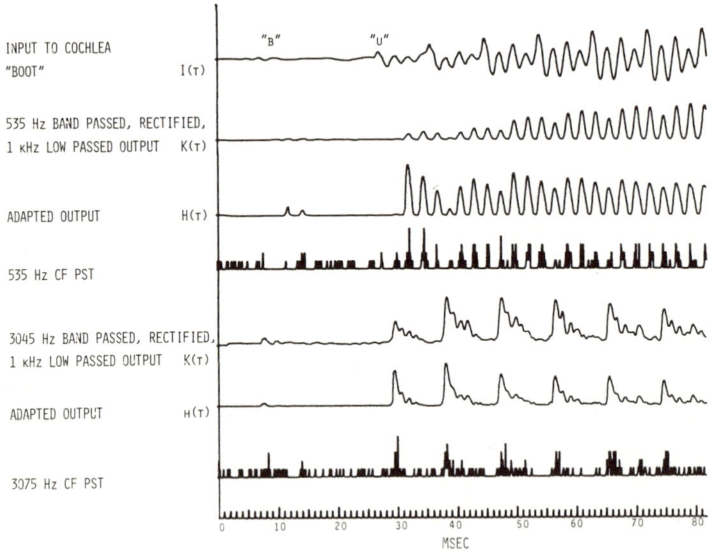

FIGURE 7. Processing model results for speech at 535 Hz and 3045 Hz. The *upper half* of the figure compares model processing at 535 Hz with the PST response of a 535-Hz CF neuron. The *lower half* of the figure compares the model processing at 3,045 Hz with the PST response of a 3,045-Hz CF neuron.

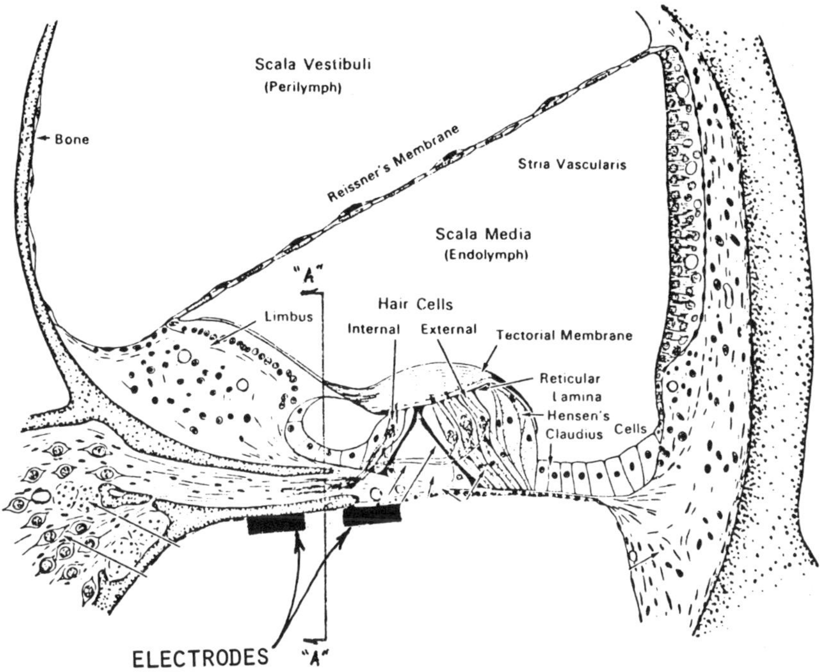

FIGURE 8. This cross section of the cochlea shows a theoretical electrode pair placement just below the basilar membrane and osseous spiral lamina. The section marked as "A–A" represents the view used in FIGURE 9 to demonstrate the electrical fields produced by this electrode placement.

electrode viewed from the interelectrode plane "A–A" of FIGURE 8 and viewed towards the modiolus demonstrates in FIGURE 9 the threshold current contours produced by various voltage levels applied to the electrode (voltages are in relative voltage units, not absolute voltage). This diagram demonstrates that as the threshold current contour reaches the neural population within the bony spiral lamina, small voltage changes will produce large changes in the number of stimulated neurons. At high voltage levels, large voltage changes produce only small changes in the number of stimulated neurons. These data have been plotted in FIGURE 10 as the number of neurons within the threshold field on the ordinate with a log scale of the stimulus voltages on the abscissa. This necessitates a moderately difficult modulation scheme with minimal voltages for small neural population responses and very large voltages for maximum responses.

FIGURE 11 demonstrates the rationale behind the stimulus generation. The very top trace (A) is the unmodulated stimulus, consisting of a biphasic square wave of 5000 Hz. We have chosen a stimulus period much shorter than the 500-μsec neuron refractory period to distribute more randomly the neural responses in time for a more physiologic pattern. This is also within the stimulus frequency range reported earlier by Loeb [8] to be most efficient in stimulating auditory neurons, as measured in charge per phase. The second trace (B) is the output of the signal processor, H(t), for the stimulating phase of a 250-Hz, a 500-Hz, and a 1000-Hz sinusoid. The amplitude of this signal is proportional to the number of neurons that we wish to respond at any point in time. The third section (C) is a plot of the neuron population in the region of the specific electrode pair. The number and location of neurons responding to the electrical stimulus is proportional to the height and location of the vertical lines. The bottom trace (D) represents the actual electrical stimulus to be delivered to the electrode. Note that the stimulus does not bear a simple monotonic relationship to the processor output, H_t.

In determining the stimulus for the first sinusoid, the generator determines the number of neurons to be discharged from the value of the processor output H(t) where o positive value of H(t) first coincides with a positive zerocrossing of the unmodulated stimulus. It then looks up the required stimulus intensity from the stimulus versus population plot (FIG. 10) and modulates the square-wave stimulus accordingly, producing the first biphasic pulse. The generator goes to the next positive zerocrossing and again determines the number of neurons to be discharged from the value of the

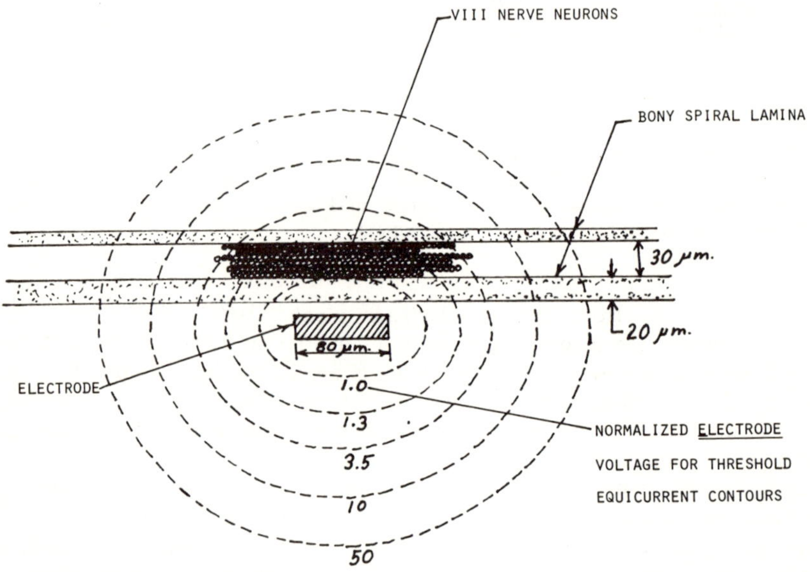

FIGURE 9. Radial view of electrode, neurons, and equicurrent threshold contours in section "A–A" of FIGURE 8. The neural population, bony spiral lamina, and electrode are viewed from an interelectrode position looking towards the modiolus. The dotted contour lines represent threshold contours produced by the labeled relative voltage levels. All neurons falling within (central to) the contour line would theoretically be stimulable by the respective voltage level applied to the electrode. These contour lines were plotted from a computer model which assumed a uniform conductivity and did not take into account the differential resistances of tissue and bone (see text).

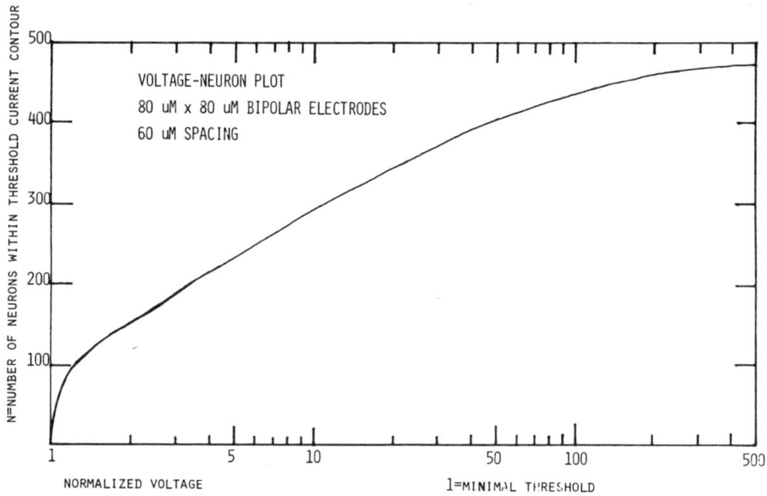

FIGURE 10. Stimulable neurons versus stimulus intensity. The number of neurons falling within the threshold contour, and therefore stimulable, is plotted on the Y axis. The normalized voltage applied to the electrode is plotted on the X axis as a logarithmic function. Results are from a computer model.

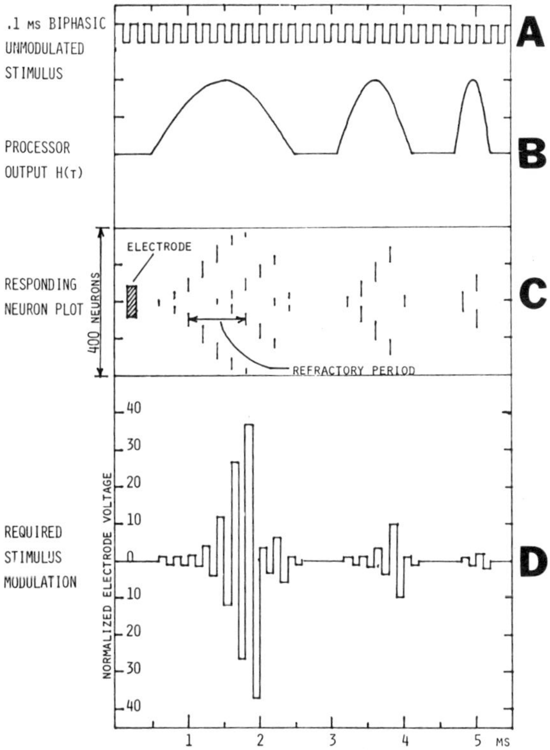

FIGURE 11. Stimulus generator rationale and output. (**A**) the unmodulated stimulus pattern that will be modulated by the stimulus generator logic to produce the pulse pattern demonstrated in (**D**). This output stimulus which consists of symmetrical biphasic pulses will then be capacitantly coupled to the implanted electrode. (**B**) represents the output of the processor, H(t), and shows the number of neurons to be discharged at any point in time. (**C**) is a diagrammatic representation of the neural population in the vicinity of the electrode. The vertical lines represent the number and positions of the neurons that are responding at any point in time. All four functions take place within the 5½-msec time scale shown on the bottom of the figure.

processor output. The number of neurons within the threshold contour must be larger than the number to be discharged, because some of the neurons will be nonstimulable since they are in their refractory period. The generator, therefore, adds the number of refractory neurons to the number to be stimulated and again looks up the required stimulus level to produce a threshold contour that will encompass this total population. It then modulates the square wave accordingly. The timing and position of the responding neurons are illustrated in FIGURE 11C. Eventually enough time will have passed for the initially stimulated neurons to recover and again be available for stimulation. This accounts for the rather unusual modulation envelope of the generator's electrical stimulus (FIG. 11D). The basic principle of this stimulus scheme is to produce an instantaneous responding fiber sum proportional to the processor output signal, in other words, the simultaneous PST histogram. All of the timing and amplitude information in the processor signal is therefore maintained.

Some differences will still exist between the neural response pattern to normal acoustic stimulation and that produced by the proposed electrical stimulation scheme. These differences are illustrated in FIGURE 12 relative to a 1-mm length of basilar membrane. The top trace is again the output of the stimulus processor. The dots in the lower section of the graph represent the

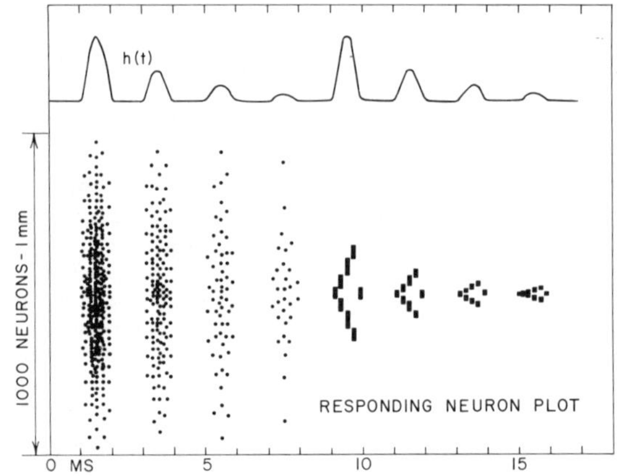

FIGURE 12. Single-neuron response patterns to acoustic stimulation compared to electrical stimulation. The top trace, H(t) represents the processor output for four sinusoids of decreasing amplitude used for acoustic stimulation (*left*) and for electrical stimulation (*right*). The *lower portion* of this figure represents diagramatically the position of 1000 neurons centered on the center frequency of the stimulus for acoustic stimulation and centered on the physical location of the electrode for the electrical stimulation. The *dots* represent the positions of the responding neurons and the timing of their discharges in relation to the time scale shown on the *bottom* of the figure. The *left* part of the figure demonstrates the probabilistic nature of the neural responses in both the time and position domains with normal acoustic stimulation. The *right* part of the figure demonstrates the deterministic response of neurons responding to the electrical stimulus code. If a PST histogram is constructed using 0.2-msec time bins for each of these responses, the PST histograms would be identical and would look like the H(t) trace at the top of the figure.

hypothesized individual responding neuron's position on the ordinate and the time of the response plotted on the abscissa. The responses to four cycles of acoustic stimulation are seen on the left and comparable responses to the electrical stimulation code on the right. There is a randomness seen for acoustic stimulation both in the time domain and in the position domain which reflects the probabilistic nature of the neuron's response to acoustic stimulation. In contrast, the response to electrical stimulation is deterministic, with very synchronous discharges of adjacent neurons locked to the timing of the stimulus square wave. The discharge rates of individual neurons will also be quite different. The rate function for individual neurons undergoing acoustic stimulation will be proportional to H_t, while those responding to electrical stimulation, especially those neurons close to the center of the neural population for that channel, will frequently be at saturation. The most important similarity between the acoustic and electrical responses is the instantaneous responding fiber sum. The number of neural pulses from a defined frequency region of the cochlea reaching the appropriate region of the cochlear nucleus will be very similar in both stimulation schemes and will be proportional to the processor output, $H(t)$. This electrical stimulation scheme using a multichannel electrode will, therefore, retain the place code for pitch, the volley code for pitch, the fine timing important to speech discrimination, and even the discrete waveform of the stimulus, as seen by different eighth nerve frequency population groups, reflecting the physiologic timing of the traveling wave of the basilar membrane.

References

1. Smith, R. L. 1979. Adaptation, saturation, and physiological masking in auditory periphery. This volume.
2. Smith, R. L., M. L. Brachman & D. A. Goodman. 1982. Adaptation in the auditory periphery. This volume.
3. Kiang, N. Y., D. K. Eddington & B. Delgutte. 1979. Fundamental considerations in designing auditory implants. Acta Otolaryngol. **87**(3–4): 176.
4. Parkins, C. W. 1979. Single eighth nerve neuron responses to speech as a model for a cochlear prosthesis. *In* Advances in Prosthetic Devices for the Deaf: A Technical Workshop. D. McPherson, Ed.: 291–301. National Technical Institute for the Deaf. Rochester, N.Y.
5. Kletsky, D. J. & J. M. Stengrevics. 1972. Estimation of the integration time constant in auditory receptor units. J. Acoust. Soc. Am. **52:** 141.
6. Mundie, J. R., J. C. Roch & A. J. Goldstein. 1973. Signal processing principles revealed by an auditory system model. *In* Cybernetics and Bionics: Proceeding of the Fifth Congress of the Deutsche Gesellschaft für Kybernetik.: 292–307. R. Oldenbourg. Munich and Vienna.
7. Walsh, S. 1979. Damaging effects of electrical cochlear stimulation. Presented at the Neural Prosthesis Workshop, National Institutes of Health.
8. Loeb, G. E., M. W. White & W. M. Jenkins. 1982. Biophysical considerations in electrical stimulation of the auditory nervous system. This volume.

CODING OF SOUND IN A COCHLEAR PROSTHESIS: SOME THEORETICAL AND PRACTICAL CONSIDERATIONS [a]

Michael M. Merzenich

Coleman Laboratory
University of California at San Francisco
San Francisco, California 94143

Introduction

The optimal strategy for coding speech as intelligible across an intracochlear multielectrode array reflects a compromise between what should be done and what can be done. That is, it reflects a compromise between simulation of the critical aspects of the representation of speech elements across the auditory nerve array and the idealization of that representation, given practical limitations of the spatiotemporal control of nerve array stimulation with applicable intracochlear electrodes.

Recent studies on the auditory nerve array representation of speech elements (especially the studies of Sachs, Young and colleagues [1–3]) coupled with parametric studies with cochlear implant devices [4–6] indicate, on a first order, what is *essential* to represent in the distributed excitation of the nerve array. Further, they reveal how high levels of speech recognition are accounted for in the distributed patterns of activation of the auditory nerve array in normal-hearing subjects driven with low-channel-number vocoders.[7] These studies suggest that the "optimal" simulation model is a special kind of channel vocoder, especially given limitations of electrical stimulation control of the auditory nerve array.

In this report, it will be argued that a distributed nerve-stimulation vocoder model constitutes a rational starting point for progressive development of a multichannel cochlear prosthesis. Nerve array stimulation control required to implement such a model is described. Some basic test results in a patient stimulated with three- and four-channel versions of such a model are described. Physical and practical limitations that impede development of more complex stimulation models are discussed. Finally, strategies for improving the simulation (reducing distortion) is such devices are briefly summarized.

Simulation Coding Models for an Auditory Prosthesis

A strict auditory nerve array response simulation strategy has been most explicitly described by Kiang and colleagues.[8] Such a device would employ an algorithm of distributed spatiotemporal firing patterns across the auditory nerve array to control excitation at distributed sites along the array. The objective would be to effect a faithful simulation of distributed sound-evoked nerve-discharge patterns.

[a] This work was supported by Grant NS–11804 and Contract NO1–NS–0–2337 from the National Institute of Health, and by grants from Hearing Research, Inc., the Saul and Ida Epstein Foundation, and the Coleman Memorial Fund.

0077–8923/83/0405–0502 $01.75/0 © 1983, NYAS

A simpler form of a simulation-based device is suggested by the recent studies of the distributed patterns of representation of speech elements across the auditory nerve array, especially by Sachs, Young, and colleagues.[3] They have shown that components of speech elements (such as the formants of vowels) are apparently represented by a spatially restricted temporal encoding of individual speech element components. Thus, to cite the simplest example, the first formant of a steady-state vowel is represented by the temporal discharges of neurons over a restricted sector (the corresponding resonance region) of the nerve array, roughly one to a few millimeters in length. The second formant is represented by the temporal discharge characteristics of neurons over a restricted, somewhat narrower, more basal sector; and so forth. Two-tone "inhibition" acts to stabilize the spatial domains of this temporal information, so that the representation of the vowel is largely independent of stimulus level and highly immune to noise across the speech reception range of loudness. Both temporal and spatial features of this representational pattern are remarkably invariant as a function of level.

Moderate-level stimulation with such a speech element (for example, just above the speech reception threshold) would lead to excitation across a relatively restricted cochlear sector extending across the frequency range of the spectrum of the speech element. Higher-level stimulation with such a speech element results in a distributed, nearly saturated neural response across the entire nerve array basal to the position of resonance of the lowest frequency component.[3, 9–11] In a strict simulation model, distributed nerve excitation would be very different in these two cases. Sachs and Young's studies indicate that critical features of the speech element are represented throughout the speech reception range across a restricted sector of the nerve array corresponding to the regions of resonance of the speech element components. Their studies strongly suggest that what is critical to simulate are the relatively spatially constant (as a function of level) and relatively narrow sectors over which distributed temporal information is most strongly representing speech element structure.

A channel-vocoder-based multichannel cochlear implant device accomplishes just that, in the sense that (if its electrodes are well designed) it can bring a series of restricted sectors of the auditory nerve array under independent temporal control. Its applicability would be limited: (1) by the ability to simulate critical *details* (both spatial and temporal) of the "temporal representation" of speech element components within these restricted sectors; (2) by the ability to distinguishably represent speech element components varying little in frequency (that is, approaching critical band distances [approaching categorical boundaries]); and (3) upon the ability to represent spatially nonstatic frequency transitions of speech elements. Given appropriate spatial electrical stimulation control, the latter two limitations should be a direct function of channel number.

As will be briefly described later, significant levels of speech recognition have been recorded with use of this kind of implant device.

Some Considerations in the Implementation of These Models

Directed evaluation of any simulation model is difficult, unless individual electrodes in multielectrode arrays operate linearly. In fact, most constructed "multiple channel" devices do not, at least in most patients. This is certainly the case for monopolar electrode arrays and for common-grounded arrays of at least most applied designs (for example, where stimulus elements are well removed from excitable structures). It is also the case for bipolar arrays in which pair elements are broadly separated.[12–15]

Even with radial bipolar stimulation with ideally located electrodes, independent control of excitation on a grain finer than a millimeter or two is not achievable, for several reasons. First and foremost, the stimulating elements of a scala tympani array are unavoidably physically separated from stimulatable targets (minimally, as in our device, 100–150 microns). Second, physical surface contact areas cannot be greatly reduced without elevating charge density (thereby compromising device safety).[15–17]

The implications that this bears on considerations of implementation of a *sim*ulation model are obvious. First, fine spatial features of temporal reponse across a resonance-peak region cannot be represented across a series of linearly operating (noninteracting) electrodes. If such fine spatial patterns of temporal distributions of discharges are important to simulate in a channel-vocoder-based device, they can only be manipulated by control of stimulus waveform on given electrode elements. That is, *the Sachs and Young phase-locked regions representing components of speech elements are within the domain of control of single electrodes.* There is no practical way to introduce and linearly control simultaneously excited electrodes *within* these relatively narrow regions.

Model "ideally" located and oriented bipolar electrodes have been demonstrated (in cats with good nerve survival) to bring appropriately restricted sectors of the auditory nerve array under independent (noninteractive) control.[12–14, 18] Recent studies in a patient believed to have good nerve survival implanted with nearly identical electrodes confirm that such electrodes bring less than 2-mm sectors of the nerve array under virtually independent control, with simultaneous stimulation of distributed elements across the speech reception range of loudness.[4] That is, regions approximately corresponding to the presumptive vowel formant zones of temporal representation in man can be brought under independent temporal control with these stimulating elements. Boundaries of speech elements correlate with critical band dimensions; and normal channel vocoders approach full intelligibility when channel separations approach the critical band distance (about 1.5 mm) in separation.[7] It is interesting to note, then, that noninteractive control can be realized on this grain. It is also interesting to note that a full range of loudness is effected with stimulation restricted spatially to 2 mm or less in a patient with apparently very good nerve survival.[4]

If spatiotemporal control around each stimulating element is adequate, a six- or seven- or eight-channel device of this type *should* provide a high level of speech recognition, equivalent to that achievable with a simple channel vocoder of higher number (higher, because these devices act like a "baseband vocoder," as frequency information below about 1 kHz is very strongly and discriminably represented by a single, appropriately located apical channel). The limitation of such devices will, again, reflect the precision with which critical spatial and temporal *details* of nerve array response are simulated.

It might be noted that spatial field summation interactions with simpler electrode arrays (such as monopolar arrays) can theoretically be minimized by using temporally nonoverlapping stimulation. Unfortunately, there are severe limits imposed by residual neural effects that severely restrict use of nonoverlapping stimuli. Thus, stimulation on one electrode will affect the territory of response to stimulation on a second electrode over about a 3–4-msec post-stimulus time.[4] This effect severely limits use of sequenced stimuli as a technique for minimizing channel interaction. In other words, if 1- or 2- or 3-mm sectors of the nerve array must be brought under separate temporal control, this can only be achieved with confidence with an array comprised of distributed bipolar elements. And again, any significant distributed nonlinear interaction of stimulated elements across the array will frustrate speech component representation simulation.

The advantages of bipolar stimulus control are especially important for patients with poor nerve survival. Such a patient has almost certainly been studied in our series. There, monopolar interaction was extraordinarily powerful. Tests indicate that with stimulation of a single element in the center of the array, for example, there was strong interaction with stimulation anywhere else (that is, over a more than 14-mm length of the nerve array) at low stimulus levels. On the other hand, bipolar pairs 4 mm apart were essentially noninteractive. If we consider a distributed excitation vocoder (baseband vocoder) model alone, representation of speech across linearly operating 3- or 4-mm sectors under independent temporal control could result in significant levels of speech recognition using distributed bipolar stimulation. Especially in the case of poor nerve survival, then, use of monopolar or common-grounded electrodes will introduce enormous complexities for implementation of a simulation model.

Strategies for Improving These Devices

Encoding of pitch in the speech frequency range would appear to involve more than detection of stimulus periodicity alone.[6] Thus, perceived pitch for stimuli above about 300 Hz is electrode-specific, and does not change as stimulus frequency is changed. This is especially interesting in the light of the fact that there appears to be strong phase-locking of discharges of electrically stimulated auditory neurons.[19, 20] For example, with sinusoidal electrical stimulation, there is a powerful representation of stimulus period for stimulus frequencies up to at least 3–4 kHz.[19]

If the representation of stimulus period at appropriate distributed (resonance) sites were to constitute a high-fidelity representation of these essential features of the distributed nerve representation of speech elements, then given the cross-species assumptions, we should be able to easily achieve levels of speech recognition equivalent to those recorded in a normal subject with a baseband vocoder with the same channel number.

Unfortunately, the detailed representation of temporal information as a function of position across restricted speech element component representational nerve array sectors also appears to be important, that is, the auditory nervous system appears to be reading spatiotemporal details across each resonance-peak region. Because we can manipulate neural activity across those restricted sectors realistically only with single stimulating elements, only somewhat limited parametric adjustments can be effected. Fine distributed temporal discharge patterns can be manipulated by varying stimulus waveform. However, temporal patterns around each electrode are invariably symmetric.[21] Higher than normal discharge saturation rates (not limited by hair-cell receptor potential saturation) are achieved. Abnormal sequential charging distortions are recorded.[4] Given these and other possible and unavoidable sources of distortion, the achievable fidelity of representation of critical neural response patterns is somewhat uncertain.

Some Results Derived in Testing a Multichannel Cochlear Implant of this Form

The basic design of a UCSF vocoder-based multichannel cochlear implant in which this model is being evaluated has the following features [22, 23]: (1) The electrode array is designed for insertion 24–26 mm into the scala tympani. (2) Mechanical properties of the intracochclear array insure (*a*) low probability of insertion trauma and (*b*) highly reliable "ideal" electrode element placement. (3) A "surgical disconnect" plug using a "rubber under pressure" sealing strategy allows for (*a*) temporary use of an external percutaneous cable, giving direct access to the multielectrode array during an experimental period; (*b*) application of an optimally coupled passive electronic receiver and removal of the temporary percutaneous cable at the end of an experimental period; and (*c*) later capability for relatively simple replacement of failed or obsolete receiving electronics. (4) Receiving electronics are sealed into a welded titanium capsule. Independent passive radiofrequency detectors are now being used. They insure high reliability, acceptable power efficiency for a limited-channel-number device, good channel isolation, and good channel bandwidth. These detectors have the disadvantages of (*a*) a relatively large foreign-body size; and (*b*) voltage-control operation (see the report of Loeb and colleagues).[15] (5) The three- or four-channel sound processor–stimulator units initially tested are channel vocoders operating like a basic baseband vocoder. Special charge filters and compressors effect the translation between sound and appropriate electrical stimulation of myelinated nerve.[14, 15, 21]

In tests with these model devices in which electrodes have been positioned at the approximate center frequency (resonance-peak) locations of vocoder channels, significant levels of speech recognition have been recorded, in both current and voltage-control modes.[4,24] (Even higher recognition scores have been obtained by Eddington [25] with a very similar four-channel device.) Different channel outputs are described by a tested patient in qualitatively the same terms as equivalent channel outputs in a baseband channel vocoder in a normal-hearing subject. The baseband (most apical) channel alone provides a strong basis for recognition of first formant information, but good distinction of first formants is dependent upon three- or four-channel operation. Significant recognition of second formant features has also been recorded, when second formant information is devolved across two or three higher-frequency channels. With even a three-channel voltage-control device, in almost every speech category (including open test material ranging from recognition of words in sentences through recognition of open, single syllables), very highly significant recognition capabilities have been recorded.

Results derived with other device configurations (such as monopolar three- or four-channel driving or single-channel driving) are limited, but suggest that distributed, independent control of separated nerve sectors following this distributed, linearly operating vocoder cochlear prosthesis model is far superior in terms of speech recognition and is the basis of recorded recognition results.

Indeed, *recognition scores achieved in this patient are not greatly different from those that might be expected with a three-channel baseband vocoder in a normal subject.* We believe that these sources reflect the fact that one of the conceptually simplest and most easily fabricated forms of a patient device—a channel vocoder nerve stimulator with effective sector-by-sector stimulation control of the nerve array—is at least crudely simulating the normal essential encoding of speech across the auditory nerve array.

Acknowledgments

All members of the cochlear implant research team at the University of California at San Francisco, but especially Mark White, Jerry Loeb, Robert Shannon, Lindsay Vurek and Earl Schubert, have contributed to the development of our applied cochlear implant models.

References

1. Young, E. D. & M. B. Sachs. 1979. Representation of steady-state vowels in the temporal aspects of the discharge patterns of populations of auditory nerve fibers. J. Acoust. Soc. Am. **66:** 1318–1403.
2. Sachs, M. B. & E. D. Young. 1980. Effects of non-linearities on speech encoding in the auditory nerve. J. Acoust. Soc. Am. **68:** 858–875.
3. Sachs, M. B., E. D. Young & M. I. Miller. 1983. Speech encoding in the auditory nerve.: Implications for cochlear implants. This volume.
4. White, M. W. 1983. Formant frequency discrimination and recognition in auditory nerve: Implications for cochlear implants. This volume.
5. Eddington, D. K., W. H. Dobelle, M. G. Mladejovsky, D. E. Brackmann & J. L. Parkin. 1978. Auditory prostheses research with multiple channel intracochlear stimulation in man. Ann. Otol. **87** (53): 5–38.
6. Loeb, G. E., M. W. White & M. M. Merzenich. 1982. A new theory of acoustic pitch perception. J. Neurosci. Submitted for publication.
7. Flanagan, J. C. 1972. Speech Analysis. Springer-Verlag. Berlin.
8. Kiang, N. Y. S., D. K. Eddington & B. Delgutte. 1979. Fundamental considerations in designing auditory implants. Acta Otolaryngol. **87:** 204–218.
9. Tsuchitani, C. 1978. Neural encoding of auditory information. *In* Advances in Prosthetic Devices for the Deaf. D. L. McPherson, Ed. NTID. Rochester,
10. Kim, D. O. & C. E. Molnar. 1979. A population study of cochlear nerve fibers: Comparison of spatial distributions of average-rate and phase-locking measures of responses to single tones. J. Neurophysiol. **42:** 16–30.
11. Kim, D. O. 1983. Spatiotemporal response patterns in populations of cochlear nerve fibers: Single and two-tone studies. This volume.
12. Merzenich, M. M. & M. White. 1977. Cochlear implants: The interface problems. *In* Functional Electrical Stimulation. F. T. Hambrecht and J. B. Reswick, Eds. Marcel Dekker. New York, NY.
13. Merzenich, M. M., M. Vivion, P. Leake-Jones & M. White. 1978. Progress in development of implantable multielectrode scala tympani arrays for a cochlear implant prosthesis. *In* Advances in Prosthetic Devices for the Deaf. D. L. McPherson, Ed. National Technical Institute for the Deaf. Rochester, NY.
14. Merzenich, M. M., M. White & M. C. Vivion. 1979. Some considerations of multichannel electrical stimulation of the auditory nerve in the profoundly deaf: Interfacing electrode arrays with the auditory nerve array. Acta Otolaryngol. **87:** 196–203.

15. Loeb, G. E., M. White & W. M. Jenkins. 1983. Biophysical considerations in electrical stimulation of the auditory nervous system. This volume.
16. Brummer, S. B., L. S. Robblee & F. T. Hambrecht. 1983. Criteria for selecting electrodes for electrical stimulation: Theoretical and practical considerations. This volume.
17. Roblee, L. S., J. McHardy, J. M. Marston & S. B. Brummer. 1980. Electrical stimulation with Pt electrodes. V. The effect of protein on Pt dissolution. Biomaterials **1:** 135–142.
18. Schindler, R. A., M. M. Merzenich, M. White & B. Bjorkroth. 1977. Multielectrode intracochlear implants. Arch. Otolaryngol. **103:** 691–699.
19. White, M., M. M. Merzenich & G. E. Loeb. 1983. Electrical stimulation of the eighth nerve in cat: Temporal properties of unit responses in the large spherical cell region of the AVCN. Ann. Otol. Submitted for publication.
20. Moxon, E. C. 1971. Neural and Mechanical Responses to Electrical Stimulation of the Cat's Inner Ear. Thesis, Massachusetts Institute of Technology, Cambridge, MA.
21. Merzenich, M. M. & M. White. 1980. Coding considerations in design of cochlear prostheses. Ann. Otol. **89:** 84–87.
22. Merzenich, M. M., C. L. Byers, M. White & M. C. Vivion. 1980. Cochlear implant prostheses: Strategies and progress. Ann. Biomed. Eng. IEEE **8:** 361–368.
23. Loeb, G. E., C. L. Byers, S. J. Rebscher, D. E. Casey, M. M. Fong, R. A. Schindler, R. F. Gray & M. M. Merzenich. 1983. The design and fabrication of an experimental cochlear prosthesis. Med. Biol. Eng. Comp. In press.
24. Owens, E., D. Kessler & M. Raggio. 1983. Results for some patients with cochlear implants on the minimal auditory capabilities (MAC) battery. This volume.
25. Eddington, D. K. 1983. Speech recognition in deaf subjects with multichannel intracochlear electrodes. This volume.

ROUND-TABLE DISCUSSION

DR. CHARLES W. PARKINS (*Division of Otolaryngology, University of Rochester School of Medicine and Dentistry, Rochester, New York 14642*): I hope that this session will serve as a vehicle to allow the faculty to express any new ideas synthesized at this conference.

First, I would like to thank the faculty members for agreeing to come and to participate, even though this has entailed a financial sacrifice for a number of persons. All are to be commended for their participation and for the excellence of the papers presented at this convocation.

Now let me turn to Dr. Kiang for any new thoughts or ideas he might have as a result of this conference and for any specific suggestions or questions he might like to raise.

DR. NELSON Y. S. KIANG (*Department of Electrical Engineering and Computer Science, Massachusetts Institute of Technology, Cambridge, Massachusetts 02139*): To describe what I find new at this conference I must first engage in a little personal historical review. In 1957, as we were setting up our laboratory to do auditory physiology, Djourno's paper came out on what must now be called a single-channel cochlear implant. I knew then that the contemplative work on stimulus coding in the auditory system would be a critical factor in further development along these lines.

Some years later the Doyles introduced a multiple-electrode implant, but they never understood the difference between multiple electrodes and multiple channels. Then came Blair Simmons' paper in the early 1960s, which, like Djourno's, confirmed that auditory sensations could be elicited in the profoundly deaf by electric stimulation, presumably of the auditory nerve.

At that time the profession of otology was not ready to accept overt human experimentation on this matter, so there was a short gap in publications for a while. The silence was then broken by Robin Michelson, who in 1971 expressed some views based on essentially "off the wall" ideas of electric tuning in nerve fibers. This gave him enough courage to publish some of the results on implantation in human subjects, which was followed quickly by a publication by Bill House, who then described some of his work.

I don't believe that anyone who has ever thought about the issue has maintained that cochlear implants will not ever work. At that time I told Dr. House that I thought that his cochlear implant would not do what he claimed it would, and I think that this remains true even today.

However one might wish for an orderly, if not informed, research on cochlear implants, the reality is that many more energetic practitioners are leaping into the field, mostly with inadequate and often with appallingly deficient backgrounds. The present conference is a fairly good example of the helter-skelter assortment of workers that now populate this field, and the situation is likely to get worse.

What do we now know?

First, I have to say that, to their credit, the surgeons have done their part. They have shown that it is possible to work in the inner ear without catastrophe, although the consequences of less-adept surgeons and long-term stimulation remain to be seen.

Second, the engineers have not quite solved the problem of electrode fabrica-

0077-8923/83/0405-0509 $01.75/0 © 1983, NYAS

tion on a large-scale basis, but I have every confidence that they will be better able to do that once the performance specifications become more refined.

Third, there appear to be a great many people who do not yet appreciate how well a clever central processor can utilize impoverished cues. In this context I am disappointed in the lack of dialogue between the basic scientists and the cochlear implant workers, and I don't think that the situation will improve until more of the implant investigators learn to read the basic literature so that they can ask the proper questions.

I am encouraged by the entry of young, trained investigators, such as Drs. Eddington, Tong, and Müller, who are taking reasonable steps in trying to determine the cues in controlling behavior in many of these cochlear implant studies. Nevertheless, it is still the case that no existing device will enable a profoundly deaf person to process free running speech using acoustic cues alone.

Having attended this conference I find no need to change the conclusions that I stated in my paper earlier. I do not believe that there will be a single optimal coding scheme for all patients, and I think that the task is to describe the variables that must be known in order to determine the best scheme for a particular patient.

As one who was not involved immediately in the cochlear implant derby, I would like to give some advice to the younger workers in the field. Please try to report your work as openly, completely, and accurately as possible. Let others persist in holding preconceived attitudes, but do your own research in as objective a manner as is within your capabilities. Examine the dogmas and the personal biases, but let the evidence speak for itself.

Unsupported beliefs, no matter how firmly stated, will not enhance one's scientific reputation, and, even worse, may actually keep you headed in unproductive lines of inquiry. I hope that the elders will start to gather more critical and assertive junior colleagues and give them more of a head because fawning sycophants do not a research team make.

Just as a specific note, I consider the idea of implanting intracochlear single-channel electrodes in young children to be indefensible at this time. I wish that Dr. House would get together with the British group and clearly articulate the disadvantages of a round-window or a promontory approach before he proceeds any further with his program.

We need more direct and candid approaches to debating such issues, and the organization and format of this conference was not successful in promoting thorough discussion of honest differences. In aiming at inclusiveness, the planners sacrificed coherence of purpose. As a forum for expounding dogmas it was inadequate for beginners and tiresome to the veterans. The cacophony produced by the different levels of sophistication, styles, and intellectual content of the presentations must be absolutely bewildering to the uninitiated. It is not even easy for those actively working in the field to sort out the complex, but valid, arguments from those that merely represent muddled thinking. So, if any of you who paid good money to attend this conference are confused, there is no need to feel inadequate.

PARKINS: Thank you Dr. Kiang. Now let me ask Dr. Sachs to address the same questions.

DR. MURRAY B. SACHS: (*Department of Biomedical Engineering, Johns Hopkins School of Medicine, Baltimore, Maryland 21205*): I would like to focus on two issues. First, I would like to clarify what I and my colleagues have and have not shown about coding of speech in the auditory nerve. And, second,

I would like to comment about what I think we can learn from those working with cochlear implants.

We have shown that in the temporal patterns, the phase-locked patterns of auditory nerve fibers, there is an exquisite representation of the spectrum of a speech stimulus. In fact, we have yet to find a feature in the speech stimulus that cannot be represented in these patterns. What we have *not* shown, and I want to emphasize this, is that the central nervous system uses these patterns. We don't know whether it does or not.

The second thing that we have not shown is that a code based on average rate cannot work. In my paper I spend an equal amount of time discussing codes based on average rate, and this is not by chance. We have not ruled out the possibility that a code based on average rate can work.

In terms of what we can learn from you, I share much of the confusion that my mentor just talked about. Nevertheless, the one fact that I come away from this conference more or less convinced of, because I saw evidence in at least two dozen slides, is that there seems to be no discrimination of rate pitch above about 300 to 400 Hz.

Now Dr. Merzenich has suggested some ways in which that result might be explained, and in our paper we have suggested other ways to explain that finding. But this finding is a pretty tough one to handle in terms of a temporal code for frequency in the auditory system. I think that we who are interested in the normal coding of speech must examine carefully that result and others from cochlear implant studies. I find it hard to understand in terms of the notions that we put forward why there is no rate pitch above 300 to 400 Hz. We can think of arguments that are testable in animal and cochlear implant studies that can help to answer some of these questions.

PARKINS: Dr. Sachs, when you are talking about a rate code are you referring to a rate code per single neuron or an ensemble rate within a frequency population of neurons?

SACHS: I am talking about a rate versus place profile. Our experimental regime uses the anesthetized cat, which is very important because in this animal there is a whole system of efferent fibers innervating the cochlea, and the only thing that we can ascribe to that bundle of efferent fibers is some sort of automatic gain control properties. What we have shown within the constraints of this experimental situation is that peaks in a rate versus place profile across the population of auditory nerve fibers disappear at high stimulus levels and in a noise background primarily because of the effects of rate saturation and two-tone suppression. In evaluating a rate–place code, we must further delineate the function of the efferent fibers. Second, we must consider the low spontaneous high-threshold fibers, which, as we have pointed out in every paper we have written, will add another 20 to 30 dB.

Some of the adaptation properties that Dr. Smith has talked about are another feature of a possible rate–place code that needs to be accounted for. I fear that because the temporal–place representation is so exquisite, too much emphasis has been given to it. Although I didn't have enough time to discuss this, we have data on rate versus place profiles for stop consonants, showing, in the range where vowels have saturated their rate–place profiles, nice formant-related structure in the rate–place profiles for consonants.

KIANG: I am happy to hear Dr. Sachs set the record straight. We have discussed this between ourselves and I think that he has unintentionally misled a great many people who have taken his writings further than he has intended them.

Parkins: I would next like to ask Dr. Merzenich to comment on his electrode design.

Dr. Michael Merzenich (*Coleman Laboratory, Departments of Otolaryngology and Physiology, University of California, San Francisco, California 94143*): Before I speak about our electrodes I would like to remark that Murray Sachs is probably in more danger of having too little attention paid to his temporal–place work rather than too much. That would be very unfortunate.

It is obvious to those who have gone through the practical experience of building electrodes, such as the Hochmairs and the groups in Stanford and Melbourne, that the critical feature of design is that the electrode be insertable without trauma. This requires, as the Hochmairs so nicely pointed out in their presentations, that the electrode be capable of being opened to initiate its insertion into the scala tympani. For maximum insertion into the scala tympani the electrode needs a memory for the spirals of the cochlea so that when the electrode is fully inserted, it is relaxed. The mechanical properties of the electrode must not drive it upward across the basilar membrane and destroy it.

This is achieved in our electrode by constructing a central rib made by stacking the flattened conductor wires with their greater diameter oriented in the plane of the modiolus. The wires vary in size depending upon where they come into the rib, that is, the finest wires come into the basal aspect of the rib and the heaviest wires into the apical aspect. This confers stiffness to vertical displacement of the electrode apically beyond what would be achieved with uniform flattened wires. This array is relatively rigid to any vertical flexion, even in the apex, and yet has a full flexibility in the plane of curvature of the cochlea. It is basically this property that confers insertability.

The surgical procedure described by Dr. Michelson is significantly modified in the implants that are being done in our other experimental project. The electrode is never hyperextended. Basically, the coil is taken out with a probe. The surgeon pushes out the tip of the electrode through the round window into the scala tympani where it rides on the inside of the spiral. The inherent flex of the array causes it to slide along on the medial aspect of the scala tympani, which prevents it from moving up into the more fragile region of the basal membrane. Then, in the final several millimeters of insertion the electrode seeks a more lateral position just beyond the margin of the osseus spiral lamina.

In tests in cadavers, this insertion is highly predictable with respect to both control of trauma, which is rarely induced by a practiced surgeon, and placement of electrodes. If the electrode is properly inserted, all of the contacts, including the most apical electrode pairs, are visible lying along the edge of the bony spiral lamina, under the basilar membrane, when the cochlea is opened for examination.

So in our case, as in the case of the Hochmairs, we believe that we have an electrode that can be inserted with acceptable risk of trauma and that has good placement of stimulating elements throughout the array. Again, that is significant if the position of the electrodes is important in terms of what they stimulate, which, of course, it is. The height of the scala tympani does not vary continuously, and the electrode's dimensions are gauged to follow the height rather than the width of the scala tympani.

Parkins: I would now like to ask Dr. Gerald Loeb to summarize briefly some of the similarities seen in electrical stimulus parameters used by the different cochlear prostheses.

DR. GERALD LOEB (*Laboratory of Neural Control, National Institute of Neurological and Communicative Disorders and Stroke, Bethesda, Maryland 20205*): I would like to discuss how these electrical parameters interact with coding. In listening to the descriptions of the varying approaches to this problem, I was struck by the number of groups who are using a relatively simple electrode with relatively sophisticated coding strategies that are obviously designed to try to overcome the limitations of the electrode. And, conversely, there are a number of groups using an electrophysiologically sophisticated electrode with what appear to be rather simple coding strategies. This leads to the question of the extent to which one can expect a coding strategy to improve upon an electrode design that is simple or sophisticated. Then we also must ask: What do we mean by simple or sophisticated? What is the potential of an electrode?

We can loosely divide all of the prostheses into three categories. First, there are those prostheses in which the electrode is not capable of producing a relatively localized stimulus. This includes prostheses with promotory electrodes, round-window electrodes, and any intercochlear electrode in which there is an extended region of electrical contact that does not provide a localized stimulus.

The next category of sophistication includes prostheses with electrodes in which there is a chance for one point of localized stimulation, such as an intracochlear electrode that is closely positioned in a reasonably small area. In fact, investigators generally have not set out to put in such a single electrode, but have used multiple electrode arrays in such a manner.

Finally, there are the most sophisticated devices, in which there are truly multiple independent signal sources, each of which is independent and each of which is capable of local stimulation.

The first point to be made is that if there is poor nerve survival and if there are no nerves to be activated locally, then all three of these prostheses devolve to virtually the same potential. On the other hand, if there is good nerve survival, one might expect that the ultimate capability of the three systems would be in ascending order of sophistication.

There also appear to be two approaches to the coding used for the electrical stimuli. First is what I would call corrective strategies. The processor must perform all those functions such as filtering, dynamic compression, and clipping necessary to modify the original acoustic signal to the limited dynamic and unusual frequency response of the auditory neurologic system to electrical stimulation. These corrective actions have to be taken by all three electrode types and obviously need to be optimized. Then there are transformations that truly transform the signal and change the manner in which the information is presented. These include such functions as formant detection and pulse-width modulation.

It is rather interesting that we do not have evidence that those three ascending classes of electrode sophistication produce the ascending levels of performance that we might have expected. In particular, when I look at the effects of the middle class of prosthesis, the one with a localized stimulus, I find that without any significant transformation of what is virtually an analog representation of the acoustic waveform, we are getting better results than we could have expected in a couple of cases. These are the miracle cases from both San Francisco and Vienna.

Such results have to be accounted for and I think that they point to the fact that analog waveforms are in some way providing more information than we would have guessed, even when they are introduced as a single channel if that channel is localized. I don't think that such effects can be achieved when the single channel is at the round window or at the promotory.

On the other hand, we have to ask ourselves the reverse question. Why have so many groups with a sophisticated electrode given up on the transforming types of processing, the formant detectors and the pulse-width modulation? Why do they seem to get poorer results than they get with relatively unadulturated analog waveforms, that is, waveforms of electrical stimulation that, if played into a loudspeaker, would be comprehensible?

These are the paradoxes that you can expect to deal with when working towards a better stimulating system.

PARKINS: Dr. White, do you have any comments?

DR. ROBERT WHITE (*Department of Electrical Engineering, Stanford University, Stanford, California 94305*): I will start by saying that the technological problems associated with the cochlear prosthesis, such as electrodes and the small electronics, are substantial, but I doubt that they are going to be the real roadblocks to the development of a truly operational cochlear prosthesis. I think that the tools and the technology are available to solve those problems.

The central problem is that of speech processing, that is, determining the appropriate electrical stimulus and delivering it to the auditory nerve in such a way that it triggers, with the assistance and consent of the central processor, the desired auditory percepts. Dr. Sachs has pointed out the central paradox of this whole problem: the question why a 3-kHz electrical sinewave stimulus placed in a localized fashion on the 3-kHz best-frequency region of the basal membrane does not produce a 3-kHz percept.

Now we have been able to retreat behind conjectured differences in patterns on the nerve stimulation. Some single-unit recording experiments have now commenced that are of central importance in clarifying that question. I pressed the two people who I know are working on that problem, Mark White and Itzhak Glass, to make more definitive statements than their data will allow, but superficially it appears that single-unit patterns resulting from electrical stimulation are rather similar to those produced by normal acoustic stimulation in the sense that the binning histogram gives the binned responses phase-locked at various interval-multiples of the driving frequency. The temporal pattern appears, on the basis of preliminary evidence (data always look clearer and simpler from a distance, when you are not responsible for them and know all the qualifiers), to be more similar to the normal ear's acoustic signal than I, for one, had always thought. Certainly, more work needs to be done in that direction. If we can learn how to control the spatial and temporal neural response pattern, we will be a long way toward understanding the acoustic-driven part of the information. Then there is another whole layer of perception, the cognitive perception, which has to be considered in this problem.

It is true that the investigators dealing with stimulation have been quite separate from the traditional auditory physiologists. Dr. Kiang is probably an exception in that he is an auditory physiologist who knows the literature of the field of stimulation. Generally these fields are quite disparate. Dr. Sachs too has become interested in bridging these fields. So we do need to bring together researchers from these disciplines so that the data bases get shared. Physiologists do not know the data base of the work in cochlear stimulation because much of it has not yet been published—it is on the back of envelopes, in the folklore, so to speak. This material isn't publicly available, a situation that should be amended.

DR. E. E. DOUEK (*Guy's Hearing Research Group, Guy's Hospital, London, England*): I think that I can speak on behalf of all the surgeons, who are perhaps bored to high heaven listening to you talking about coding. I can assure you that we are not stupid. If what you are saying is not getting through to us, it is because it is not clear in your own minds. We can advise you to talk among yourselves. It may be that you haven't achieved a point where you can say something meaningful to us, just as we may not have achieved something surgically acceptable to you These meetings, perhaps rightly, tend to be dominated by discussions of coding and psychophysics, but it certainly gives us a sense of the unreal.

When we actually deal with patients, I sometimes have to ask my colleagues to stop psychophysical testing on these patients because they are driving them to tears, and go on to speech tests, which the patients enjoy because they see themselves making some progress.

I am going to talk in terms that may not make sense to you, but they make sense to the patients and to me. There may be more to speech than what you are looking for; and there may be more to communication than you are even touching upon. We have a patient, Mrs. I. H. from Liverpool, whose accent was from Newcastle, which is in the north of England. When she heard her children speak she said, "My goodness, I didn't realize they talked posh." "Posh" meant the southern English accent, which was more like that heard on the BBC. What was it that she heard? Was it the consonants? Was it the phonemes? Was it this? Was it that? This is an important part of communication.

I went to visit Dr. Michelson on one occasion, and I asked his patient whether he thought I was American. He said "No," and in fact was able to place my origins better than many of you. He picked up something in my accent. It is an important part of communication to be able to tell whether the chap to whom you are talking is not one of your compatriots.

Another point, which is of crucial importance, is this: In discussion, we continually divide the subjects into those with single-channel electrodes and those with multichannel devices Of course, we would prefer to insert the multichannel device, but we sometimes have reasons for not doing so.

What is most important to surgeons is that they be able to distinguish which patients have enough neurons to benefit from a multichannel system and which do not. Those who do not would perhaps do quite well with some simple, single-channel extracochlear arrangement. There is great need for developing techniques of diagnosis to help make these decisions. I therefore put it to you that perhaps this is a much more important field for those of you who are interested in coding and measuring electrical responses.

DR. ADRIAN J. FOURCIN (*Department of Phonetics, University College London, London, England*): While Dr. Douek is the surgeon for our team, I am one of the people who are behind the scenes dealing with the patients once they have been operated upon, and indeed before they have been operated upon.

It is important for surgeons to realize that, metaphorically speaking, their active paternity is fleeting and often involves scant responsibility. The treatment of the patient afterwards with regard to introduction to the speaking world is long and painful and requires careful thought and long nurturance. One has to consider whether or not the patient can even possibly benefit from all the training that is going to be supplied by the speech therapists and the psychologists, and others of the supporting team. For example, it seems almost immoral to provide information that is severely reduced in terms of speech patterns to persons who are congenitally deaf and in their middle years. They are not going to be able to learn the contrasts in speech patterns that the postlingually deaf person can perceive so easily.

Surgeons and those who are concerned with speech coding must adopt a common language, although given the nature of human affairs, this probably won't happen. As Nelson Kiang suggested, we will have to rely on the new generation, who possess a more unbiased attitude, and a surer foundation than now exists. I am making a plea for greater cooperation, even though I think that it will come only from the young.

The lesson that I have learned, which is especially poignant for me since I started working on the problem in New York 25 years ago and first heard temporal pitch binaurally, is that there is an enormous gulf between what we can provide for our patients and what we know we ought to be able to do. It is perfectly possible for all of you as hearing individuals, especially if you've got two viable ears, to put yourself in the position of someone who has only temporal information neurally transmitted and hears pitches clearly up to 1 kHz. It is also possible, although you may not know this, to hear timbre changes. You can do astonishing things by moving the timbre around in your head binaurally as a lateralization trick with 5-msec interaural delays and you can hear different pitches, but the same timbre simply on the basis of the neural transmission of temporal information. If we can do this, then we should be able to help our patients immensely. It may be that a few patients are doing this willy-nilly, and the thing that speech people know is that every person has his own ways of understanding speech and he uses an individual set of emphases with regard to the processing of speech. We are all different in respect to the way we process pattern elements. It may be that a few individuals in this large population of patients we've come across can indeed extract spectral and temporal information from the scant temporal clues that we provide them with single-channel stimulation. We have to find out why and we have to do it cooperatively.

PARKINS: As a surgeon who is also deeply involved in the single-neuron physiology and in the coding question, I am quite dismayed to see this split developing between the surgeon, who wants results now, with which I can sympathize, and the basic scientist, who wants to nail every little pin in its proper place.

Both approaches have some validity, but it is very important that the two groups continue to talk to each other and that the scientist doesn't say that the surgeon is "all wet" and ignore his results because they don't represent "basic science" or that the surgeon not ignore the necessity of careful experimental design and data analyses because progress is not rapid enough. Successful development of the cochlear prosthesis for patient use requires close collaboration between scientist and surgeon.

DR. JUERGEN TONNDORF (*Department of Otolaryngology, College of Physicians & Surgeons of Columbia University, New York, New York 10032*): In response to Dr. Douek, I would like to pursue the analogy of the development of the morse code. Samuel Morse realized rather quickly that one could not speak along the telegraph wires which were being strung throughout the country, and so he had to devise a code that was impervious to the shortcomings of these new channels, which were of narrow width. That is how the morse code came about. There is a lesson to be learned in this. When Morse devised his dot–dash code, he didn't just do it out of hand. He went to a printer's office and examined the frequency of letters in the English language and found out that E and T occur most frequently, and that Q and a few others are less frequent. In those days stock-market reports were not necessary, and numbers were used infrequently. So, he made the code economically. He assigned the shortest symbols, the dot and the dash, to E and T, and the longer symbols to those letters that are less frequently used.

This is a marvelous achievement and is what we mean by coding. We have an incomplete channel here and we try to make the best out of it by finding a code that is suitable to the occasion.

LOEB: I'd like to make a general comment. Because I design devices that are used by people, I see a lot of specifics every day that I don't report because I can't put the whole schematic up on the board. I am sure there are other designers here, like Erwin Hochmair, Mark White, and others, who have built devices and have had to make their own subtle decisions that are not represented in the block diagrams we generally see. Now I wonder whether all these subtle decisions are important. Can we just ignore these things and say that as long as we have five block diagrams representing the processing scheme, that's all that is necessary? Do these subtle design changes make a difference?

MERZENICH: I would like to note that we don't know too clearly the significance of relative nerve survival. We have seen two patients, one of whom had relatively poor nerve survival and the other the opposite condition, that is, relatively complete nerve survival. A variety of experiments with these two patients indicate that we are farther away from the elements we are stimulating in the patient with poorer nerve survival.

I think it is possible to distinguish these two patient populations with an appropriate electrode and, therefore, predict what can be achieved in the two cases.

When there is less nerve survival there is less spatial control of stimulation; it gets more difficult to get close to the neurons that you are exciting So, while you can control the neural population within a critical distance (frequency region) with an electrode like ours, this segment may contain a large number of neurons in the patient with good nerve survival and only a few or no neurons with poor nerve survival.

Nevertheless, with a simple, limited-channel vocoder kind of device, the descriptions of the channel-by-channel percepts of these subjects are not that different, and I would not be surprised to see results with relatively simple devices that are not very different. The limitation in the instance of nerve survival is that when we employ devices that approach channel vocoders that could give high intelligibility (if that model turns out to work), there will still be a limitation in resolution. I think that this direction in the design of devices might be the best for both of those populations.

DR. MAXWELL ABRAMSON (*Department of Otolaryngology, College of Physicians & Surgeons of Columbia University, New York, New York 10032*): In reference to Dr. Kiang's comments, I would like to ask whether another one of the experts wants to comment upon new ideas engendered by the multidisciplinary aspect of this conference.

DR. DONALD K. EDDINGTON (*Division of Artificial Organs, Institute for Biomedical Engineering, University of Utah, Salt Lake City, Utah 84112*): Let me respond: One of the benefits to me, a contributor, was to learn more precisely what's going on in areas far away from the United States, such as Australia and Vienna and London. It was very helpful for me to actually sit down and talk with these workers.

DOUEK: It might interest you to know that it is quite extraordinary for Dr. Spillmann, and Professor Chouard, and the Hochmairs and us to meet in New York because we have never met together before.

DR. ROBERT REMEZ (*Department of Psychology, Barnard College, New York, New York 10027*): In view of the wide range of performance that different subjects achieve with the same or nominally the same system, the same implant, the same coding, and so on, I would like to ask the panel to describe what they view as a scenario for progress in this field. How do you know that progress is being made?

MERZENICH: As implanters, we are fundamentally interested in interpatient comparisons. We are comparing the results of different devices implanted in different patients, and trying to determine the differences due to the devices themselves. We gauge progress using individual comparisons on how a patient's performance can improve or change as a function of device change. Of course, any time there is a fundamental change in the configuration of the device, such as a change of the electrode system, we are leaping across an abyss (and presumably such a decision will be made on the basis of rational consideration), but fundamentally we are dealing with interpatient comparisons.

LOEB: This is part of a large philosophical question which asks: do we have to implant a specific device in hundreds of patients so that we can determine statistically whether or not this device has an advantage?

So far, one of the prosthetic devices available has, in fact, been used in hundreds of patients. As a result we now have a good understanding of its limitations and advantages. Furthermore, I believe that those limitations were apparent long before 200 patients were implanted with the device. Nevertheless, none of the claims of any of the groups working in the field are going to be believed until relatively large numbers of patients have been studied with some degree of consistency.

A problem that may arise with rapidly increasing the number of teams and devices in this field has been alluded to earlier. If these new investigators are not adequately experienced, supported, and funded, their data may not be comparable to the present data base, thereby being a scientific waste. There also may not be enough technically qualified people available to fill the positions created. Very few people really understand the magnitude of the investment needed just to get a single device of any degree of sophistication working and the effort it takes to get from an experimental physiology (one at a time) device fabrication to something that can produce scores of devices, at least. At the same time, each implanted patient must be closely followed using sophisticated testing much more complex and extensive than that the House group is currently using. This is an enormous undertaking. I don't know how many groups can afford to pursue this course in parallel, at least until someone has shown a significant way of simplifying the problem so that one or two cases for each group's device would produce reliable results fully describing the capabilities of that approach. That's a big problem and obviously I cannot provide an answer for it.

EDDINGTON: Before we go on with this discussion, let us define progress. The deaf person's idea of progress is probably measured as "how well can I understand?" So to make progress in that area we must determine why some devices provide more or less understanding than others. We must ask: What are the cues? What are the attributes of those devices that the patient uses to perceive speech or attain good recognition scores. I think that in trying to leapfrog to processing without determining the attributes that work in the system you are now using will only add to the confusion So, if we assume that speech communication is the goal of these devices, we should study a particular scheme, determine its attributes, and discover what cues the patients are using to recognize speech with that device. Then, perhaps an intelligent decision can be made on what needs to be changed to increase recognition with any device.

DR. C. H. CHOUARD (*Laboratory of Oto-Rhino-Laryngological Research, University Hospital, Paris-Saint-Antoine, Paris, France*): Let us enumerate the devices for cochlear implantation currently available. First, we have the devices of the group from Melbourne, those of Clark and Tong. Second, we have the device of Burian and Hochmair-Desoyer. And, third, we have the device of Michelson. The device of House and of Douek make five. Progress will come if a large number of patients are implanted with these devices, which are able to provide some hearing. Maybe the results will not be as good as those produced by the next generation 10 years from now. If, in the next 2 or 3 years, we implant the device in a couple of hundred patients, then, first, these patients will be able to hear—a very important point; and, second, we will be able to make statistically significant comparisons between these devices and stimulation schemes. The best way to advance is to implant. We have the devices available; now we have to implant them.

EDDINGTON: I disagree. How is implanting more patients going to increase their scores? I don't think that implanting more of House's devices, my devices, or anyone else's devices is going to increase the quality of those devices or increase the scores that patients can obtain with these devices. At this point it is basic understanding that is going to advance this field. Implantation should only be done if it is going to increase this basic understanding. I don't see much evidence of an attempt to understand why the 2 or 3 or 200 patients that have already been implanted are attaining good scores or bad. Until that can be explained, I don't see what implanting more patients is going to do.

CHOUARD: The more patients you implant, the better you understand what they hear, and your progress will be made from one patient to the next. If you have certain results with the first ten patients, you can then improve the device. We did this 5 years ago with our system, and I believe that Burian did the same.

DR. ERWIN S. HOCHMAIR (*Department of Electrical Engineering, Technical University of Vienna, Vienna, Austria*): With the device we are presently using we can already help the patient, so we have to divide our effort into two areas. One is to improve speech quality, which is of more academic interest, and the other is to help the subject to hear and to improve his life. The patient cares not only how well he understands with his device, but also how easy it is to wear. And there are probably many other things that are important to the patient. I predict that within 2 years we will have a device that works on electrical stimulation which is as small as a behind-the-ear hearing aid. The patient will also be able to wear it behind the ear. This will represent a very large improvement for the subject who is almost totally deaf.

EDDINGTON: I agree with Dr. Hochmair. To answer the question of the logistics of progress in this area, I reiterate: You don't make progress by multiplying what you now have without understanding it.

MERZENICH: It is a reasonable strategy to design the implant device so that it can be easily upgraded. Presumably there will be products of our research, and therefore there are aspects of the device that must be capable of improvement, at least in the short term. For example, an 8-channel electrode array must be designed so that it can function as a 3-channel or a 4-channel device now, but there must be the capability for gaining control of all eight channels of that array if an 8-channel driver may be available in the future. There must also be a component replacement strategy. In our case it is a connector disc replacement. Bob White has also worked on such a system, as have several other people. Such a strategy is also important because we all know that devices are prone to failure. So, we must have a way to replace components in failed devices that should not necessitate removal of functioning electrodes. It is very important to provide those limited number of patients whom we are implanting with a device that is upgradable so that they can benefit from the improvements derived from the fruits of our research. Also, the driving systems that we use should be relatively transparent, that is, we must not use some artificial coding scheme that limits our later manipulation as the external driver becomes modified.

It is of critical importance that we have the capability of applying what we learn in coding studies to the patients that we are treating at this time.

PARKINS: I will now invite questions and comments from the audience.

DR. RICHARD S. TYLER (*Department of Otolaryngology, University Hospitals, Iowa City, Iowa 52242*): One underlying theme of this conference is the lack of a common thread among the results from different patients using similar implants or the lack of a common thread among those using different implants. One important reason for this is, of course, that they are simply different patients I believe that if we hope to make important strides in learning what these individual differences are, extensive psychophysical information must be gotten from each patient who receives an implant. I know that some groups are already pursuing this avenue of research. However, I want to support Dr. Eddington in his observation that data from 500 people aren't going to help us if all we know is a few things like the threshold and uncomfortable-loudness levels. I would like to see the groups proceed a little more slowly and provide more comprehensive results for each patient.

MERZENICH: You also can't ask a patient to dedicate the rest of his or her entire life to your study. Dr. Eddington has a very good relationship with a couple of patients and has been able to study them intensively over a number of years. But you must remember that these patients are volunteers, and you can only ask for so much of their time.

In our case, we ask the patient to dedicate 4 to 5 months of his time to our studies, but then we feel that we must provide him with a device that he can wear. I am sure that the Hochmairs as well as the Stanford group have also faced this problem. So, you don't need a large number of patients, but you do need to give the patient a break so that he can spend the rest of his life using the device.

DR. GREG R. BOCK (*MRC Institute of Hearing Research, University of Nottingham, Nottingham, England*): Along with a lot of other people at this meeting, I came here to find out which device works best, and I am going to leave the conference with no answer to that question because all of the researchers seem to use a different test and to assess their success in different ways. So I would like to know why you can't all get together, at least the English-speaking groups, and agree on some standard universal tests. These tests would not preclude your own favorite particular tests, but at least you would be able to present comparable data so that the rest of us can decide who is doing best.

I have another question: There is one potential use of the cochlear prosthesis that has not yet been mentioned at this meeting—use of this device for suppressing tinnitus. Does anybody have any experience with this?

PARKINS: I would like not to get into that now—it is another complex question that will just muddy the waters at this point.

CHOUARD: But the question of tinnitus is important and where it occurs with total deafness, it has been totally suppressed by the implant.

PARKINS: But it has not been investigated to the point where we can draw valid conclusions. While I know that there are some investigators here who are very much interested in this, I would prefer to defer its discussion so that we can pursue the topics already raised.

LES ATLAS (*Applied Electronics Laboratories, Stanford University, Stanford, California 94305*): I would like to address the testing issue. This has come up over a number of years, especially at the conferences on the West Coast, where the groups from San Francisco, Stanford, and Los Angeles have all tried to compare devices. A recent development over the last year or so from a speech perception standpoint has been the MAC battery. This test is too recent to have been extensively used with the deaf population, but the basic principles of the battery are solid. At this conference, I presented results from the MAC battery, as did Dr. Owens and the group from Stanford. The group from San Francisco mentioned data from some tests within the battery. So we can see that a significant step forward has been made in trying to standardize testing for comparison of data across groups.

EDDINGTON: One test that is common to all groups, even non-English-speaking groups, is open-set, two-syllable word recognition, and I believe that those data are available for comparison.

MERZENICH: It should also be mentioned that the Austrian group uses basically corresponding test material. Despite language differences, the tests are basically of the same design and allow the same kind of comparison. I urge everyone to get this material If you contact Dr. Elmer Owens, we can try to provide it for the cost of reproducing the tapes. These can be used as a basis for comparison, if appropriate.

ATLAS: This material is commercially available through Autotech.

DR. LAUREL J. DENT (*Division of Otolaryngology, Stanford University School of Medicine, Stanford, California 94305*): The groups in London, Vienna, and Australia are all using the consonant in a two-syllable frame where the vowel on either side is an "a". This is a stimulus that we can all use regardless of the language, even though the consonants would differ from dialect to dialect. I don't see any of the American groups initiating an effort to make a videotape like the one that the London group has of "a-consonant-a," a stimulus that we can play for our patients as a standard. Perhaps someone in this audience would be interested in making such a tape available.

PARKINS: The test battery has to accomplish two different things: It must first measure how well the device functions so that valid comparisons between devices can be made. It must also determine what types of errors in communication occur so that these errors can be analyzed and the device or coding scheme modified to prevent these errors.

R. WHITE: If Dr. Bock is disappointed, he should have been present a year ago at any one of these meetings. Enormous progress has been made toward standardization. As scattershot as it seems to be, there is at least the will to move toward the MAC test, toward certain confusion matrices. It is quite true that it is hard to know which is the best device; the question seems unanswerable at present. But there is a movement towards standardization of tests, which is very gratifying because it was even harder a year ago than it is now to make any sense out of what was being reported.

DOUEK: Another reason why we all don't get together and come to a decision about which device is best lies in the lack of confidence that we all have or should have regarding the present state of our own art. A good example of this is the Viennese group. Within that one group one technique is tested and then another, and their work is outstanding. So, if within your own group you have not yet decided what you are going to offer, you can hardly get together with other groups to choose just one device. If we did that, we would be excluding lots of ideas that may be much more productive than anything any one of us is doing right now.

HOCHMAIR: It is very important that one group tests several different strategies—single-channel, multichannel—because of the very difficult comparison from one group to the other. So, within one group with the same tests you can study different strategies with almost the same patients. This is one of the reasons why we have tried from the beginning to make our implant as transparent and as flexible as possible.

DR. CAROL DE FILIPPO (*National Technical Institute for the Deaf, Rochester, New York*): In reports of evaluation schemes it seems to be recognized that, except to the deaf–blind person, there is information in speech represented not in the acoustic portion of speech, but in the visual portion. A distinction has also been made by workers in tactile devices between communication aids or lipreading aids· and sensory substitution devices. I am wondering whether a clear goal is in mind, particularly among the designers in the group. Are you looking for a sensory substitution device? Are you looking for a communication aid, a lipreading aid? Is it a worthy enough goal to develop a lipreading aid? Or should we go all the way to obtain sensory substitution and not bother with the interim goal of just a lipreading aid, which may mean different coding?

SACHS: Let me answer that question from my own standpoint. A subject we've had for about 5 years is a tremendous lipreader, and if we were to compare results of lipreading only with lipreading plus electrical stimulation, we wouldn't see much change, because with lipreading only, this patient's performance is almost perfect. So we would like to give him the kind of aid that would not be just an aid to lipreading, but rather the kind of device where he could possibly talk on the phone or get more from watching TV.

HOCHMAIR: It is very important for the patient to have a sensory aid and not just a communication aid so that he can hear environmental sounds.

PARKINS: In other words, you are working towards a sensory substitution aid.

EDDINGTON: Dr. De Filippo's point is well taken. From the comments made so far I get the impression that a lot of people working in the field don't have a clear idea of what they are working towards and why. The fact that some lipreading help can be gotten with these devices is a nice side-effect, but the decision about whether to build a sensory aid or a sensory substitution device seems to be muddled. If these goals could be well defined, it would probably change our ways of approaching the problem.

I believe that the development of a sensory substitution device is the goal. The "fallout" from this work done so far is that the patients can use the devices as a sensory aid, but since that was not the goal previously established it's not the direction of our maximum effort.

DR. SAMUEL W. ANDERSON (*Department of Psychiatry, College of Physicians & Surgeons of Columbia University, New York, New York 10032*): As for sensory substitution, I can't resist saying something in response to this question that was slowly building in my mind from what I heard before. I think that there are about three models that have been implicit in everyone's presentation, not that everyone has adopted, or even necessarily understood, all three; but there seem to be about three basic theoretical approaches here.

One of them is the neurophysiology model, which projects as its natural application the sensory threshold techniques of classical psychophysics. Second, we have the speech reception model, or, as I would prefer to call it, the speech comprehension model, about which we have heard little since the first session. Finally, as I suddenly realized from the comments of Dr. Tonndorf and Dr. Douek, is the good old communication channel model of Shannon, which appealed to many of us as a useful and rigorous way to combine the other two. I think that perhaps the surgeons here may especially like this view. But I believe that the notion of sensory substitution is not a very revealing way to look at the different communicative functions of the senses. They are not simply equivalent channels that can be switched in and out, one substituted for another like a spare tire if one goes bad. Attention and memory, for example, are handled differently in vision and hearing.

It is my view that in designing an implant we are trying to restore whatever we can of what is in fact the primary line for normal speech communication, to reestablish an acoustic link for which there is no equivalent substitute at all. This is true even among patients who have mastered lipreading or Ameslan and make the most of these sensory substitutes. However effective they become, these communication systems are not fully equivalent alternate channels. Just as vision complements hearing in normal speech, a complementary composite should be available to the patient with an implant.

Those who remember the work of Shannon and Weaver know that all of the hard mathematics that they solved for us deal with the properties of a single idealized channel. You have to discover all the properties of the channel, after which the theory will allow you to know the optimal code for that channel. But you can infer nothing from this about the properties of the human being as a message source or receiver or what flexibility may exist or not with respect to the coding and decoding operations that we can expect the brain to be able to perform. It is the receiver's code that we have to understand when we deal with the person who may or may not be helped by a cochlear prosthesis, and we may know more than we need to about coding for telephone lines, morse code, or the printed page. All of these things have yielded impressively specific mathematical solutions in terms of information theory, but I am convinced from what I've heard that one reason why we can't apply it very well to implant design is because when we deal with patients we deal with people whose neurological condition is unknown—both in the normal and in the pathologic sense: in the cochlea itself, we don't even know how many functioning cells may remain.

Therefore, even if we can know what kind of implant we've achieved, we have great difficulty in deciding how effective the system might be in advance. I'm not sure how the other two models can help; I think the neurophysiologists would surely call for studies on normal cochleas. You could implant a normal cochlea and see what would happen. I realize, of course, that there are ethical limitations on this and that the surgeons would not do it, but that, I think, would be the physiologist's solution.

I think that sensory psychophysics yields the least help in understanding how speech can be successfully transmitted by means of implants. This view presents us with a very interesting paradox, in fact. We have discovered that patients who report no sense of tonality through their implants at frequencies higher than 300 Hz or 500 Hz nevertheless can discriminate between speech sounds that are distinct only at higher frequencies, showing that speech features up to the F2 range inputs are being processed. I am curious as to whether Dr. Remez's sinusoidal formants would improve the sense of tone or accuracy of speech detection, but I think we must treat these as independent questions.

The brain is a very wonderful thing, and I believe that we have been assuming correctly that we are dealing with normal brains, which, however poorly they can hear, remain at least normally good, and possibly better, at multimodal communication. We can also assume that these brains all learn how to use what we know about the world and about what we've just understood in order to help decode each particular word or sentence as it comes in. I think that Dr. Cooper made that point rather eloquently.

DR. Y. C. TONG (*Department of Otolaryngology, University of Melbourne, Victoria, Australia*): I don't think that sensory substitution aids and lipreading aids ought to be thought of as mutually exclusive in the sense that a compromise may be obtained. I agree with Dr. Eddington that our final aim is to provide sensory substitution, but in the meantime, if it is not within our understanding of psychophysics or speech perception, an intermediate type of aid can be used. As far as I can see, all the cochlear implant devices used at present are lipreading aids, not complete sensory substitution aids. So, the compromise here is to try to handle single variables that are manageable within the cochlear implant domain.

Also, do we know the supplementary nature between hearing and lipreading? Do we know which are the characteristics that would give a perfect lipreading aid? I don't think we do. So we must make sure that we can manipulate the variables and make sure that the speech-processing scheme is manageable, in terms of both a lipreading aid and a sensory substitution aid.

LOEB: That is really the question. We don't know what an optimal lipreading aid would be because nobody has asked the question.

EDDINGTON: The Fourcin group has.

LOEB: That is very interesting: For the first time we have a group that has actually thrown its energies behind a device that they knew to be limited in its capabilities and have therefore adapted their strategy to the best performance of that device. So far almost every other group attempted to build a prosthesis based on doing it all—replacing speech, eliminating the need for lipreading aids—and, then, having developed such a device, admitted that it could not be used for speech recognition alone, but was just an adjunct for lipreading. This is the point at which most researchers in neural prosthetic projects have found themselves—not building devices for patients, but rather building the devices the *investigator* thinks the patient might want.

While most of us have been working on the assumption that patients want to hear speech without the need for any kind of visual aid, we may be shortly confronted with the fact that that may not be possible or may only be possible in a rather limited number of patients. Therefore, the devices we are going to have to develop can't just be accidental spinoffs of devices built to provide speech perception; rather they will have to be intentionally designed to optimally complement speech recognition from lipreading.

EDDINGTON: Right; that was the good point drawn from the question. There is one group—Fourcin's and Douek's—who has declared their motivation from the outset to provide a lipreading aid, and because of that, because their goal was well defined, they are proceeding in a very scientific manner. This group is deciding what is needed for lipreading and determining how it can be implemented, while many others are fuzzy on their goals. . . .

LOEB: They are not fuzzy; they have just had to retreat.

EDDINGTON: But I don't see them falling back into a position very scientifically; these groups seem to be falling back in the manner they have always operated on, and then said, *ex post facto,* well now we have a lipreading aid.

DE FILIPPO: Dr. Eddington, we are very close to delineating the requirements for an effective lipreading aid. Speech perception in the severely hearing-impaired has been studied and seems to indicate what might be needed from the acoustics in order to supplement or complement or add redundancy to the visual information. All we need to learn is the appropriate display, and I think you people have it; we have coding.

MERZENICH: You shouldn't go away with the idea that you cannot generate differences in pitch above 200 or 300 Hz. There is an electrode-specific pitch, and there is no fundamental reason to believe that the pitch generated around any electrode is encoded in any different way than pitch encoded at that site by the corresponding acoustic stimulus encoded normally. When you vary the electric stimulus frequency to a specific electrode, you are obviously not changing the center of the resonant position or the position on the cochlear membrane where the traveling wave would reach its maximum in acoustic stimulation. It should therefore not be surprising that increasing the electric stimulus frequency above 300 Hz to a specific location (electrode) on the basilar membrane does not produce a higher pitch sensation. What you must do is change the location of the stimulus on the basilar membrane and, more importantly, the responding neural population. In small-channel devices, and to a certain degree in monopolar multichannel stimulation, this neural population does not change.

DR. D. W. AIRD (*University Hospital of Wales, Cardiff, Wales*): As a clinician I am interested in obtaining more specific diagnostic help. It is all very well to ask what the patient would like, but it is not entirely a question of what the patient wants—it's what he has in the basket, so to speak. How are we to determine which patients are most likely to benefit from the device?

How can we assess the degree of nerve survival preoperatively as a predictor of postimplantation performance? We can only compare the performance of devices if the implanted patients have comparable nerve survival.

PARKINS: We agree with that. Dr. Simmons' paper on the ABR is one approach to this question, and I think that we will continue to look for ways to determine the amount of surviving neurons or whatever else correlates with the good or spectacular results achieved in certain implanted patients.

CHOUARD: From this point of view, it is necessary to have a sufficient number of patients to make a statistically significant correlation between the parameters you study and the clinical results you obtain.

DR. ROBERT SMITH (*Institute for Sensory Research, Syracuse University, Syracuse, New York 13210*): I hope that you will forgive me for getting back to specifics—the coding problem. I would like to reiterate a point I tried to make earlier concerning adaptation. If we use the neural physiology model, we are stimulating the auditory nerve, trying somehow to simulate the response of the nerve fiber array. Yet in most of the devices described it is the hair cell array that is being simulated because adaptation has been largely ignored. While it might not be important, I am wondering whether there isn't a simple way to look into adaptation in some of these devices.

I don't think that the automatic gain control (ACG) system, as I've heard it described, is the same as additive adaptation. Is there an empirical way to investigate whether or not the adaptation effect is of any importance in this whole business?

PARKINS: Your point about adaptation is very important. With the devices that have given exceptional speech perception results there is an AGC with a very short attack time constant in the system that is doing some of this adaptation coding emphasizing onset phenomena. It is not identical to the adaptation model, but has some similar results.

MERZENICH: Several investigators have studied this, including Mark White and Bob Shannon in our laboratory, as well as Don Eddington. You need to know such things as the growth of loudness as a function of signal duration. In this case, it turns out that that is not so different from normal. The functions are quite remarkably similar to normal in our patients and therefore no particular compensation seems to be required. You also need to know whether or not there is poststimulus depression of the sort that occurs in the normal running signal. Amazingly enough, contrary to contemporary ideas in auditory physiology, there is such a depression. There are the kind of forward masking phenomena that are very much like normal, with a time course much like the normal. In a gross sense, at least, what is happening temporally in terms of suppression appears to be remarkably like the normal. Therefore, at least on a gross level, these functions would not seem to require particular compensation.

Of course, this is just looking at things on a first order. Many implant groups are studying parameters like this that relate to temporal sequencing and adaptation effects.

SMITH: Are these temporal forward masking effects across channels or within a channel?

MERZENICH: Both within a channel and across channels, if the channels are interactive. In other words, you can use forward masking in a cochlear implant just like you can use it in normal sound, but it requires that the masker affect the region of the probe. It works just the same way, and the time course is very similar.

Contemporary neural physiologists believe that the forward masking is dictated by events and suppression occurring in the eighth nerve. Implant experiments strongly indicate that while that parallelism is unquestionable and may be really what dictates the function and detail, there is at least a central nervous system function that crudely approximates it with a very similar time course and a very similar depth of effect.

SMITH: I am glad to hear that. In all of my publications I try to refrain from using the term "forward masking" because that is a term describing psychophysical phenomena which clearly are central nervous system phenomena that may have peripheral components.

SACHS: I would like to expand on your remarks about AGC, Dr. Smith. Over the last two days I have heard three different definitions for AGC, and I am confused now as to what is really meant. I imagine that the definition depends on who built the processor and what he decided AGC should really do. Since your results do not imply an AGC type of system, what kind of system do they imply?

SMITH: On the single-fiber level, it depends upon what time scale the analyzer is using. The properties of the system that I described reflect the analysis that I used. I hope that I made that point clear. The basic system is what I would call an additive system, that is, there is a sort of compression, but it is an instantaneous compression which is followed by a subtractive effect. Adaptation builds up and reduces the response, but anything that is added simply adds on in the same way as if there hadn't been any adaptation. However, in an AGC type of system, as adaptation built up, there would be either a proportional reduction in response or a shift in the operating range for its higher intensities. Again, this is just at one station, and I am sure that other things happen more centrally.

I would like to speculate on the functional unit in the periphery. As Nelson Kiang mentioned and Charles Liberman has shown, the hair cell is innervated by 20 or 30 auditory nerve fibers. Perhaps they form more of a functional unit than any single fiber. In particular, if there is a spread of thresholds among those fibers, then you have to add up these functional units that I was describing to get the overall functional unit. So, this composite functional unit may extend a response from one hair cell over a wider dynamic range than the data that I described for any single fiber in the group.

SACHS: Then I propose that someone come up with a good analytical model of what you just described to guide us in deriving this function.

PARKINS: Since there are no further questions I will close by noting that I am amazed that this audience has stayed so faithfully to the very end of this long, tiring 3-day conference. If there is confusion in the field, it is because the results are confusing at this time. Bear with us. We have to sort this out. I think that uniformity of reporting is an extremely important constraint, as is uniformity of testing and uniformity of reporting stimulus levels and electrodes. Let us hope that we will continue to work on those problems so that in another 5 years, when we have another conference, we can present data that even Dr. Kiang will agree are valid and not representative of "muddled thinking."

CLOSING COMMENTS

Charles W. Parkins

Division of Otolaryngology
University of Rochester
School of Medicine
Rochester, New York 14642

Samuel W. Anderson

Department of Psychiatry
College of Physicians & Surgeons of
Columbia University
New York, New York 10032

The preceding round-table discussion was originally conceived to express, develop, and discuss new ideas pertinent to stimulus coding for the cochlear prosthesis. Although partially successful in this purpose, it also expressed some of the philosophic questions regarding the cochlear prosthesis today and therefore serves as a fitting conclusion for this book. The discussion demonstrates a rather classic triangle, whose vertices are the scientist, the physician, and the patient. We like to think that the scientist and physician share a common base, and we agree that the patient should be the apex. The viewpoints fundamentally differ in how each formulates the problem of deafness, the approach to its solution, and the acceptability of solutions offered.

The scientist's basic goal is to discover some previously undiscovered "truth," a previously unrecognized order of things that provides an incremental leap in our ability to understand, explain, and recreate an ideal system. For the auditory physiologist, the primary goal is documenting and understanding the intricate function of the auditory system. Towards this end, he is very concerned with the meticulous design of experiments in which he must ask clear questions that have definite answers, answers beyond which there is no longer need for further speculation. His highest priority is to serve the needs of logical thinking, and his devotion to telling an unrefutable story endows him with endless patience. The practical application of his findings is usually of less importance to the scientist than are his discoveries. This is not to say that he is indifferent to the practical significance of his work, for, as has been demonstrated here, the scientist is often very much concerned about the application and misapplication of his findings in which patients would be harmed or benefitted suboptimally by his discoveries. The scientist, with his very disciplined approach to the problem, frequently has no patience for the physician's less disciplined and more intuitive approach to the problem. Because of his concentration on the problem and the investigative method, the scientist may lose sight of the potential patient for whom his findings are extremely important indeed.

The view from the physician's vertex of the triangle is of a disease state, in this case deafness, for which he must find a treatment. The physician is trained to care for patients, and this frequently entails making very important decisions which are sometimes a matter of life and death, and making them quickly, often on the basis of very imperfect or inadequate clinical and scientific knowledge. The physician is trained to obtain as much information regarding the patient's condition as he can within a reasonably restricted time frame, evaluate it in terms of his general or recently acquired knowledge, make his decision, and act accordingly. The physician, then, tends to use this same approach in developing a cochlear prosthesis to treat the problem of deafness. He is willing to accept less complete and less detailed information regarding the basic functioning of the auditory system. He will also make intuitive decisions based on the best available information in developing implant design and stimulation schemes. This has the advantage, at times, of bypassing minor knowledge-gaps and resulting in gigantic strides forward. But it may also lead to ideas and treatment procedures that are poorly founded, and if tenaciously held, become ultimately counterproductive. The physician frequently grows impatient with the slowness of the pace at which the meticulous scientist makes progress. He recognizes a trade-off between providing immediate, although limited, benefit to his patients from a suboptimal prosthesis available today and waiting for the ideal prosthesis to be developed some time in the future. Questions that must be answered are: What are the real benefits from the suboptimal prosthesis and how valuable are they to the patient? Which patients will be most benefitted from the suboptimal device? And how are they to be selected? Treatment now must not preclude treatment with a better device in the future. In his preoccupation with stamping out the disease, the physician may also lose sight of the real needs of the patient.

The patient's view, from the apex, arises from the very personal experience of deafness, which is a total communication problem with the hearing world. The problem begins with the loneliness of silence in a world devoid even of simple alerting sounds such as the ring of a telephone, the knock on a door, the footsteps of an approaching person, the warning of a car's horn. The problem is even more profound for the prelingually deaf patient, who usually ends up, if no effective treatment is possible, with no more than a restricted oral communication skill and a degree of native language development that does not surpass the normal grade-school level. The postlingually deaf patient usually does not have retardation of language development, but does have a significant oral communication deficit. Both types of patients have problems with speech production as well as reception, in that they have no feedback mechanism to allow them to moderate the intensity and composition of the sounds that they are uttering.

What does the patient want? Stated simply, the patient wants help with his communication problems. His definition of help may extend from the ideal of total restoration of auditory input, which would allow him to experience all of the intensity, frequency, and timing parameters enjoyed by persons with normal hearing, across a gamut of decreasing capabilities, extending through full speech discrimination to less complete auditory signals that could function as an aid to lip (speech) reading and finally to the detection of simple environmental sound and acoustic rhythm information. Individual patients differ a great deal in their need for and satisfaction with these varying degrees of help, so that each case must be individualized. It is very important for the scientist and the physician to address the definition of their goal in terms of help for the patient in designing their cochlear prosthesis project.

Patients will not receive the help they deserve unless scientists and physicians can work together on a prosthesis project, each respecting the value and necessity of the other's approach and selecting the best attributes of each. It is the responsibility of both to protect the patient from injurious procedures and overzealous application. In the end, we must recognize that medicine is an imperfect art, and that a single, perfect prosthesis will probably never be developed. We believe that it is possible to develop a cochlear prosthesis that will provide excellent speech discrimination for a significant number of implanted patients without the use of visual cues and that such a device will be available within the next ten years. Further development and refinement of this device, however, will continue far into the future as a search for that perfect prosthesis.

Index of Contributors

(Italicized page numbers refer to comments in the Round-Table Discussion)